APPLIED PHYSIOTHERAPY

Practical Clinical Applications with Emphasis on the Management of Pain and Related Syndromes

APPLIED PHYSIOTHERAPY

Practical Clinical Applications with Emphasis on the Management of Pain and Related Syndromes

Paul A. Jaskoviak, DC, FICC
and
R. C. Schafer, DC, FICC

Arnold E. Cianciulli, DC, MS, FICC
Development Director

Produced by
Associated Chiropractic Academic Press
for

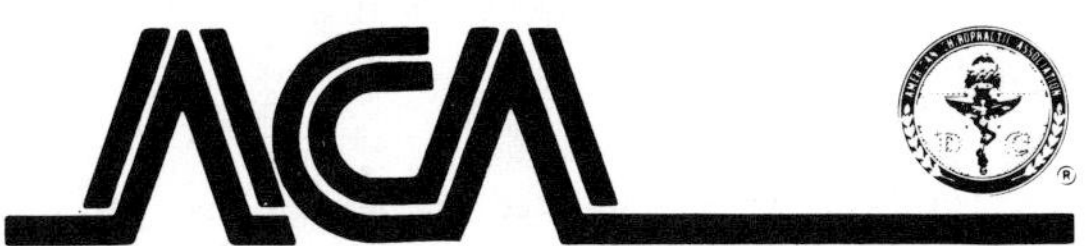

THE AMERICAN CHIROPRACTIC ASSOCIATION
1916 Wilson Boulevard, Arlington, Virginia 22201

Library of Congress Catalog Card Number: 85-71674

ISBN: 0-9606618-2-4

1916 Wilson Boulevard
Arlington, Virginia 22201

Printed in the United States of America

FOREWORD

As we explore the field of adjunctive therapy, we find a fair number of texts, with most of them specializing in one or another mode of therapy. Few give us the "complete" picture required by the doctor of chiropractic.

This text written by Drs. Jaskoviak and Schafer not only affords the doctor of chiropractic a complete volume on therapy, but it is written with clarity and practical application in mind. It will assist the doctor in developing viable treatment programs and provide him or her with the rationale necessary for insurance and narrative reports.

The American Chiropractic Association is to be complimented for developing the concept and commissioning two of our most astute academicians to author it.

Frank T. Langilotti, MS, DC, DABCN

PREFACE

This manual is written with both the practitioner and therapist in mind. In reviewing many of the texts on physical therapy, it became apparent that they either emphasized the physics of the modalities described or they related application only to named conditions. Although these are important considerations, it is the contention of the authors of this book that physiotherapeutic modalities are not geared toward affecting diseases; rather, they are designed to affect the symptomatic features of pathophysiologic disorders in specific ways. Thus, this book on *applied physiotherapy* will be found to be unusually practical in that it supports this assertion by emphasizing how each modality affects pain, muscle spasm, edema, inflammatory processes, stiffness, and other symptoms and signs often associated with musculoskeletal complaints.

The subject of physiologic therapeutics is a rapidly advancing product of modern technology. To benefit from this, each chapter draws upon scores of excellent texts currently on the market and points out the findings of recent research and the technical advances that are of vital interest to the field.

This manual may be used as a text for training in the applications of the modalities or as a frequent reference guide for the practicing physician or technician. Each chapter describes a particular modality or group of modalities that fall under a general category by offering (1) a brief review of the historical implications and (2) a comprehensive, but not weighty, explanation of the underlying physics, physiologic effects, indications and contraindications, and practical application of each.

Without question, the field of physiologic therapeutics has advanced because of both scientific and empirical findings of multiple minds seeking answers that have the potential of relieving pain and enhancing healing. This quest, by far, has not reached its full maturity. Thus, readers are encouraged to submit to the authors information for use in future editions such as unusual case histories or ways in which they have found certain modalities or techniques to be of benefit that are not presently described.

Paul A. Jaskoviak, DC, FICC
R.C. Schafer, DC, FICC

ACKNOWLEDGMENTS

Professional Consultants

Larry L. Hill, BS, DC
Lecturer in Physiological Therapeutics,
National College of Chiropractic

William J. Hogan, DC
Chairman, Clinical Science Division,
National College of Chiropractic

John Humphrey Merrick, RPT, MS, DC
Private practitioner,
New Hampshire

Robert F. Metcalf, BS, DC
Instructor, Physiological Therapeutics,
National College of Chiropractic

James F. Ransom, DC
Lecturer, Physiological Therapeutics
National College of Chiropractic

Linda L. Zange, BA, DC, DABCO
Lecturer, Acupuncture
National College of Chiropractic

Cooperating Organizations

American Chiropractic Association
Associated Chiropractic Academic Press
Behavioral Research Foundation
Chattanooga Corporation
Contour Comfort Company
Flex-Wedge Company
Fluidotherapy Corporation
Gebauer Chemical Company
Ohio Chiropractic Equipment & Supplies
Rich-Mar Corporation
Smith Truss Company, Inc.
VRB, Inc.
Widen Tool & Stamping, Inc.

Photography Credits

Many of the photographs reproduced herein were taken at the facilities of the National Chiropractic College.

The patient model shown in several photographs of Chapters 4—10 is Kim Alters, a student at National Chiropractic College.

CONTENTS

Chapter 1

The Rationale Of Physiotherapy In Chiropractic

Within the chiropractic profession following World War II, increasing interest developed in the theory and practice of adjunctive therapy. A major basis for this was the recognition that in all but the most simple and acute disorders, proper case management requires a multitherapy approach. This fact is apparent by noting the weight of professional papers and the large number of postgraduate seminars offered by accredited institutions on advances within the realm of physiologic therapeutics.

INTRODUCTION

Chiropractic physiological therapeutics encompasses the diagnosis and treatment of disorders of the body, utilizing the natural forces of healing such as cold, electricity, exercise, traction, heat, light, massage, and water. To utilize these forces on a rational basis, the practitioner must have knowledge of their actions and an understanding of their predictable effects on the tissues and pathophysiologic processes involved.

The word *physiotherapy* is generally considered to be a shortened form for *physiological therapeutics:* treatment by physical or mechanical means.

The term *physical therapy* is used in reference to the application of specific modalities such as rehabilitative procedures that are concerned with the restoration of function and prevention of disability following disease, injury, or loss of a body part.[1] To improve circulation, strengthen muscles, improve joint motion, and normalize other functional imbalances, for example, the therapeutic properties of the natural forces of healing described above are applied.

The Council on Physiological Therapeutics of the American Chiropractic Association defines *chiropractic physiotherapy* as the therapeutic application of forces and substances that induce a physiologic response and use and/or allow the body's natural processes to return to a more normal state of health.[2]

A wide variety of therapies has proven to be effective. The most common clinical applications include the therapeutic use of cold, electricity, exercise, heat, light, massage, nutrition, oriental therapies, rehabilitative procedures, supports, traction, trigger point therapy, vibration, and water. See Table 1.1.

PREMISE

As long as people have been thinking, feeling, creating, and deciding, they have sought relief for their discomforts. Their first source and recourse was to those natural agents and forces within their surrounding environment; viz:

1. Heat such as derived from the sun, hot mineral springs, and warm mud or clay packs.

2. Actinic rays such as the ultraviolet effects of sunlight.

3. The cleansing effects of water proper

Table 1.1. Common Types of Physiological Therapeutics

Application	*Definition*
Actinotherapy	Treatment of disease by rays of light, especially actinic (rays of short wavelength occurring in the violet and ultraviolet parts of the electromagnetic spectrum) or chemical light.
Cryotherapy	Treatment by means of cold; eg, the application of ice packs to a body part to relieve swelling.
Electrotherapy	The treatment of disease by means of electricity.
Hydrotherapy	The treatment of disease by using water; eg, a Hubbard tank or a sitz bath.
Mechanotherapy	The treatment of disorders using active and passive exercises; eg, traction (intermittent or sustained), braces, shoe lifts, and casts or other supports.
Meridian therapy	The evaluation and treatment of disorders using the Oriental method.
Nutritional therapy	The use of nutritional planning, dietetics, and special food or nutritional supplementation.
Rehabilitative therapy	The treatment and training of the patient that is geared toward attaining maximum potential for normal living physically, psychologically, socially, and vocationally.
Trigger point therapy	The stimulation of trigger points on the body surface by manual or other means.
Vibrational therapy	The therapeutic use of soft-tissue manipulation and massage.

(both internally and externally) and the varieties of mineral water.

4. The force of moving or running water.

5. The energy and nutrition of certain foods and supplements.

6. The encouragement and counsel of an understanding attitude and a positive mental outlook.

7. The privileges of rest and relaxation.

8. The extension effect of tractional forces.

Hence, the application of physiological therapeutics precedes any and all schools of healing. Its use is generic within the healing arts; thus, such natural methods and forces are the common property of all practitioners who are duly recognized by society and its laws to treat human ailments.

HISTORICAL BACKGROUND

The application of physiological therapeutics in chiropractic at the National College of Chiropractic was firmly established in approximately 1914. However, the forces of nature have been utilized throughout history as a means of facilitating the body's healing processes.

During early recorded civilization, both Eastern and Western cultures had much to do with building the foundation of the healing arts. The Babylonians gave us our first key to the nature and prevention of communicable diseases. The early Jews originated public hygiene and developed a weekly day of rest for recuperation.

In the Chinese *Kong-Fou,* written almost 4700 years ago, the popularity of massage is well documented. The Chinese, as far back as 2838 B.C., offered advances with their development of manipulation, massage, anthropometry, acupuncture, the moxa, pulse diagnosis, and herbs. Records are also clear that manipulation, massage, and acupuncture were practiced by the Japanese at least as early as 600 B.C. Early Chinese and Hindu writings also included exercise therapies.

The Egyptians developed skill in manipulation and the use of natural forces as far back as 2500 B.C. There is evidence that heliotherapy in the form of light and water sunbaths in the temple of Aesculapus (the sun god) were used to treat rheumatism and muscle wasting in 1400 B.C. By 770 B.C., treatment within Aesculapion sanctuaries was essentially based on bathing, fasting, drugs, and suggestion. The temple priests also stressed the importance of massage (amid an atmosphere of hypnotic-like suggestion and incantations) in the treatment of epilepsy, dizziness, and headaches.

The early Greeks used a multitude of mechanical devices for stretching the spine and setting dislocations. See Figure 1.1. A wide variety of crude traction devices were invented. Hippocrates, in 450 B.C., contributed to physiologic therapeutics by recording his observations of the effect of hot and cold on the body. Among his many recordings, he also wrote *Manipulation and Importance to Good Health* and *On Setting Joints by Leverage.* See Figure 1.2.

Herodicus, a contemporary of Hippocrates, is often called the first great drugless healer: "The one who laughed at the use of tonics." He was a great athlete who achieved wide fame by curing diseases by correcting abnormalities in the spine, which he did in the relatively healthy through therapeutic exercise and in the weak by manipulations with his hands.[3] He was criticized by Aristotle because "He made old men young and thus prolonged their lives too greatly."

In later Greece, Claudium Galen (130—200 A.D.) became the most distinguished practitioner of his time. He was the first to teach the proper positions and relationships of the vertebrae and the spinal column, the examination of urine in certain diseases, the value of specific foods during illness, the critical days of fever, the significance of the pulse and arteries, and many other features of health and disease. Among his many recordings, Galen is attributed with 16 books on exercise and massage, and his many findings influenced physicians for centuries. See Figure 1.3.

Documents disclose that heat and hydrotherapy (eg, hot springs) were used in America as a general body heating technique in 1706. It was not until 1745 that the first book on electrotherapy was published—wherein it suggested the use of torpedo fish to treat gout. By 1870, the practice of electrotherapy had greatly advanced. Galvanism and ultraviolet light were commonly used as therapeutic measures prior to 1900.

For centuries, the use of sun rays, mineral spas, therapeutic exercise and massage have been popular in both Eastern and Western Europe. However, the use of physiologic-therapeutic devices was initiated and developed within America by the nonallopathic professions, with pioneer chiropractors offering some leadership in both application and development.[4] The various applications were originally described as actino-therapy, electro-therapy, hydro-therapy, mechano-therapy, etc.

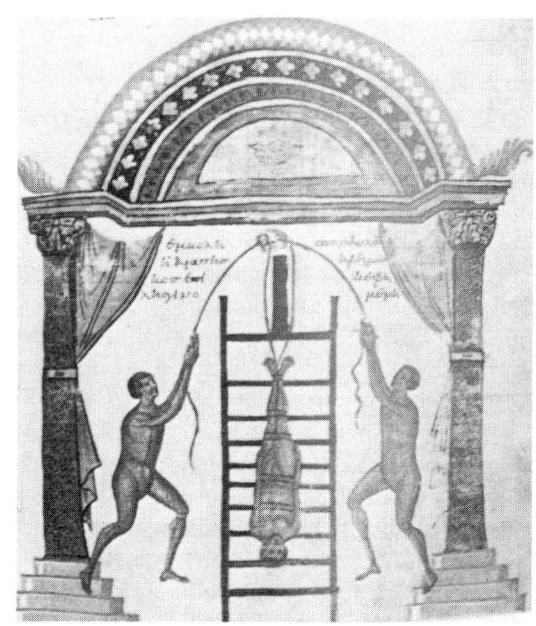

Figure 1.1. Reduction of vertebral dislocation or subluxation by inverted succussion and traction during the time of Hippocrates (courtesy of Behavioral Research Foundation).

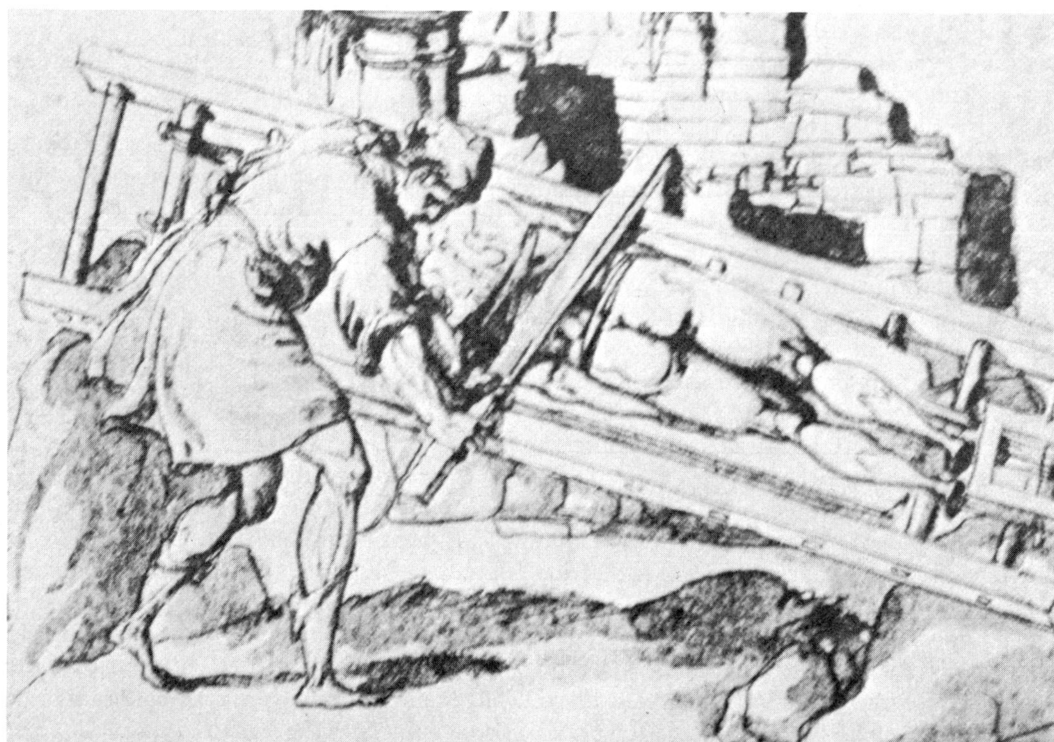

Figure 1.2. Demonstration of a crude method of reduction of spinal curvatures by using traction and leverage pressure as described by Hippocrates in *Articulation,* XLVII (courtesy of Behavioral Research Foundation).

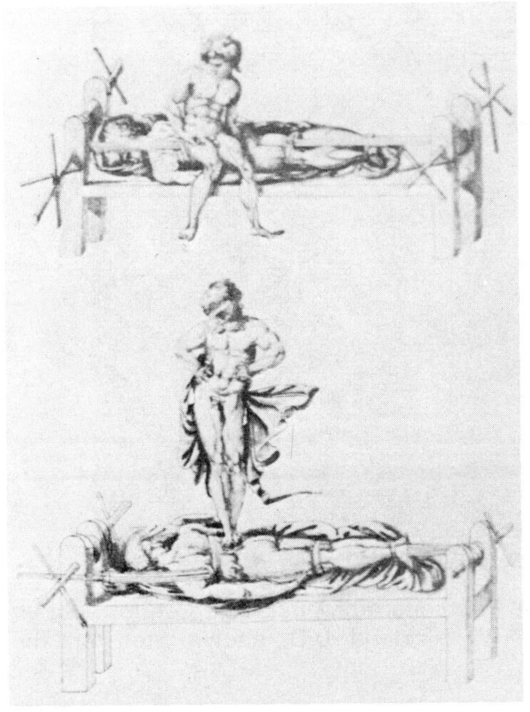

Figure 1.3. Old engravings showing reduction of a spinal lesion by use of traction combined with sitting or standing on the spine by Paracleus during the early 1500s A.D. (courtesy of Behavioral Research Foundation).

Spinal analysis and adjustment have always been emphasized within the practice of chiropractic, but they have never constituted the sole scope of therapy used by the majority of practitioners. For example, a chiropractor patented an automated "traction couch" in 1914. See Figure 1.4. Drs. A. L. Foster and W. C. Schultz of the National College wrote extensively on the physiology of the nervous system and reflex therapies during the early part of this century. In the 1920s, Dr. J. S. Riley made frequent mention of various peripheral reflex techniques in vogue within chiropractic at that time.

Physical therapy and the many modalities we know today did not become generally accepted by the allopathic medical community at large until the period around 1914—1918, during World War I, when their use was demanded by the Armed Services.

CONCEPTUAL ROLE

The role of physiological therapeutics within the practice of chiropractic can best be appreciated via the answers to four basic questions:

1. *What role and place does physiological therapeutics play in the practice of chiropractic?* The agents and forces of nature in their basic state, but controlled, represent therapeutic aids and privileges that belong to all the healing arts. Within chiropractic, these concepts represent a significant adjunct to manipulative therapy.

2. *What is the relationship between physiological therapeutics and the chiropractic adjustment?* The answer to this question is fourfold:

First, solely the structural adjustment of a patient cannot always be considered to effect

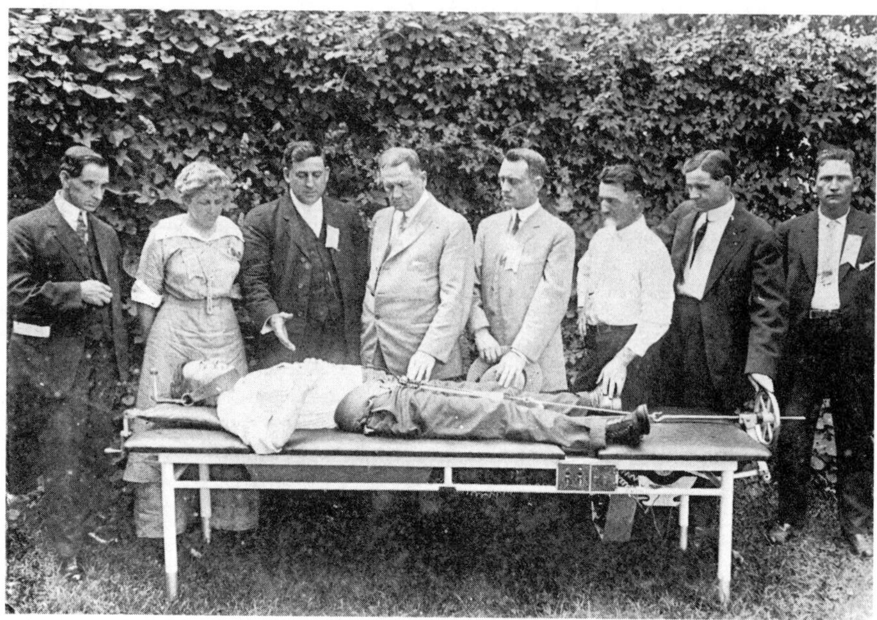

Figure 1.4. Historic photograph depicting a 1914 demonstration in Davenport, Iowa, of an automated "traction couch" by its inventor, D. W. Riesland, D.C., shown third from the left (courtesy of ACA Council on Orthopedics).

adequate case management by a responsible physician. Rest, exercise, diet, temperature control, sensory stimulation, and proper elimination are a few of the other important factors of health that must be addressed.

Second, physiotherapeutic procedures often enhance and augment the structural adjustment by means of physical agents and forces. Heat tends to relax engorged tissues, thus making them more receptive to manipulation. Certain forms of diathermy and galvanism often soften indurated tissues, allowing a corrective adjustment to hold a more favorable position for a longer period. When applicable, joint traction applied before and an orthopedic support applied after structural manipulation takes advantage of the biomechanical forces of intrinsic stress relaxation and creep. Both of these properties are a function of time that is difficult to achieve manually.[5]

Third, when physiological therapeutics are properly applied, the humeral, chemical, and cellular elements of the body are more competently readied and conditioned to allow for a more effective response to the structural adjustment.

Fourth, total body function is enhanced. Physiotherapy aids proper elimination, promotes proper nutrition, and affects the mental and emotional status of the patient in a constructive manner.

3. *What is the major objective in the utilization of physiological therapeutics?* At all times, the primary purpose is to bring the body to homeostasis, to health, as effectively as possible. A secondary objective is to help the body to normalize or adapt to the abnormal processes of a diseased state. An incorrectly applied physiotherapeutic measure, however, may worsen the condition.

4. *What are the general actions of physiotherapy and, basically, how do they work?* Any form of energy applied to human tissue exerts a primary physical (physiochemical) action. This action, in turn, initiates secondary

physiologic or cellular alterations, either locally or systemically, that lead to therapeutic changes.

The efficiency of physical therapy in the treatment of injury and disease depends to a great deal on (1) the direct reflex effects of the stimulating agent employed and (2) the influence of these agents exerted through the autonomic centers. The typical procedure and the force of a physical modality are applied through the skin. In addition to protection, the skin is the greatest neural sensorium of the body—being responsible for perception, absorption, excretion, and temperature regulation functions. Stimulation of cutaneous receptors brings about numerous vascular changes; eg, dilation, increased permeability of vascular walls, and increased circulation. Sundry reflexes are also initiated that have numerous nociceptive and autonomic implications.

SCOPE OF APPLICATION

The scope of clinical application is directed by customary utilization based upon scientific and empirical evidence, the physiologic effects of the agent or modality used, and the individual patient and pathophysiologic needs at hand.

Physiotherapy Utilization

Most basically, the common procedures of physical therapy on a clinical level may be classified into several categories. Typical considerations include cryotherapy, diathermy, exercise, hydrotherapy, interferential current, low frequency current, meridian therapy, rehabilitative therapies, and thermotherapy. See Table 1.2.

Common Physical Agents and Their Effects

Each of the common physical agents utilized has more or less specific primary effects and secondary effects. Heat from any source, for example, has a primary thermal effect with secondary effects in hyperemia, sedation, and attenuation of microorganisms. Cold from any source offers a hypothermal primary effect with secondary effects of decongestion, ischemia, and sedation.

Photochemical and electrochemical effects are seen with some physical agents. For example, sunlight, heated metals, and carbon or mercury-vapor arcs present primary photochemical effects and secondary effects of erythema, pigmentation, and activation of ergosterol. Galvanic current offers a primary electrochemical effect and secondary polarization and vasomotor effects.

Kinetic and electrokinetic effects are seen with other physical agents. For instance, vibration, massage, traction, and therapeutic exercise offer primary kinetic effects with secondary actions of muscle stimulation, increased venous and lymph flow, stretching of tissue, and reflex stimulation. Electric currents (eg, low-frequency, alternating, interrupted, sinusoidal) present primary electrokinetic effects with secondary effects of muscle stimulation, increased venous and lymph flow, tissue stretching, and reflex stimulation. Ultrasound therapy is unique in that it offers primary mechanothermochemical effects with secondary effects of intracellular massage and thermal sedation.

A brief summary of common physical agents and their effects are shown in Table 1.3.

Note: Occasionally, a claim to a third party (eg, insurance company) is rejected on the basis of duplicated therapies billed on a unit basis for a disorder treated during a particular visit. For example, hot water, hot air, radiant heat, heat lamps, diathermy, and microwaves all have a primary thermal effect and all have secondary effects of hyperemia, sedation, and the tendency to weaken microorganisms. Thus, application of more than one of these modalities during the same patient visit would appear to be a duplication of effort unless an unusual factor is involved.

Table 1.2. Basic Forms of Physiotherapeutic Applications

1. Thermotherapy
   a. Hot moist packs
   b. Infrared
   c. Heating pads
   d. Ultraviolet
   e. Paraffin
   f. Fluidotherapy

2. Cryotherapy
   a. Ice
   b. Cold packs
   c. Vapocoolant sprays
   d. Clay compresses
   e. Cold therapy
   f. Cold immersions
   g. Cryokinetics
   h. Alternating heat and cold

3. Diathermy (high frequency)
   a. Short wave
      (1) Induction or coil field
      (2) Condensor field
   b. Microwave
   c. Ultrasound

4. Interferential current (medium frequency)

5. Low frequency currents
   a. Direct current, eg low voltage galvanism
   b. High voltage current
   c. Alternating current
      (1) Sine wave
      (2) Faradic current
         (a) TENS
         (b) Muscle stimulators

6. Hydrotherapy

7. Exercise therapy

8. Rehabilitative therapy

9. Meridian therapy
   a. Pressure techniques
   b. Acupuncture
   c. Auriculotherapy
   d. Ryodoraku

10. Vibratory therapy

11. Traction and stretching

12. Bracing and supports

Table 1.3. Brief Resume of Common Physical Agents and Their Effects[6]

Physical Agent	***Primary Effect***	***Secondary Effects***
Hot water, hot air, radiant heaters, incandescent lamps, diathermy, microwaves	Thermal	Hyperemia, sedation of sensory or motor irritation, attenuation of microorganisms
Cryotherapy (vapocoolants, ice)	Hypothermal	Sedation, decongestion, ischemia
Ultraviolet (sun, heated metals, carbon arc, mercury vapor arc)	Photochemical	Erythemia, pigmentation, activation of ergosterol
Ultrasound	Mechanical, thermal, chemical	Cellular massage, heat, sedation

Table 1.3, continued

Physical Agent	*Primary Effect*	*Secondary Effects*
Low voltage galvanic currents	Electrochemical	Polar, vasomotor
Low frequency, interrupted current, sinusoidal current, other alternating currents	Electrokinetic	Muscle stimulation, increase of venous and lymph flow, reflex stimulation
Vibration, massage, traction (intermittent), therapeutic exercise	Kinetic	Muscle stimulation, increase of venous and lymph flow, tissue stretch, reflex stimulation

When such duplication is necessary, justification should be explained in the submitted report and noted in the patient's records.

General Considerations for All Treatments

The rational application of modalities requires a basic knowledge of the actions and effects on pathophysiologic processes. Any therapeutic agent possesses a potential for effectiveness and a potential for danger. Each modality has its indications and contraindications, and certain precautions must be observed if the modality is to be applied safely and effectively in line with the biophysics and physiologic responses involved.

When properly applied, benefits are gained in normalizing function, preventing and minimizing pain and deformities, and maintaining what has been gained in treatment. The physician-operator must be well acquainted with the physics involved and the underlying application fundamentals to properly prescribe or utilize an appropriate modality, as well as be skilled with the technique of application, its intensity and duration, and to effectively analyze the anticipated effects.

The widespread considerations for all treatments are described in Table 1.4.

ASSISTING NATURAL HEALING PROCESSES

The primary intent of chiropractic physiological therapeutics is to assist the body in adapting to and/or normalizing the aberrant processes within an abnormal state. The abnormal process existing at the time of therapy determines the particular type of therapy applicable. Any injury or disease state comprises a number of abnormal physiologic reactions depending upon its state of healing or adaptation. Thus, therapy *must* be varied according to the process at hand to assist the body in normalizing or adapting to the condition. The therapeutic goal is usually to stop or reverse a noxious reaction that is preventing or delaying normal healing processes.

Table 1.5 lists the major criteria and rules regarding physical therapy.

No inflammatory process (traumatic or nontraumatic) is static. It continues to produce harmful effects on the patient until either the inflammatory process or the individual's defensive powers are defeated. As these effects may be systemic as well as local, the response to injury is also both systemic and local. For this reason, functional and pathologic disorders and their effects must be evaluated from the standpoint that the physiology of the whole person is disturbed and not

Table 1.4. General Considerations for All Treatments

I. Preparation of the patient

A. Check the following data:
1. Diagnosis
2. Correct area
3. Correct modality and usage
4. Contraindications
5. Special instructions
6. Vital signs.

B. Determine the procedure to be used:
1. Type of modality
2. Method of application
3. Patient position
4. Timing.

C. Check the unit's use and operation:
1. How it works
2. How to explain how it works
3. Know how to use it
4. Be sure it is working correctly
5. Check the connections
6. Properly ground the unit.

II. Starting the treatment

A. Give the patient your name —be sure he or she knows it.
B. Know exactly what you are doing and how to do it.
C. Be calm and reassuring —act with confidence.
D. Explain the procedure to the patient by discussing:
1. What you are going to do.
2. The sensation the patient should feel (test it on yourself).
3. How long the treatment will be.
4. How the patient can signal for aid if there is a problem (have a bell handy).
E. Instruct the patient to remove necessary clothing. Offer assistance if it might be necessary. Give clear directions.
F. Position the patient carefully.
G. Inspect the patient. Check skin and skin sensitivity to the modality.
H. Start the treatment and set the timer. Make note of starting time.
I. Monitor the patient frequently.

III. Terminating the treatment

A. Turn off the unit.
B. Dry and check the patient's skin.
C. Check the patient for dizziness, nausea, and faintness.
D. Ready the patient for the adjustment, make them comfortable prior to another procedure, or instruct the patient to dress.

IV. Precautions and complications

Immediately note any signs of burns or any other problems and take appropriate action.

V. Schedule the patient's next appointment.

Table 1.5. General Criteria and Rules Regarding Physical Therapy

1. Be sure you know what you are confronted with (ie, symptoms, conditions, pathophysiology involved).
2. Choose a modality that is best suited for the presenting complaint.
3. Guard against insufficient or excessive treatment.
4. Intervals of long duration between treatment will result in failure. Generally speaking, treatments scheduled once per week are of little or no value.
5. Don't "overtreat" with certain modalities.
6. Explain to the patient what to expect; eg, long-term results, temporary results, the anticipated number of treatments necessary, etc).

---

from the view that an otherwise well-off person is afflicted with a local defect or that only a part of the total system is affected.

The Stages of Healing

A musculoskeletal injury exhibits a classic example of the healing process. Following either extrinsic or intrinsic trauma, there is at first a variable degree of hemorrhage and edema. This is usually obvious, but in some cases it may be hidden or at the microscopic level (eg, deep spinal or hip sprain or strain). The adverse effects of this initial stage of bleeding and swelling can be minimized by the use of cold, pressure, elevation (when logical), and rest.

Resolution begins after bleeding stops to organize minute thrombi to form the richly vasculated granulation tissue that allows: (1) The *inflammatory stage* where white blood cells dissolve extravasated blood elements and tissue debris, characterized by swelling and local tenderness. (2) The *reparative stage,* where the network of fibrin and the fibroblasts begin the reparative process, characterized by local heat, redness, and diffuse tenderness. (3) The *toughening stage* of fibrous deposition and chronic inflammatory reaction, often characterized by palpable thickening and induration in the area of reaction, with tenderness progressively diminishing. Invariably, the greater the bleeding, the more acute and diffuse the inflammatory state, and greater induration and fibrous thickening can be anticipated.

Since the effects of injury and the body's efforts to defeat them are constantly changing, the doctor cannot rely on one observation or one major symptom in evaluating the condition of the patient, especially one seriously injured or ill. Repeated observations must be made and indications of the patient's circulatory condition, temperature, blood pressure, pulse, respiration, color, and vitality must all be considered to obtain as clear a picture as possible of the patient's condition and the treatment required at the moment the particular observation is made. Pain, tenderness, local swelling, spasm, ranges of motion, neurologic findings, weakness, vital signs, and the psyche are the doctor's primary indices for evaluating the progress of recovery.

Procedural Applications Relative to Pathogenesis

Whether a tissue becomes primarily injured through frank trauma or microtrauma, or is undergoing a change such as a secondary reaction to a pathologic process initiated elsewhere, four stages usually occur.[7] See Table 1.6 The best approach is to anticipate each step in the healing process and provide the opportunity for natural processes to express themselves. This is not to say that if a variation is seen at one of the normal stages of healing that treatment should not be varied accordingly. Increased local swelling and tenderness during a later stage typically indicate an infectious process.

While these stages and their processes usually exist in varying degrees within tissues simultaneously, one process usually dominates. Treatment should be directed primarily at the dominant process and altered as the dominant feature changes. In this context, the presence of a coexisting neuropathy must be realized and the area of therapy should be considered as not only at the site of local symptoms, but also at the neuromere or spinal segment directly or indirectly involved.

Nothing should be done during the complicated healing stages that might disrupt the natural process or restimulate bleeding or swelling. The injury itself is all the local stimulation necessary for maximum response. Direct massage, heat, hydrocollators, whirlpool baths, ultrasonics, enzymes, hormones, and other extrinsic stimulants are usually contraindicated as they only add additional irritation to an already maximally stimulated part.

Basic Rehabilitation Concerns

Once the stage of likely recurrent bleeding and swelling has passed, a gradual rehabilitation program can be initiated that encourages the inflammatory reaction of resolution to pass quickly and reduce fibrous thickening of tissues. This program may be accelerated once the stage of fibrous thickening, noted through inspection and palpation, is exhibited. A great deal of atrophy, muscle weakness, and fibrous induration can be eliminated by applying progressive rehabilitative procedures as soon as possible. Naturally, timing must be coordinated with the type of injury; eg, bone injuries require longer support and rehabilitation procedures than do soft-tissue injuries.

When necessary, continuous support during the resolution stage must be provided by external measures without impairing the natural healing process. The common means are through tapes, bandages, splints, and foam-type braces. However, while extensive and prolonged immobilization assures a painless recovery in most instances, it always carries with it a degree of related fibrosis and atrophy. On the other hand, quickly initiated and gradual rehabilitation speeds the reduction of swelling and tenderness, and minimizes fibrosis and atrophy. Thus, a compromise must often be made.

CLOSING REMARKS

Physiotherapeutic procedures can often enhance and augment specific structural adjustments by means of physical agents and forces. The goal is to assist the body in adapting to and/or normalizing the aberrant processes within an abnormal state. In each application, the primary purpose is to bring the body to homeostasis as effectively as possible.

While the stages of healing and their processes usually exist in varying degrees within tissues simultaneously, one process usually dominates. Treatment should be directed primarily at the dominant process and altered as the dominant feature changes, keeping in mind that each of the common physical agents has more or less specific primary effects and secondary effects. Nothing should be done during the complicated stages of healing that might disrupt the natural processes.

Table 1.6. Modalities Related to the Physiologic Stages Involved in Healing[8]

I. **Stage of Hyperemia or Active Congestion**
   1. *Ice packs:* vasoconstrictive effects.
   2. *Galvanism:* vasoconstrictive, hardening of tissues effects.
   3. *Pulsed ultrasound:* dispersing effects; increased membrane permeability effects.
   4. *Rest,* with possible support: prevents irritation and further injury.

II. **Stage of Passive Congestion**
   1. *Alternating hot and cold applications,* preferably in a 3:1 ratio every few hours: revulsive effects.
   2. *Light massage,* particularly effleurage: revulsive effects.
   3. *Passive manipulation:* effects of revulsion, maintenance of muscle tone, freeing of coagulates and possibly early adhesions.
   4. *Mild range of motion exercise:* effects same as 3.
   5. *Alternating current stimulation,* of a surging nature: effects same as 3.
   6. *Ultrasound:* increase in gaseous exchange, dispersion of fluids, liquefaction of gels, and increased membrane permeability effects.

III. **Stage of Consolidation and/or Formation of Fibrinous Coagulant**
   1. *Local moderate heat,* preferably of a moist nature: mild vasodilation, increased membrane permeability effect.
   2. *Moderate active exercise:* revulsive effects, freeing of coagulant and early adhesions, maintenance of tone, and ligamentous and muscular integrity effects.
   3. *Motorized alternating traction:* effects same as 2.
   4. *Moderate range of motion manipulation:* effects same as 2.
   5. *Ultrasound:* hyperemia, liquefaction of gels, dispersion of gases and fluids, increased membrane permeability, and tissue-softening effects.
   6. *Sinusoidal current,* surging or pulsating: effects same as 2.

IV. **Stage of Fibroblastic Activity and Fibrosis**
   1. *Deep heat,* prolonged (eg, diathermy): prolonged vasodilation, increased membrane permeability, increased chemical activity effects.
   2. *Deep massage* (eg, petrissage or other soft-tissue manipulation: tends to break down fibrotic tissue and create more elasticity.
   3. *Vigorous active exercise,* preferably with slight traction or at least without weight bearing: maintains muscle and ligamentous integrity, stretches fibrotic tissues, breaks adhesions, and creates greater elasticity.
   4. *Motorized alternating traction:* effects same as 3.
   5. *Negative galvanism,* particularly with an antisclerotic (eg, potassium iodine): vasodilation, softening, liquefaction, and antisclerotic activity effects.
   6. *Ultrasound:* effects causing softening of tissues as previously mentioned.
   7. *Active joint manipulation:* reduction of muscular spasm, breaking of adhesions and fibrotic tissue, and restoration of physiologic motion effects.

—Adapted from 1975 report of the ACA Council on Physiotherapy

Undertreatment or infrequently administered therapy will undoubtedly fail to bring about the results desired. On the other hand, overtreatment, whether it be of time or intensity, may counteract the beneficial effects desired. In any particular stage of physiologic activity, a misapplied or too vigorous application may be an insult to the lesion as well as to adjacent healthy tissues, causing a return to active inflammation.

REFERENCES

1. Thomas CL (ed): *Taber's Cyclopedic Medical Dictionary,* ed 14. Philadelphia, F.A. Davis, 1981, p 1098.
2. ACA Council on Physiological Therapeutics: Physiotherapy guidelines for the chiropractic profession. *ACA Journal of Chiropractic,* June 1975, p IX, S—65.
3. Schafer RC: *Chiropractic Health Care,* ed 3. Des Moines, IA, The Foundation for Chiropractic Education and Research, 1978, p 14.
4. Ibid: pp 31-32.
5. Schafer RC: *Clinical Biomechanics.* Baltimore, Williams & Wilkins, 1983, pp 356-357.
6. ACA Council on Physiological Therapeutics: Physiotherapy guidelines for the chiropractic profession. *ACA Journal of Chiropractic,* June 1975, p IX, S—66.
7. Schafer RC: *Chiropractic Management of Sports and Recreational Injuries.* Baltimore, Williams & Wilkins, 1982, pp 168-169.
8. Ibid: p 197.

Chapter 2

Pain Suppression In The Twentieth Century

This chapter describes the basic concepts and patterns of pain as seen in the clinical setting, and explains the role of endorphin and enkephalin production in its control. Specific phenomena associated with pain such as muscle spasm, edema, inflammation, restricted ranges of motion, neuralgia, and psychic-related factors are reviewed from the viewpoint of pain suppression and alleviation. The management of musculoskeletal complaints, a vital part of chiropractic practice, is outlined for the management of both acute and chronic disorders. The chapter concludes with a practical summary of the steps involved in evaluating a patient in pain, including how to examine a patient to deduce the cause of pain and determine the pathophysiologic problems involved.

This chapter is by no means a complete study on the subject of pain. Much of it is an updated summary of a monograph prepared a few years ago and material yet to be published.[1,2] A vast library of information exists from which our sources have been chosen to present this practical compendium. They are authorities who have done reputable study of the subject and are widely accepted for their knowledge.

INTRODUCTION

In this chapter, our goal is to examine this vast subject from a practical clinical standpoint. Hopefully, the reader will be given some new insight into the physiologic basis of pain, how and why we perceive it, what causes it, and how it differs from one part of the body to the next.

Definitions of Pain

Pain is one of mankind's most basic responses—an everyday experience to varying degrees. It is an advantage in health and a disadvantage in disease.

Pain can be defined as any sensation of severe discomfort, suffering, or distress because of sensory receptor provocation that is difficult to ignore. It is the result of central interpretation arising from an abnormal condition within the human body or from an external stimulus that has a detrimental effect upon the body. It is a feature of physical as well as psychological illness, and its perception may vary from mild discomfort to excruciating, intolerable agony.

Stedman's Medical Dictionary doesn't appear to do justice to the sensation when it defines pain simply as "an unpleasant sensory and emotional experience...."[3] *Webster's Dictionary* more accurately states that it is "a basic bodily sensation induced by a noxious stimulus, received by naked nerve endings, characterized by physical discomfort (as pricking, throbbing, or aching), and typically leading to evasive action."[4] Yet, this also is poorly descriptive.

Regardless of its official definitions, pain is a quality to which everyone has a personal concept. A stimulus that doesn't cause a hurt or ache for one individual, may produce excruciating torment for another. Thus, while pain to many people may mean different things, its common denominator is *suffering*, whether it be physical or mental (eg, grief, guilt).

Two of every three patients seeking help of a physician do so because of pain, it is the complaint from which relief is most desired, and its alleviation is the primary criterion on which the patient judges the success of treatment.[5]

Although sensory responses often overlap, the response to pain is distinctly different from that to heat, cold, touch, or pressure. Its threshold, however, is somewhat the same for everyone, but how each individual grades pain and responds to it can differ greatly from one person to another. Pain, therefore, may be considered the subjective accompaniment of a set of bodily responses aimed at protection and withdrawal from noxious and destructive stimuli. Pain contributes a perceptual impetus for immediate avoidance behavior, and for anticipation and escape from disagreeable situations in the future. In fact, most psychologists view all animal behavior, including human life, as simply the goal-oriented product of seeking pleasurable and avoiding painful experiences, actual or imagined.

Pain, however, is more than these definitions imply. It can make many misleading contributions such as referred pain and phantom limb pain, and it can become an overwhelming disorder in its own right. It can actually become a type of physiologic juggernaut that disrupts normal somatic and visceral regulatory processes and dominates all aspects of perception, judgment, and action.

Historical Background

Concepts involving pain localization and its mechanisms have been expressed since the earliest records of health-care practice. Plato thought pain was the effect of disturbed elements (ie, air, earth, fire, and water) on the soul. Aristotle viewed the heart as the center of sensation, receiving ripples from the periphery and referring them via the blood vessels.[6]

A more rational insight of the mechanisms of pain did not manifest until the 19th Century, even though the central nervous system was discovered in 300 B.C.[7] It was the discovery that the dorsal nerve root was a specific organ of sensation that led to the theory that singular neural pathways carried particular sensations. This led to the search for the "pain pathway," which was aided by physiologists demonstrating the electrical activity of individual nerve fibers and surgeons studying the malfunction of severed pathways.

Pain Control Perspectives

A great deal remains to be accomplished in the field of pain control. So far, there has been only moderate progress toward understanding the regulatory processes of pain in health and disease. In fact, there has been only a modest gain in understanding the workings of human nature insofar as knowledge is concerned. The physician, therefore, is in a key position to contribute to mankind's well-being on an individual and collective basis. By analyzing and sharing clinical experiences, physicians can contribute to humanity's further understanding of self and of the many opportunities we have for constructive adaptation upon this magnificent spaceship that we call Earth.

In this context, therapy should be geared toward an attempt at restoration of normal sensory input signals from any affected part—for it is observed that *normal input conditions normal output.* To return input to normal tends to restore exaggerated reflexes to their usual regulatory levels and thereby decrease the number of sites of origin of painful signals. To return input to normal also affords corrective assistance to whatever higher centers have started to become self-sustaining sources of abnormal pain perception.

Obviously, early detection is always a benefit to case management. In all cases, the treatment of any and all sources of pain (primary and secondary) is indicated.

BASIC CONCEPTS

Pain can be elicited by means of noxious stimulation in normal individuals, and it is also the outstanding symptom in many disease processes. Pain gives us information about biologic status; but, unlike other sensations, it does not tell us about the nature of the stimuli. With normal afferent pathways, pain results from tissue damage; but with hypersensitive receptors, non-noxious stimuli may also evoke pain.

It is literally impossible to define pain in words that would make sense to anyone who has not experienced it. It is an extremely subjective entity, even though it may be accompanied by measurable physiologic responses such as reflex withdrawal, antalgic postures, changes in vasomotor tone, and other reactions that will be described later in this chapter. In addition, inasmuch as pain is a highly unpleasant experience, it has a large emotional (affective) accompaniment to it.

Neurophysiologic Principles

To experience any sensation (eg, pain, temperature, sight, touch, smell, hearing, taste), it is necessary that: (1) the sensory receptors are intact, (2) the sense-conveying organs are normal, (3) the sense-interpreting centers are active, and (4) the associative memory centers of consciousness are intact. All pain is mediated by the nervous system, yet only some pain originates from neuropathology. Any type of nociceptor will register pain when irritated or overstimulated, and any somatic, visceral, or mental stimuli that are harmful to the well-being of the organism can provoke pain.

In general, the poorly adaptable sensation of pain has four components: (1) reception of the pain stimulus by the pain receptors, (2) conduction of the pain impulses by sensory nerves, (3) perception of pain in the higher brain centers, and (4) reactions to pain such as physical, emotional, and psychologic responses. Thus, pain is a complex "mind-body" experience involving the total person rather than only the mind or the body; ie, the mental and physical experiences of pain are inseparable.

To better appreciate the neurophysiologic basis of pain, a review of the function of the pain receptors and the spinal tracts that mediate pain impulses is helpful.

SIGNIFICANCE OF LOCALIZATION

The localization of pain depends on whether or not the source of the pain is superficial or deep. Pain can be localized only because most of the stimuli that excite pain receptors (nociceptors) also excite touch, pressure, or stretch receptors at the same time. See Figure 2.1. Thus, localized pain arises only because more than one type of receptor is activated. If it were not for this important fact, pain would be practically impossible, if not completely impossible, to localize.

Tenderness. Tenderness is a frequently encountered sensory symptom that can be defined as pain upon pressure. *Rebound pain* or *rebound tenderness* refers to the sensation or intensification of discomfort when pressure is released; eg, rebound pain at McBurney's point is a classic symptom of acute appendicitis.

NEURORECEPTORS

Special nerve endings for specific sensations were isolated just before the turn of this century. It was Von Frey, a German scientist, who in 1895 showed that pain spots could be identified that did not involve other sensations (eg, light touch). But it was not until 1940 that it was shown that responses to painful stimuli were produced by the irri-

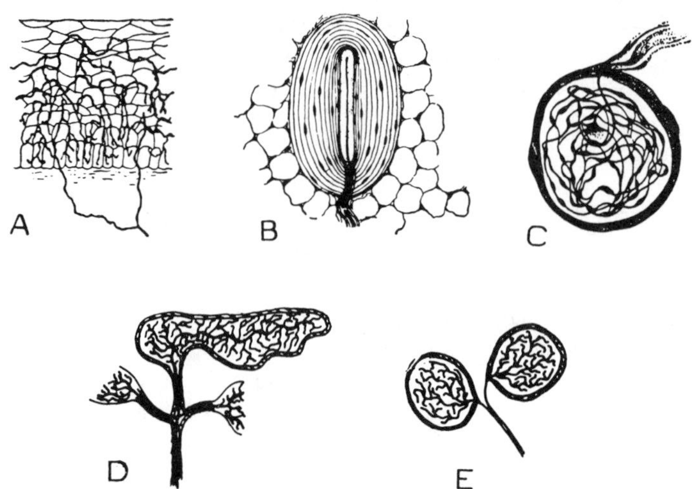

Figure 2.1. Various types of sensory receptor end organs. *A,* diffuse distribution of free, naked nerve ending in stratified squamous epithelium. *B,* a Pacinian corpuscle, a rapidly responding receptor situated in the deep layer of the skin and near tendons and joints. They are highly sensitive to movement, pressure, and vibratory stimuli. *C,* a Meissner corpuscle, involving many terminals, found just beneath the dermis. They send patterned signals of touch necessary for precise discrimination and integrative processing. *D,* a flower-spray Ruffini end organ. These slowly responding receptors, located in joint capsules and the midlayer of the skin, signal messages of joint position and possibly of heat. *E,* a Golgi-Mazzoni corpuscle, a small flower-spray pressure-sensitive organ containing an afferent neuron. They are found near joint capsules (courtesy Associated Chiropractic Academic Press).

tation of free endings of nonmyelinated and finely coated nerve fibers located in the deep layers of the skin.[8] Although free nerve endings are receptive to noxious stimuli, they are not exclusive in this function. For example, it is controversial whether temperature perception is related to a specific end organ. While it is known that pain and temperature stimuli are conducted along the same tracts, some authorities believe that specific pain receptors must exist because some fibers that have been isolated respond only to specific types of noxious stimuli.[9]

During development, reflexes appear early in response to painful stimuli. Pain receptors are, in fact, the most primitive of all neuroreceptors, being free, naked, unembellished terminations of peripheral nerves that have sprayed out among the deeper cells of the epidermis and are distributed quite uniformly over the body surface.

The locations for pain receptors include the following:

1. Skin
2. Periosteum
3. Vascular walls
4. Joint structures (eg, articular cartilage, synovial membrane, capsules, para-articular soft tissues)
5. The falx and tentorium of the cranial vault
6. Deep tissues diffusely distributed throughout the body.

Generally, it can be said that pain is a dynamic response. While damage is taking place, severe pain may be experienced by the patient. However, after an insult has occurred to the body and damage has been done, pain is not perceived unless a self-perpetuating focus has been established.

In 1972, it was demonstrated that subdermally infused prostaglandin increased sensitivity to both bradykinin, histamine, and slight pressure over the injected site.[10] A year earlier, it had been shown that aspirin inhibits prostaglandin synthetase, thus preventing the formation of prostaglandin. This offered for the first time an explanation of the mechanism of action of such peripherally acting analgesics as aspirin.[11]

NERVE FIBERS

Stimulation of free nerve endings leads to an excitation of pain fibers that synaptically activate neurons in the dorsal gray matter of the spinal cord. Not until 1946 was it learned that specific sensory fibers were related to characteristic diameter sizes. Bishop found that the transmission of pain signals was primarily by way of the small caliber fibers, which he designated as A8 and C types.[12]

Type A Fibers. Type A fibers are essentially large diameter fibers. An A fiber may be anywhere from 1 to 20 microns in diameter, with a spike duration of 0.5 milliseconds. As a group, A fibers are subdivided into small delta and gamma types, with transmission rates of from 6 to 40 meters/second. Thus, they have a relatively rapid conduction velocity. These myelinated fibers are mostly dual motor-sensory nerves that innervate the peripheral areas of the body. Their endings are located primarily in the skin, conveying afferent impulses that are perceived as touch and pressure. The smallest of these fibers, however, do convey pain impulses.

The largest A fibers are essentially comprised of muscle afferent and efferent axons, while most touch, pressure, and vibration sensations from the skin and joint-position receptors are conveyed by somewhat smaller diameter fibers. Many of the smaller diameter A afferent fibers convey "stinging" or "bright" pain, although others of this category mediate temperature, light touch, or other sensory modalities.

Type C Fibers. The Type C fibers are less than 1 micron in diameter, and they have a spike duration of about 2 milliseconds. They are unmyelinated autonomic post-ganglionic nerve fibers. Transmission through C fibers is slower than that of A fibers: approximately 0.5—2.0 meters/second. C fibers convey a vague, inaccurate sense of location, are allegedly related to common pain transmission, and are found predominantly in deep somatic and visceral tissues. Thus, it can be generally said that peak pain activity is found in C and small A fibers. However, to confuse the picture, these fibers are not wholly specific for the sensation for pain. Some C fibers, for example, also respond to light touch.[13]

PERTINENT SPINAL TRACTS AND COLUMNS

The major structures that appear to be involved in the transmission and detection of pain are the dorsal root, the lateral spinothalamic tract of the spinal cord, the thalamus, parietal cortex, and the prefrontal cortex. This has been learned by carefully mapping the effects of severe accidents and surgical data.[14] It should be noted, however, that lesions in these structures greatly modify pain (+ /–), but they rarely abolish it. Thus, much more is to be learned, especially about the associated role of the sympathetic nervous system.

In the spinal column, almost all pain impulses are transmitted within the spinothalamic tract. The importance of this fact will be described later. At this point, a review of what specifically occurs is in order.

Pain impulses are perceived by free nerve endings and transmitted to the dorsal roots of the spinal cord. See Figure 2.2. The cell bodies of the dorsal root ganglia are of the small unipolar variety. These processes that

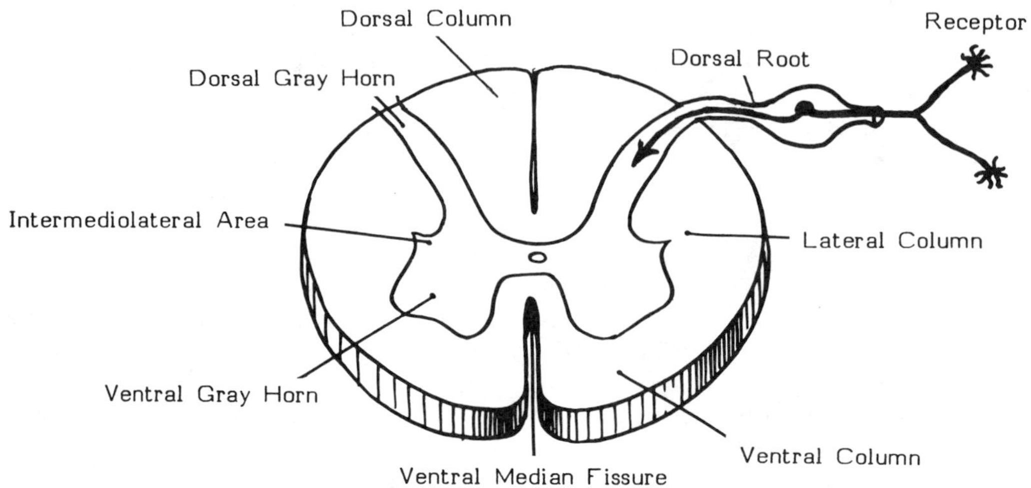

Figure 2.2. Schematic representation of the neural connection between a sensory receptor and the dorsal root of the spinal cord.

extend or approach the cord are afferent neurons—afferent because they travel *to* the spinal cord. Once they reach the cord, they enter (from the dorsal root of the spinal nerve) the dorsolateral fasciculus (Tract of Lissauer). Within this fasciculus (bundle of nerves), the nerve bifurcates and some of the fibers ascend and some descend, superiorly and inferiorly, within the cord from about one to six spinal segments. See Figure 2.3. These fibers end in the posterior horn of the cord's gray matter, in the portion called the substantia gelatinosa of Rolando. Neurons in this region have axons that cross over to the opposite side of the cord in the anterior commissure, and then ascend to the brain via the lateral spinothalamic tract. See Figure 2.4. Most of these pain fibers terminate in the hindbrain, but some pass to the thalamus and terminate in its lateral nuclear group. Neurons in the ventral posterolateral portion of the thalamus receive input from the spinothalamic tract and project it onward to the somatosensory portion of the cerebral cortex. See Figure 2.5. The conscious perception of pain apparently results when spinothalamic stimuli activate certain ventral posterolateral thalamic or cortical neurons, or both.

This brief explanation portrays how pain impulses travel. In summary: (1) noxious stimuli irritate naked nerve endings, which are widely distributed; (2) pain impulses, after a fashion, are transmitted up the spinal cord via the spinothalamic tract; and (3) once arriving at the thalamus, the perception of these impulses is finally achieved by the transfer of impulses to the somatosensory area of the cerebral cortex.

THE GATE THEORY

The "gate" theory was first proposed by Melzack and Wall in 1965. They hypothesized that an anatomical gate was situated in the cells of the substantia gelatinosa of the dorsal horn and that central transmission to higher centers via "T cells" could not be made until impulses pass this gate.[15] This theory serves to explain several phenomena associated with the mechanisms of pain.

It is known that pain is essentially mediated by the C and small A groups. Both A and C fibers send communicating branches to cells in the substantia gelatinosa, and the final discharge of T cells is controlled by the relative activity in the C and A fibers. When

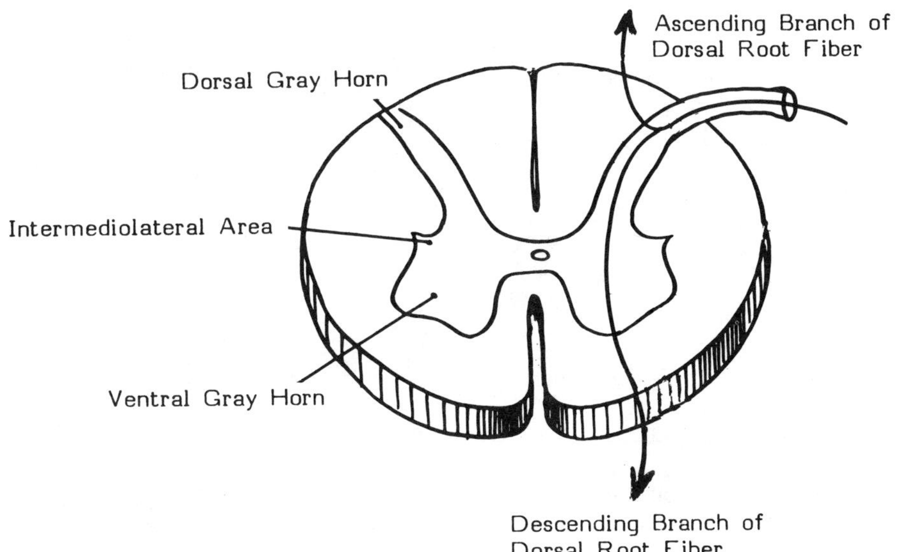

Figure 2.3. Schematic representation of the ascending and descending branches of a dorsal root fiber.

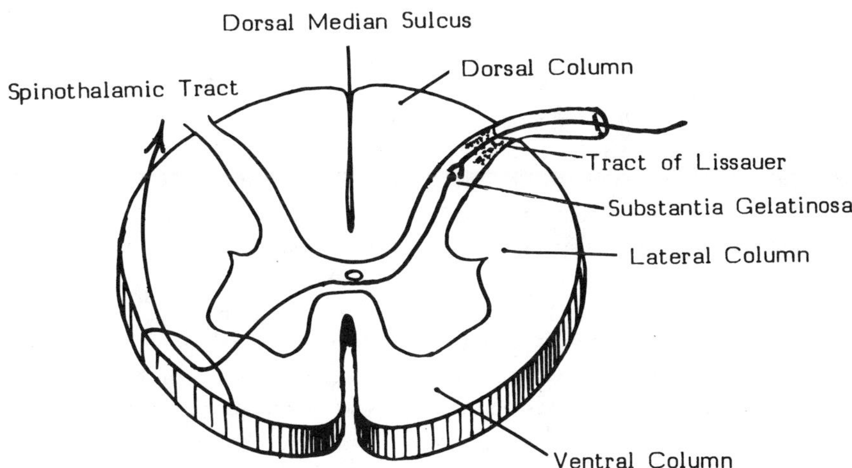

Figure 2.4. Schematic depicting the contralateral course of ascending and descending pain fibers prior to becoming part of the lateral spinothalamic tract.

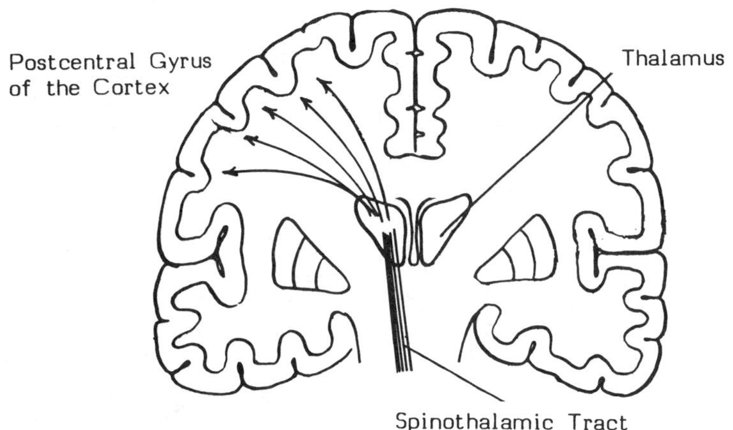

Figure 2.5. Schematic depicting how impulses are conveyed from the spinothalamic tract, to the thalamus, and then to the postcentral gyrus of the cortex for central interpretation.

A-fiber activation is high, the effect is initial pain, partial closure of the gate, and then a diminishing of the pain. Associated reflexes include crying out, withdrawal, and/or rubbing the part—and instinctive rubbing, scratching, and vibration of an injured part appear to increase A-fiber discharge and thus reduce pain. That is, volleys of small-fiber impulses seem to be initially effective in stimulating groups of T cells in the cord (open gate), but this activation can be diminished by an inhibitory mechanism produced by volleys of large-fiber impulses (eg, touch).

This same principle can be used therapeutically. Practical application of this theory was furthered in 1967 when it was found that threshold stimulation of peripheral nerves (assumed to activate only the A fibers), abolished the ability of local pressure to cause pain.[16] That is, impulses from the slower conducting C fibers found the "gate" closed. It was also demonstrated that a large destruction of A fibers produces an "open gate" where severe pain may be caused by a slight touch (eg, herpes zoster).[17] Thus, the gate theory is a useful hypothesis and provides an anatomical framework for further study. It should be noted, however, that several authorities have questioned its complete validity after finding conflicting evidence.[18,19]

It is thought that the (theoretical) gate is normally held open by tonic activity of the small A fibers even though noxious stimulation is absent. While this results in maintaining a constant state of defensive readiness, it also predisposes that pain can be produced via the higher centers (eg, anxiety, suggestion) in the absence of peripheral pathology or noxious stimulation. Thus, a central control mechanism was proposed; ie, sensory signals are transmitted centrally via the dorsal columns and, after processing, the effect can influence the gate via descending tract impulses. That is, higher center activation stimulates descending efferent fibers that tend to influence conduction (+/−) at the T cells within the segmental levels of the cord.[20] Thus, an explanation is provided as to how higher centers affect pain (eg, in emotional states, conditioning, hypnosis).

Direct Causes of Pain

Four major theories have been put forth as to what actually causes pain: (1) a chemical cause, (2) tissue ischemia, (3) muscle spasm, and (4) postexertion conditions.

CHEMICAL CAUSES

For many years, several investigators were of the opinion that some chemical substances are released from the cells of the body or are formed in damaged tissue. These chemical substances, it was believed, could excite free nerve endings.

It was demonstrated in 1964 that there were specific chemosensitive pain receptors. Keele and Armstrong showed that some naturally occurring substances were capable of inducing pain at extremely low concentrations.[21] Some examples are bradykinin, which is involved in acute inflammatory processes, acetylcholine, histamine, hydrogen and potassium ions, various peptides, and 5-hydroxytryptamine. This was not true, however, for epinephrine or norepinephrine. More recently, evidence suggests that prostaglandin E_1 can sensitize free nerve endings to certain chemical mediators and other stimuli (eg, pressure) even though it is not a pain-producing substance except in extremely high concentrations.

TISSUE ISCHEMIA

Another widely mentioned and accepted theory deals with tissue ischemia. In an experiment that demonstrates how this works, a sphygmodynamometer cuff is placed on the arm of a subject after which the forearm is run through a bout of active exercises. When the exercise is completed, the individual will experience pain within 15—20 seconds. With the cuff inflated and no exercise is performed, the subject will experience pain within 3—4 minutes. If this experiment is repeated in a part with poor blood flow and a low metabolic rate, then pain will be perceived within 20—30 minutes.

Ischemia, then, has been demonstrated to cause or give rise to pain. When a relative ischemia occurs, it has been found that large amounts of lactic acid are formed. This is probably because of the anaerobic metabolism that takes place in the absence of tissue oxygen (exercise anoxia). Ischemia, it is postulated, may also give rise to pain because it may possibly allow or facilitate the release of histamine and bradykinin.

MUSCLE SPASM

A third theory, which is interwoven with the previous two, has to do with muscle spasm as being a frequent factor involved with the onset of pain. Muscle contraction restricts circulation, and this, in turn, leads to ischemia. In addition to this, an active muscle is in a state of increased metabolism and the levels of irritating by-products (eg, lactic acid) tend to increase if they cannot be removed rapidly enough by the area's circulation.

POSTEXERTION PAIN

Further insight into the significance of these theories is found in examining postexertion pain of muscular origin—a common syndrome seen in chiropractic practice. There are two types: immediate and delayed. They may be found most anywhere in the body but are more common to the lumbar area.

Immediate Pain. Immediate pain can persist for hours. This is largely attributed to diffusible metabolic end-products (eg, potassium and lactic acid) acting on pain receptors within the involved muscle(s). De Sterno states that an isometric contraction of only 60% of maximum strength results in almost complete occlusion of the blood vessels that supply muscle tissue. This results when the pressure of the contracted muscle exceeds systolic arterial pressure. Such contraction and vascular compression reduces oxygen supply, reduces the removal of metabolic ash, lowers muscle pH, increases receptor-irritating lactic acid, and increases the osmotic pressure within the muscle—all of which contribute to pain, fatigue, decreased contractility, and a breakdown in tissue homeostasis.[22]

Delayed Pain. Delayed pain is characterized by localized spasm and soreness that does not appear for 24—48 hours (often called exercise myositis). While the same mechanisms involved in immediate pain can explain some of the etiology of delayed pain, two other explanations can be put forth. One involves spasm and the other fatigue.

1. *The spasm theory.* There is no doubt that exercise to the level where capillaries are occluded by muscle contraction produces intrinsic ischemia and potassium leakage into extracellular tissues which, in turn, elevate osmotic pressure. This increased pressure irritates pain receptors that initiate a reflex tonic contraction which, in turn, enhances the ischemia. Thus, a pathologic cycle is created.[23] See Figure 2.6.

2. *The fatigue theory.* Repeated contractions with short rest intervals (1—2 seconds) produce a decrease in contraction amplitude accompanied by fatigue. This results in an inability to achieve complete relaxation and leads to spasm.

OTHER CAUSES OF PAIN

Mechanical causes of pain include stretching, displacement, and pressure involving various tissues of the body. It has been described previously that spasm causes pain when contractions are sustained. In addition, any direct pressure on a nerve will give rise to pain in the distribution of the nerve. Pressures can arise from hard tissue such as bone; but, edema, inflammatory exudates, adhesions, gaseous distention, visceroptosis, and muscle tension have all been known to bring about mechanical pressure or tension on nerves in certain instances. Distention of the venous system can also cause pain if the back pressure is sufficient and maintained.

It should be recognized at this time that any generalizations made or any that will be made are just that, generalizations. Such broad statements may at first seem slightly confusing to the reader; but, tissues often behave in certain characteristic ways and certain facts are worth mentioning because they often enable the clinician to identify the source of pain. For example, the pain arising in fatty tissues (eg, in panniculitis) can be localized precisely because the fat is near the surface and it can often be picked up separately from underlying muscle tissue. Squeezing the involved fatty tissue will evoke a highly painful response, while squeezing fatty tissue elsewhere will not elicit such a pain—unless, of course, a generalized disease is present (eg, adiposa dolorosa).

General Etiology of Physical Pain

Pain can be generally classified into two general divisions: objective pain and subjective pain. Objective (physical) pains are those which arise from some foreign agent or condition that is abnormal to the area in which it is located. Objective pain can be further divided into central objective pain and peripheral objective pain. Central pain is that for which no peripheral cause exists at the time the pain is perceived by the patient. Subjective pains are those that have no organic cause; rather, they arise primarily through a mental process. See Table 2.1.[2]

CENTRAL OBJECTIVE PAIN

Central pains are mainly due to lesions in the optic thalamus. The common cause of a thalamic pain syndrome is a thrombosis (usually of a branch of the posterior cerebral artery perfusing the thalamus), which causes transient paralysis, marked loss of position, abnormal vibratory and touch sensations on half of the body, and moderate loss of pinprick perceptions that are followed by severe painful dysesthesias. The second central le-

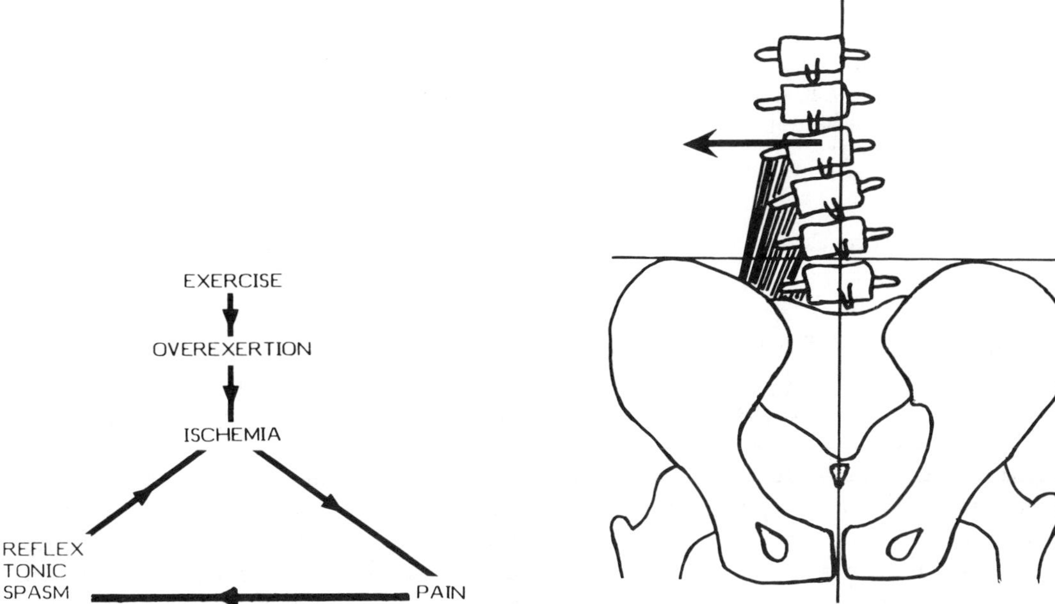

Figure 2.6. *Left,* the pathologic cycle as commonly seen in acute lumbago following overexertion. *Right,* schematic of painful erector spinae reflex spasm following postexertion irritation. Arrow indicates direction of effected scoliosis (courtesy of Associated Chiropractic Academic Press).

sion that can cause extremity pain is secondary to paralysis from either a loss of spinal cord or corticospinal tract function that is always related to immobilization of a joint or spasticity. It is differentiated from thalamic pain in that there is no dysesthesia, and movement of an extremity, especially of the proximal joints, increases the pain.

Causalgias, phantom limb pains, and central pains are sometimes referred to collectively as central pain syndromes even though their etiologies differ. Causalgia from injury to a peripheral nerve is sometimes listed separately from central pain and from lesions within the central nervous system (CNS) that affect pain pathways, but the fact remains that causalgia, phantom limb pain, and central pain are all related.

PERIPHERAL OBJECTIVE PAIN

This type of pain may be either intrinsic or extrinsic.

Peripheral Pain of Intrinsic Origins. A sprained joint is an example of an abnormal condition in the body creating pain. In a sprain, the ligaments are stretched. There are sensory impressions constantly arising from this abnormal condition. These impressions reach the brain, are interpreted, and then efferent impulses are referred to the point from which the impression originated. The sensation of pain, however, occurs in the brain. Other examples of intrinsic pains include the parenchymatous type that arise from inflammations, masses, colic contractions, or displacements.

Table 2.1. General Classification of Pain

1. Objective pain
   a. Central objective pain
   b. Peripheral objective pain
      (1) Intrinsic
      (2) Extrinsic
2. Subjective (psychic) pain
   a. Emotional pain
   b. Habitual pain
   c. Hysterical pain
   d. Occupational pain

Peripheral Pain of Extrinsic Origin. A pin prick is an example of pain arising from an external stimulus. Pain is adaptive to prevent further use of the injured part until it can be properly and naturally repaired. If the skin should be pricked with a pin, an impression is immediately sent to the brain where it is interpreted as pain and motor impulses are sent back to the muscles, which causes them to contract and withdraw from the injury. Other examples of extrinsic pains are those that register from functional pressure upon nerves or nerve terminals such as new growths, swollen organs, tensed tendons, stretched ligaments, and contracted muscles.

Assessing the Origin of Pain

In evaluating pain, it is frequently not possible to subjectively determine how much of a patient's pain is due to pathologic excitation and how much is caused by an emotional factor. In most circumstances, however, some qualified judgments can be made of how large or small a contribution is made by mood and how much is made by the quantity of the stimuli to the overall experience. In this respect, pain differs quantitatively and not qualitatively from other sensory states that may be involved.

The assessment of pain should begin with the recognition that it is a subjective experience, so it is invariably a psychological topic. That is, it is something that happens in the mind, although it is described in terms of events that we perceive as originating in the body. This means that our knowledge of pain is subjective; but, we ordinarily attribute it to physical events affecting the body (eg, the forehead, the right foot, the left arm, etc).

There may be times when pain arises from purely physical disorders, but it is made worse by emotional factors. At other times, pain may be only from psychic origins. Chronic pain invariably causes emotional disturbances and is strongly colored by it. All measurement of pain has to take into account the fact that people subjected to physical pain are more than likely to also be in a somewhat disturbed emotional state.

To further approach the subject of clinical pain, several other principles will be considered in later sections of this and other chapters. For example, the ability to diagnose pain depends on:

1. The different qualities of pain reported.
2. A knowledge of how pain can be referred.
3. A knowledge of how pain can spread from its initial site.
4. What caused or continues to cause the pain.

Purpose of Pain

Pain, most importantly, is a protective mechanism for the human body. When tissues are being damaged, for example, it causes the victim to react reflexively to remove himself/herself or the harmful agent from contact.

The individual who sits for a long time in

a chair has considerable pressure placed in the region of the ischia. This gives rise, after a time, to a reduction in circulatory flow within the lower buttocks. When the situation becomes uncomfortable (consciously or unconsciously), the person involved will normally shift body weight to relieve the annoying signals. If, however, the person has sustained a spinal cord injury that has destroyed sensory feedback from the area, he may fail to shift his weight and a decubitus-like ulcer can form.

The human organism, like any animal, instinctively avoids pain. An example of this may be found in Chicago's Science and Industry museum. An exhibit there consists of a round flattened object that radiates a red glow. A sign above the exhibit states, "Do Not Touch." The fact is, however, no heat comes from the object. The exhibit serves merely as an example of our innate protective mechanism to avoid pain, for it takes a strong conscious effort to reach down and touch the object without first carefully determining if, indeed, the object is hot.

Pain warns the body that something is amiss. It alerts the body that something is immediately wrong, and once this datum is stored in our memory bank, it serves to remind (condition) us that the painful stimulus is to be avoided in the future.

Qualities of Pain

Various qualities have in the past been ascribed to pain. When considering the quality of pain, remember that pain is always subjective. While the effects of pain can be measured in the office, it is clinically impossible to measure in itself. We must generally rely on the communicative ability of the patient in order to assess the nature and degree of pain being experienced.

We are obliged to evaluate and judge each patient as an individual, as a new and entirely different case. To do so properly, we must first know, understand, and appreciate the qualities in question. We should have a working knowledge of the types of pain characteristically produced by the different types of tissues and by varying disease processes and their stages.

Pain may be a prickling sensation, like a needle prick or knife cutting skin. It may burn or be a dull ache, perceived deep under the surface. It may be a throbbing, cramping, nauseous, or sharp sensation. Thus, the three basic qualities attributed to pain are: sharp, dull, or burning.

INTENSITY

Pain also has a certain intensity, and this can also be difficult to evaluate. One possible way is to have the patient rate the pain on a scale from one to ten, extending from no pain (one) to almost unbearable pain (ten). On each visit, beginning with the physical examination, the patient should report the present level of pain. This offers a somewhat consistent gauge as to progress from visit to visit.

Another technique frequently used by allopathic physicians is to have the patient relate the pain to the effect of aspirin or other drugs. Here the patient is asked whether or not the medication alleviates or modifies the pain and, if so, how much. If no analgesic, regardless of logical dosage, relieves the pain short of producing unconsciousness, it is likely that the pain is not of a physical origin. In such a case, some underlying psychogenic cause should be considered. However, a few pathologic conditions frequently exhibit intractable physical pain such as certain malignancies, cluster headaches, or the passage of a kidney stone.

The intensity of pain is one of the most difficult qualities to assess because it is, as explained, purely subjective and because individual responses vary so greatly. The personality of the neurotic patient accentuates the pain, for example, while the Spartan-like mind appears to diminish it.

The intensity to which a patient is suffering pain can often be closer appreciated by noting pertinent complaints and findings that are associated. See Table 2.2.

The general behavior of a patient in pain can give us a fair measure of its intensity and the patient's ability to cope with it. If the patient is able to concentrate on something else, or if he completely forgets about the pain when asked something unrelated, then the pain is probably not severe. If the patient is able to continue normal activities (eg, working, sleeping), then the pain may be a nuisance but it would not be considered severe even if the patient may relate it in terms reflecting "unbearable agony." Through actions, words, gestures, facial expressions, and voice tones and inflections, the patient slowly, and often indirectly, gives us a picture of how much suffering is occurring.

Writing in a broad, general sense, Janse reminds us that the acuity of interpreted pain is greatly dependent upon the degree and clarity of consciousness possessed by a particular individual; ie, the greater the degree of mentality, the greater degree of estimating and interpretive capacity of the individual. The more keenly the mind is developed, the more pain sensitive it becomes. People in the sciences and skilled professions show a much greater degree of pain symptoms than those in the physical trades where less intellectual activity is required. Other factors that determine pain sensitivity are an individual's ethnic disposition, temperament, the general integrity of the nervous system, attitude and circumstance, age, and other factors affecting an individual's pain threshold.

THRESHOLD

A patient's pain threshold is often defined as the lowest intensity of stimulus that will excite the sensation of pain even when the stimulus is applied continuously. However, Beecher's 1957 definition is also widely quoted. He described it as "the first barely perceptible pain to appear in an instructed subject (usually revealed by a verbal statement) under given conditions of noxious stimulation."[24] Thus, a literature search will reveal widely diverse definitions of *pain threshold.* In fact, they span the extremes: (1) the pain threshold is a physiologic phenomenon akin to the electrical threshold of isolated nerve fibers, or (2) a pain threshold does not exist.[25]

After testing hundreds of subjects, it has been found that most people will perceive pain when skin temperature reaches 45 °C. It is at this temperature that tissue damage first begins to occur because of thermal injury. Almost all subjects perceive pain before the temperature reaches 47 °C. Thus, *it is almost never true that some people are unusually sensitive or insensitive to pain.* However, this is not to say that different people do not react differently to the same intensity of pain.

Table 2.2. Complaints and Findings Commonly Associated with Pain

Antalgic posture	Guarded movements	Rapid eye blink
Apprehension	Hyperesthesia	Redness or blanching
Clenched jaw or fists	Hyperhidrosis	Restlessness
Cramps and spasms	Hypertension (early)	Sobbing and moaning
Delirium (late)	Irritability	Shock
Dizziness	Nausea	Splinting
Facial grimacing	Nervousness	Swelling
Fearful expression	Paresthesia	Sympathicotonia

Some investigators have found a remarkable similarity of pain thresholds among themselves and other subjects, while other investigators, using the same methods, found wide variations.[26,27,28] Several studies have shown wide response variations among different individuals but fairly constant thresholds within the same individual at different times within a span of hours, days, or a few weeks.[29,30,31]

There is no doubt, however, that noxious stimuli undergo complex central processing. This has been tested by altering the intensity to evoke a painful response. When considering threshold, individual reactions to pain must be considered. Conditioning impulses entering the sensory areas of the central nervous system from various parts of the cerebrospinal and peripheral nervous systems can determine whether incoming sensory impulses will be transmitted extensively or weakly to other areas of the brain.

Pain causes or brings about various reflex motor reactions such as pulling away from a hot surface, together with psychic reactions that include anguish, anxiety, crying, depression, nausea, and neuromotor hyperexcitability.

Tickling and itching seem to be forms of or graduations of pain. Apparently, they are caused by weak, barely threshold stimulation of nociceptors. Some authorities state that a weak stimulation will give rise to a tickling sensation and a stronger stimulation of pain receptors will cause itching. This precept, however, is highly controversial for there must be another element between tickling, itching, and pure pain besides the force of the stimuli and the number of receptors involved.

It has been found that the perception of pain may be strongly modulated according to an individual's past experiences and his direction of attention and intentions. Since our past experiences, expectations, and motivations cannot be equivalent, present perceptions are not likely to be the same except in areas where general experiences overlap. Even then, two people will rarely report a simultaneous experience in the same terms or with the same emphasis. Therefore, the same event, as determined by sensory data reaching consciousness, may be experienced as distinctly different events in different people. Furthermore, custom and human values may be deeply embedded in these mechanisms of central control of perceptual processes. Naturally, differences in perceptual processing will be the greatest when the gulf of differences in past experiences (psychic conditioning) is the greatest.

DISTRIBUTION AND PERIODICITY

Two other qualities of pain are its distribution and periodicity. These subjects will be described later in this chapter, but it is well here to mention the crux of the problem: What causes the differences in the quality of pain? It seems that differences in quality are due to: (1) different patterns of stimulation of nociceptors, (2) different locations in the body, and/or (3) simultaneous stimulation of other types of receptors along with pain receptors. At this time, we can say that distribution refers primarily to the myotome, dermatome, or sclerotome area in which the pain may be perceived to be located or referred.

Concerning the periodicity of pain, it should be noted that various factors may influence whether the pain is worse or better at certain times of the day or night, or following certain activities. It should also be noted if some factors intensify or diminish the discomfort.

Measuring Individual Sensitivity Levels to Pain

Pain can be measured clinically (1) to determine the integrity of pain pathways, (2) to evaluate the level of patient sensibility, and/or (3) to determine the patient's pain threshold.

Pricking, pressure, heat, cold, electricity, and vascular occlusion are the methods used most often. The degree of sensibility measured can be recorded as *analgesia,* a complete absence of sensitivity to a painful stimulus; *hypalgesia,* a diminution of sensitivity to a painful stimulus; or *hyperalgesia,* an exaggerated sensitivity to a painful stimulus. Regardless of the actual method used, the procedure should afford a clear perception of painful stimulus, control, convenience, measurability, minimal tissue damage, and reproducibility.

Some of the applications described here can be used clinically, while others are more applicable only to the research laboratory and described here for their background significance. A patient's threshold of the pain is frequently determined clinically by (1) pricking the skin with a pin or (2) pressing an area of tender tissue.

METHODOLOGY

Pricking. The simplest means of evaluation is by means of a pin prick. Here the patient attempts to evaluate the different stimuli that the physician applies with a pin.

Pressure. Another technique, and one not as crude, is the use of a solid object or probe pressed against a muscle or protruding bone with a measured force. Various procedures have been used by investigators such as applying the pressure of horse hair brushes of varying hardness, pressing the mastoid processes with a thumb or an object, using a cheese grater concealed within a sphygmomanometer cuff, or using an *algesiometer.*

Algesiometers have been used since the Victorian period in an attempt to measure an individual's sensitivity to pain. A typical application has been a blunt rod where one end is placed on the patient (eg, forehead) and the other end is attached to a coiled spring and scale (calibrated in ounces) that indicates varying degrees of pressure applied to the body part. In other instruments, a measured blow is made to a site favored for testing deep pain sensation (eg, just anterior to the lateral border of the Achilles tendon).

Heat. Measured amounts of heat can also be applied over an area, and an evaluation of the reaction can be recorded. A thermal stimulus with various intensities at a constant time or a constant intensity at various exposure times can be used.[32] However, changes in environmental temperature and the effects of repeated stimulation are often difficult to control.

Cold. Extremes of cold as well as those of heat are well known to cause pain. One technique is to immerse a subject's hand in warm water for a measurable time, then quickly transfer it to an ice water bath and record the reaction time.[33]

Electricity. Electrical stimuli have been used by researchers to measure pain sensitivity since the Civil War period. In recent techniques, brief shocks are applied to an area less subject to external influences (eg, tooth pulp). Such techniques, obviously, have little clinical value except to the dentist to determine the effect of an analgesic.[34]

Vascular Occlusion. It has been previously described that a tourniquet can be applied to the arm while the subject alternately makes a fist at a constant rate. The time taken to produce pain is then recorded.[35,36]

Ultrasound. An ultrasonic generator can be used to apply micromassage and heat to measure individual pain sensitivity.[37] For example, a subject's thumb can be kept in contact with an applicator, noting the initial perception of pain and the point of unbearable pain (ie, withdrawal).

PAIN TOLERANCE AND RELATED FACTORS

In most testing methods, the patient is asked to say "pain" when a painful sensation is first felt and say "stop" when the sensation becomes unbearable. This gives the points of (1) threshold and (2) end-point. The span between these points is a measure of tolerance. As with pain threshold, an exact definition of pain end-point and tolerance is controversial.

During research studies, three arbitrary

phases are often recorded: (1) When the intensity of a noxious stimulus is slowly increased, there comes a point where pain is experienced by the subject and reported (initial verbal complaint). This can be considered the individual's *low pain threshold.* (2) If the intensity is continued to be increased, it reaches the degree where it "hurts a lot." This can be considered the individual's *severe pain threshold.* (3) If the intensity is still increased, it reaches a point characterized by a rapid pulse increase and automatic withdrawal. This can be considered the individual's *upper pain threshold.*[38,39,40,41]

Pain tolerance, thus, is the quantity of painful stimuli that a subject can bear voluntarily between low and upper pain thresholds. However, there does not appear to be a definite correlation between the tolerance of pain (reaction interval) and its threshold.

FACTORS AFFECTING PAIN TOLERANCE

An individual's response threshold of pain may be altered by many factors. A listing is shown in Table 2.3.

RECORDING DEGREE OF COMPLAINT

The most common methods of recording a patient's degree of pain between office visits in a general practice is by a numerical descriptive rating scale. An example is shown in Table 2.4.

PATTERNS OF PAIN

Various regions of the body and certain body tissues have their own characteristic pain patterns. It is well to review them and see how they relate to the type of pain that is reported in the patient's complaint.

Spinal Pain

Spinal pain is usually felt in the vicinity of the spinal column and can arise in the following ways:

1. By mechanical irritation of any pain-sensitive structure
2. By reflex spasm of the paravertebral muscles
3. By mechanical irritation of the nerve roots
4. By chemical irritation of any pain-sensitive tissues by constituents of an inflammatory process or metabolic by-products (eg, stasis)
5. By edema and vascular distention
6. By referred pain from viscera.

RADICULALGIA

There is also the pain of spinal root disease, which arises from the posterior roots. It is due, primarily, to direct impingement of one or more nerve fibers at the intervertebral foramen (IVF). The causes, which are quite varied, include cord tumors, spinal tuberculosis, trauma, osteoarthritis, vertebral lipping, intervertebral disc (IVD) protrusion, etc. Although unlikely, uncomplicated spinal misalignment may also give rise to radiculalgic syndromes.

Radicular pain is felt in the distribution of the nerve root itself. The pain is sharp, knife-like, or even lancinating in character. It is aggravated by any maneuver (eg, Valsalva's) that increases intraspinal pressure. Thus, coughing, sneezing, or straining at the stool will aggravate the pain of spinal root disease. While not dermatomal in its referral, the pain will follow the anatomical course of the nerve that is involved. Sensory changes such as hyperesthesia and abnormal reflexes may also accompany spinal root disease.

Muscle Pain

Muscle pain also has its peculiar characteristics. The pain that arises from an injury to

Table 2.3. Typical Factors Affecting Pain Tolerance

Factor	*Threshold Level*
Age	Rises with age.[26,41,42]
Anxiety	Lowers with fear of pain, domestic distress, and other anxiety states.[41,43,94]
Distraction	Rises with external distraction (eg, noise.)[29]
Fatigue	While physical fatigue does not appear to influence pain threshold, mental fatigue often lowers the threshold.[41]
Laterality	Lowers on dominant side for physical pain.[43] Reports differ whether psychic pain is increased on the nondominant side.[44,45]
Life-style	Lowers in patients confined to bed or home with little to occupy their minds.[94]
Nausea	Lowers.[46]
Pain elsewhere	Hippocrates as well as recent investigators have noted that when pain is produced simultaneously in two places, the lesser tends to be obliterated by the greater.[47]
Pathology	Lowers if tissue damage is present at the site of measurement, thus such a site should not be used to test general threshold.[29,39,48]
Personality	Lower with a history of severe, prolonged childhood pain (eg, beatings).[37,49]
Placebos and direct suggestion	Increases.[29,34,37]
Race	Lower in Blacks, Hebrews, and Mediterranean races. Higher in East Indian and North European peoples.[38,41,50]
Sex	Lower in women with electrical stimuli, but reports conflict with heat or mechanical pressure.[26,29,41,42,51,52,53]
Skin temperature	Lowers when skin temperature is warmed.[29,54]
Miscellaneous conditions	Rises with carbon dioxide retention, impaired judgment, peripheral vasoconstriction, and respiratory depression.[46]

Table 2.4. Numerical Descriptive Rating Scale for Patient Pain

( ) 1. No pain.
( ) 2. Alternates between no and slight pain.
( ) 3. Slight but constant pain, awareness of pain without distress.
( ) 4. Alternates between slight and moderate pain.
( ) 5. Moderate constant pain, distracts attention from routine activities.
( ) 6. Alternates between moderate and severe pain.
( ) 7. Severe pain, constantly fills mind and makes me feel physically ill.
( ) 8. Alternates between severe and agonizing pain.
( ) 9. Agonizing pain, causes restlessness, groaning, constantly tormenting movements.

muscle tissue may be elicited by making the muscle contract against resistance without allowing it to shorten; ie, preventing movement of adjacent joints. This test, although it may be of help in differentiating myalgia from the pain of other etiologies, is not absolute because it is not always possible, even with great care, to avoid some indirect pressure or tension on adjacent structures. An additional feature is that the pain which arises from a chronic contraction of the involved muscle is not increased by contracting the muscle further.

Pain that is due to sustained muscular contraction is ischemic in character. Lewis, a prominent researcher in the neurophysiology of pain, has shown that pain develops if exercise is carried out when local circulation is occluded; but as soon as the circulatory flow is restored, the pain will disappear. Apparently, some "P" substance forms in the muscle and this is oxidized by the blood when the circulation to the area is restored. During sustained contraction, relative ischemia develops because, as a rule, blood flows freely only during relaxation. Sustained contraction impedes the blood flow so that P substances (amino-acid peptides) form and pain ensues. This is the probable explanation for the pain of myofibrositis in which some fibers are in a chronic state of contraction.

Tendon Pain

Pain in damaged tendons usually arises when the attached muscle is contracted. The tendon fibers that are torn will usually not cause pain when the muscle is relaxed; but, with the least muscle shortening, pain ensues. The pain of true tendinitis is often superficial, resulting from a tenosynovitis. It is evoked by passively moving the tendon to and fro within its sheath.

Ligamentous Pain

Pain is elicited from irritable ligaments by stretching and deep pressure. Para-articular ligaments, and even deeper ones, can be stretched by passive movements of the related joint to the limit of the range of motion (ROM). When accessible to palpation, an irritated ligament will be tender; and if it can be squeezed, pain will be evoked. For example, when inflamed interspinous ligaments are squeezed between palpating fingers, pain will be produced.

Painful Adhesions

Adhesions do not in themselves contain nociceptors. During movement, however, pain arises when they stretch or occlude adhering, connecting, or congruent pain-sensitive tissues (eg, periosteum, vascular walls, joint or visceral capsules). The cause may be from direct compression or tensile forces or be the product of ensuing stasis, ischemia, or distention.

The most common situation encountered is the painful adhesions that develop after surgery or major trauma. However, adhesions may develop intrinsically. In adhesive capsulitis of the shoulder (frozen shoulder), for example, the joint cavity can be infiltrated with a local anesthetic that will reduce the pain of stretching, but only partially so, because there may be extracapsular adhesions present that are not reached by the anesthetic. A similar situation can be found in forms of septic or rheumatoid arthritis.

Cartilaginous Pain

As with adhesions, pain arises from most cartilaginous tissues only when they are displaced or swollen and stretch or pull is applied upon adjacent pain-sensitive receptors. One exception to this is intervertebral fibrocartilage, whose posterior periphery is infiltrated with a few sensory fibers. The menisci of the knee and jaw also contain nociceptors.

A cartilaginous loose body (eg, in the knee) will produce pain if it is caught between two apposing articular surfaces (joint block). Cartilaginous thickening and chondrophytes at articular sites are often impregnated with sensory fibers; thus, pain will arise when they are compressed. If adjacent tissues are inflamed, then both compression and tensile forces will give rise to pain.

Bone Pain

When considering bone-originating pain, we must recall whether the structure is compact or cancellous and whether or not any increased pressure is involved. Compact bone is, for the most part, insensitive to painful stimuli. Most of the pain sensitive fibers within the medullary portion of bone are those few located within vascular walls. The periosteum, however, is richly supplied with pain receptors, and it is from them that most bone pain originates.

Visceral Pain

Visceral pain is characterized by a diffuse dull ache that is entirely unrelated to posture. There are, generally, no *articular* signs of muscle guarding (splinting), blocked motion, or sharp pain during movements of the part, unless somatic soft tissues are also involved (eg, peritonitis).

Viscerally produced pain is indistinguishable, for the most part, from deep somatic pain except for colic. A distended viscus can produce intermittent regular pain, sometimes of an extreme degree, which is characteristic and quite unlike the intermittent pain produced by somatic structures.

In general, visceral organs have sensory receptors only for pain, especially nociceptors sensitive to tensile (stretching) forces. For example, a ruptured, ulcerated, or severed viscus is not painful in itself, but one distended by gas or a space-occupying mass (eg, tumor, aneurysm, swollen gland or capsule) is. Receptors for light touch, compression, heat, and cold are either not found within visceral walls or are very sparsely distributed. It is for this reason that highly localized types of damage to an internal organ rarely gives rise to pain. However, any stimulus that causes diffuse stimulation of nociceptors throughout a viscus can cause pain that may be extremely severe. An occlusion of the blood supply can also do this. Thus, any stimulus that excites pain receptors in diffuse areas of a viscus can elicit visceral pain.

TRUE VISCERAL PAIN

The major causes of true visceral pain are:

1. *Ischemia.* Anoxia gives rise to a buildup of lactic acid, histamine, and bradykinin, which irritate free nerve endings. The result is usually a vague, sometimes burning, deep-seated ache.

2. *Chemical Irritation.* The peritoneum contains a few chemoreceptors. Thus, substances leaking out of the gastrointestinal tract into the abdominal or pelvic cavities may give rise to pain when extensive areas are involved because of the presence of irritating substances (eg, blood, gastric or pancreatic juices, bile, fecal matter, urine, toxins).

3. *Smooth Muscle Spasm.* True visceral pain may be indirectly due to spasm of a sphincter or wall of a hollow viscus. Such a spasm can cause or give rise to a diminished blood flow to the involuntary muscles associated, which, in turn, increases the metabolic demands initiated by the ischemia/anoxia. The visceral pain produced by such a situation is characterized by rhythmic abdominal cramps every few minutes because of smooth muscle contractions (autonomic syndrome). This syndrome is often seen associated with such disorders as gastroenteritis, perforated ulcer, colitis, and spastic constipation. The associated distention above (and infrequently below) the spastic blockage will also contribute greatly to the severity of the syndrome. It is well to keep in mind that it is often difficult to differentiate between a local spasm (eg, ileocecal valve), an obstruction (eg, gastric tumor), or a lumen constriction caused by an adhesive band (eg, chronic appendicitis).

4. *Distention.* Acute distention of a hollow viscus is probably the most frequent cause of true visceral pain. The major cause is the stimulation of tensile receptors in visceral walls or capsules, but occlusion of blood vessels within the walls of a hollow organ or a capsule of a solid organ will also contribute an ischemia/anoxia factor. Such a syndrome is often seen associated with acute indigestion (bloating), gallbladder disease, food poisoning, peritoneal gas gangrene, neoplasms, biliary tract obstruction, urinary or intestinal tract obstruction, large abscess or cyst development, most gastrointestinal inflammatory processes, hepatitis, pancreatitis, acute hepatomegaly or splenomegaly, and parturition.

It should also be mentioned that there are some visceral structures that are entirely insensitive to pain. That is to say, no pain is produced when they are irritated, pulled, stretched, cooled, or heated. Such structures include the parenchyma of the liver, the aveoli of the lungs, and the uterine endometrium.

PARIETAL REFLEXES

Visceral pain may also have an underlying parietal cause or contribution. Some pain sensations are transmitted from the viscera to nerve fibers that innervate the parietal peritoneum, pleura, and pericardium. These are primarily spinal cord arcs (viscerosomatic reflexes). The parietal surfaces of visceral cavities are supplied mainly by sensory fibers that penetrate centrally from more superficial branches. Thus, parietal pain is due to this extension innervation. It is frequently sharp and pricking in quality but may be perceived as a burning sensation or a dull ache.

Visceral pain is, as a rule, quite difficult to localize. It is not uncommon for the pain of a viscus to be referred to an area of the skin a great distance from the site of the focal stimulus.

True visceral pain can often be distinguished from parietal pain in that the pain of the latter is usually localized directly over the involved organ. This can create problems in diagnosis, especially when both the parietal nerves and one or more visceral structures are involved.

The location in the spinal cord to which visceral afferent fibers pass from each organ depends almost entirely on the segment of the body from which the organ developed embryologically. For example, the heart, which initially buds from the neck and upper thorax, sends pain impulses to C3—T5 cord segments. The stomach's afferent fibers originate from T7—T9 segments of the embryo, thus its pain impulses flow into this area of the spinal cord. The topographic location of referred pain on the surface of the body represents the dermatome of the segment from which the viscus was originally derived during embryologic development.

To reiterate for the parietal fibers, the pathway for transmission of abdominal and thoracic pain is found to be through the skeletal nerves overlying the parietal peritoneum and pleura. Thus, it is quite possible to have a situation with dual innervation such as the appendix. The body of an inflamed appendix will refer pain through visceral fibers T11—T12. If the process involves the congruent parietal peritoneum, it is perceived as local pain (sensed directly at the site of irritation) and almost never referred.

Recurrent Pain

Acute pain or a dull ache recurring at nonspecific intervals is a common characteristic of chronic visceral disease. It is expressed in those segmental dermatomes that are supplied by neurons whose cell bodies lie adjacent in the cord to the cell bodies of the afferent neurons from a viscus which is or has been the site of distress. See Figure 2.7. This pain may occur when there is no other evidence of pathology, and it is often precipitated at a time of psychic stress or hormonal change (eg, grief, worry, fatigue, menstruation, weather changes, etc).

Pottenger felt that the cause of recurring pain is often a hypersensitive viscerosensory reflex (ie, a functional cord conditioning lowering the threshold response) established by a previous visceral pathology and initiated by a stimulus that would be insufficient to produce overt malfunction under normal conditions.[55] If this hypothesis is true, then a somatosensory reflex from an old musculoskeletal injury could produce a similar effect. Several examples of this will be described later.

Referred Pain and Tenderness

Referred or *heterotopic* pain and tenderness are distressful sensations that are perceived to arise from an area other than its origin. In contrast, distress sensed at the point of injury is called *homotopic* pain.

BACKGROUND

Pathologic conditions in many organs of the body have been noted to exhibit painful symptoms that are directly related to specific cutaneous zones. These skin areas have been noted to be so characteristic that they have come to be quite useful to the physician in clinical diagnosis. Although pain has been known to be referred from one visceral structure to another (viscerovisceral reflex), pain is most often referred from a visceral organ to the periphery. In fact, many visceral ailments exhibit no other sign except that of referred pain.

In some cases, a paravertebral inflammatory reaction need not be of infection but of irritation from malfunction in a part of the gastrointestinal tract that reflexly produces vasospasm in the para-articular tissues and hence pain. Thus, we must be aware that irritation produced by malfunction of a viscus can produce many signs and symptoms that confound the diagnostician.

Some types of pain are caused by reflex muscular spasm. For example, many back pains and certain types of headaches appear to be caused by muscular spasm, with the spasm originating reflexly from much weaker pain impulses originating elsewhere in the body. Examples of this are the severe cluster-like temporal headaches associated with gastric ulcers or the migraine-type headaches associated with the premenstrual syndrome (such migraine, of course, may also be hormonal-vascular related). Another example is the pain associated with a ureter, which can result in reflex spasm of the lumbar muscles.

It seems that when visceral pain fibers are intensely stimulated, especially by overdistension or an impaired blood supply (eg, gas, spasm, appendicitis, ischemia or infarction, respectively), the intense stimulation produces such a bombardment of impulses to the cord that some spill over to affect synapses

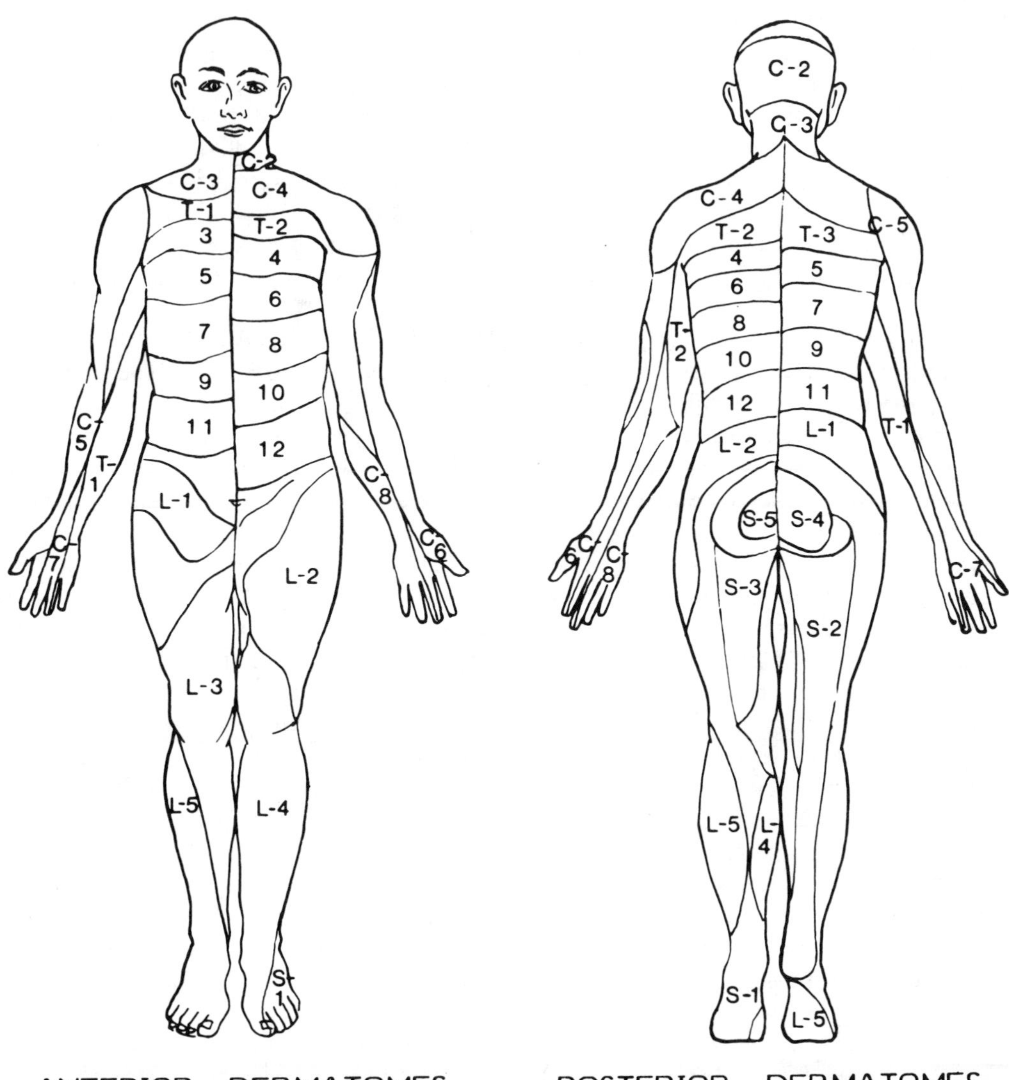

Figure 2.7. Anterior and posterior cutaneous sensory zones. These figures illustrate dermatomes supplied by each of the dorsal root ganglia, and each segment indicates an area of possibly altered sensation. The sensory root field of a particular dorsal root ganglion overlaps that of the dermatomes supplied by adjacent ganglions (from Gray's).

that connect with cutaneous afferents from the skin and subcutaneous tissues, producing overlying hyperesthesia and referred deep tenderness. The victim then has the feeling that the sensations are originating in the peripheral structures.

NEUROLOGIC IMPLICATIONS OF REFERRED PAIN OR TENDERNESS

Afferent fibers from visceral receptors usually accompany the visceral motor system all the way to the spinal nerve trunk. This is especially true in the thoracic, upper lumbar, and mid-sacral regions of the spine. The brain, then, is only able to give interpretation of the stimulus as if it were occurring at the body surface in the neighborhood of the receptors belonging to those nerve trunks which the visceral fibers join and in the dorsal roots of which they pass. For example, afferent fibers from the heart enter T1—T5 segments, afferents from the liver and gallbladder enter T7—T9 segments, and so on down the spine. These levels may vary slightly in different individuals. See Table 2.5.

Both somatic and visceral afferents act on common pools of spinal cord neurons that are subject to summing up, enhancing, and inhibiting effects. Irritation from either pathologic or traumatic processes can refer pain and/or tenderness locally, distally, or both. Because tenderness can be referred, some examiners are misled into believing that the site of irritation must be at the site of palpable tenderness. This can lead to misdiagnosis. The richly innervated posterior joint facets especially may send signals above, below, and outward from the focal site of irritation.

Visceral pain radiates to distant parts of the body depending upon the intensity of the stimulus, amplitude of the afferent impulse, and the excitatory state of the spinal cord at the level into which the noxious impulses enter. These phenomena are of utmost importance in interpreting the sensory manifestation of disease in the central nervous system.

Care must be taken in the differential diagnosis of visceral disease and referred pain from somatic structures on the basis of pain and muscle rigidity alone. Referred symptoms from lesions in widely separated groups of structures can often be practically identical. The symptoms of many diseases can be mimicked by spinal lesions, and vice versa.

MUSCULOSKELETAL DISORDERS MIMICKING VISCERAL DISEASE

Just as visceral disease can exhibit solely as signs of a somatic nature, musculoskeletal disorders can mimic visceral disease. Several examples are described below.

Chest pain. Chest pain points to acute or chronic coronary insufficiency, dissecting aneurysm, or it may be of esophageal or pleural origin. However, chest pain may also be the result of somatic rib cage dysfunction, costochondral or costovertebral strain, or be referred from the gallbladder, stomach, duodenum, or pancreas.

Chest Pains Associated with Cough. In chest pains associated with a cough, acute and chronic pulmonary infections, pneumonia, lung abscess, and chronic bronchitis are usually suspected, along with pleuritis and lung or pleural tumors. Bronchial tumor, pulmonary embolism, broncholith, bronchiectasis, postnasal discharge, or the inhalation of irritants should also be considered. Reflex considerations would include costovertebral dysfunction, costochondral dysfunction or separation, or costal fracture. Reflexes from clavicular strains affecting recurrent laryngeal nerves, cervical subluxation, or cerumen impaction should not be overlooked.

Headaches. Headaches, the most frequent symptom in America today, are usually attributed to tension, migraine, abnormal sinus, tumor, vascular disorders, or hysteria. Often neglected causes are overall postural strain and trauma to the cervical spine, and headaches caused by viscerosomatic reflexes from the gallbladder, stomach, and duode-

Table 2.5. Classic Locations of Segmental Pain

Priority Suspect Nerve(s)	*Area of Localized Pain*	*Priority Suspect Nerve(s)*	*Area of Localized Pain*
Trigeminal	Anterior head and face	T5—12	Peritoneum
C1—2, T7—12	Occiput	T6—10	Pancreas, spleen
C2—3	Forehead	T7—9	Ascending colon
C3, T1—5	Neck	T8—9	Gallbladder
C3—4, T1—3	Aortic arch	T9—10	Small intestines
C3—4, T1—5	Heart	T9—11	Transverse colon
C3—4, T1—8	Head and face	T10—11	Umbilical area, ovary, testicle
C3—4, T3—5	Lungs	T10—12	Crown of head, scrotum, lower limbs
C3—4, T6—7	Stomach, cardiac aspect	T10—12, S1—3	Prostate
C3—4, T8—10	Stomach, pyloric aspect	T10—L1	Kidney, uterine body
C3—4, T7—9	Liver	T11—L1	Urethra, epididymis
C4	Shoulder girdle, temple area	T11—L2	Bladder neck, descending colon
C5	Deltoid area	T11—L1	Suprarenal area
C6	Thumb	T12—L1, S1—4	Uterine neck
C7	First or index finger	T12—L2	Ureter
C8	Fourth finger	L1	Groin
T1	Fifth finger	L1—3, S1—4	Bladder body, rectum, genital organs
T1—4	Thorax	L3	Knee, medial aspect
T2	Nipple area	L5	Great toe
T2—4	Bronchi	S1	Fifth toe
T2—5	Upper limbs	S2	Thigh, posterior aspect
T2—12	Pleura	S2—4	Cervix
T4—5	Mammae bodies		
T4—7	Thoracic aorta		
T5—8	Esophagus (caudal)		

Note: Authorities differ somewhat as to exact levels, and variances of a segment above or below are commonly stated by different authorities. The above data are a composite of the findings of Pottenger, Firth, Head, and Harvey, et al (Courtesy of Associated Chiropractic Academic Press).

num are much more common than suspected. Nausea or vomiting with headaches is usually considered to have a neurologic basis of a vascular nature; however, a vagal disturbance due to upper cervical malfunction may be the cause.

Respiratory Symptoms. Several common chest symptoms may indicate visceral disease or may often reflect referred musculoskeletal problems. Ventilatory impairment is usually suspected in dyspnea or of metabolic origin, but it may be the result of rib cage dysfunction, spondylitis, or paravertebral muscle spasm and pain. Air hunger at rest is a cardinal sign of anxiety, and it is often seen in chronic obstructive pulmonary disease. However, it is also a reflex sign of rib cage dysfunction of a musculoskeletal nature.

Upper Extremity Symptoms. Several diseases may refer pain to the shoulder or arm. This is seen often in disorders other than those of the gallbladder such as coronary artery disease, empyema, pneumothorax, pericarditis, mediastinal lesions, peptic ulcer, diaphragmatic hernia, perisplenitis, and subphrenic abscess. Pain radiating to the arm may be referred from coronary disease. It may also be a reflex from brachial neuropathy caused by dysfunction or degenerative disease of the cervical spine. The referred scapular pain of gallbladder disease and other visceral disorders has been mentioned. Frequently overlooked is the gallbladder reflex causing cardiac arrhythmia. Pain, numbness, or tingling in the hands is seen in a number of neuropathies. However, the cause may be musculoskeletal in origin such as degenerative disease or somatic dysfunction of the cervical spine, brachial plexus entrapment due to clavicular and upper rib dysfunction, or carpal tunnel syndrome.

Vertigo. Vertigo makes basilar insufficiency or Meniere's syndrome suspect; but vertebral artery ischemia due to upper cervical dysfunction or an atlanto-occipital subluxation may be the reason. In blackout spells of an unexplained nature, epilepsy and arterial occlusive disease are suspect; but somatic dysfunction involving the cervical ganglia may be the cause.

In probing the history of any visceral problem, one must consider the sympathetic and parasympathetic innervation to the viscera and the structures related to the viscera. Next must be considered the somatic and visceral reflexes that affect other visceral or somatic tissues. Visceral disease or dysfunction frequently refers pain to the spinal segments supplying the involved viscera and also alters the function of other viscera sharing the same nerve supply. In addition, the probability should be considered of somatic dysfunction occurring in segmentally involved areas causing visceral disease or dysfunction or of other somatic structures sharing the same nerve supply.

THE DIFFERENTIAL DIAGNOSIS OF PAIN

The diagnosis of the cause(s) of pain depends on the skillful interpretation of its often subtle features. Almost 90% of all diseases either begin with pain or have pain as a prominent symptom at some time during their course. Thus, a correct diagnosis can hardly be made without an intensive study of the many symptomatic expressions of pain.

There are many ways of discussing and differentiating the various types of pain or severe discomfort in addition to the two major classifications of subjective and objective pain previously described. For example, pain may be referred to in terms of: (1) *time of occurrence* as in posttherapy pain; (2) *duration* or length of time experienced as in acute or chronic pain; (3) *intensity* such as in mild pain or severe pain; (4) *location* as in superficial, deep, or central pain; (5) *mode of transmission* as in referred or projected pain; (6) *ease of transmission* as in inhibited or facilitated pain; (7) *manner experienced* as in sharp, burning, throbbing, or dull pain; (8) *general causative agent* as in self-inflicted pain, spontaneous, organic, (9) *direct source* as in gallbladder or sacroiliac pain; or (10) *autonomic relationship* such as related to sympathetic or parasympathetic origin. These ten differentiating factors can be classified under four major headings: differentiation of pain by (1) duration and intensity, (2) mode of production, (3) quality, and (4) source of input.[2]

Differentiation of Pain by Duration and Intensity

• A *continuous dull spontaneous pain* indicates expanding inflammation or muscle strain.

• A *continuous sharp pain* suggests a neuritic pain if it is accompanied by paresthesia.

• An *exacerbative or paroxysmal pain* is usually of a vasoconstrictory sympathetic nature.

• An *intermittent sharp pain with paresthesia* is found in neuralgia.

• An *intractable pain* that is almost impossible to relieve is typical of metastatic invasion or an obstructed duct.

• A *remittent pain* that features temporary abatement of severity is typical of colic and neuralgia.

Differentiation of Pain by Mode of Production

• *Pain produced by external pressure* suggests trigger points, traumatic lesions of sensitive subdermal tissue, or the development of a deep-seated inflammation or accumulation.

• *Pain produced by gravitational stress* is witnessed when the strain involves articular and periarticular structures and/or the musculature; ie, structures engaged to provide the body equilibrium which the locomotor act demands. The result is pressure and tension stress.

• *Pain produced by immobilization* is caused by the stasis produced in muscle and related soft tissues by reflex contracture, which is responsible for a dull ache and feelings of stiffness (eg, arthritis).

• *Pain produced by passive motion* is almost invariably a sign that either the joint or structures in its immediate vicinity are involved. Impingement pain is characteristically induced by certain forceful passive movements. The patient usually protects himself against these painful movements by a protective muscle spasm. This is often so complete that it abolishes all passive movement of the joint as in the so-called frozen shoulder. In all inflammatory diseases, pain is greatly increased upon motion because the dry and inflamed surfaces come in contact with each other and the friction thus induced produces intense pain.

• *Spontaneous pain* occurs from direct irritation of pain receptors at any site.

Differentiation of Pain by Quality

• An *acute paroxysmal pain* is common in the neuralgias, neuritis, gastric ulcer, rheumatism, and the lightning pains of tabes dorsalis.

• An *acute sharp pain* usually indicates a severe inflammatory condition of nerves, nerve sheaths, serous or synovial membranes, or an acute pressure irritation of nerves without inflammation. It is sometimes described as a cutting or lancinating pain. Good examples are witnessed in peritonitis, pleurisy, arthritis, pericarditis, posterior root inflammations, appendicitis, and cystitis. Both acute and dull pain may be intermittent.

• An *agonizing pain* reflects an intense torturing state of either the mind or the body. It is a typical feature of angina pectoris, aortic aneurysm, coronary thrombosis, mediastinitis, and during the passage of a kidney stone. In milder forms, it is characteristic of the direct pain of asthma or tracheobronchitis, or the referred pain of diaphragmatic hernia, gallbladder disease, intestinal obstruction, pancreatitis, or a perforated gastric ulcer.

• A *diffuse pain*, as its name implies, is scattered over an entire region or a large portion of the body, not being localized in any one organ. It is common during the initial period of the acute febrile diseases and rheumatism. When diffuse pain is located in the head, it is spoken of as a general headache (eg, a "hangover").

• A *dull or aching pain*, as found associated with a bruise, is found in acute inflammation of mucous membranes or chronic inflammation of serous membranes. Dull pain is also found in pharyngitis, gastritis, tonsillitis, acute catarrh, pyelitis, and prolapsed organs. A constant dull aching, often accompanied by a continuous mild throbbing, usually arises from the body wall or a viscus.

• A *dull boring pain* indicates a deep seated lesion, usually of bone but it may also indicate increased tension of soft tissues.

• A *dull paroxysmal pain* is usually produced by some irritant coming in contact with a chronic condition of some type such as food in contact with chronic inflammation of the stomach wall or the passage of feces in intestinal ulceration.

• A *generalized aching* is often experienced in infectious diseases such as influenza, myalgia, rheumatic fever, smallpox, and various toxic headaches.

• A *girdle pain* resembling the sensation of a constricting cord around the waist occurs in certain spinal cord diseases.

• A *gnawing, burning or itching* pain nearly always takes place in the mucous membrane lining the abdominal viscera where the sensory nerves are less numerous. It is characteristic of cancer and may be located in any area in which cancer could appear.

• A *sharp, burning, or stinging pain with paresthesias* suggests trauma to a peripheral nerve including sympathetic fibers such as a direct blow to a superficial nerve (eg, elbow) or the neuralgic constriction of a spinal nerve in the IVF involving the spinal recurrent nerve.

• A *searing pain* is seen in lacerations, sharp pressures, nerve insults, or degenerations of the nervous apparatus.

• A *shifting pain*, which seems to arise from different areas from time to time, is typically associated with hysteria, locomotor ataxia, and rheumatism.

• A *throbbing pain* usually arises from the vascular system, in or out of a viscus wall or muscular structure. It is usually influenced by the pulsations of the vascular tree. It is characteristic of dental caries, phlegmonous inflammations, suppuration, arteritis, migraine, and temporal and orbital headaches. Pain arising from arteries themselves increases with the systolic impulse, thus any process that would increase pulse pressure or systolic pressure will increase the severity of the pain (eg, alcohol, coughing, exercise, fever, forward flexion, abdominal contraction, etc).

• An *imperative pain* that is persistent in character occurs in psychasthenia.

Differentiation of Pain by Source of Input

Peripheral pain can be divided into the two broad categories of superficial pain and deep pain syndromes.

SUPERFICIAL PAIN

Superficial pain is relatively uncomplicated since it is directly perceived and can be readily localized. It usually has a sudden onset. In terms of location, the pain is often experienced as a point, spot, or line that is well localized on the surface of the body. The quality of pain is a sharp, prickling, or burning sensation felt superficially. The intensity correlates with the intensity of stimulation as seen in familiar surface injuries. The pain is intensified by contact and alleviated by gentle stimulation in adjacent areas. The patient guards the area involved, and often presents a history involving the application of warmth, cold, or soothing and counter-irritation agents. Its duration is typically shorter than that for deep pain, and localization tends to be more precise than that for deep pain.

Associated symptoms may include hyperalgesia, paresthesia, analgesia, tickling, or itching. It may also be associated with brisk movements, a quick pulse, and a sense of invigoration. Hyperalgesia of a primary nature may occur at the site of the original noxious stimulation. Nausea is rarely, if ever, associated.

DEEP PAIN

Deep pain arises from structures deeper than the surface. It usually has a slow onset. Localization is often diffuse over a fairly broad area. The pain may remain confined to the original spinal segment, but it frequently spreads into one or more neighboring skin segments. The quality of pain is primarily dull, aching, but it may be boring, crushing, throbbing, or cramping. And, in mild cases, soreness or hurting may be perceived. The duration is often quite long.

The associated symptoms of deep pain are those of autonomic response as sweating, nausea, vomiting, and at times low blood pressure, bradycardia, syncope, faintness, and perhaps shock. Muscle contraction and tenderness often occur. Quiescence and abdominal muscular rigidity may be associated. Nausea is found with renal disorders, intestinal colic, and angina. A superficial hyperesthesia, secondary in nature, may occur at a distance from the original noxious site of referred pain.

Three varieties of deep pain may occur:

1. True visceral (splanchnic) and deep somatic pain, which is felt at the point of noxious stimulation and may or may not be associated with referred pain. True visceral pain comes from a diseased organ. Deep somatic pain is characterized by its segmental distribution and originates from a lesion of vertebra, muscle, or other neuromuscular origin.

True visceral pain is located deep, segmental, poorly localized, and often radiates or is referred to the surface as is deep somatic pain. Its intensity correlates with the intensity of stimulation. It is described as a gripping, cramping, aching, squeezing, crushing, stabbing, burning pain. It is intensified by motor activity or compression of an involved viscus which correlates with secretory or motor rhythms of the involved viscus. The patient presents a trial-and-error behavior attempting to relieve the pain, which is often based upon past experience.

Deep somatic pain is also located deep, segmental, poorly localized, and often radiates or is referred to the surface. Its intensity also correlates with the intensity of stimulation. The pain has a vague, aching, dull, heavy, boring, or pounding character that is intensified by movement, compression, pulsation (artery), and alleviated by rest and inactivity. The patient avoids movement, pressure, and presents awkward motions because of the protective spasm associated.

To differentiate visceral from musculoskeletal pain, Kirby recommends that the examiner should press, squeeze, move, or stress that portion of the body giving the painful signals. If this maneuver intensifies the discomfort, the trouble most likely lies in the musculoskeletal system rather than in an underlying viscus. If the discomfort is not intensified, the viscus must be tested by prodding or probing if the organ is available to these procedures.

2. Referred deep pain, which is pain experienced at a site other than the area of stimulation. It is projected from a viscus or other structure deep to the surface of the body. The neuromechanisms (usually autonomic) are similar to those of cutaneous zone manifestations but transverse deeper.

3. Pain from secondary skeletal muscle contraction; ie, pain from the spread of excitation within the spinal cord (eg, prevertebral and/or perivertebral musculature).

Three other subtypes of pain that can be differentiated at their source of input are neurogenic, autonomic, and psychogenic pains.

Neurogenic Pain. Neurogenic pain is situated within neural distribution, on the surface or deep, and it radiates. There is an excessive response to stimulation. It is difficult for the patient to describe its character as it is unlike any other type of pain and usually is a combination of painful sensations. It is provoked by any peripheral stimulation in the involved zone, and stimulated trigger points cause spontaneous paroxysms. The patient vigilantly guards the involved part and shows great apprehension.

Autonomic Pain. The overt and covert signs and symptoms of autonomic pain can be divided into two groups: those that are essentially of sympathetic or parasympathetic origin:

1. Pain sympathetic in origin occurs with the vital functions stimulated. A basically sympathetic response occurs with pain of low—moderate intensity or superficial pain. Observable signs and symptoms include pallor, elevated blood pressure, dilated pupils, skeletal muscle tension, and increased respiratory and heart rates. Bodily defenses are mobilized and the patient assumes a "fight or flight" attitude.

2. Pain parasympathetic in origin occurs with the vital functions depressed. A basically parasympathetic response manifests with pain of severe intensity or deep pain. Observable signs and symptoms also include pallor but it is related to hypotension, contracted pupils, nausea and vomiting, weakness and fainting, prostration, and possible loss of consciousness. In the body's prolonged attempt to minimize the effects of the threat, bodily defenses may collapse.

Psychogenic Pain. Psychogenic pain is located according to body image or appropriate to a fantasy. It may be superficial or deep, well or poorly localized, and may or may not radiate. It is described with vivid, elaborate imagination correlated with ideas of suffering, punishment, and torture that is inconsistent in the re-telling. There is a clinical discrepancy between the patient's appearance and the intensity of pain reported. The history may show guilt, a reward from past pain, depression, a recent loss, or other psychic motivations.

SUPERFICIAL VS DEEP PAIN

Pain that is superficial can be better localized and is generally sharp in character. If someone were to pinch a portion of skin at some spot on our back, we should be able to localize the area with some measure of accuracy even though the area is not seen. This is, of course, because of the simultaneous stimulation of touch and pressure receptors that are also involved. Deeply produced pain, on the other hand, is less well localized and is generally of a duller quality, although its intensity depends on the severity and cause of its source.

Deep pain may be best compared with strong squeezing of a normal muscle, although the sources of deep pain are quite varied. While superficial pain is often felt at the site of origin, deep pain is appreciated in the dermatome, myotome, or sclerotome with which it is segmentally connected. Thus, deep pain is generally poorly localized and often felt at some distance from its source. The distribution of this referred pain is segmental no matter what the source of the deep pain may happen to be.

Deep pain arising from somatic structures can rarely be distinguished from pain that is derived from the viscera if the sources are linked with the same segment. Deep pain may give rise to variations in sudomotor, visceromotor, and myotomic activity; but, it does not cause a loss of muscle strength, a loss of normal reflexes, or a loss of sensory perception (eg, light touch, pressure, temperature, position, two-point discrimination).

ENDORPHINS AND ENKEPHALINS

During the past 10 years, literally thousands of articles and technical papers have been written on physical therapy and its use in the treatment and management of pain. Formal texts concerning physical therapy, however, have displayed, for the most part, information that was compiled prior to

World War II. It was this need for current data that this book was developed.

Background

Most of the current articles and research have applied to the subject of this section: how to trigger the body to produce morphine-like *endorphins* and *enkephalins* by stimulation of the skin and subcutaneous receptors. Subsequent chapters will deal solely with the practical application of this research.

The discovery of endorphins and enkephalins was a research off-shoot of two diverse areas of interest in pain control: (1) Melzack and Wall's "gate" theory, and (2) attempts to place the principles of Far-Eastern acupuncture on a scientific basis.

The Gate Theory, in review, postulates that large myelinated nerve fibers of the skin, when stimulated, have an inhibitory effect on the small pain bearing fibers that enter the same segment of the spinal cord. Mayer's studies in Virginia found that all humans have opiate receptor sites. In Canada, Cheng studied small animals and found that their pain thresholds could be increased by electrical stimulation or the use of thin needles inserted into specific subdermal sites. See Figure 2.8. Many others have continued this work, and recent reports indicate that long-duration running, extended exercise, and manipulation can trigger the intrinsic production of endorphins.

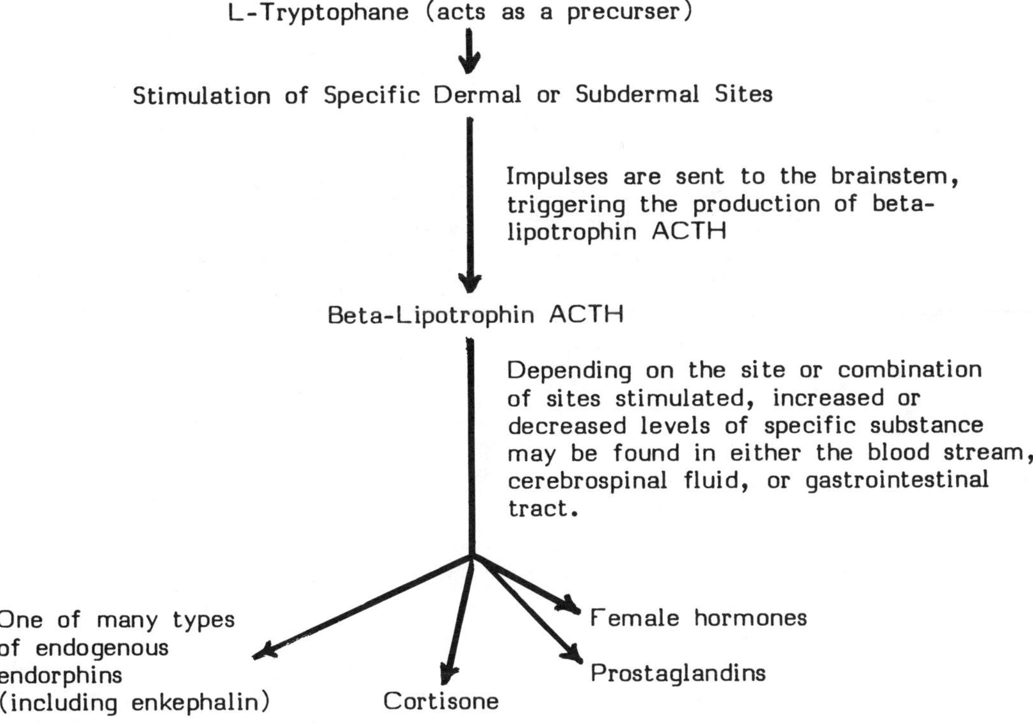

Figure 2.8. Supposed mechanism in the production of natural pain suppressors.

Some of the more recent studies have expanded the use of acupuncture into such areas as behavioral modification,[56] the relief of symptoms associated with drug withdrawal,[57,58] and stimulation of the immune system.[59] These studies seem to have a link with aspects associated with those neuropeptides that are generally referred to as the endorphins.

Historical Perspective

In 1931 England, Von Euler and Gaddum isolated a powder that they called Substance P. They demonstrated that this substance, later learned to be an amino-acid peptide, caused vasodilation and contraction of nonvascular smooth muscle. It also appeared necessary for the transmission of sensory nerve impulses. This established the concept of physiologic transmitters being produced at the synapse that were necessary for the next neuron to fire. Later, in 1936 England, Loewi and Dale demonstrated that nerve impulses traveled across a neuron similar to a wave of electric current. They also found that agents (acetylcholine, norepinephrine) were released at nerve endings which activated neuroexcitable tissue (eg, muscle).

Several years later in 1964 at Berkeley, Chou Hao Li isolated the peptide beta-lipotropin (B-LPH), which was apparently manufactured in the same pituitary cells as the adrenocorticotropic hormone (ACTH) because the two substances were always released together. The function of B-LPH, however, was unknown at that time.[60]

Drug addiction in the United States had reached almost epidemic proportions by 1960. Because of the social concern, federal funding for research in this area of concern and for a cure became available. Goldstein at Standford University began studying morphine and its two forms—the so called "right-handed" and "left-handed" molecules. It was determined that it is the left-handed form that produces effects in the body similar to those of the opioid narcotics. The implication in this finding was that if morphine can affect the CNS, there must be an anatomical receptor site(s) present to elicit its effects. However, another important question was raised as to why the human nervous system would have receptors for extracts of poppy seeds. Thus, it was theorized, the body must produce some substances that are similar or equivalent to morphine. These, then unknown, substances were called *endorphins* (morphine from within).[61]

Recent Research Findings

It wasn't until 1973 that Tirenius in Sweden and Snyder at John Hopkins University demonstrated that a substance was indeed bound to cells of a synaptic area and that specific sites in the synapse were receptors for that substance.[62,63] Also in 1973, other researchers were experimenting with pain relief by using electrical stimulation of the periaqueductal gray matter near the dorsal raphe nucleus. One of these scientists, Huda Akil, demonstrated that electric currents could inhibit pain signals in a manner similar to that of morphine and that the effects would gradually diminish, as do those of morphine. Dr. Akil's breakthrough came when she discovered that naloxone, a drug that counteracts the pain-killing effects of morphine, also counteracted the effects of electrically produced analgesia. The conclusion reached in her paper was clear: Electrical stimulation somehow produces a morphine-like substance in the brain.[64]

Another member of Akil's team, David J. Mayer, presented a paper in 1975 at the First World Congress on Pain, which suggested that acupuncture worked through a central control system.[65] Later, he showed that acupuncture analgesia was also reversed by naloxone and therefore must involve endorphins.[66]

Tangible proof of the existence of endorphins was indirect until scientists began to isolate the substance. This occurred when a team of Scottish scientists utilized literally tons of pig brains to achieve this goal. It was reported by Kosterlitz in 1975 that brain extracts were refined and purified, and then applied to electrically stimulated tissue. After thousands of separations, only one extract was found to deaden this tissue response—and it was called *enkephalin*.[67]

Further analysis by mass spectrography showed that enkephalin was a two-linked pentapeptide.[68] It was then able to be synthesized. Equally important was the discovery that a pituitary peptide, beta-lipotropin, contained the enkephalin peptide sequence.

Since these initial discoveries, tomes of research findings have been published. Most of this effort has been directed toward (1) identifying the endorphin family and the specific neurophysiologic effects of each member, (2) localizing the specific sites of endorphin production, and (3) determining those stimuli that result in endorphin mobilization. Attention has also been frequently focused on three specific peptides: (1) leucine enkephalin (leu-ENK), methionine enkephalin (met-ENK), and the C-fragment of B-lipotropin, beta-endorphin (B-END).

Although B-lipotropin does not have an analgesic property, its C-fragment was shown to have much stronger analgesic qualities than morphine itself.[69] It was determined by Feldberg and Smyth's work in England, and to the surprise of many, that B-END has an analgesic potency near 200 times that of morphine.[70] In addition to analgesia, other effects were produced such as chills and fever, mydriasis, pinnae vasodilation, restlessness and hyperexcitability, signs of catalepsy, tachypnea with bouts of panting, vocalization, and widely opened eyelids. In other words, symptoms associated with severe shock and psychosis. B-END was also found to be like morphine in that it was strongly hyperglycemic. It was also discovered that potent peptides like B-END were long-lasting but in short supply. In the same series of tests, met-ENK was found to have an extremely weak and short-lasting analgesic effect. This was proved to be due to a rapid enzymatic breakdown of enkephalins within the body.[71]

The Receptor Sites

Much attention during this development stage has been directed toward localization of the opiate receptor sites. Early work was done by autoradiographic identification of the binding sites of stereospecific (^{3}H) diprenorphine, which is a strong antagonist to opium.[72] By utilizing this method, it was found that opiate receptors were highly localized within:

1. Layers of I (marginal cell zone) and II (substantia gelatinosa) of the dorsal horn of the spinal cord.
2. Areas of the substantia gelatinosa of the spinal trigeminal nucleus.
3. Components of the vagal system, including the vagus nerve and the nuclei ambiguus, commissuralis, intercalatus, originis dorsalis vagus, and tractus solitarius.
4. The area postrema, which is located in the lateral wall of the inferior recess of the 4th ventricle (one of the few loci in the brain where the blood-brain barrier is lacking.)

It can be readily appreciated that these receptor sites are strategically placed to modulate noxious stimuli, and their discovery helps to explain some of the visceral side-effects of opiate administration. Through this research, it has also been discovered that a neuron produces and releases more than one transmitter substance, and that these neurotransmitters are not stored, produced, or released in the same manner.

Clinical Significance

By 1977, studies relating these findings to acupuncture and other forms of stimulation-produced anesthesia had proliferated. All of these studies, and the volumes of data left in the background, support the following basic conclusions of Albert Fields:[73]

1. Endorphins and enkephalins are the body's own natural opiates, and they are produced in certain tissues (eg, pituitary gland) in response to pain, stress, acupuncture, electrical stimulation, and other stimuli, either centrally or peripherally. Hundreds

of types have been discovered, and each affects pain in a *different* region or regions of the body.

2. In the CNS and other tissues of the body, there are specific receptor sites designed to accept endorphins and enkephalins when they are not blocked by other substances (eg, naloxone).

3. Acupuncture, TENS, and other forms of electrical stimulation can be effective in the management and treatment of acute and chronic pain, in part at least, through the biologic activation of neurohormonal, neurotransmitter systems. See Figure 2.9.

Most authorities feel that endorphins are about 200 times more potent than morphine. Some types of endorphins (eg, dynorphin) are thought to be 730 times more potent than L-enkephalin. Although it is difficult to ascertain pain relief in humans, it can be stated with some certainty that if the correct procedure is followed, then pain relief will be dramatic and significant.

Mechanisms for Stimulating the Production of Endorphins

Stimulations of the skin with a needle or an electric impulse triggers the brainstem to increase levels in the blood stream, cerebrospinal fluid, and the gastrointestinal tract. In this context, three points should be noted:

1. Levels build up within 30 seconds; however, clinical results are often not appreciated by the patient until 12—24 hours later.

2. *The site of stimulation determines the type of endorphin that is released and the area of the body that it will affect.* Thus, endorphins are *site specific* in their effect.

3. Since an active endorphin is a circulating hormone, the side of the body (when bilateral points exist) stimulated makes little or no difference (other than psychological).

According to recent research findings, the production of endorphins may be stimulated by acupuncture needles or electrical stimulation placed at specific sites. These sites are the subject of the next chapter. For now, it is well to list the following rules that apply when electrical stimulation is used:

1. A small diameter electrode, no larger than a dime, should be used. See Figure 2.10.

2. Most research indicates that from 1 to 10 pulses per second (Hertz) for the frequency of stimulation is appropriate. However, recent evidence seems to indicate that the best results occur at 4—6 Hz.

3. Stimulation must be to the exact site. See Figures 2.11 and 2.12. Combinations of sites may trigger endorphins that affect pain in various areas of the body.

Mechanisms for Stimulating the Production of Enkephalins

Stimulating the production of enkephalin is primarily by means of electrical stimulation to the skin. The following general rules of application apply.

1. Dampened sponge electrodes, 3 or 4 square inches in size, are commonly used. Firm skin contact is essential. Stiff electrodes that do not readily conform to the shape of the surface make poor conductors and greatly limit the depth of impulse penetration.

2. Research appears to indicate that pulse rates of 70—130 Hz when using high-volt modalities and 90—100 Hz when using interferential units are most valuable. Some studies with interferential tend to indicate that modulation of frequency is valuable because it limits accommodation.

3. Although almost all modalities have some analgesic properties, low frequency spiked-wave therapies (eg, TENS) are preferred.

4. Careful placement at the segmental level of involvement is essential.

5. With patients in acute pain (eg, IVD syndrome), it should be made certain that the intensity of the stimulation is just to the level where the patient barely perceives the current. In this manner, the physician is able to achieve effective sensory stimulation with-

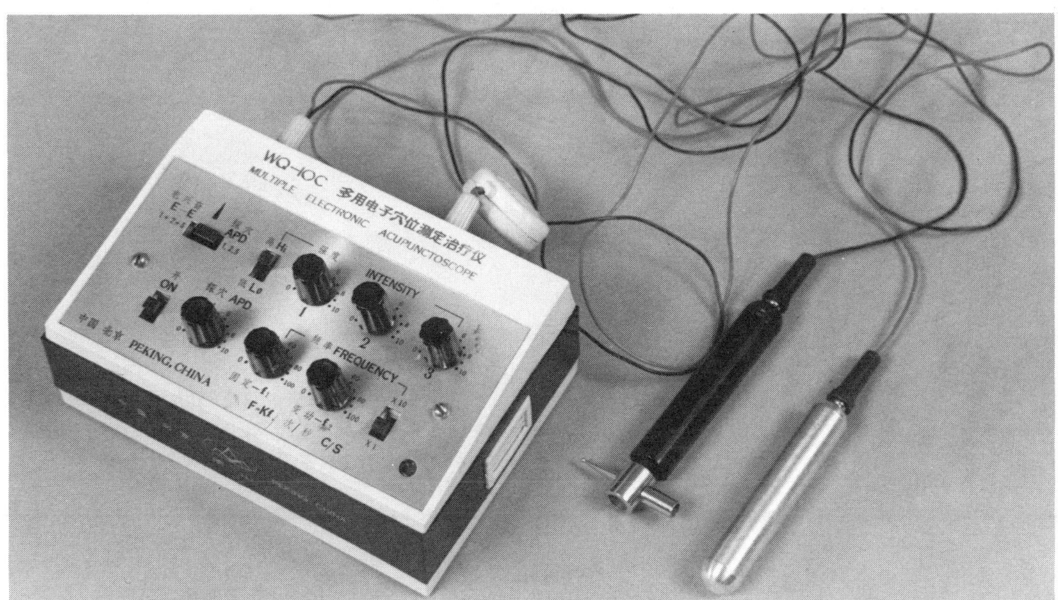

Figure 2.9. The WQ-10C electronic acupunctoscope. Small, relatively inexpensive, portable, battery-operated units such as this are often as efficient as more expensive devices.

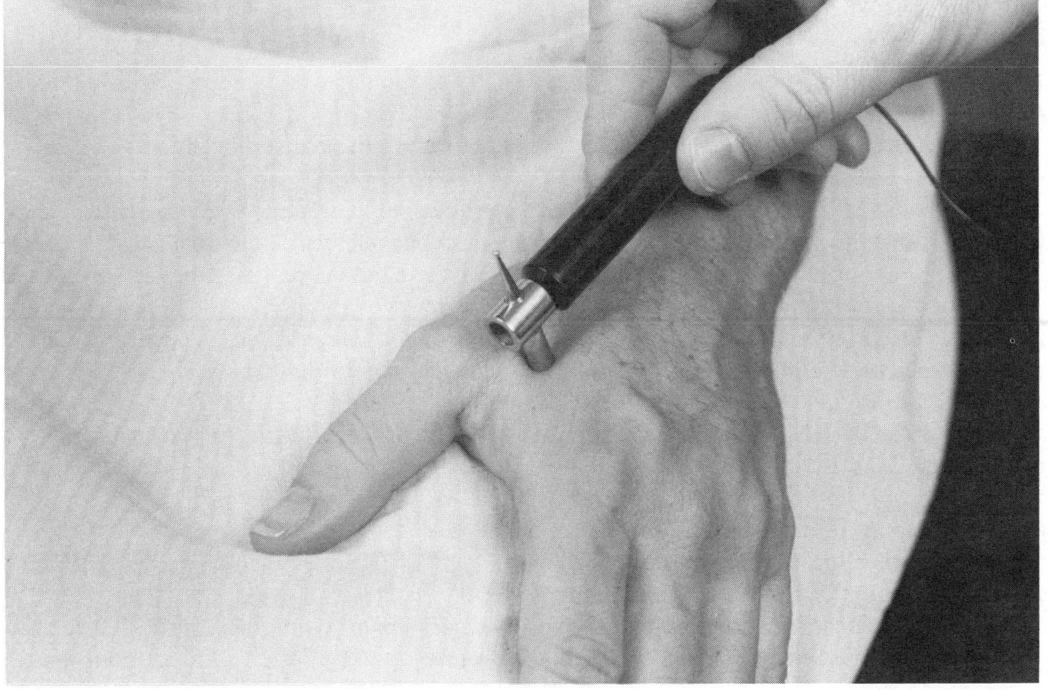

Figure 2.10. The small applicator head, approximately $\frac{3}{16}$-inch OD, being utilized to stimulate point LI-4 is hollow so that an inserted cotton plug (eg, Q-tip) may be soaked in a saline solution to assure adequate conduction.

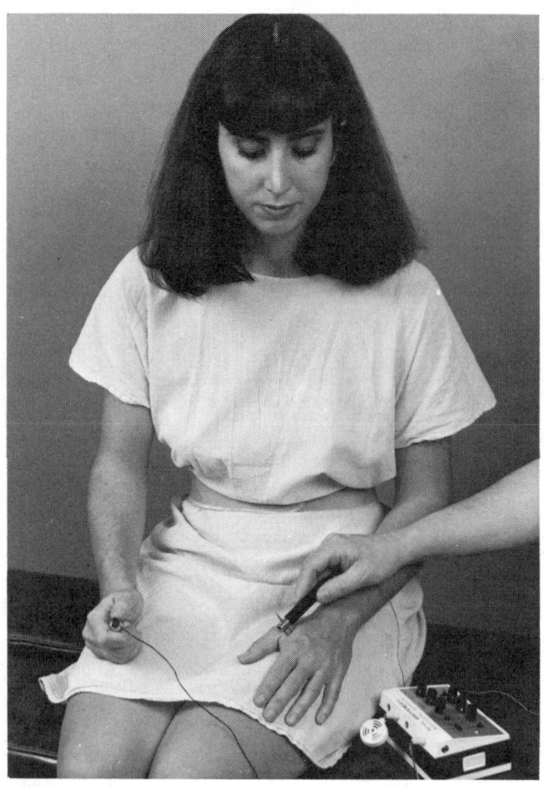

Figure 2.11. In this photograph, point LI-4 is being stimulated to relieve pain in the upper extremity, anterior neck, face, or scalp.

out aggravating the patient's complaint by producing muscle contractions.

Closing Remarks

The principles of acupuncture are still treated as experimental methods in many circles within the Western health-care professions. The undisputed findings in endorphin and enkephalin research should now lay outdated skepticisms aside. While there are still specific questions to be answered, there is no longer a need to defend the efficacy of acupuncture by needling or electrical stimulation as modalities for the control of pain. Bioenergetic and biochemical mechanisms can be clearly demonstrated in response to acupuncture-induced stimuli.[74]

Health according to Chinese philosophy is the result of body, mind, and spirit being in harmony with the environment. Only by treating all these diverse elements as a *single, balanced energy system* can harmony and wellness be maintained. A student of chiropractic history will note that such a philosophy is parallel to that expressed by D. D. Palmer throughout his initial text.[75]. A student of contemporary science will note that it parallels the findings of such noted physical scientists as Einstein, Rosen, and Podolsky, whose work was primarily at the microscopic level.[76,77]

MUSCLE SPASMS AND PAIN

Acute pain syndromes with a history of overexertion are often muscular in origin. This overexertion may be from (1) continuous contractions of long duration in a normal physiologic state, (2) vigorous jerky movements of short duration, or (3) a combina-

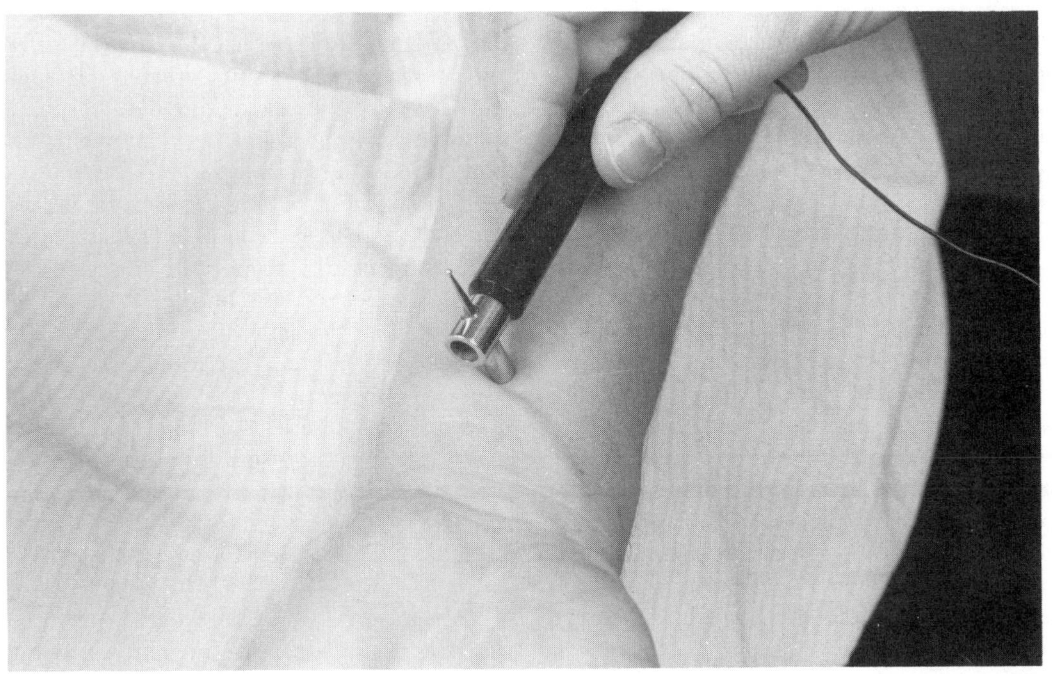

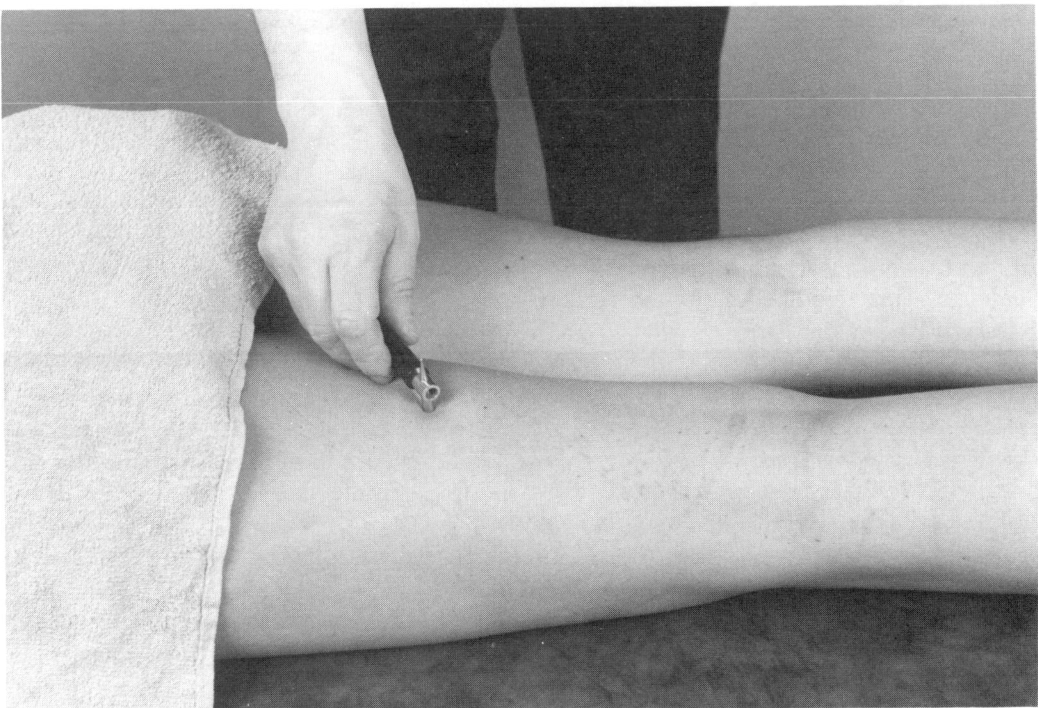

Figure 2.12. *Top,* stimulation to point HC-6 to relieve thoracic pain; *bottom,* stimulation to point BL-51 to relieve low back or lower extremity pain. Pertinent meridian points will be more thoroughly described in Chapter 3.

tion of stretch reflex and relaxation reactions if fibers have been stretched to an abnormal length. It has been shown that repeated stress can produce more soreness if a short rest interval is allowed between movements (eg, shoveling).[78]

Clinical Considerations

Once the difference between the normal and the abnormal is well understood, changes in posture, muscle tone, and movement offer fundamental clinical clues to diagnosis and therapy. And once the biomechanical mechanisms involved are appreciated, painful effects can often be reproduced or relieved at will. Knowing exactly *where, when,* and *how* motion increases or decreases pain are the major clues that lead the examiner to find and correct the fault whether it be functional or structural.

Observing how the body moves offers the best clues to muscle trouble. The patient will invariably assume an antalgic position. In low back spasm, for example, the posteriorly rotated pelvis, the flattened lumbar area, and the slight flexion of the knees and hips, bilateral or unilateral, are unconscious attempts to lessen the tension of the involved sciatic nerve and/or to reduce intradisc pressure. Antalgic muscle spasm is extremely common to acute lumbar dysfunction. The greater the pain, the greater will be this "semi-squat" posture in the upright position.

Note: Whenever muscle tenderness is found, the examiner should keep in mind that the sensory innervation of muscle follows the motor innervation and not that of the cutaneous zones.

GENERAL SPASMS

General spasm of the spinal muscles guarding motion in the vertebral joints can be tested by watching the body attitude (eg, stiff, military carriage) and by efforts to bend the spine forward, backward, and to the sides. If we are familiar with the average range of mobility in each direction at different ages, this test is usually easy and rapid. Care should be taken to differentiate phasic spasm (usually antalgic) from frequently exhibited reflex hypertonicity.

It is one thing to find muscle spasm present and another to determine if it is protective, compensatory, hysterical, or a causative factor. Careful analysis of gait is an important method of gaining differential clues. Limitations of motion due to muscular spasm are seen with special frequency in joint pathology and subluxation-fixations, but they may occur in almost any form of joint trouble, particularly in the larger joints.

THE STRETCH REFLEX

Keep in mind that the myotatic stretch reflex uses a single sensory neuron and is initiated by elongation of the muscle spindle's annulospiral receptors. The effect is a protective contraction designed to protect against further stretch so that the muscle may maintain a constant length. This reflex action is many times more severe if initiated by a sudden stretch (eg, dynamic thrust) than by a slow stretch. In addition, inhibitory impulses are transmitted to the motor neurons of the antagonists (reciprocal inhibition) and facilitating impulses are transmitted to the synergists—both of which enhance the response.

The stretch reflex is not normally initiated by voluntary contraction. If there is spasm present after trauma, the irritating focus can usually be attributed to irritating ischemia initially and blood debris later.

PAINFUL SPLINTING

Muscle splinting is another factor frequently associated with pain. Striated muscles, especially the erectors, go into a painful splinting spasm when fatigued. The result is muscular dysfunction. In time, trophic changes occur and tone is lost. Muscle splinting is seen as active, often involuntary, muscle contraction that immobilizes the part. It differs from muscle spasm in that relaxation of the affected muscles occurs at rest. Prolonged pain from bone, muscle, tendon, and joint lesions with resultant long-term muscle splinting or pseudoparalysis may lead to eventual osteoporosis in affected and possibly adjacent bones. Joint contractures may also develop. This is another example, similar to a psychic conversion symptom, wherein a sensory symptom may lead to definite structural changes.

PAINFUL CRAMPS AND SPASMS

A cramp is a painful muscular contraction. Abdominal cramps are common and frequently associated with gastralgia and enteralgia in which there are spasms of the muscles of the stomach, intestines, and sometimes of the abdominal wall. *Windedness* is an acute cause of abdominal pain and is associated with a diaphragmatic cramp. Musculoskeletal disorders are also frequently characterized by associated muscle cramps or spasms. These are powerful involuntary muscular contractions shortening the flexor muscles that result in extreme, often incapacitating, pains stimulated by ischemia and hypoxia of muscle tissue. They are commonly associated with myositic, fibrositic, and articular disorders.

Any type of excessive motor fiber stimulation results in pathologic, involuntary, and painful muscle spasm. This may be the result of toxic irritation of the anterior horn cells; encroachment irritation of the nerve root; irritation, stretching, or pressure upon a nerve trunk or plexus; irritation or pressure upon peripheral nerve branches; muscle spasm secondary to trauma of an adjacent structure; primary muscle spasm from direct irritation or trauma; or psychogenic muscle spasm.

It has been estimated that from 50% to 60% of the pains and discomforts that the average ambulatory patient has are the direct or indirect result of involuntary muscle contraction. Thus, the physician is compelled to consider the relationship of muscle contraction to pain symptoms in both diagnosis and therapy.

MUSCLE ENLARGEMENT

Hypertrophy and spasm must be differentiated from the muscular enlargement that follows exercise. The increase in muscle bulk following exercise is caused by two factors: (1) the opening of capillaries during activity that are closed during rest; and (2) prolonged activity, which appears to increase the size of individual muscle fibers. This latter point is thought to be from an increase in sacroplasm. A few authorities believe that even the quantity of myofibrils may increase during increased exercise over several weeks.

MUSCULAR PAIN FROM LYMPH DYSFUNCTION

Pain of muscular origin is often a complex problem. Although skeletal muscle tissue lacks an intrinsic lymph supply, a muscle's connective-tissue sheath and tendons are richly endowed with lymphatic vessels. During the normal physiologic exchange of fluids through capillary walls, the quantity of fluid leaving the capillary is usually greater than that entering the venule. The related lymphatic network takes up this excess and eventually delivers it to the venous system. It is this process that allows a continuous exchange of tissue fluids and maintains a constant pressure of interstitial fluid.

The flow of lymph is increased during activity as is capillary circulation, but this flow can be restricted by excessive pressure exerted by a constantly hypertonic or phasic contracted muscle. De Sterno shows that inhibited lymph drainage contributes to muscular pain during prolonged activity by (1) causing a buildup of interstitial fluids that increase hydrostatic pressure and (2) encouraging the accumulation of metabolic waste products that would normally be drained by the lymphatics and venules.

Management of Muscle Spasm

Attention directed toward the relief of muscle spasm depends on the stage of the patient's complaint. Although we will divide this category into two sections, the mechanisms for management must be primarily based on the doctor's clinical evaluation of the patient.

PATIENTS WITH PAIN

After the most acute stage of pain has passed (usually after 48 hours), therapy should be directed at relaxing muscle spasm. We prefer a tetanizing current that can be adjusted to provide pain relief. High voltage and interferential units appear to be best for this purpose, although several low voltage modalities are often effective.

The intensity should be slowly increased to a tetanizing pulse rate up to patient tolerance. The ideal situation is to alternately tetanize and then relax those muscle groups involved in an effort to break the spasm.

PATIENTS WITHOUT PAIN

After modulation of the pain has been achieved, therapy should be directed toward those modalities that relax muscle tissue and promote healing. Any modality that will produce controlled heat in specific muscle groups can be utilized.

Some general examples are shown in Table 2.6.

EDEMA

When physical therapy modalities are utilized, the reduction of edema is enhanced most effectively by pulsating currents that tend to apply a "milking" action on the tissues involved. Pulsed diathermy, pulsed ultrasound, or pulsed alternating currents (eg, muscle stimulators) can all be of some benefit when patients present with edema of a musculoskeletal origin.

It is also both helpful and necessary to give patients with edema home instructions,

Table 2.6. Basic Muscle Function, Dysfunction, and Rehabilitative Therapy

Function	*Dysfunction*	*Primary Therapy*
Strength	Weakness	Exercises against resistance
Physiologic elasticity	Spasticity	Thermotherapy, ultrasound, autosuggestion, biofeedback therapy, postural correction, relaxing exercises
	Spasm	Pain relief, "gate" blockage techniques, relaxing exercises, heat
	Tension	Relaxing exercises, hydrotherapy, biofeedback, hypnotherapy, psychotherapy
Physical elasticity	Contracture	Stretching exercises, joint mobilization, ultrasound, thermotherapy
Coordination	Incoordination	Strengthening and relaxation exercises, coordination training and practice.

including specific advice not to apply heat. Many patients have been known to aggravate their conditions by injudicious use of heat as a home remedy.

INFLAMMATION

Although specific modalities are not recommended for the management of inflammatory situations, we can not stress too strongly how important it is to *not* use heat in any form when acute inflammation is present. There is considerable evidence that heat will actually accelerate the progression of the patient's condition in acute situations (eg, rheumatoid arthritis).

RESTRICTED RANGE OF MOTION

Attention will be given in future chapters to exercise and those modalities that are aimed at increasing ranges of motion. However, a few points are pertinent to mention here.

In arthritics, stroke victims, or patients with deformities or generalized stiffness, fluidotherapy, paraffin, and hydrotherapy followed by or combined with exercise have proven to be most useful. The most important factors are to:

1. Set objectives and specific goals for the patient
2. Combine office therapy with a specific home management program
3. Assess progress at regular intervals.

The goals established must be realistic and slowly progressive (step by step) with achievement rewards and frequent positive reinforcement included or the patient may quickly lose interest and possible benefits will never eventuate.

With patients who have sustained musculoskeletal injuries, muscle stimulating currents with surge settings should be combined with a vigorous and well-defined exercise program for maximal rehabilitation. Whenever possible, it is recommended that some exercise be applied simultaneously with the therapy.

NEUROLOGIC SYMPTOMS AND COMPLAINTS

Neurologic findings such as sciatica, foot drop, numbness, paresthesia, neuritis, etc, should be carefully evaluated, and then the therapy can be specifically directed so as not to aggravate underlying conditions or produce adverse side-effects.

Certain neurologic diseases have specific therapy contraindications, and these should always be considered. Two examples are heat in patients with multiple sclerosis or a suppurating infection, or massage and electrical stimulating to involved muscles in patients with muscular dystrophy.

Nerve Root Pain

It is well to keep in mind that areas of sensation on the skin supplied by one dorsal root are called dermatomes or skin segments, and pain limited in distribution to one or more dermatomes is called radicular pain. Myotomes are groups of muscles innervated by a single spinal segment. Evaluation of the integrity of the neurologic levels rests upon the examiner's knowledge of dermatomes, myotomes, sclerotomes, and reflexes. See Figure 2.13 (also refer to Figure 2.7).

Determination of the lesion site is often aided by noting the distribution of pain along the course of the involved nerve and the areas of cutaneous sensory disturbance. The pain may be localized below the site of involvement or it may be widespread as a result of referred or reflex pain.

Pain can be perceived in the vicinity of the spinal column by a number of factors such as (1) mechanical irritation of the nerve roots, (2) mechanical irritation of any of the involved pain-sensitive soft tissues, (3) edema and vascular distension, (4) reflex spasm of the paravertebral muscles, (5) chemical irritation of any of the involved pain-sensitive tissues by the effect of inflammatory exudates, (6) referred pain from viscera or distant structures, and (7) psychic mechanisms.

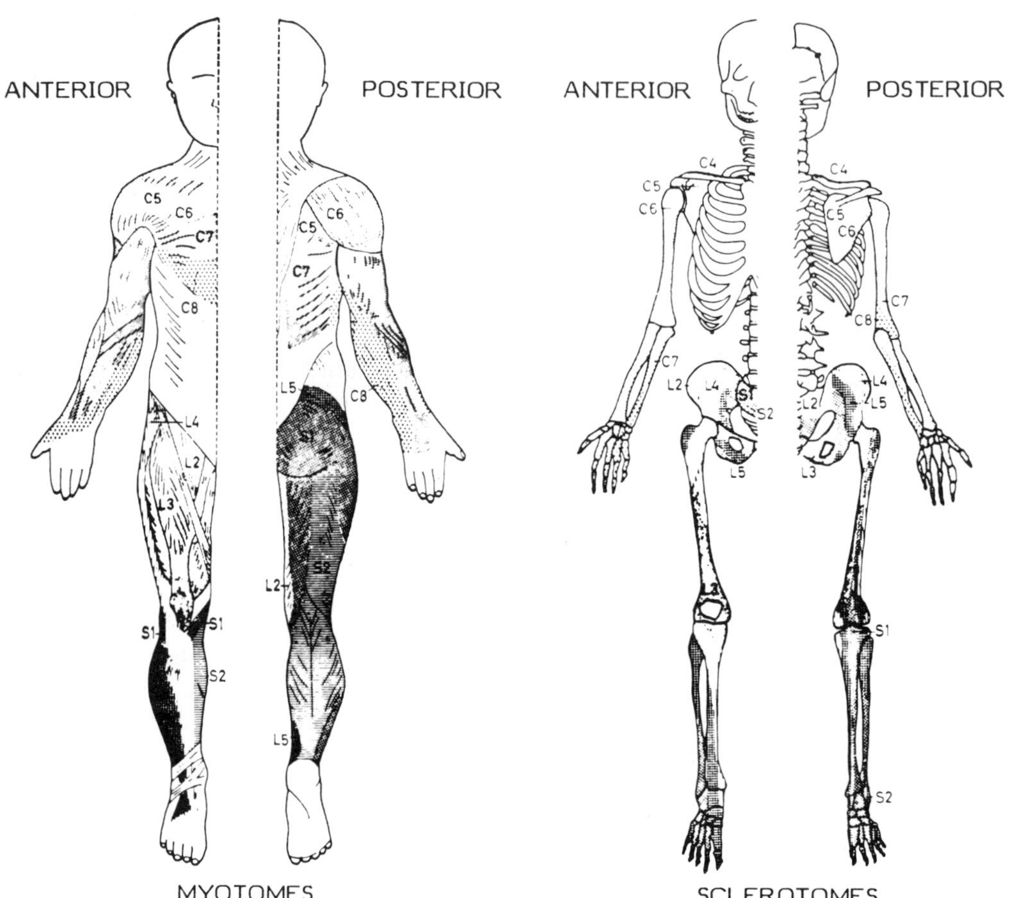

Figure 2.13. *Left,* illustrations depict major anterior and posterior muscle innervation from a single spinal segment (myotome). It should be noted that the distribution of the motor nerves from the various segments does not coincide with the distribution of the cutaneous nerves (dermatomes, Fig. 2.7). Sensation is supplied to the muscles by sensory nerves that correspond in origin with their motor nerves. *Right,* illustrations depict the area of a bone innervated by a single spinal segment. In regard to area and depth, the position of pain or anesthesia can indicate which nerve root may be involved, particularly symptoms of distal distribution (after Maitland).

Inflammation or a grating compression of dorsal nerve roots irritates nociceptive fibers and commonly produces pain that is felt along the anatomic distribution of the roots affected. The pain radiates to the periphery, is usually deep-seated, and is directly related to muscle tension enhanced by any movement that would cause stretch or contraction of the involved muscle(s).

The origin of nerve root lesions can often be traced during the history to trauma, herniated discs, IVF narrowing, cord traction, hypertrophic changes in the vertebrae, neoplasms, and inflammation of the nerve root (eg, subluxation, pyogenic processes, herpes zoster, Guillain-Barre syndrome). Peripheral nerve disease will sometimes indicate a history of an entrapment neuropathy (eg, median nerve at the wrist, ulnar nerve at the elbow, digital nerve between metacarpal heads, meralgia paresthetica). Nutritional disorders may result in a polyneuropathy because of unfavorable metabolic activities within the neural apparatus.

The two most common painful peripheral neuropathies are diabetic neuropathy and alcoholic neuropathy. Diabetic neuropathy is seen as either a mononeuropathy or a symmetrical distal polyneuropathy. Toxic neuropathies are the result of ingestion of heavy metals (eg, lead, arsenic), exposure to organic solvents, or excessive insecticide contact. The two most common painful familial neuropathies are interstitial hypertrophic neuropathy (Dejerine-Sotta's disease) and progressive peroneal muscular atrophy (Charcot-Marie-Tooth syndrome).

Painful Peripheral Nerve Disorders

Pain associated with somatic peripheral nerves is generally due to (1) irritation or pathology of somatic nerves, (2) a disorder within tissues innervated by somatic nerves, or (3) referral to a somatic dermatome.

Irritation or Pathology of Somatic Nerves. Examples of this common disorder arise in a large variety such as carcinomatous nerve or root involvement, herpes zoster, IVD syndromes, IVF deposits, large nerve neuromas, nerve entrapment syndromes, neuron compression or tension, and last, but not least, vertebral subluxations.

A Disorder Within Tissues Supplied by Somatic Nerves. These disturbances are primarily caused by trauma, secondarily by disease processes. Trauma can cause tissue damage supplied by a particular somatic nerve, producing by-products that can irritate nociceptors. In carcinoma, for example, pain may travel to involved somatic nerves serving that dermatome (eg, a neck tumor radiating pain down the arm).

Referral to a Somatic Dermatome. Pain may be referred along a somatic dermatoma because of visceral inflammation, ischemia, or a tumor (eg, the shoulder/arm pain associated with myocardial infarction or angina). Such pains have two major features in common: (1) their distribution is limited to an anatomical dermatomal pattern, and (2) interruption of the nerve's function by any means will alleviate the symptoms, at least temporarily.

Neuralgia

Neuralgia is a general term that refers to any sharp, severe, stabbing, paroxysmal, remittent pain with temporary abatement in severity that travels along the course of one or more nerves. The pain is usually associated with tenderness along the course of the nerve and violent episodic spasms in the muscles innervated. In contrast, the term *neurodynia* is often used to describe a similar pain that is less severe, ie, a deep ache.

Although the term *neuralgia* is nondiagnostic, it is often used in situations where the exact etiology and pathology involved are not known (idiopathic). Morphologic changes cannot usually be detected early in a pure neuralgia or neurodynia. The cause of neuralgia can frequently be traced later to nerve trauma, pressure on a nerve, neuritis, toxicosis, early carcinomatous invasion, nerve malnutrition (local or general), or a rheumatic origin.

A classic sign of neuralgia is *Brodie's pain*: When the skin is folded near a joint affected with neuralgia, pain is produced in the joint area.

Severe neuralgias are often seen in practice. Pain of this type rarely subsides spontaneously, and it is often so severe that the victim becomes totally incapacitated and frequently addicted to narcotics.[79] Depression is a common associated factor, and suicidal tendencies are not infrequently seen. The typical causes for such pain are listed in Table 2.7.

Hyperalgesia

Hyperalgesia literally means an excessive sensitivity to pain. A painful tenderness produced by external pressure frequently results from trigger points, traumatic lesions of sensitive subdermal tissue, the development of a toxic accumulation, or a deep-seated inflammatory irritation. Note that an extremely "ticklish" person is one whose superficial reflexes (skin and muscles) are very lively, thus a low pain and temperature threshold can be anticipated.

Pottenger points out that hyperalgesia of soft tissues is not uncommon in the areas that have been the seat of reflex sensory pain. For example, subcutaneous soreness within the shoulder and upper arm muscles is often associated with inflammatory diseases of the lungs. Pottenger also reports that cutaneous hyperalgesia is a common finding in visceral disease. For example, hyperalgesic skin frequently overlies an area of pleurisy, a tubercular cavity, a peptic ulcer, or an inflamed ovary.

HEAD'S LAW

During the differentiation of visceral pain with hyperalgesia, it is well to keep in mind that visceral distress is manifested in two ways: (1) an uneasy discomfort in the viscera itself, and (2) a truly painful sensation on the surface of the body. Head's law states that "When a painful stimulus is applied to

Table 2.7. Examples of the Potentially Severe Neuralgic Conditions

Arachnoiditis of caudal roots
Atypical neuralgia
Cardioaortic pain
Causalgia and allied conditions
Coccygodynia
Disseminated diseases with widespread pain
Facet syndromes
Gastrointestinal distress
Glossopharyngeal or vagal neuralgia
Idiopathic dysmenorrhea
Intercostal neuralgia
Intermittent claudication
Intervertebral disc syndromes
Lightning crisis of tabes dorsalis
Local scarring of spinal nerves
Nervus intermedius neuralgia
Neuroma of large nerves
Occipital neuralgia (cervico-capital neuralgia)
Periodic migrainous neuralgia (cluster headaches)
Postamputation neuralgia
Postherpetic neuralgia
Posttraumatic sensory root entrapment
Posttraumatic peripheral nerve entrapment
Residual pain after lumbar disc surgery
Sciatica
Temporal arteritis
Terminal stage of cancer
Trigeminal neuralgia (tic douloureux)
Tunnel syndromes
Vasospastic states

a part of low sensibility (eg, viscus) in close central connection with a part of much greater sensibility (eg, skin), the pain produced is felt in the part of higher sensibility rather than in the part of lower sensibility to which the stimulus was actually applied."

NERVE TRACING

There may be a condition that would cause tenderness if pressure would be exerted, but no abnormal sensation will be felt if there is no pressure. It is upon this fact that *nerve tracing* is based. Nerve tracing is the palpable act of following the course of tenderness over nerves that are irritated or impinged that will usually assist in locating the focus of pain, tenderness, or headache. It is a diagnostic art that is used more in chiropractic than any other healing art.

Zones of hyperalgesia (often associated with cutaneous vasoconstriction and hypermyotonia) are more commonly associated with acute and subacute visceral disease rather than chronic disorders. The afferent fibers occupying the pre- and post-ganglionic pathways of the autonomic system from soma and viscera have a general segmental arrangement. Refer to Table 2.5.

Selected Pain-Related Disorders

CAUSALGIA

Causalgia refers to an agonizing burning pain, usually associated with severe trauma, that is essentially a reflex vasomotor sympathetic dystrophy. It consists chiefly of sympathetic phenomena, invariably following trauma, involving one or more limbs. It is often followed by organic changes such as bone atrophy and mottling, resulting from persistently recurring nutrient artery spasms as well as skin and muscle dystrophy and atrophy. The vasospasm produces an excruciating, diffuse, burning pain that may involve either or both the lower or upper extremities.

The major characteristics of causalgia include:

- Burning sensations
- Cutaneous coolness
- Discoloration of skin
- Hyperhidrosis
- Perceptions of heat or cold
- Redness or pallor
- Severe pain
- Swelling
- Trigger points

Joint immobility with or without pain, scleroderma, and contractures may occur. Emotional disturbances are often associated. Any slight thermal, tactile, sensory, or even psychic stimulus may result in an explosive attack.

COLIC

Colic is a nondiagnostic term that refers to any symptom complex whose major feature is acute paroxysmal pain. There are several common clinical forms:

- *Abdominal colic,* due to abdominal distress. Pottenger feels that the cause can be traced to something that overly excites the abdominal vagus. The result is spastic constriction of a gut lumen at irregular intervals, resulting in pockets of gas, slowed peristalsis, inhibited intestinal function, and colicky pains. Travell feels that many cases of abdominal colic in adults can be traced to trigger points in the periumbilical rectus abdominis.
- *Biliary colic,* due to passage of a gallstone through the bile duct.
- *Gastric colic,* due to a stomach disorder (eg, perforating ulcer).
- *Infantile colic,* a form of gastrointestinal colic occurring during the first few months after birth that features irritability, crying episodes, and apparent abdominal pain. Incompatibility with commercial milk is a common cause.
- *Menstrual colic,* a synonym for dysmen-

orrhea. Lumbar subluxations and trigger points in the lower rectus abdominis area should be a musculoskeletal consideration.

• *Mucous colic,* a synonym for chronic colitis.

• *Renal colic,* featuring agonizing loin pain that radiates around the abdomen, into the groin, and toward the thigh, is due to embolism or dissection of the renal artery, intrarenal mass lesion, passage of a kidney stone, renal infarction, or thrombosis of the renal vein.

• *Salivary colic,* due to a salivary calculus (eg, submaxillary).

• *Vermicular colic,* due to a catarrhal inflammation that blocks the outlet of the appendix or a functional spasm of the ileocecal valve.

CLUSTER HEADACHES

This disorder, sometimes called periodic migrainous neuralgia, is characterized by severe unilateral burning pain in the temple/forehead area that sometimes radiates to the suboccipital area, lower face, and/or neck. It is most often seen in adult males (30—60 years). Patients have been known to bang their heads against a wall, just to change the pain being experienced. Attacks usually awake the patient at night and usually last for several hours. Unpredictable intervals (hours or months) may intersperse attacks. Associated symptoms and signs include intracranial arterial dilation, tearing, facial flush, injected conjunctiva, and sometimes autonomic signs (eg, Horner's syndrome).

EXTREMITY PAIN

A careful history will frequently indicate that pain situated in various parts of the extremities will reveal the point of origin by its peculiar location and quality. The cause may be of mechanical, chemical, thermal, toxic, nutritional, metabolic, or circulatory origin, or a combination of some of these factors, depending upon the nature of the pathologic process involved. See Table 2.8. The most important clues toward determining cause—type of pain, its distribution, and its associated symptoms—are the result of a carefully taken case history.

Pain in the extremities may originate in muscle, skin, bone, joints, arteries and veins, and in lesions of the nervous system. Muscle etiologies commonly include trauma, systemic infection, alteration in blood supply, inflammation, and neoplasms. Pain from lesions of the nervous system may originate from (1) central nervous system lesions, (2) spinal root and plexus lesions (eg, nerve root lesions, lesions of the brachial or lumbosacral plexuses), or (3) peripheral nerve disease from trauma, entrapment neuropathies, reflex sympathetic dystrophy, or peripheral neuritis. Thus, limb pain may be the result of any structural disorder of the extremities or a disturbance elsewhere where the sensory phenomena are referred to the limbs.

When an inflammatory process (eg, neuritis) involves sensory fibers, pain (neuralgia) is frequently present along the total nerve course. For example, in median nerve entrapment (carpal tunnel syndrome), pain is rarely localized in the wrist. It often extends into the upper arm and shoulder.

GLOSSOPHARYNGEAL-VAGAL NEURALGIA

Intense bursts of throat pain are characteristic of this syndrome. The pain extends from the back of the tongue to the larynx and sometimes refers to the area of the ear. It can be triggered simply by chewing, swallowing, yawning, or sneezing, and it sometimes complicates trigeminal neuralgia. Rarely, cardiac arrest, convulsions, and syncope are associated when impulses spread to the carotid sinus and affect the vagus.

INTERMITTENT CLAUDICATION

Claudication manifests as a cramping sensation or a severely distressing pain that is

Table 2.8. Typical Causes of Extremity Pain

PAIN IN THE UPPER EXTREMITIES

Musculoskeletal Causes
- Joint pain
  - Arthritides
  - Sprain
  - Subluxation
  - Various orthopedic disorders
- Bone pain
  - Bone tumor
  - Osteomyelitis
- Muscle pain
  - Bursitis
  - Fibrositis
  - Strain
- Tunnel syndromes

Neurologic Causes
- Polyneuritis
  - Infectious
  - Nutritional
  - Toxic
- Radiculitis
  - IVD protrusion
  - IVF entrapment
  - Spinal cord tumor
  - Spondylosis
- Referred pain
  - Angina pectoris
  - Articular fixation
  - Gallbladder disease
  - Hepatic disease
  - Myocardial infarction
  - Trigger point

Vascular Causes
- Raynaud's disease
- Vascular disease
  - Arteriosclerosis obliterans
  - Embolism
  - Thromboangitis
  - Thrombosis

PAIN IN THE LOWER EXTREMITIES

Musculoskeletal Causes
- Joint pain
  - Arthritides
  - Sprain
  - Subluxation
  - Various orthopedic disorders
- Bone pain
  - Bone tumor
  - Certain hematologic disorders
  - Generalized bone diseases
  - Osteomyelitis
- Muscle pain
  - Cramps
  - Strain
  - Myositis

Neurologic Causes
- Mononeuritides
  - Meralgia
  - Metatarsalgia
  - Neuralgia
  - Paresthetica
  - Sciatica
- Polyneuritis
  - Infectious
  - Nutritional
  - Toxic
  - Diabetic
- Radiculitis
  - IVD protrusion
  - IVF entrapment
  - Osteoarthritis
  - Tabes dorsalis
  - Spinal cord tumor
- Trigger point

Vascular Causes
- Sudden peripheral artery occlusion
  - Causalgia
  - Embolism
  - Thrombosis
- Intermittent claudication
  - Thromboangitis obliterans
  - Arteriosclerosis obliterans
- Thrombophlebitis
- Chronic venous insufficiency

due to exercise-related ischemia in the upper or lower extremity muscles. It is commonly related to atherosclerosis and predominantly affects elderly males who are heavy cigarette smokers. It is also related to a number of conditions characterized by vascular insufficiency such as thromboangitis obliterans (Buerger's disease), embolism, vascular compression, arteriospasm, or a vascular anomaly. Intermittent claudication is often seen in atherosclerotic occlusive disease.

Claudication symptoms arise distal to a major lesion when local circulation becomes insufficient to meet the needs of active muscles. The pain comes on after a certain degree of exercise, and it leaves with rest of the muscles involved when the involved artery supplies enough blood for rest but not for prolonged action. The condition is more common to the elderly male, usually involving the calf muscles. As occlusion advances, pain or ache may be present at rest (especially at night), skin ulcers may appear, and limb gangrene may rarely result from the lack of cellular nutrition. A femoral artery block is found in 80% of the cases.

The patient's history will help determine the site of major arterial obstruction to the affected distal muscles. For example:

- Occlusion of the aortoiliac segment results in hip and buttock pain.
- When the iliofemoral segment is involved, thigh pain registers.
- A superficial femoral segment obstruction results in calf pain.
- A tibial segment obstruction produces foot pain.

Leriche's syndrome is a complex of symptoms denoting involvement of the major pelvic muscles. As a result of internal iliac insufficiency, there is buttock claudication and an inability to achieve an erection. This syndrome is commonly used to denote distal aortic occlusion, affecting either the posterior iliac artery or the common or anterior iliac artery.

NERVUS INTERMEDIUS NEURALGIA

This episodic syndrome involves the nervus intermedius, a small sensory nerve containing secretory fibers that arises from its geniculate ganglion and accompanies the facial nerve. Attacks usually occur during youth and middle age, especially in males. The pain is usually brief but intolerable. Its major distribution is in the anterior tongue, soft palate, auricle canal, and tympanic membrane area. A trigger point is often found in the aural canal.

NEUROMAS OF LARGE NERVES

Any axonal or end-bulb neuroma can become a source of disabling pain. The fairly persistent pain is usually associated with posttraumatic degenerating or partially regenerating, well-myelinated, rapidly conducting axons that conduct proprioceptive and tactile sensations. The slower conducting C fibers are infrequently involved.

OCCIPITAL NEURALGIA

This syndrome, sometimes called cervicocapital neuralgia, is characterized by lancinating pain with a suboccipital focus (with point tenderness) that often radiates down the neck and sometimes into the shoulders and/or to the vertex and often over the scalp into the retro-orbital area. It is typically unilateral, and cervical extension usually aggravates the pain. Suboccipital spasm and upper cervical root irritation (especially C1—C2) are invariably involved. Afferent impulses from the upper cervicals involve the descending trigeminal tract.

This syndrome is often associated with occiput, atlas, or axis subluxation, and is sometimes related to basilar impression, fibrotic nodules in the tendon of the trapezius entrapping the greater and/or lesser occipital nerves, or "whiplash" trauma. Rarely is osteoarthritis the cause, regardless of extensive roentgenographic evidence of its presence.

POSTHERPETIC NEURALGIA

As the herpes virus has a predisposition to produce gliotic lesions in the posterior spinal root ganglions and entry structures to the cord, severe intercostal neuralgia and later scarring entrapments can be expected. As an aftermath of shingles, supraorbital neuralgia is sometimes expressed as the result of herpetic invasion of the trigeminal fibers in the Gasserian ganglion and the brainstem. It is characterized by a continuous burning facial pain associated with numbness to touch.

TEMPORAL ARTERITIS

This syndrome features severe persistent temple pain, related to thick tender branches of the temporal artery. The onset is frequently acute, often with fever. Typically associated are an increased sedimentation rate, hypochromic anemia, and a rise in serum globulin.

TRIGEMINAL NEURALGIA

Tic douloureux exhibits as severe, sudden, stabbing pain in one or more divisions (mandibular, maxillary, supraorbital) of the trigeminal nerve. Although the trigeminus has three branches, as its name implies, involvement is almost invariably in only one or two branches. In the rare bilateral variety (3%), the flashes of pain occur only unilaterally at any one time. The onset is usually in the second half of life and triggered by minor stimuli such as from brushing the teeth, eating, shaving, speaking, or touching the face. There is no neurologic deficit. Thus, if corneal or cutaneous hypesthesia manifests, the pain is continuous, or distribution does not correspond to that of the trigeminus, another cause must be sought.

VISCERAL NEURALGIAS

While it is thought that sympathetic fibers do not transmit pain from the extremities, it has been well established in recent years that the cardioaortic and splanchnic nerves serve as pathways for visceral sensations. It has been shown that while the internal organs are insensitive to cutting, burning, or pricking, they can react intensely to distension and ischemia.[80,81]

The axons involved in transmitting visceral sensations are part of the somatic afferent system, with impulses transversing the visceral plexi, the paravertebral sympathetic ganglia, and then entering the cord via the posterior nerve roots from T1—L2. The afferent sensations of pain from the bronchi, trachea, and esophagus are carried by the vagus, and those from the bladder, cervix, and rectum traverse the inferior hypogastric plexus and enter the cord via the lower sacral nerves.[82] Cardiac pain is transmitted by two distinct routes: (1) cardiac sympathetic nerves arising from the three cervical ganglia, and (2) smaller thoracic rami, from the upper three thoracic sympathetic ganglia, that contain sensory fibers.[83,84]

It can thus be appreciated that sympathectomy to relieve pain in intractable disorders is only effective if the cause is within the visceral capsule. It is ineffective if the condition (eg, a malignancy) invades neighboring tissues supplied by somatic nerves.

MISCELLANEOUS CAUSES OF NEURALGIA

Atypical Facial Neuralgia. This unusual facial neuralgia is characterized by continuous pain where no evidence of an organic cause can be demonstrated. Local cold often aggravates the pain, suggesting a vasomotor involvement.

Caudal Root Arachnoiditis. Severe low back trauma is sometimes followed by a harsh persistent lumbar pain, especially in injuries to the cauda equina with constrictive arachnoiditis of the spinal roots. This syndrome is usually the result of a penetrating wound, thus rarely seen in general practice.

Coccygodynia. Coccygeal pain usually follows coccygeal subluxation, dislocation, or fracture. The associated pain is aggravated by sitting, even when using a rubber ring to relieve the lower sacrum of compressive forces.

Intercostal Neuralgia. Radicular pain that follows the course of ribs is not an infrequent complaint. TENS will usually afford relief until the cause can be found and corrected or until the disorder heals spontaneously.

Local Scarring of Spinal Nerves. Adhesions of the pia-arachnoid or epidural scarring frequently produce radicular pain, usually unilateral, as a complication to vertebral fracture or spinal surgery, even though no cord damage is present.

Residual Pain Following Lumbar IVD Surgery. Epidural scarring is the most common cause of post-IVD surgery. The result is duplication of the original complaint.

Tunnel Syndromes. Carpal tunnel and tarsal tunnel syndromes are characterized by a painful tingling paresthesia, often waking the patient at night.

Vasospastic States. Painful vasospasms of extremity vessels are not uncommon. They may have an embolic, a posttraumatic, or an idiopathic etiology.

PSYCHOLOGIC PAIN-RELATED FACTORS

This is a complex subject, yet the patient's psyche and attitude must always be taken into consideration. Attitude is always important in how a patient relates to the therapy prescribed and to his or her progress. Every effort should be made to alleviate patient fears that may exist regarding diagnosis, therapy, rehabilitation, and prognosis.

The two components of pain, perception and reaction, were differentiated at the turn of the century.[85,86] Prior to that time, it was thought that pain was simply caused by a stimulus sufficient to activate a pain-sensitive structure and send the message to the brain. There was no knowledge at that time of the *reaction component*—central modification of peripherally generated impulses that causes conscious perception that is not necessarily in proportion to the intensity of the peripheral stimuli.

Emotional Responses to Pain and Injury

Pain itself has different manifestations in different people. A patient may exhibit excruciating pain before an audience, but none upon private examination. A quickly reduced subluxation may disable one person for 3 minutes, another for 3 weeks. One patient may be silent with severe pain, while another reacts with pain and tears far disproportionate to the injury. One patient may want to return to work with a severe whiplash, while another will go into shock over a sprained finger. Even during the early 1800s, it was noticed that great wounds may be painless and small wounds highly painful.[87,88] While people differ in their response to injury and pain, each individual has a more or less predictable pattern which is soon learned by family, friends, physician, and co-workers.

Some people like to play the "wounded hero" role. A patient may present absolutely no lameness in the office, yet "gimp" awkwardly out of the office. The rewards of special attention and sympathy from this role encourage a delay in returning to strenuous work and foster poor cooperation during the recovery program. While some people are overly anxious to return to normal daily activities, others may refuse the slightest effort until all symptoms are eliminated.

A patient will occasionally be met who desires (consciously or unconsciously) to remove himself from a certain activity because of a minor injury. This is the type who secretly dislikes a certain role, has previously entered a situation because of social, parental, or occupational pressures, and finds an injury or discomfort a guiltless means to relieve the burden. Astute counsel and a good rehabilitative program will allow such an individual an opportunity to face the problem.

Psychological Mechanisms Involved in Pain Control

Pain is a universal experience and a normal, continual protective mechanism of the body in response to noxious stimulation. Its cause may be trauma, disease, a thalamic or peripheral nerve lesion, a psychosomatic conversion manifestation (eg, dysphagia, dyspnea), or it may have a purely psychogenic origin (eg, anxiety, hypochondriasis) in which an organic explanation cannot be found.

During World War II, Beecher noticed that some patients with great but painless wounds could feel a clumsy venipuncture, suggesting that the perception mechanism was intact but noxious stimuli were being modified.[88] It was theorized that this was the reason why soldiers often do not notice their wounds until after battle and why athletes often fail to recognize injuries until after they were out of competition.

The reaction component can be affected in many ways. Emotional states, placebos, suggestion, and hypnosis are a few examples. Lobotomy can be considered a surgical lesion of the reaction component. Even analgesic narcotics act upon the reaction component, for light touch and temperature stimuli are still preserved. Thus, pain as typically exhibited is a complex process in which the intensity of the focal stimulus plays only a part. Much of the perceived sensation is determined by central processing mechanisms, and this, as previously described, may include those factors explained in Melzack and Wall's Gate Theory.

At this point, it should be remembered that psychic "pain" can be just as painful as physical distress; if not, it would not drive some people to suicide. People free of physical disease often suffer from the most intractable types of pain. From the standpoint of the patient, there is no such thing as "psychogenic pain"—pain is pain. An unconscious person does not suffer, regardless of the intensity of noxious stimuli applied, but autonomic manifestations are retained.

Human emotions are obviously much more than simple stimulus-response reactions. Emotions do not "happen to a person." They are not just sensations in response to physical phenomena; rather, they are experiences of the "conscious" organism.[89,90] Thus, in most doctor-patient relationships, the physician is confronted with two problems: the *complaint of pain* and the *painful person* (homo dolorosus) who has unique experiences and relationships, hopes and fears. This takes an appreciation of the patient's perspective, not the doctor's. Even monomaniacal hypochondriacs do not choose a "career" of pain unless they see no other alternative.

Two types of patients commonly frustrate many physicians: the type that complains of a great deal of pain and no organic cause can be found, and the type that exhibits great damage and makes no complaint. Proper management can only result when the two components of pain, the mechanisms of perception and reaction, are understood and fully appreciated.[91]

THE MANAGEMENT OF PAINFUL MUSCULOSKELETAL COMPLAINTS

Basic Investigative Approach

Two factors should be considered in problems of faulty body mechanics: structural tension and nerve irritation:[2]

1. Pain produced by gravitational strain, resulting in tension stress, involves not only articular and periarticular structures but the musculature as well. The pain may be slight or excruciating depending on the severity of tension within structures containing nerve endings sensitive to stretch such as those found in muscles, tendons, ligaments, and capsules, especially those of and adjacent to joints. Piriformis, tensor fascia lata, and lumbago syndromes are examples of nerve irritation associated with abnormal muscle, fascia, and tendon tautness and stress.

2. Pain may also result from nerve irrita-

tion, or grating pressure on nerve roots, trunks, branches, or endings from some adjacent structure such as bone, cartilage, fascia, scar tissue, taut muscles, or swelling from congestion, edema, or a mass. Examples of nerve root pressure pain would include dynamic osseous encroachments of a subluxation or tunnel syndrome, facet syndrome, enlarged capsular ligament, or protruded IVD.

General Etiologic Picture

Musculoskeletal pain may result from faults in posture, disturbed spinal dynamics, articular stress, off-centering of the vertebral segments within their motor beds, asymmetrical muscle tension, postural fatigue, articular instability arising from developmental defects, myofascial plane adhesions, viscerospinal reflex muscle spasms, overstress, strain, and degenerative proliferative changes following trauma.

Janse reminds us that when a vertebral segment or several vertebral segments (eg, a lumbosacral articular complex or sacroiliac mechanism) are traumatized or deranged in its articular bed, there is always an irritation of the relating sensory bed. This irritation projects onto the initiating motor centers of the motor bed leading to the muscles that move the articulation. Most frequently, therefore, subluxations are commonly attended by asymmetrical painful spasm of the relating musculature that leads to further articular strain and derangement.

Another consideration is that of trigger-point foci of stress or inflammation, resulting in binding cobweb adhesions that incarcerate sensory nerve endings to produce sharp demarcation of pain, especially on pressure. Such trigger points are usually found in the "stress-sites" of the myofascial planes of the erector muscles of the neck, shoulder girdle, back, abdomen, and extremities.

Associated Complaints and Findings

Nagging musculoskeletal pain causes the patient to be restless and to change position frequently. The patient also attempts to protect the anatomical region in which the pain arises by either muscle splinting or pseudoparalysis. Pseudoparalysis mimics paralysis but is not accompanied by loss of sensation.

Depending on the constancy involved, postural and mechanical faults may exhibit severe pain in what appears to be mild postural defects and manifest little or no pain in obvious cases of severe postural deficit. Minor postural deficits are often associated with considerable joint stiffness, and a very faulty posture may be seen in a very flexible subject whose body positions change readily. It is also observed that cumulative effects of constant or repeated small stresses over a long duration can give rise to the same difficulties as severe sudden stress.

No clear picture can be drawn of pain associated with postural faults. In some cases only acute symptoms may appear; some cases have an acute onset that progresses into chronic symptoms; some cases exhibit chronic symptoms that exhibit acute phases; and others remain in a chronic condition. Regardless of the clinical picture, it must be kept in mind that no matter where the stimulus may arise, the sensation of pain is conducted only by those nerve fibers affected by the biomechanical factors involved.

Clinical Approach

This section will summarize those symptoms and signs commonly associated with musculoskeletal complaints and describe how certain modalities can alter their overt and covert features. We have found that rather than study the physics of a particular modality and then learn a list of diseases that respond to treatment with that modality (as has been done traditionally in texts on this subject) that it is better to study how each modality affects the pathophysiologic processes involved.

Musculoskeletal complaints can be divided into two major categories of study, acute and chronic disorders, each of which is approached differently when we refer to management with physiotherapy.

ACUTE DISORDERS

When the expression "an acute condition" is used, a situation is implied to be occurring for the first time; eg, the first time a person strains a shoulder or the first instance that a particular patient suffers a case of torticollis. Such patients are not concerned with the long-range sequela. Their primary interest is to rid themselves of the associated pain. Thus, the initial therapy should be primarily directed toward the alleviation of the pain.

There are three basic stages in the approach to the patient with an acute musculoskeletal disorder:

1. *Acute Phase.* During the initial 24 hours after onset, measures should be directed toward sedating the area. If an electrotherapy modality is used, then it should be gradually turned to an intensity where the patient barely feels it. In others words, sensory stimulation only. Heat should never be used during this phase. The primary objective at this stage of care is to only trigger the production of endorphins and enkephalins.

2. *Subacute Phase.* After the first 24—48 hours, the regimen can be expanded. Procedures can be used to remove edema, break muscle spasm, and further reduce the inflammatory process. Heat can now be used, based on the clinical evaluation of the patient's status. This is the phase when healing begins.

3. *Rehabilitation Phase.* Just because pain and swelling have reduced, it doesn't mean that the patient should be discharged. After pain, swelling, and muscle spasm have been resolved, it is now necessary to develop strength in those muscles, tendons, and ligaments that were involved. As healing progresses, we can gear the therapy towards this strengthening process—rehabilitation, if we wish to label the process by that name.

Each of these three phases represent a different approach to patient care. As such, the modalities utilized will be different for each stage. For example, continuous ultrasound may be indicated for the second phase, but, certainly, it would be of minimal use in the first or third phases of the patient's complaint.

The therapeutic phases enumerated above are not fixed points to be memorized. Rather, they should be appreciated as rational approaches to the stage of healing at hand. After any severe strain or sprain, for example, there is undoubtedly a degree of soft-tissue microhemorrhage. Resolution begins after bleeding stops to organize minute thrombi to form the richly vasculated granulation tissue that allows the normal healing process. See Table 2.9.

The best procedure is to anticipate each step in the healing process and provide the opportunity for natural processes to express themselves. This is not to say that if a variation is seen at one of the normal stages of healing that treatment should not be varied accordingly. For example, increased local heat and tenderness during a late stage of a musculoskeletal injury usually indicates a secondary infectious process.

Good care during healing requires repeated inspection and sometimes external support. Periodic and regular appraisal can usually be made simply through inspection and palpation. When dealing with many injuries, one becomes astute in seeing and feeling the various stages of healing. Continuous support during the resolution stage may be provided by external measures without impairing the natural healing process.

CHRONIC DISORDERS

The chronic case can be subdivided into two basic categories, each of which has its own particular approach: (1) the acute exacerbation of a chronic complaint and (2) what is referred to as the truly chronic case.

Table 2.9. The Stages of Healing in a Typical Strain or Sprain

The inflammatory stage	White blood cells dissolve extravasated blood elements and tissue debris. Swelling and local tenderness are present.
The reparative stage	The network of fibrin and the fibroblasts begin the reparative process. Local heat, redness, and diffuse tenderness are present.
The toughening stage	Fibrous deposition and chronic inflammatory reactions occur. Palpable thickening and induration in the area of reaction are present, with tenderness progressively diminishing.

ACUTE EXACERBATIONS OF A CHRONIC DISORDER

This type of situation is best exemplified by patients who have repeatedly injured the same sacroiliac joint, disc, shoulder, knee, etc. An important point to remember is that regardless of how many exacerbations there have been, each should be treated as a new complaint. To avoid prejudgment leading to false conclusions, the doctor should approach the patient as if he or she has never seen the patient before.

Although this type of patient might have acute pain, the patient should be dealt with quite differently from a patient with an acute disorder. This type of patient has had a similar problem before, and they are more likely to understand that just because the pain is gone it does not mean that the problem is gone. It's also more likely that the problem will be complicated and exacerbated by adhesions from one or more previous injuries.

There are four stages to be considered in the approach to the patient with an acute exacerbation of a chronic musculoskeletal disorder:

1. *Acute Phase.* Attention to acute pain relief can generally be reduced in time with the patient who has had a similar problem previously. With some patients who present injury without severe pain, Phase 2 treatment procedures can be initiated immediately, directing attention toward signs of muscle spasm or restricted ranges of motion.

2. *Subacute Phase.* As with an acute case, therapy in this phase should be designed to reduce inflammation, edema, spasm, etc. Heat may be used judiciously, as may other forms of therapy. Because the complaint has occurred before, the treatment time will undoubtedly be of longer duration than that of an acute case. In fact, with some cases, it might not be possible to achieve total relief. If so, therapy must be directed toward achieving as much healing as possible under the circumstances.

3. *Rehabilitation Phase.* This stage is approached as with the acute case; however, it is essential to continue rehabilitation to another, a 4th, phase.

4. *Home Care.* More time must be directed to healing and strengthening than that utilized within the doctor's office. If such patients are to avoid further exacerbations, it is essential that they be given a program that will keep their bodies in optimum condition. For example, if the problem is complicated by weak muscles or obesity, then prescribed exercises or dietary regimens are essential.

CLASSIC CHRONIC DISORDERS

The truly chronic case represents, by far, the most common type of situation seen in general health-care practice. Some studies have indicated that two of the most common reasons that patients are absent from work are arthritis and neurologic problems. In most of these two major groups, a cure is unlikely and therapy must be directed accordingly.

There are seven guidelines to be considered in the approach to the patient with a chronic neuromusculoskeletal disorder:

1. Be thorough in the examination. Each exacerbation of a musculoskeletal complaint should be attended to as a new complaint.

2. When dealing with the chronic arthritic, be aware of the many systemic complications that may be a contributing factor in the overall status of the patient. Since many musculoskeletal disorders may be aggravated by or associated with visceral complaints, steps should be taken to address these complaints if they can be treated within the practice or by referral.

3. The specific type of arthritis must be determined to avoid those types of therapies that may aggravate the condition; eg, the use of local heat in acute rheumatoid, tubercular, or septic arthritis. Likewise when treating chronic neurologic conditions, certain types of therapy may aggravate the patient's complaint; eg, intense heat in multiple sclerosis and massage or electrotherapy in muscular dystrophy.

4. Set appropriate objectives for case management. In many chronic cases, the objective might be to inhibit further progression of the disorder. In post-stroke cases, the objective may be to provide increased mobility. In establishing objectives, the doctor should be certain that the patient is aware of and in agreement with the objectives.

5. Set realistic case management goals. Setting unrealistic goals too high gives a patient false hope that may prove later to be counterproductive. It may be necessary to emphasize that the problem will always be with the patient to some degree. Thus, the goal is not curative, but to help the patient better cope with the problem(s).

6. Part of the treatment program should be the responsibility of the patient. When necessary, emphasis must be placed on diet, nutrition, exercise, and proper rest. Failure to emphasize necessary acts and changes in life-style places an unrealistic burden on the attending physician. The usual result is symptomatic care only, with no concern for any factors that might improve the overall well-being of the patient.

7. Establish a problem/solution-oriented approach. That is, each active problem (complaint, symptom, sign) should be listed, coupled with a therapeutic approach, and carefully monitored until resolution.[92]

It should be underscored in the management of musculoskeletal complaints that modalities should be used in such a way that they will primarily affect those symptoms causing the patient's complaints. Thus, during doctor-patient communications, the treatment of disease is not emphasized; rather, how each modality will help to reduce the patient's pain, spasm, inflammation, etc, is explained. This only takes a summary of how the problem(s) can best be resolved.

PAIN, POLARITY, AND TRIGGER POINTS

Pain impulses tend to occur in an alkaline area and, in chronic situations, in association with a blood calcium deficit. In contrast, trigger points are hypersensitive spots of acidity, relative to the surrounding area. Because the area under a positive electrode (eg, in galvanic therapy) becomes acidic, a positive polarity is usually recommended when treatment is applied over areas initiating great pain. If, however, the trigger point itself is treated, then a negative polarity is recommended because the site is acidic.

PAIN AND TEMPERATURE

Most studies of recent vintage indicate that heat should not be used during those periods when the patient is experiencing severe pain, especially of an acute physical nature. The primary reason for this is that some degree of swelling is invariably present that would be aggravated by heat. Cold is recommended at least for the first 48—72 hours or until evidence of acute inflammation and edema has disappeared.[93] Added to this should be the stimulation of endorphin and enkephalin production whenever pain, anxiety, and systemic homeostatic imbalances are present.

REST, SUPPORT, AND EXERCISE

Because use is aggravating, a severely painful joint must be rested until the acute symptoms subside. Such appliances as braces, canes, collars, crutches, orthopedic pillows, special mattresses, etc, should be prescribed whenever they would be of benefit to the patient. However, because excessive rest encourages fibrosis, stasis, and mineral deposits, massage and passive/active exercises should be judiciously incorporated, up to tolerance, as soon as it is possible. These procedures are especially effective following postacute thermotherapy and during warm hydrotherapy.

Special Concerns in Rheumatic and Related Disorders

Approximately 160 different degenerative, infectious, inflammatory, or traumatic entities can be placed under the broad classification of rheumatism.[94] They are all painful and usually relentlessly so. Some are acute, some are self-terminating, some abate gradually, and some have remitting-relapsing episodes. Many however, are persistently chronic and feature unremitting pain that drains the strength of the suffering victim.

These many different types of rheumatic disorders can be grouped into three major divisions: (1) backache syndromes, (2) osteoarthritis, and (3) rheumatoid arthritis and other sero-negative arthropathies. Several selections of these are briefly described below.

THE CHRONIC BACKACHE SYNDROMES

As with most all chronic musculoskeletal conditions, a complaint of chronic back pain may arise from primary, secondary, referred, or reflex etiologies.[95,96]

1. *Primary disorders.* In primary situations, the pain can usually be traced to one of two general etiologies: mechanical or chemical irritation of intravertebral or extravertebral pain-sensitive tissues.

2. *Secondary disorders.* Pain derived from secondary sources are typically the afferent impulses of the dorsal roots and their branches that serve the receptor systems in the dura and epidural mater, spinal ligaments, vertebral periosteum and related soft tissues (eg, tendons, fascia), fibers that pierce the posterior aspect of the IVD, walls of the arterioles supplying the centrum, and walls of the paravertebral and epidural veins.

3. *Referred disorders.* In cases of referred back pain, the cause is typically found in some focus of irritation of pain receptors distributed throughout the abdominal and pelvic regions that are segmentally innervated by the dorsal roots.

4. *Reflex disorders.* Reflex backache is usually the result of splinting; ie, a reflex spasm of paravertebral muscles, which, in turn, causes irritation to nociceptors in walls of the arterioles within the involved intramuscular tissues. Splinting may also apply compression or traction forces on the underlying nerve roots and periosteal receptors.

With these general categories in mind, the diagnostic process must be narrowed further to a specific entity to arrive at a diagnosis. Some considerations are shown in Table 2.10.

Table 2.10. Typical Disorders Associated with Spinal Pain (Acute/Chronic)

Type	*Examples*	
Degenerative process	Apophyseal osteoarthritis Cauda equina disorders Disc degeneration Hyperostosis Joint instability	Nerve root compression Spinal cord disease Spinal stenosis Spondylolisthesis Spondylosis
Developmental deficit	Hypermobility Kyphosis Lordosis Scoliosis	Short-leg syndrome Spondylolisthesis Various anomalies (eg, hemivertebrae)
Iatrogenic origin	Ill-advised manipulation Misplaced spinal tap Myelography	Poorly fitted support Postsurgical adhesions Prolonged use of support
Infective arthropathy or neuropathy	Actinomycosis Brucellosis Icterohemorrhagica Influenza Leptospirosis Meningitis Osteomyelitis Paratyphoid fever Poliomyelitis	Smallpox Staphylococcal infection Subarachnoid hemorrhage Syphilis Syringomyelia Tetanus Tuberculosis Typhoid fever
Inflammatory arthropathy	Ankylosing spondylitis Fibrositis Focal sepsis Muscular rheumatism Osteochondritis Panniculitis Polarteritis nodosa Polymyalgia arteritica	Psoriasis Regional ileitis Rheumatoid arthritis Reiter's disease Secondary spondylitis Systemic lupus erythematosus Ulcerative colitis
Metabolic deficit	Gouty rheumatism Hyperparathyroidism Osteomalacia	Osteoporosis Paget's disease
Spinal malignancy	Myelomatosis	Secondary carcinoma
Trauma	Disc protrusion Dislocation Facet syndrome Fracture Obesity Postural fault	Short-leg syndrome Spondylolisthesis Sprain Strain Subluxation

Table 2.10, continued

Type	*Examples*	
	REFERRED SYNDROMES	
Abdominal focus	Ascites Enteritis (chronic) Malignant lymphadenopathy Pancreatic carcinoma	Pancreatitis (chronic) Peptic ulcer(s) Pyelonephritis Renal carcinoma
Cervical focus	Malignant lymphadenopathy Subarachnoid hemorrhage	Vertebral artery deficit
Pelvic focus	Aortic obstruction Colon cancer Disseminated sclerosis Ectopic pregnancy Endometriosis Endometritis Hip disease Ileocecal stenosis	Iliac artery obstruction Malignant lymphadenopathy Ovarian cyst/tumor Prostate carcinoma Prostatitis Rectal carcinoma Uterine carcinoma
Thoracic focus	Aortic aneurysm Bronchial carcinoma Cardiac enlargement Coronary artery disease Esophageal carcinoma Gallbladder disease	Herpes zoster Hiatus hernia Malignant lymphadenopathy Mediastinal mass Pancoast tumor Pulmonary disease
Psychic focus	Anxiety Camptocormia Compensation neurosis	Depression Hysteria Malingering

MECHANICAL AND CHEMICAL FACTORS OF TRAUMATIC LOW BACK PAIN

Pain experienced after trauma (eg, a primary disorder) can be the result of mechanical factors, chemical factors, or both, according to the differentiation used by McKenzie.[97,98]

Characteristics of Mechanical Pain. Normal mechanical force applied to normal tissue does not produce pain. However, abnormal mechanical deformation occurs whenever (1) abnormal stress is applied to normal tissues (eg, postural pain), (2) abnormal stress is applied to abnormal tissues, or (3) normal stress is applied to abnormal tissues (eg, soft-tissue shortening). Pain from mechanical causes is typically sharp, acute, and occurs immediately. If mechanical pain does not occur until several minutes or hours after an activity, it is most likely that the position assumed following the activity is the cause of the pain rather than the activity itself.

Mechanical pain may be intermittent, appearing and disappearing, or vary in intensity according to aggravating and beneficial circumstances. It is usually intermittent because of increased and decreased mechanical deformation forces. *In cases of pain of mechanical origin, the examiner should always be able to reproduce the patient's symptoms by test movements.* Unrelenting pain from constant mechanical deformation (eg, irreducible disc protrusion) is always possible but not common. The rule to remember is that *pain of mechanical origin is always affected by movement,* for better or worse.

The motion that eases pain the most (reduces mechanical deformation) usually determines the plane of traction or adjustive therapy. An exception to this would be the pain produced by motion that stretches shortened tissues. This type pain subsides immediately when passive tension is removed and the joint returns to its neutral position.

Characteristics of Chemical Pain. Chemical irritants accumulate in damaged tissue soon after injury. As soon as nociceptive receptor activity is enhanced, pain will be experienced. Chemical irritation can be the result of any inflammatory, infectious, or traumatic process of sufficient degree. It can also be the result of any abnormal metabolic by-product, especially that of ischemia, of sufficient concentration to irritate free nerve endings in involved tissues.

In contrast to pain of mechanical origin, pain from chemical causes is constant, dull, and aggravated by normal movements as long as the chemical irritants are present in sufficient concentration. It may not occur until several minutes or hours after an injurious event has taken place. Chemical pain subsides during the natural healing process as scar tissue forms. Rarely does chemical pain from trauma extend pass 15—20 days after the accident.

GOUT

An acute case of gout is frustrating agony for the patient. Immediate attention must be given to the inflamed, swollen, tender, and tense joints and periarticular tissues. With proper control measures and rapid care, an attack is usually of short duration and severe joint crippling can be held to a minimum. Poorly controlled cases entering a practice at a late stage are most difficult to manage.

OSTEOARTHRITIS

The general degenerative changes associated with aging are rarely overtly painful unless the area is bruised, but pain may be associated with the cardinal signs of stiffness, articular fixation, restricted ranges of motion, soft-tissue atrophy, fibrosis, bone spurring, thinning IVDs, subluxation/fixations, initially hot Heberden's nodes, and weakness. Progressive, but highly variable, disability is associated. Some cases show great tissue destruction during roentgenography and have little pain, and some exhibit minor changes that are severely painful. The painful syndromes often have a genetic link.

PAGET'S DISEASE OF BONE

Osteitis deformans is a chronic disease of unknown etiology. It is characterized by abnormal bony changes in texture and shape, hypervascularization, a reduced cortex, spontaneous fractures, and hypercalciuria leading to kidney stones. It may involve the skull, spine, pelvis and/or extremities. It is usually asymptomatic in its early stages. Later, a dull nagging persistent ache appears, which is slowly progressive and sometimes episodic. The final stage features osteogenic sarcoma and persistently severe pain.

POLYMYALGIA RHEUMATICA

This disease has recently been renamed *polymyalgia arteritica* because it is usually an articular manifestation of giant cell (cranial, temporal) arteritis. The painful syndrome features a high sedimentation rate, early morning stiffness in the shoulders and hips, possible visual impairment, and roentgenographic signs of degenerative joint disease. Early therapy is crucial to offer optimal relief and prevent possible blindness.

RHEUMATOID ARTHRITIS

The discomfort suffered by a victim of rheumatoid arthritis is complex. There is pain on movement because articular tissues have become disorganized, and there is even pain during rest because of swelling and stretching of inflamed tissue, which is at its worse upon arising in the morning. In fact, most of the pain in rheumatoid arthritis is due to tissue swelling. Joint capsules and tendon insertions are richly endowed with free nerve endings. When inflammatory processes subside, there still is incapacitating pain because of destroyed tissues attempting to move against tough contractures and jagged deposits.

Overt and covert systemic illnesses are also usually associated. They are often reflected in anorexia and weight loss, anemia, arterial occlusion, unnatural fatigue, Felty's and Sjogren's syndromes, feverishness, pericarditis, palpitations and tachycardia, pleurisy, diffuse aching, subcutaneous hemorrhages, and general weakness.

In long-standing cases, overtones of iatrogenically related blurred and impaired vision, blood disorders, cerebral paresthesiae, constipation, Cushing's syndrome, diarrhea, dyspepsia, dysuria, headaches, osteoporosis, and necrotizing papillitis are frequently seen. It is the rare patient under allopathic care that has not been prescribed analgesics, anthranilates, antidepressants, choroquin, codeine, corticosteroids, corticotrophin, indomethacin, phenylbutazone, oxyphenbutazone, tetracosactrin, tricyclic depressants, and large doses of salicylates.[99] As the result of these medicinally-induced side-effects, symptoms of anxiety and depression are often exhibited. It should come as no surprise that many of these patients seek chiropractic care.

THE ANKYLOSING SPONDYLARTHROPATHIES

This group of entities closely resembles rheumatoid arthritis in many respects. It includes idiopathic ankylosing spondylitis, Reiter's disease, psoriatic arthropathy, and the arthropathies associated with ulcerative colitis, Behcet's disease, Crohn's disease, Still's disease (late), Whipple's disease, etc. Each progresses to diffuse spinal stiffening, bony tenderness, and involvement at some time of the hips, sacroiliacs, and shoulders rather than the smaller peripheral joints.

The Articular Receptors

When manipulation, traction, deep vibration, etc, are applied to any joint, changes in muscle, tendon, capsule, and ligamentous tension stimulate mechanoreceptors embedded within the affected tissues.[100]

TYPES AND FUNCTION

The apophyseal joints of the spine contain three of the four types of sensory mechanoreceptors that are stimulated by tissue tension. The four types are described by Wyke as follows:

Type I: These are globular corpuscles, thinly encapsulated, embedded in three-dimensional grape-like clusters of 3—8 corpuscles. They are found in the outer layers of joint capsules, originating from small myelinated nerve fibers. These very low threshold, slowly adapting biologic transducers are stimulated by slight increases in both static and dynamic local tissue stretching. They readily respond during active and passive manipulation. Their firing frequency, occurring even during joint rest and immobilization from static tension, is increased during capsule tension and decreased during capsule relaxation. Thus, their degree of activity is proportional to and signal the velocity, direction, and amplitude of joint movement (ie, tissue stretch).

Type II: These consist of conical receptors, thickly encapsulated, found individually or in clusters of 2—4 corpuscles. They are located in the deep subsynovial layers of joint capsules and articular fat pads, originating from medium-size myelinated nerve fibers. They have a low threshold as do Type I receptors but adapt readily to dynamic tension changes and do not fire during joint rest. These receptors signal that joint motion has been initiated, but offer no information as to joint velocity, direction, or amplitude of movement. During the ipsilateral tissue stretch of activity, they produce only short bursts of impulses that blend into Type I impulses; while simultaneously, impulses from the contralateral relaxed ligamentous fibers are greatly reduced in the Type I tonic nerve fibers. During axial traction, however, Type I discharges remain proportional to the tension force.

Type III: These are relatively large fusiform receptors, thinly encapsulated, found individually or in clusters of 2—3 corpuscles. They are sited at the surface of extremity joint ligaments, collaterally and intrinsically, originating from large myelinated nerve fibers. These high threshold receptors are *absent* in intrinsic vertebral ligaments but are affected indirectly within the extremities during spinal motion. They adapt slowly to dynamic changes in tissue tone but fire continuously when activated by severe dynamic changes of tissue tone.

Type IV: These are the nociceptive receptors, and they have two subtypes:

1. One subtype consists of the three-dimensional plexuses of unmyelinated nerve fibers found embedded in joint capsules, articular fat pads, and the outer coat of joint blood vessels, but this type is absent in menisci and discs, synovial tissue, and articular cartilage. These receptors comprise the articular nociceptive system that is normally inactive during joint rest but activated during joint motion or chemical irritation (eg, inflammation), thus they provide the major source of joint pain.

2. The other subtype is the free unmyelinated nerve endings found weaving between collateral and intrinsic joint ligament fibers of both axial and appendicular joints.

Both forms originate from tiny myelinated and unmyelinated nerve fibers, are of extremely high threshold, are nonadapting, are highly sensitive to abnormal tissue metabolites, and have an intimate morphologic relationship with other types of joint receptors.

CENTRAL EFFECTS

The afferent discharges from Type I and II capsule receptors especially offer important effects during professional manipulation, traction, and deep percussion. Wyke describes reflex, pain suppression, and position perception effects.

Reflex Effects. The afferent nerve fibers of articular receptors transmit polysynaptically with fusiform motor neurons within the CNS. Connection with alpha neurons is absent. The circuits contribute to the activity messages produced at the fusiform muscle spindle receptors, thus affecting muscle tone and the stretch reflexes of voluntary muscle. Specific joint manipulation affects muscle activity both locally (ipsilateral and contralateral) and remotely because the afferent nerve fibers from the mechanoreceptors involved give off collateral branches that are distributed both segmentally and intersegmentally. Thus, joint manipulation, traction, etc, produce reflex muscle tone changes (via motion unit facilitation and inhibition) so often seen in clinical application of various techniques.

Pain Supression Effects. If Type IV receptors are involved in a joint disorder involving the capsule or ligaments, polysynaptic afferent impulses are transmitted to alpha fibers of the local muscle motor pools to produce abnormal reflex activity. Pain is simultaneously manifested by neural synapses within the basal nucleus of the spinal cord's gray matter to ascending tracts that end in the limbic areas of the cerebral cortex. As previously described, this spinal "gate" can regulate the central flow of nociceptive transmission if affected by inhibitory peripheral receptor impulses.

A short review of this point is pertinent here: Type I, II, and III receptors offer fibers within the dorsal roots that enter the posterior horns of the cord. They synapse with neurons of the apical spinal nucleus that connect with presynaptic terminals of the nociceptive afferent fibers located in basal nuclei. Because the apical interneurons release an inhibitory transmitter substance at the synapse, nociceptive impulses are inhibited. Thus, muscle stretching and joint manipulation (as well as compression, cold, acumassage, and deep vibration) produce peripheral receptor stimulation that creates presynaptic inhibition of nociceptive activity in the basal nucleus to dampen the central perception of pain.

These pathways are more active during youth than old age, and this possibly explains why certain manipulative techniques are more effective in the young than in the elderly. Regardless, the relief of pain through reflexogenic mechanisms provides an important therapy in nonsurgical case management by utilizing manipulative and cutaneous electronic stimulation techniques.

Positional Effects. Messages from Type I receptors make a significant contribution to postural and kinesthetic perception. They arise from the dorsal and dorsolateral columns of the spinal cord and finally are relayed through complex synaptic relays to the parietal and paracentral regions of the cerebral cortex. It is for this reason that loss of Type I receptor activity (spinal or extraspinal) from traumatic, inflammatory, or degenerative joint processes manifests in abnormalities of posture, gait, and specific joint movement because of inhibited kinesthetic perception.

THE CERVICAL SPINAL RECEPTORS

The apophyseal joints of the cervical spine are richly innervated with mechanoreceptors and afferent fibers. In fact, they are endowed more than any other spinal region. Activity from the cervical articular receptors exerts significant facilitatory and inhibitory reflex effects on the muscles of the neck and both the upper and lower extremities.

Wyke points out that the patterns of "normal cervical articular mechanoreceptor reflexes are profoundly distorted when cervical articular nociceptive afferent activity is added to that derived from the normally functioning cervical mechanoreceptors." To underscore this point, he states that (1) manipulation of the head on the neck can produce coordinated flexion and extension movements on the paralyzed arm and leg of a hemiplegic patient, (2) arm movement control in the absence of visual aid is considerably affected by rotation of the head, and (3) induced unilateral local anesthesia of the cervical joints in healthy subjects produces severe postural instability, dizziness, nystagmus, and muscular incoordination. These signs and symptoms are similar to those experienced by some patients who suffer from cervical spondylosis, ankylosing spondylitis, gross fixations, and some while wearing an orthopedic cervical collar.

THE LUMBAR NOCICEPTIVE RECEPTOR SYSTEM

Static postural support of the lumbar spine in the prolonged relaxed erect or seated postures is provided essentially by the passive elastic tension of the involved ligaments and fascia rather than the spinal muscles whose roles can be considered insignificant during a state of relaxation. This shifting of support from the muscles to the ligaments, however, occurs slowly over a period of several minutes before significant EMG activity can be considered absent.

The lumbar ligaments and fascia are richly innervated by nociceptive receptors. When the lumbar spine is in a relaxed neutral position, its nociceptive receptor system is relatively inactive. However, any mechanical force that will stress or deform receptors, with or without overt damage, or any irritat-

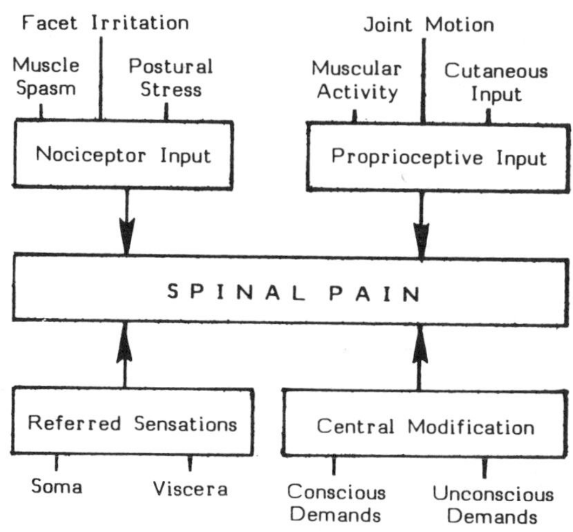

Figure 2.14. Common factors that influence spinal pain.

ing chemical of sufficient concentration will depolarize unmyelinated fibers and enhance afferent activity. See Figure 2.14.

EVALUATING THE PATIENT IN PAIN

In approaching the examination of the patient as it relates to pain processes (only a segment of the total examination), our concern in this section will relate primarily to musculoskeletal problems of the spine for such cases represent an extensive volume of concern in clinical practice.

As the patient is examined, the physician should be conscious of the patient's actions and reactions. A mental picture should be drawn of how much each patient is suffering. It is axiomatic that, if a person is to appreciate the pain of another, it must have been personally experienced. It should not be assumed that a patient does not suffer because its description is stated in light-hearted terms or the pain appears to be of a nonphysical nature. Sympathy for the patient is never misplaced except in overt malingering.

Suffering is not the same as physical distress. The degree of pain from a fracture may be greater than that of angina; but the suffering is greater with angina because the patient is terrorized of what the future might hold, whereas the patient with a fracture knows that the pain will cease in time and that recovery is not in doubt.

Severe pain produces several noticeable signs, and we should be cognizant of them. With severe pain, there is an increase in pulse rate, respiratory rate, perspiration, and vasomotor tone. There is also an initial rise in blood pressure and possibly nausea and vomiting.

Interviewing Techniques

Although pain is almost always present in patients with musculoskeletal problems, it must not be *assumed* to be present. Patients must be allowed to describe the symptoms in their own way, even if the words may be somewhat misleading initially. For example, numbness is frequently used incorrectly, and if one asks the patient if absence of sensation is implied, the usual reply is "No, I don't mean that. I mean a dull ache."

It is inevitable that most patients will have difficulty in describing their pain because there is no objective yardstick to which it can be measured. The most common subjective comparison is the toothache, on the assumption that everyone has suffered from this. When describing pain, picturesque and dramatic phraseology often reflects an underlying neurosis.

Questions relating to pain should fall around four major areas: (1) the *onset* of the pain, (2) the *nature* of the pain, (2) the *location* and *radiation* of the pain, if any, and (4) whether or not certain *positions* tend to enhance or diminish the pain.

THE ONSET

It should be determined whether or not the onset of the pain is sudden or insidious. By a sudden onset, it is implied that the pain arose suddenly during some type of motion. Several conditions will characteristically give rise to a sudden onset of pain. Among them we have acute joint fixation or locking, subluxations of a sacroiliac joint, whiplash injury, a tendon rupture or a capsule tear such as might occur during a sudden lift or split, a ruptured muscle, and, finally, the common traumatic IVD syndrome.

Next we have the insidious onset, which may be acute or chronic in nature. ''Insidious'' means that there was no overt precipitating factor(s) involved. An onset of pain that is acute and insidious should make us think of a systemic problem. During the diagnostic process, it is best to eliminate the common causes first (eg, the flu, visceral disease) before we progress to the less common causes (eg, epidural abscess, early osteomyelitis). Chronic disorders having an insidious onset of pain will mainly fall in the category of bone or joint disease. However, we must also consider distant irritable pathology with referred pain or possibly a neoplastic process.

THE NATURE

The next step is to evaluate the nature of the patient's pain. ''What is the pain like when you get up in the morning?'' Pains of joint disease or muscle injury are not improved much by rest. In fact, overstressed spinal muscles tend to stiffen with rest. The patient who has severe night pains in the spine is a special concern because this symptom is characteristic of a neoplasm.

''Do certain movements or postures (positions) relieve or aggravate the pain?'' Sacroiliac dysfunctions may be relieved by a tight belt or girdle. The patient might state, ''I start to feel lousy soon after I get home and get into some comfortable clothes.''

Lumbosacral dysfunction is at its worst when the patient assumes a semistooped (partially flexed) posture (eg, washing dishes, ironing, leaning over a workbench). These types of back problems are often relieved by sitting on a high stool that has a backrest.

THE LOCATION AND RADIATION

The physician must be especially concerned with the location of pain and whether or not it has any radiation to another area of the body. Pain that is unilateral frequently indicates simple joint dysfunction or subluxation. Bone or joint disease will usually give rise to a bilateral distribution.

It is good practice to have patients point a finger at the area of worst pain. When requested to do so, they will generally say something like, ''Oh, it's right in here.'' Then you can mark that spot with a skin pencil and record it in your notes for future reference. Without such a reference, it might be difficult on future visits to determine if the focal point of the pain is shifting or if the patient is malingering.

THE POSITION

The next consideration involves the relationship of pain to position. Symptoms will often vary with a change in position, and this strongly suggests that the problem has a mechanical origin involving the musculoskeletal system rather than due to some visceral disorder. In fact, positional pain that has been present consistently for years without exacerbation is invariably considered to be of mechanical origin.

Mechanically produced pain arises from stretching or compressing a sensitive structure. If the pain increases during compression, it suggests that the tissue being compressed is tender. Compression may be nothing more than normal weight bearing, or it may be from the tissue squeezing that occurs in lateral flexion or extension of a joint. Pain that develops when tissues are stretched suggests that the tissues being elongated by tensile forces are tender. Thus, pain that develops during side bending is either of compression or tension. If the pain arises on the opposite side of the lateral flexion, then the stretching action is the aggravating factor (eg, torn or tight tissues). If the pain occurs on the side of lateral bending, then, obviously, compression of tender structures is the problem (eg, subluxation, thinned IVD, jammed joint, tissue entrapment).

Stretch Pain. Spinal pain that is produced by standing and relieved by movement and rest suggests that there is some type of IVD compression, with concomitant bulging of the posterior longitudinal ligament. Disc herniation is often suggested when the patient can extend and laterally bend without much difficulty but forward flexion severely aggravates the pain. If forward flexion causes pain only after a delay of some minutes, ligamentous weakness is suggested. This sign is referred to as *delayed stretch pain*.

Pain that arises on prolonged forward bending is usually muscular in origin and referred to as *fatigue pain*. Myalgia due to fatigue is not at all uncommon. General fatigue after a busy day can accentuate any pain as can anxiety because both tend to lower the pain threshold. Backache of muscular origin (eg, that of a weekend gardener) that is due to unaccustomed physical effort and unusual positions tends to abate rather quickly. Muscular pain or rather the aching stiffness in muscles that follows unusual exercise sometimes arises from what appears to be trivial overstress. This should lead the examiner to suspect that an underlying focal sepsis or metabolic fault might be present (eg, increased serum uric acid level, electrolytic imbalance).

Spinal pain that occurs with forward flexion which is followed by pain during the return extension to the upright position indicates an unstable joint and weakened ligaments (eg, lumbopelvic rhythm deficit, usually due to weak pelvic stabilization). Spinal pain that is seen only when the patient is bending backward in extension suggests a jamming of facets or spinous processes or compression of the pars interarticularis—typical of the lordotic syndrome.

Stretch pain occurs most commonly with adhesions. The pain in this situation is immediate in onset and not delayed as when the ligaments are relaxed. Another diagnostic clue is the fact that there is a pronounced hypomobility when adhesions are present.

If the patient is unable to extend freely from the Adams position, then weak extensors, a disc lesion, or possibly a hip disorder is involved. An IVD lesion is particularly suspect if there is also acute pain during forward flexion because of the stretch placed on splinting muscles. When spinal movement is painful in all ranges of motion, it is likely that a nerve root is riding over a herniated disc. Spinal pain that is sharply increased by sneezing or coughing indicates abnormal disc pressure, characteristic of an eccentrically compressed IVD.

Spinal pain that is relieved by traction indicates that there is opposition to normal IVD hydration. This is especially common with degenerative disc disease such as seen in spinal osteoarthritis and certain rare (usually genetic) carbohydrate metabolism deficits. In spinal osteoarthritis, the characteristic *arthritic cycle* can usually be elicited by alert questioning. Osteoarthritic pain increases with rest so that the patient feels worse in the morning upon arising. After being up and around for a while, the pain tends to ease but a good deal of stiffness remains. After more activity, the pain increases in intensity and rest is sought. This is why it is called a cycle. Thus, pain plus stiffness after rest is almost pathognomonic for some arthritic conditions, and this pain is probably due to some sustained reflex muscular guarding of the involved joint(s).

The influence of activity can also be of some value in the differential diagnosis of vasomotor syndromes. Pain that develops only with exertion and disappears immediately with rest points to claudication or some other type of intermittent circulatory insufficiency. The discomfort is the result of the relative ischemia (anoxia) during the activity demand for more oxygen. As the vascular disorder progresses, further impairment of circulation may cause pain on trivial activity and even at rest during the late stage (where the danger of gangrene is a threat). Thus, a thorough case history is always a necessity in such cases.

Pain that develops with rest and is relieved by activity is not so easily explained. It might well be of a vascular origin in so far as the rest might lead to circulatory stasis, especially on the venous side, and an accumulation of metabolites. This is a possible explanation why the pain of gout is worse during the morning hours.

Ligamentous Pain. Ligamentous pain arises gradually. It is the type of pain that develops when a joint is under extremely prolonged stretch (tension). A hypomobile joint should be the first suspicion in such cases. Generally, ligamentous pain comes on slowly after assuming some posture in which the joint is held at a limit of motion. A common example is the individual who curls within an arm chair to watch some lengthy movie on television. Because there is no support for the lumbar spine, tensile forces gradually overstretch the ligamentous straps. An ache arises from the irritation of the intraligamentous and periosteal receptors. Another common example is the "flat-footed" individual who is prone to painful plantar ligaments and fascia after standing for lengthy periods. In both of these examples, the pain eases as soon as the tension is removed from the stressed tissues.

Pain originating from adhesions and tightened capsules occurs at once when the capsule is stretched. If adhesions are stretched further, a sharp pain may ensue, leaving the surrounding muscles flaccid. The intensity of such a pain varies with the site and size of the adhesion(s). For the most part, pain arising from adhesions is only momentary because motion is quickly halted as soon as the sharp pain is felt.

Neuralgic Pain. Pain intrinsically arising from a nerve or nerves is always a consideration. Pain that is accentuated by heat suggest neuritis. In contrast, pain that is relieved by heat suggests something producing abnormal muscular tension. Pain of intrinsic neurologic origin is generally accompanied by paresthesiae and root signs. When throbbing pain is present, vascular congestion, crush syndrome, a vasomotor disturbance, or possibly Paget's disease should be the first suspicions.

Constant Pain. Persistent pain that is relatively unaffected by activity, rest, or position is likely to have a visceral, obstruction, or neoplastic origin. There are some exceptions to this, of course, such as most headaches, toothaches, earaches, etc. A psychologic origin may be a consideration, but psychogenic pain is unrelieved by analgesic-producing therapies unless the patient is highly receptive to suggestion. There are also certain forms of intractable pain that fail to respond to analgesics, but in these cases, there are usually other indications of the severity of the pain upon which a judgment can be based.

Nocturnal Pain. As previously described, nocturnal pain that is relieved during the day may have a positional explanation or be the effect of gout or a bone disease. Anxiety states that are worse at night often increase physical pain of other origins during the evening hours.

Other Orthopedic and Neurologic Signs. Last, but not least, should be consideration of the objective signs that depend on position as opposed to the subjective symptoms that have been described. For example, Lasegue's straight-leg-raising (SLR) test may elicit pain when a certain point of elevation has been reached. Further tension on the sciatic nerve roots can be supposedly increased by dorsiflexion of the ankle during the maneuver. When SLR induces pain contralaterally, many clinicians feel that this is an indication that lumbar torsion is part of the pressure mechanism. When pain is produced by bilateral SLR, the cause may be due to anything from tight hamstrings to an IVD lesion.

The Management of Pain

Perhaps the most important factor in developing a successful practice is the efficient management of pain syndromes. People have, from the earliest times, devised ingenious methods in an effort to weaken pain: from trephination to remove evil spirits, to acupuncture to restore Chi, to drugs and surgery to hide or excise the problem, etc. Chiropractic physicians have a key role to play, and this has been enhanced now that meridian therapy is coming into the forefront. We now have an additional tool that can modify pain patterns while we restore the health and well-being of the patient.

Before describing specific ways in which pain can be controlled and managed, the subject of subsequent chapters, it would be well to review some of the neurophysiology involved. It has been described how pain (protopathic) impulses travel to the cortex via the spinothalamic tracts. Thus, we must find a way to block or compromise these noxious stimuli if pain relief is to be achieved.

For many years, Ben-gay and other analgesic preparations have been utilized to lessen the everyday aches and pain of life. It is now believed that such counterirritants operate by sending impulses through the substantia gelatinosa of the dorsal columns to the brain so that the cord ''gate'' closes. That is, pain signals that would normally ascend the spinothalamic tracts are blocked from traveling to the higher centers.

This is much the same way that the Dorsal Column Stimulator works, which was developed by a neurosurgeon named Fox. This device provides a continuous stimulus to the dorsal columns of the cord to inhibit the ascent of nocireceptor initiated impulses. It can be surmised that the same process occurs in acupuncture and spinal manipulation; ie, transmitting a signal through the dorsal columns to the brainstem which, in turn, closes the ''gate'' and blocks the sensory impulses. The pain is then abated. Unfortunately, the impulses that are provided by the doctor or a counterirritant may not be of sufficient intensity to keep the pain from returning. Thus, patients with intractable pain must resort to surgical intervention for relief. In recent years, however, it has been found that acupuncture has proved to be an adequate substitute for previously utilized drugs and surgery—giving the patient a pain-free existence without the traumatizing effects of surgery or the dangerous complications so often associated with chemotherapy.

A LOOK BACK

Generally speaking, the management of pain in Western cultures has been best accomplished by: (1) operant conditioning, (2) biofeedback procedures, and (3) drugs and/or surgery. While pain control procedures generally fall into one of these categories, a growing interest is taking place in the subject of meridian therapy.

The most common entity encountered when a musculoskeletal complaint is discussed is the myofascial pain syndrome. Myofascial syndromes are characterized by the presence of so-called trigger foci in muscular tissue that lead to pain, spasm, tenderness, stiffness, motion restriction, and at times, autonomic dysfunction. Chiropractors have for years utilized trigger-point therapeutics on these tender sites. Medically, these areas have been treated by repeatedly inserting a syringe needle into the trigger point, infiltrating the site with a local anesthetic (eg, xylocaine), or spraying the overlying skin with some type of vapocoolant. Although these techniques have proved effective in many instances, they are highly painful to the patient involved and have usually provided only temporary relief. When the anesthetic effect wanes, the pain returns.

Chiropractic management of trigger points has been extensively studied by Nimmo and others. In contrast, the most widely used device to alleviate pain in the allopathic office has been the analgesic. The analgesic of choice for any given patient is dictated by the origin, quality, intensity, duration, and distribution of the pain. Once the dosage has been optimized, close observation is necessary to detect possible iatrogenic side-effects or drug dependence.

Although the use of potent narcotics and sedatives to control severe pain should be limited to acute diseases or to patients with inoperable or recurring cancer, this is not always the practice. Long-term use of analgesic drugs in chronic pain syndromes generally produces more distressing complications than the pain it was designed to eliminate. The same is true for many tranquilizers and muscle relaxants.

A LOOK AHEAD

At this point, it is well to review what Matsumoto has to say about pain.[101] He brings out various factors in the management of pain. He emphasizes that underlying the control or management of pain is the removal of the causal factor. This may mean that a system of pain control should be utilized while the body heals itself. In other instances, pain may be managed by the control of chemical reactions at the receptor site and by reduction of receptor sensitivity. Nerve block initiates pain management by the interruption of impulses or pathways. One might also change the pattern with time and frequency of stimulation from peripheral nerve to the CNS. Electro-stimulation therapy represents such a mechanism, as does specific acupuncture. Another means of controlling pain, according to Matsumoto, is the interruption of the pathway of stimulation in the spinal cord and brain. Implied here is neurosurgical intervention such as rhizotomy, chordotomy, and tractotomy. Finally, the control of pain might be by the use of sedatives and tranquilizers.

Matsumoto, though, is mainly concerned with acupuncture and stimulation therapy. Acupuncture is one mode of stimulation therapy that changes the pattern of impulses flowing to the CNS. Although any method of stimulating an acupuncture (meridian) point may be used (eg, moxibustion, cupping, actapotement, etc), the most commonly applied procedures utilize needle insertion, electrical stimulation, and auriculotherapy.

There is no doubt that acupuncture stimulation blocks pain. For example, the pain of a toothache in the lower jaw may be rapidly lessened by the stimulation of the Large Intestine #4 point (ho-ku). Studies conducted in Europe have shown that stimulation of this point removes tooth pain in approximately 90% of those tested.

It can therefore be concluded that needling procedures, with and without electrical stimulation, seem to offer the fastest relief for pain syndromes. By way of the cutaneo-visceral reflex and through the gate control hypothesis, an understanding of how pain may be attenuated can be readily appreciated. Thus, the utilization of such procedures as a mechanism for pain control should be considered, especially for the management of pain prior to corrective manipulation.

This chapter has described how peripheral stimulation techniques are efficient in the control and management of pain. Knowing where to apply such techniques is another concern, and this is the subject of the next chapter.

REFERENCES

1. Jaskoviak PA: *Pain Syndromes and Their Management.* Clinical Mongraph Series, 6541-A. Lombard, IL, National College of Chiropractic, 1976.
2. Schafer RC: *Symptomatology and Differential Diagnosis: A Conspectus of Clinical Semeiographies.* Arlington, VA, American Chiropractic Association. Prepublication manuscript, scheduled for publication in 1985.
3. *Illustrated Stedman's Medical Dictionary,* ed 24. Baltimore, Williams & Wilkins, 1982, p 1015.
4. *Webster's New Collegiate Dictionary.* Springfield, MA, G & C Merriam, 1980, p 817.
5. Suchman E: in *Journal of Health and Human Behavior,* 6:114, 1963.
6. Keele CA, Armstrong D: *Substances Producing Pain and Itch.* Baltimore, Williams & Wilkins, 1964.
7. Hart FD (ed): *The Treatment of Chronic Pain.* Philadelphia, F.A. Davis, 1974, p 1.
8. Woodward HH, et al: in *Journal of Anatomy,* 74:413, 1940.
9. Iggo A: in Janzen R, et al (eds): *Pain.* London, Churchill Livingstone, 1972.
10. Ferreira SH: in *Nature New Biology,* 240:200, 1972.
11. Vane JR: in *Nature New Biology,* 231:232, 1971.
12. Bishop MR: in *Physiology Review,* 26:203, 1946.
13. Douglas WW, Ritchie JM: in *Journal of Physiology* (London), 139:385, 1957.
14. McCarty CS, Drake RL: in *Mayo Clinic Proceedings,* 31:208, 1956.
15. Melzack R, Wall PD: in *Science,* 150:971, 1965.
16. Wall PD, Sweet WH: in *Science,* 155:108, 1967.
17. Noordenbos W: in Soulairac A, et al (eds): *Pain.* New York, Academic Press, 1968.
18. Schmidt RF: in Janzen R, et al (eds): *Pain.* London, Churchill Livingstone, 1972.
19. Iggo A: in Janzen R, et al (eds): *Pain.* London, Churchill Livingstone, 1972.
20. Hart FD (ed): *The Treatment of Chronic Pain.* Philadelphia, F.A. Davis, 1974, p 4.
21. Keele KD: in *British Medical Journal,* 1:670, 1968.
22. De Sterno VD: The pathophysiology of TMJ dysfunction and related pain. In Gelb, H (ed): *Clinical Management of Head, Neck and TMJ Pain and Dysfunction.* Philadelphia, W.B. Saunders, 1977.
23. Schafer RC: *Clinical Biomechanics.* Baltimore, Williams & Wilkins, 1983, pp 406-407.
24. Beecher HK: in *Pharmaceutical Review,* No. 9, 1957.
25. Hart FD (ed): *The Treatment of Chronic Pain.* Philadelphia, F.A. Davis, 1974, p 8.
26. Huskisson EC, Hart FD: in *British Medical Journal,* 4:193, 1972.
27. Gaensler EA: in *Journal of Clinical Investigation,* 30:406, 1951.
28. Keele KD: in Keele CA, Smith R (eds): *The Assessment of Pain in Man and Animals.* London, Livingstone, 1962.
29. Hardy JR, et al: *Pain Sensations and Reactions.* Baltimore, Williams & Wilkins, 1952.
30. Chapman WO, et al: in *Archives of Neurology and Psychiatry,* 57:32, 1947.
31. Seevers MH, Pfeiffer CC: in *Journal of Pharmacology,* 56:166, 1936.
32. Beecher HK: in *Pharmaceutical Review,* No. 9, 1957.
33. Wolff BB, et al: in *Clinical Pharmacology and Therapeutics,* 10:217, 1969.
34. Beecher HK: *Measurement of Subjective Responses.* New York, Oxford University Press, 1959.
35. Hewer AJH, Keele CA: in *Lancet,* 2:683, 1948.
36. Smith GM, Beecher HK: in *Clinical Pharmacology and Therapeutics,* 10:213, 1969.
37. Gelfand S, et al: in *Journal of Nervous and Mental Disease,* 136:379, 1963.
38. Sternbach RA, Tursky B: in *Psychophysiology,* 1:241, 1965.
39. Merskey H, et al: in *Journal of Mental Science,* 108:347, 1962.
40. Hazouri LA, Mueller AD: in *Archives of Neurology,* 64:607, 1950.
41. Chapman WP, Jones CM: in *Journal of Clinical Investigation,* 23:81, 1944.
42. Hall KRL, Stride E: in *British Journal of Medical Psychology,* 27:48, 1954.
43. Wolff BB, Jarvik ME: in *American Journal of Psychiatry,* 77:589, 1964.
44. Edmonds EP: in *Annals of the Rheumatic Diseases* (United Kingdom), 6:36, 1947.
45. Huskisson EC, Hart FD: in *Medicine and Hygiene,* 29:2054, 1973.
46. Hart FD (ed): *The Treatment of Chronic Pain.* Philadelphia, F.A. Davis, 1974, p 15.
47. Hardy, et al: in *Journal of Clinical Investigation,* 19:649, 1940.
48. Notermans SLH: in *Neurology,* 17:38, 1967.
49. Collins LG: in *Perceptual Motor Skills,* 21:349, 1965.
50. Zborowski M: in *Journal of Social Issues,* 8:16, 1952.
51. Kennard MA: in *Journal of Clinical Investigation,* 31:245, 1959.
52. Dundee JW, Moore J: in *British Journal of Anesthesia,* 32:396, 1960.
53. Merskey H, Spear FG: in *British Journal of Social Clinical Psychology,* 3:130, 1964.
54. Wells HS: in *Archives of Physical Medicine,* 28:135, 1947.

55. Pottenger FM: *Symptoms of Visceral Disease,* ed 6. St. Louis, C.V. Mosby, 1944.
56. Berger PA, et al: Behavioral pharmacology of the endorphins. *Annual Review of Medicine,* 33:397-415, 1982.
57. Clement-Jones V, et al: Acupuncture in heroin addicts: changes in met-enkephalin and B-endorphin in blood and cerebrospinal fluid. *Lancet,* 2:380-384, 1979.
58. Wen HL: Clinical experience and mechanism of acupuncture and electrical stimulation (AES) in the treatment of drug abuse. *American Journal of Chinese Medicine,* VIII(4):349-353, 1980.
59. Wei LY: Scientific advance in acupuncture. In Kao FF, Kao JJ (eds): *Recent Advances in Acupuncture Research.* Garden City, LI, Institute for Advanced Research in Asian Science and Medicine, 1979, pp 49-71.
60. Li CH, Chung D: Isolation and structure of an untriakontapeptide with opiate activity. *Proceedings of the National Academy of Sciences,* 73:1145-1148, 1965.
61. Goldstein A: Opiate receptors, implications and applications. *Science,* 189:708-710, 1975.
62. Terenius L: Characteristics of the receptor for narcotic analgesics in synaptic membrane fractions from rat brain. *Acta Pharmacology* (Sweden), 33:377-384, 1973.
63. Snyder SH: The opiate receptor. *Neurosciences Research Program Bulletin* (Supplement), 13:1-27, 1974.
64. Akil H, et al: Antagonism of stimulation produced analgesia by naloxone, a narcotic antagonist. *Science,* 191:961-962, 1976.
65. Mayer DJ, et al: Acupuncture hypalgesia evidence for activation of a central control system as a mechanism of action. *First World Congress on Pain,* Abstract 276, 1975.
66. Mayer DJ, et al: Antagonism of acupuncture analgesia in man by the narcotic antagonist naloxone. *Brain Research,* 121:368-372, 1977.
67. Parsons JA (ed): *Peptide Hormones.* New York, MacMillan, 1976.
68. Hughes J, et al: Identification of two related pentapeptides from the brain with potent opiate agonist activity. *Nature* (London), 258:577-579, 1975.
69. Guillemin R, et al: The endorphins, novel peptides of brain and hypophyseal origin, with opiate like activity: biochemical and biologic studies. *Annals of the New York Academy of Science,* 197: 131-157, 1979.
70. Feldberg W, Smyth DG: C-fragment of lipotropin, an endogenous potent analgesic peptide. *British Journal of Pharmacology,* 60:445-453, 1977.
71. Schwartz JC, et al: Minireview: biological inactivation of enkephalins and the role of enkephalin-dipeptidylcarboxypeptides ("enkephalinase") as neuropeptides. *Life Science,* 29:1715-1740, 1981.
72. Atweh SF, Kuhar MJ: Autoradiographic localization of opiate receptors in rat brain, I. Spinal cord and lower medulla. *Brain Research,* 124:53-67, 1977.
73. Fields A: Acupuncture and endorphins. *International Journal of Chinese Medicine,* 1(2):10, June 1984.
74. Research Group of Acupuncture Anesthesia; Peking Medical College: Effect of acupuncture on pain threshold on human skin. *Chinese Medical Journal,* 3:151-157, 1973.
75. Palmer DD: *Text-Book of the Science, Art and Philosophy of Chiropractic.* Portland, OR, Portland Printing House Company, 1910.
76. Zukav G: *The Dancing Wu Li Masters.* New York, William Morrow, 1979.
77. Capra F: *The Tao of Physics.* Boulder, CO, Shambhala Publications, 1975.
78. Schafer RC: *Clinical Biomechanics.* Baltimore, Williams & Wilkins, 1983, pp 406.
79. Hart FD (ed): *The Treatment of Chronic Pain.* Philadelphia, F.A. Davis, 1974, p 113.
80. Hertz AF: On the sensibility of the alimentary canal in health and disease. *Lancet,* 1:1051, 1911.
81. Sutton DC, Lueth HC: Pain. *AMA Archives of Internal Medicine,* 45:827, 1930.
82. Learmouth JR: Neurosurgery in the treatment of diseases of the urinary bladder, II: Treatment of visceral pain. *Journal of Urology,* 26:13, 1931.
83. Mitchell GAG: *Cardiovascular Innervation.* London, Livingstone, 1956, p 356.
84. White JC, et al: Cardiac innervation: experimental and clinical studies. *AMA Archives of Surgery,* 26:765, 1933.
85. Marshall HR: *Pain, Pleasure and Aesthetics.* London, Macmillan, 1894.
86. Strong, in *Psychology Review,* 2:329, 1895.
87. Guthrie GJ: *A Treatise on Gunshot Wounds.* London, Burgess and Hill, 1827.
88. Beecher: in *Annals of Surgery.* 123:96, 1946.
89. Achelis: in Buytendijk JJ: *Pain: Its Modes and Functions,* translated by E. O'Shiel. Chicago, University of Chicago Press, 1943, p 115.
90. Sartre J-P: *Sketch for a Theory of the Emotions,* translated by P. Mairet. London, Methuen, 1939, p 28.
91. Szasz TS: The psychology of persistent pain. In Soulairac A, et al: *Pain.* London, Academic Press, 1968, pp 93-113.
92. Neelon FA, Ellis GJ: *A Syllabus of Problem-Oriented Patient Care.* Boston, Little, Brown, 1974.
93. Schafer RC: *Chiropractic Management of Sports and Recreational Injuries.* Baltimore, Williams & Wilkins, 1982, pp 166-167, 197-198.
94. Huskisson EC, Hart FD: *Joint Disease: All the Arthropathies.* Bristol, John Wright, 1973.
95. Wyke BD: in *Annals of the Royal College of Surgeons,* England, 41:23, 1967.

96. Wyke BD: in *Rheumatology and Physical Medicine,* 10:356, 1970.
97. McKenzie RA: *The Lumbar Spine.* Upper Hutt, New Zealand, Spinal Publications Ltd, 1981.
98. Schafer RC: *Clinical Biomechanics.* Baltimore, Williams & Wilkins, 1983, pp 400-401.
99. Hart FD (ed): *The Treatment of Chronic Pain.* Philadelphia, F.A. Davis, 1974, p 64.
100. Schafer RC: *Clinical Biomechanics.* Baltimore, Williams & Wilkins, 1983, pp 247-249, 300, 399.
101. Matsumoto T: *Acupuncture for Physicians.* Springfield, IL, Charles C. Thomas, 1974, pp 19-20.

Uncited References

Bishop B: Pain: its physiology and rationale for management. Part I, neuroanatomical substrate of pain. *Physical Therapy,* 60:13-20, 1980.

Bishop B: Pain: its physiology and rationale for management. Part II, analgesic systems of the CNS. *Physical Therapy,* 60:21-23, 1980.

Elton D, Burrows GD, Stanley GV: Clinical measurement of pain. *Medical Journal of Australia,* 1:109-111. 1979.

Lamb DW: The neurology of spinal pain. *Physical Therapy,* 59:971-973, 1979.

Leavitt F, Garron DC, Whisler WW, Sheinkop MB: Affective and sensory dimensions of back pain. *Pain,* 4:273-281, 1978.

LeBars D, Chitour D: Do convergent neurones in the spinal dorsal horns discriminate nociceptive from non-nociceptive information? *Pain,* 17:1-19, 1983.

Ray CD: Electrical stimulation: new methods for therapy and rehabilitation. *Scandinavian Journal of Rehabilitative Medicine,* 10:65-74, 1978.

Wall PD: Gate control theory of pain mechanisms: a re-examination and re-statement. *Brain,* 101:1-18, 1978.

Chapter 3

Commonly Used Meridian Points

This chapter describes the theoretical basis of meridian therapy and explains how specific acupuncture points may be found and treated in the management of pain and various functional disorders. Within the context of physiologic therapeutics, the location, primary indications, and precautions associated with the major points (ie, those most commonly used) are delineated.

Both Western and Eastern cultures have effectively proven that they can relieve a large degree of human suffering. It is hoped that future generations will be able to integrate the best of each into a single healthcare delivery system for the world.[1]

THE THEORETICAL BASIS OF MERIDIAN THERAPY

Forms of stimulation to specific sites on the skin have been utilized for at least 3000 years. However, it is only within the last 20 years that comprehensive studies of acupuncture as a legitimate therapy have been seriously undertaken in this country. The fact that meridian therapy has a beneficial effect on the control of disease processes seems evident today on the basis of empirical evidence; ie, it has become accepted in much the same way as the efficacy of adjustive therapy and various drugs (eg, aspirin) were established through the years.

Theoretical Concepts

Although it generally matters little to patients as to why they get well under a certain therapy, they do, however, expect that the doctor rendering that therapy has an acceptable explanation of the biologic mechanisms that are probably involved. That is, the patient has a natural tendency to believe that their doctor selects a particular procedure of treatment for their condition on the basis of his or her knowledge of the nature of their problem, and the knowledge of the underlying principles behind a particular method of therapy. Also, since the study and effective application of meridian therapy require some basic knowledge of its theoretical scientific basis, the need for this explanation is established.

In the case of meridian therapy, a number of theories have been advanced that generally fall under the headings of "Neural" or "Nonneural" concepts. These concepts attempt to explain the scientific basis for the biologic effects of meridian therapy in terms of our present understanding of human anatomy and physiology. Although scientific verification of the concept of "vital energy" as a physiologic probability and the "meridian" system as an anatomical fact have yet to be conclusive, verification for some of the effects of meridian therapy does exist on the basis of these concepts.[2]

The Nonneural Theories

One of the most commonly mentioned nonneural concepts attempts to explain the meridian system by proposing an elaborate conducting system of what is referred to as "Bong Han Ducts and Corpuscles." This theory, put forth by a North Korean physiologist and acupuncturist, Kim Bong Han, is a histological description of elongated tubular cells lying deep within the skin. Han also thinks that a "unique" fluid circulates through these channels, which contains a high concentration of ribonucleic and other amino acids. Han believes that this fluid travels slowly through the meridians, completing a cycle each 24 hours.[3,4]

Han's theory, however impressive as it might be, has for all practical purposes been refuted by other investigators. Kellner has shown that some of this theory is based on artifacts occurring in preparation of the histological slides, and other attempts at duplicating the work of Han reveal that he was probably describing the lymphatic channels of the body.[5,6]

Various other theories have attempted to explain acupuncture and the existence of the meridians.[7] For example, magnetic fields, quantum mechanics, contraction waves of skeletal muscles, discharging of electrical potentials, and the release of histamine and epinephrine by stimulation of points have all been put forth as possible mechanisms. Others have likened the pinprick in the body to the electrical discharge of a condenser. At one time, Felix Mann proposed a theory based on the lateral line system in fish. These theories, along with others, have now been dismissed in favor of one of the neurologic explanations.

One of the most recent theories has been postulated by Koyo Takase in Japan who concluded that the so-called Chi energy circulating through a "meridian" in acupuncture therapy is actually extravascular sodium.[8] His studies involved the use of radioisotopes.

The Neural Theories

It is generally conceded that the mechanisms of acupuncture are similar to but not identical to those of the nervous system, but there are many questions that need answering.[9]

When an acupuncture point is stimulated, it has been observed that the patient will often experience a change within seconds and this change frequently occurs at the opposite end and contralateral side of the body from the point stimulated. The exact mechanism of this action is not yet fully understood, although certain aspects appear to be based on established neurophysiologic concepts. This indicates that some type of nerve conduction occurs, as nerve fibers transmit impulses at an extremely rapid rate through their pathways. Such a rapid speed of conduction excludes the blood and lymphatic systems as possible mediators of this response.

THE CUTANEOVISCERAL REFLEX

Acupuncture is founded on the premise that stimulation of the skin has an effect on distant internal organs and functional mechanisms of the body. Various experimental data tend to support the involvement of a *cutaneovisceral* reflex.[10-13]

Proof for the existence of such a reflex has strong scientific support. In a series of experiments, Kuntz and Hazelwood stimulated the skin on the back of rabbits and rats and noted changes in various parts of the gastrointestinal tract that were related to the dermatomal segment stimulated.[14,15,16] In Germany, Wernoe stimulated a small segment of the skin of fish and amphibians with silver nitrate and, after a delay of several months, demonstrated vasoconstriction of the part of the intestine dermatomally related.[17] After these experiments, he deduced that vasodilation was mediated by a spinal reflex and that vasoconstriction was mediated by a postganglionic sympathetic reflex. Travell and Rinzler found that complete and prolonged relief resulted when trigger points on the front of the chests of patients with angina pectoris or acute myocardial infarction were infiltrated with procaine or cooled with ethyl chloride.[18] Thus, the cutaneovisceral reflex is of prime importance in acupuncture. It is strongly believed that, by its mediation, an acupuncture needle placed in the correct part of the skin is able to influence the related organ or diseased part of the body.

New hypotheses are being brought forth rapidly. For example, it has been established for years that the ear is a hologram of the body as a whole, and this is the basis of auriculotherapy. However, Dale has recently proposed an elaborate hypothesis that most any part of the body is a hologram of the body as a whole.[19]

THE VISCEROCUTANEOUS REFLEX

Next, an explanation of how a visceral problem can relate to areas of the skin should be given. One method is by postulating the *viscerocutaneous reflex.* The importance of such a reflex rests in two primary areas: (1) diagnosis and (2) lowering the threshold of stimulation required in treatment with acupuncture.[20]

Various researchers have attempted to show that visceral problems may refer to the skin and give rise to trigger points, acupuncture points, and/or subluxations.[21,22,23] Diagnostically, certain superficial areas have long been known to relate to an underlying visceral condition such as pain at McBurney's point in appendicitis, in the left arm in angina pectoris, and of the right shoulder in gallbladder disease. It is often noted clinically that a disease in an internal organ will produce pain, tenderness, hyperesthesia, or hypesthesia, etc, in some area of skin. The viscerocutaneous reflex is thought to be mediated by unknown pathways of the sympathetic chain.[24]

The *Head-McKenzie Sensory Zone,* as described by Judovich and Bates, shows how visceral pain can radiate to certain parts of the skin. A familiar example is cardiac ischemia with radiating pain to the left arm.[25,26] In this context, Wernoe stimulated the rectum of a decapitated plaice electrically and found that the skin became pale. He also stimulated areas of the gastrointestinal tract of the eel and cod and noted that in each case the skin became lighter over an area of several dermatomal segments.[27] It can therefore be readily appreciated that a visceral problem can exhibit in a specific dermatomal segment via a viscerocutaneous reflex and that the stimulation of the skin can have a distinct effect on a related visceral area via a cutaneovisceral reflex.

SEGMENTAL AND INTERSEGMENTAL EFFECTS

Most of the reflexes used to explain the effects of acupuncture are segmental and follow specified dermatomal patterns.[28,29,30] Others, however, are intersegmental. For instance, stimulation of acupuncture points of the foot have been shown to affect organs over 10 dermatomes away.[31,32] A possible explanation of this phenomenon is via the long reflex of Sherrington.[33,34] In contrast, those reflexes that fit into the dermatomes are segmental reflexes, often referred to as Sherrington's short reflexes. The scratch reflex of a dog is a good example of an intersegmental cutaneomotor reflex.

NEAR AND DISTANT EFFECTS

One of the most perplexing problems is that some of the effects of acupuncture cannot be explained neurologically by either segmental or intersegmental mechanisms. For example, the effects of stimulating the acupuncture points of the head cannot be readily explained. However, some research has shown that a distinct reflex may probably exist between the nose and the heart or between the turbinates and the sexual organs.[35,36] Some scientific explanation for this is therefore likely.

The scientific proof for these reflexes is important, but it does not fully or even adequately explain exactly what happens according to the empirical results obtained. The Chinese for many years have attempted an explanation in the philosophical terms of Taoism with reference to Yin/Yang (law of opposites) and to the circulation of biologic energy (life force, Chi).

THE GATE CONTROL THEORY AND ITS CLINICAL SIGNIFICANCE

The next consideration is the more recent *Gate Theory,* as described in Chapter 2. Although this theory, originally set forth by Melzack and Wall, has been amended to some extent, it is basically the same as originally proposed, and it would be well to summarize it here.[37,38,39]

The gate theory holds that the large myelinated nerve fibers of the skin have an inhibitory effect, when stimulated, on the small pain-evoking fibers that enter the same segment of the cord.[40] The large, rapid-conducting, alpha and beta fibers of the skin conduct impulses via the dorsal columns to the brainstem and from here to the cerebral cortex. Small diameter, slow-conducting C fibers convey protopathic or pathologic and traumatic pain signals of the small fibers that arise from the deeper tissues of the body. If this were not so, the body would be in a constant state of pain. The stimuli from the dermis specifically produce inhibition in the cells of the substantia gelatinosa of Rolando, which is found in the dorsal horn of the spinal cord. It is believed that the dermal stimulus depolarizes the cells here, which renders them incapable of receiving and transmitting pain signals. Thus, painful stimuli are blocked (eg, the "gate" is closed), according to Melzack and Wall. If, however, the small fiber system is excessively stimulated by some disease process, the small fiber system then gains dominance and the patient perceives pain. It is then said that the pain gate has been opened by the increased stimulation from the small fibers of the deep somatic and visceral tissues.

This theory has many practical applications in clinical practice. For example, let us suppose that the "gates" are open and the patient is in severe pain. What can be done to relieve this suffering? Studies have shown that the inhibitory effects are enhanced when the large diameter fibers of the skin are sufficiently stimulated and the pain gate in the dorsal horn may be closed. In addition, these fast-conducting fibers may also arouse inhibitory responses in the brainstem that produce a downward projection of impulses to various levels of the spinal cord that further inhibit the transmission of pain signals that would normally progress to the brain.[41] It is by way of this system of inhibitory projections that the full value (ie, relief from pain) can be realized.

Surgical research on patients with intractable pain has shown that the implantation of a dorsal column stimulator (ie, TENS) can often completely block the transmission of painful or protopathic impulses.[42,43]

SCIENTIFIC EVIDENCE

Meridian therapy with needles, moxa, electrical stimulation, or by means of other modalities most likely work by such a mechanism; viz, by blocking pain signals in or to the brain by projecting inhibitory impulses to the thalamus and/or cerebral cortex and ultimately to the cord, and finally, by blocking noxious stimuli through the pathophysiologic reflex and thus producing muscular relaxation. Therefore, it should be noted that acupuncture, like adjustive procedures, is veiled in empirical evidence. Obviously, then, current scientific proof for acupuncture explains only in part much of what happens with articular manipulation.

Although the Melzack-Wall theory explains how pain pathways can be blocked, it does not adequately explain any possible localized tissue changes that are known to occur. By extension of this theory, however, local tissue changes may be postulated on the basis of localized vascular changes; ie, improvement in the local microcirculation.[44]

Recent studies, several without a credible basis, have been advocated. In France, ECG readings on heart patients showed improvement after acupuncture treatments.[45] In Russia, a sensitive stethoscope supposedly noted different sounds over acupoints. The Russians also noted a difference in the skin temperature over acupuncture points.

Much research still needs to be performed. It appears to be that there are demonstrable entities called acupuncture points, but scientific verification for chartable meridians connecting these points is still wanting at this writing. However, according to a 1985 paper from Russia referring to research being conducted at the Department of Neurology of the Kiev Institute for Physicians, Macheret and his associates have shown the existence of complex functional relationships between various parts of the human body and the internal organs. Their findings appear to support the existence of "channels" that are identical to those that the Orientals call *meridians*. "The 'body channels' in their peripheral link are connected with somatic and vegetative conductors running both independently in the form of nerve trunks, and like plexuses that get around the vessels and the muscles and reach the 'root' spinal cells and truncus sympaticus nodes from which the corresponding segmental associations pass to the internal organs." According to these researchers, the channels in their central link constitute the conductive pathways of the spinal cord and the brain.[46]

EMPIRICAL EVIDENCE

The volume of recently acquired empirical evidence cannot be denied. To mention just a few for example, Fields has shown that acupuncture, through the stimulation of endorphins, is an effective modality in the treatment of pain, behavior modification, relief of the symptoms of drug withdrawal, and stimulating the autoimmune system.[47] After treating just one point for acute dysmenorrhea in 10 patients, Slagoski found complete effectiveness in the resolution of the pain syndrome.[48] Tseung and Vazharov describe case after case of musculoskeletal disorders, anxiety and depression, growth problems, primary infertility, impotence, induction of labor, episcleritis, chronic asthmatic bronchitis, and canker sores (aphthous stomatitis) that responded to acupuncture after failing to respond under Western medical treatment.[49,50]

Kitzinger, a medical doctor, believes that even if acupuncture may achieve good, even spectacular, results by itself, he recommends combining it with neural therapy (electrical), manipulative therapy (chiropractic), and other standard physiotherapeutic modalities when vertebrogenic disorders are treated. He states that "Combining acupuncture with manipulative therapy for a blockage is not only feasible, but also in some cases, the only correct procedure to achieve a therapeutic breakthrough."[51] Shafshak compared the effectiveness of electroacupuncture to that of standard physiotherapy in the treatment of tension myositis: 93.3% responded completely to the electroacupuncture and 90.9% recovered completely in response to the physiotherapy.[52]

While acupuncture per se has not been as effective in treating disorders of purely a psyche nature as it has in relieving physiologic disturbances, Odell reports that when it is used in conjunction with hypnosis and visualization techniques, it has shown to be a consistent and invaluable tool in a behavioral reprogramming technique.[53] See Figure 3.1.

MERIDIAN TRIGGER POINTS AND THEIR PALPATION

Standard Methods of Stimulation

Acupuncture points are commonly stimulated by several methods:

1. Using 30-, 32-, or 34-gauge, ½- to 1½-inch stainless steel needles that are inserted into carefully selected sites for durations ranging from a few seconds up to 20 minutes or sometimes more.
2. Using electrical stimulation with any modality designed for this purpose. An economical unit was shown in Figure 2.9.
3. Using a specially designed blunt instrument (teishin).
4. Using finger or thumb pressure.
5. Using a helium neon or infrared laser (controversial).

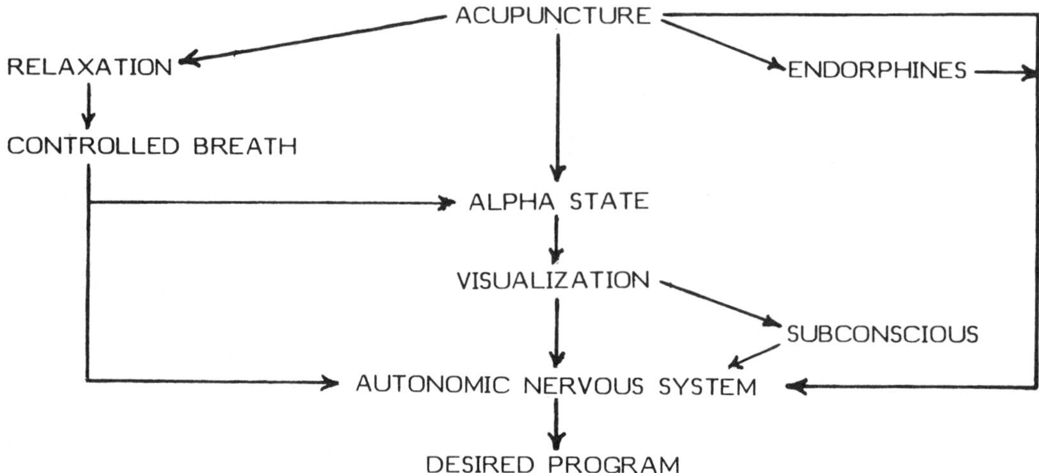

Figure 3.1. Acupuncture-related reprogramming technique of Odell.

When acupuncture sites are stimulated by means of electrical current, several factors should be kept in mind: (1) the exact location of the site must be stimulated; (2) a small diameter electrode must be used; (3) the correct frequency must be selected; and (4) the correct duration must be determined. It should be noted that many of these factors are also important when other methods are used.

Site Location

Acupuncture points are usually tender to the touch and located in palpable depressions under the skin. Although most pertinent sites are usually tender, there are many situations where a lack of normal tenderness at a site may also be diagnostic.

As previously described, recent evidence suggests that acupuncture works by means of an extravascular transport mechanism. This means that the points will be located at a certain depth below the skin surface. Some research studies indicate that stimulation is to the nervi vasorum (autonomic fibers congruent with the blood vessels), and this further lends credence to the location of specific depths.

Locating Points

Of prime importance in meridian-trigger point therapy is the proper palpation and localization of the acupuncture point. But first, arriving at a specific definition of a meridian point should be attempted.

Felix Mann states that in all diseases, physical or mental, tender areas are present at certain points on the surface of the body—points that disappear when the illness is cured. He calls these points acupuncture points. In the Chinese literature, we find descriptions of over a thousand of these points. The more common 365 points are located on certain fixed lines or pathways called meridians. It is our opinion that an acupuncture point is, in many instances, identical to the trigger point described by Travell or the *paraviose* described by Matsumoto and Hiyodo in their writings.

In locating pertinent acupuncture points and meridian dysfunction, one technique involves systemic palpation (ie, of the alarm points) of the body at predetermined sites. These points will be described later in this chapter.

BACKGROUND

The palpating hands of the examiner normally contain sensitive nerve endings that are quite perceptive to changes in tissue tone, temperature, texture, surface humidity, etc. The fingertips are particularly well supplied with touch and pressure receptors, while the dorsal surface of the hand is especially endowed with heat receptors. For these reasons, both the fingertips and the back of the hand should be utilized during the evaluation procedure.

Acupoints will often be found that are spontaneously tender. For instance, a patient with appendicitis will point to McBurney's point as being exquisitely painful. Individuals with headaches often relate a spontaneously tender area on the nuchal line of the occiput. In other cases, areas will be painful only when pressure is applied. Many of the points above the ankles and in the hand and wrist belong to this category. A third type of acupoint is not tender even when moderate pressure is applied. Many acupuncture points are of this type.

PREPARATION

In searching for the acupuncture point, the patient must first be positioned in a comfortable position. The patient should be disrobed in such a fashion that the points are readily accessible to palpation, and care must be taken in all cases to preserve the modesty of the patient. As during a regular physical examination, it is generally best to have the patient undress and then robed in a gown that ties in the back. The waist band of the patient should be loosened for comfort and to afford free access to points of the pelvic area.

Most examiners find it convenient to begin the examination with the patient seated on a low stool, and then transfer the patient to a comfortable cushioned table for examination in the prone and supine positions. Prior to searching for acupuncture points, the doctor should remove any jewelry that might scratch or irritate a patient. Personal hygiene, as always, is of utmost importance. The examiner's hands should be thoroughly washed before and after each examination.

TYPES AND CHARACTERISTICS OF ACUPUNCTURE POINTS

Several types of acupuncture points or lesions might be discovered:

1. *Fibrositic nodules.* Most commonly, the fibrositic nodule will be the point located. This area feels like a small node or mass of tissue several millimeters in diameter. It will be tender to pressure and often spontaneously painful. It is similar to the fibrositic rheumatoid nodules often located at the back of the neck, in the shoulders, or in the lumbar area. See Figure 3.2.

2. *Indurated areas.* In many instances, a hard (indurated) area will be found. Instead of a nodule, the palpator might feel a localized area of tense muscle fibers within a muscle. See Figure 3.3.

3. *Atrophic areas.* In other cases, the acupuncture point might be characterized as a localized swollen and discolored area or an atrophied area of tissue. See Figure 3.4.

ELECTRICAL ANALYSIS

The examiner might be unable to locate acupuncture points by palpation. In these cases, it may be of value to make use of one of the many electric devices available for their detection. These instruments measure skin resistance to an electric current, showing areas where the resistance is altered (+/−). Once a point is localized, whether manually or with an electric device, it should be carefully marked with a skin pencil or felt-tipped pen and then charted in the patient's records so that a comparison can be made from one visit to another.

In Japan, Nakatani mapped out areas of altered skin resistance into pathways correlating to the meridian pathways. He treats the

Figure 3.2. Palpation of a fibrositic nodule (acupuncture point).

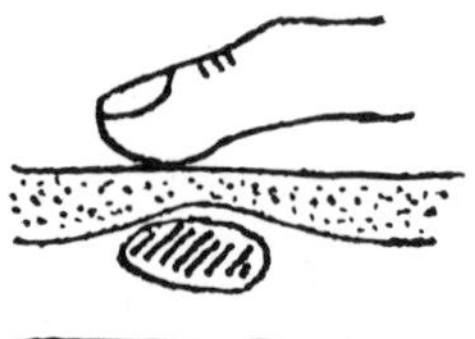

Figure 3.3. An indurated nodule.

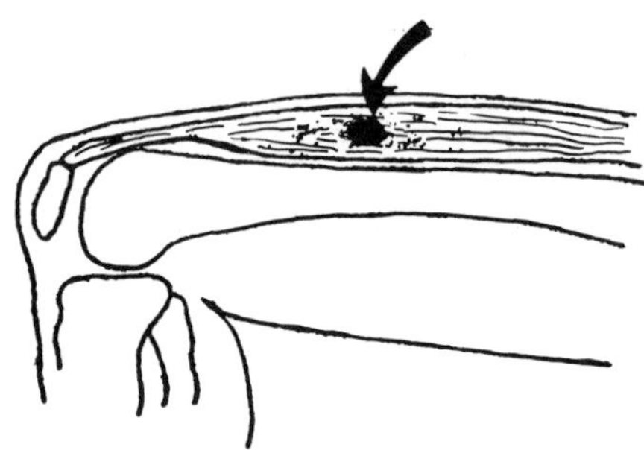

Figure 3.4. Palpation of a localized area of atrophy.

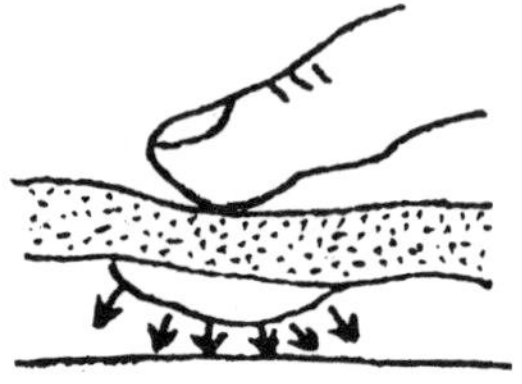

most altered points. This system is termed *Ryodoraku.*[54]

The fact that an acupuncture point exhibits altered electrical resistance allows an examiner to determine specific sites by using any instrument that measures (objectively with an ohmmeter or subjectively by sound) skin resistance at a localized point. It is presently thought that sites that are reactive (ie, involved in a complaint), especially when we are dealing with a musculoskeletal complaint, are more conductive than surrounding tissue. These points are usually more tender and conduct current more readily (less resistance to an electric current). Chinese physicians refer to these sites as *ah shi* (ouch) points; American physicians usually refer to them as trigger points.

If the correct site is chosen for stimulation, the most common reaction will be hyperemia (histamine reaction) around the point stimulated. Also noted, especially when needles are used, will be a sensation of tingling or numbness radiating or referred distally from the site stimulated. This sensation is called *Taechi.* A lack of hyperemia or Taechi appears to correlate with poor results, thus indicating that the proper site was not treated.

In 1984, studies conducted by Y. M. Sin showed that acupuncture stimulation not only gave good symptomatic relief in inflammatory disease but also suppressed the underlying progress of the disease.[55] See Figure 3.5.

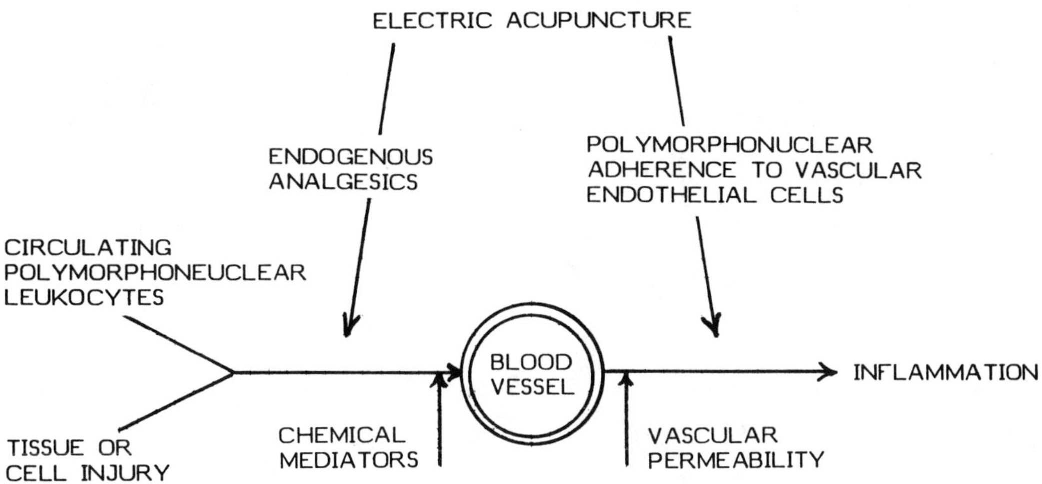

Figure 3.5. Effect of electric acupuncture stimulation on inflammation, as depicted by Sin.

The Human Inch

Besides palpation and measuring electrical resistance, charted acupuncture points can be located by using a topographical system of anatomical measurement. The unit of measure is called the *human inch* or a *cun,* and the system of measurement utilizes the patient's own anatomical proportions to establish the parameters to be used in (1) locating points and (2) determining the depth of needle insertion.

The human inch for a particular patient can be determined by measuring the distance between the patient's two joint creases of the volar surface of the middle phalanx of the middle finger when it is flexed. It can also be determined by measuring the width of the patient's thumb. See Figure 3.6. Either hand can be used unless one thumb has been deformed by trauma or disease.

Once the human inch is known, various portions of the patient's body may be measured lengthwise or transversely and that measurement may be divided into a certain number of human inches. Because a human inch is a proportional measurement for a specific individual, the number of cuns on a body part (eg, a forearm or leg) is approximately the same whether the patient is young or old, tall or short, or lean or obese.[56] The only exception to this is where obvious growth, surgical, or pathologic asymmetries are present (eg, disproportionate limb-trunk dwarfism). See Figure 3.7.

MAJOR POINTS: LOCATIONS, PRIMARY INDICATIONS, AND PRECAUTIONS

As the result of millions of observations of patient responses over several centuries, Oriental physicians have charted over 300 major points on the body and have attributed certain related functions to these locations. As a general rule, however, it is thought that any localized point in an area of musculoskeletal pain can be stimulated to inhibit pain in that location.

In 1984, Peter Eckman, M.D., Ph.D., developed a schematic model of the general effects of acupuncture.[57] See Figure 3.8.

In the following sections, we will attempt to describe the most common sites of stimulation and the indications for treatment as

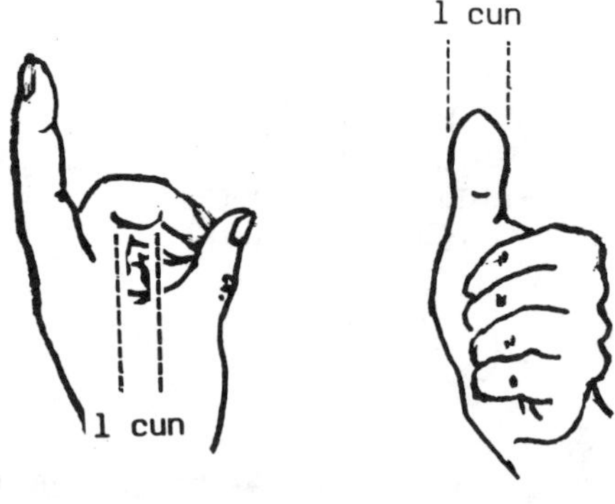

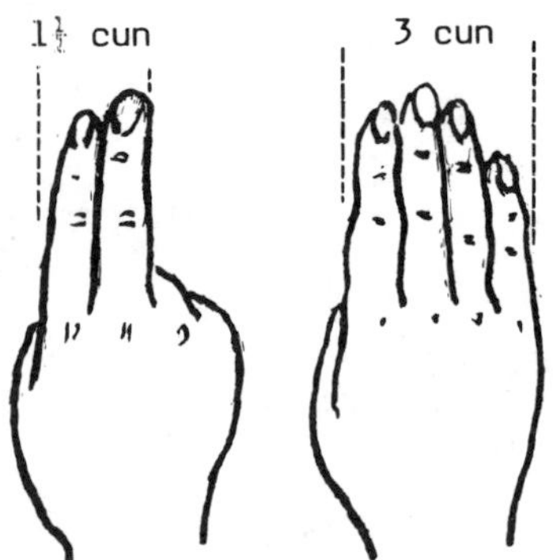

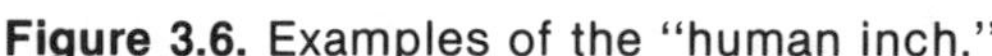

Figure 3.6. Examples of the "human inch."

cited by various authorities. We must state unequivocally, however, that little or no scientific verification has been done in the West to substantiate these projected effects. Thus, the reader is cautioned to utilize every possible diagnostic tool available necessary to evaluate the patient's complaints and to use this chapter as a reference to those sites used by Oriental physicians. The complete validity of the effects described must await further research substantiation.

Points on the Lung Meridian

The major points on the lung (LU) meridian are LU-1 and LU-7.

LU-1

Location. The site of this point (zhongfu) is found on the anterior lateral aspect of the chest. Using your finger, palpate below the clavicle and seek a tender spot in the space between the first and second rib, approximately 6 cun lateral to the anterior midline of the chest. See Figure 3.9.

Indications. This point is the *alarm point* for the lung meridian, thus it may be tender in any condition related to the lung meridian. This site is primarily used for chronic respiratory complaints as it is the major point that influences the lungs. Stimulation may also be made at this site for shoulder disorders, especially those exhibiting painful adduction.

LU-7

Location. This point (lieque) may be found just lateral to the radial artery at a spot 1.5 cun from the transverse crease on the volar aspect of the wrist. To find this site on yourself, interlock the webs of your hands, and, without bending the wrist of the hand you are grasping, the index finger of the upper hand will extend to a site just proximal to the styloid process of the radius. Under the tip of the index finger, a slight depression marks the site of LU-7. See Figure 3.9.

Indications. This is one of the seven *master points* of the body. Its primary indication is in the reduction of localized edema of a musculoskeletal origin.

Points on the Large Intestine Meridian

The major points on the large intestine (LI) meridian are LI-4, LI-11, and LI-20.

LI-4

Location. When the thumb and index finger are brought together, such as when

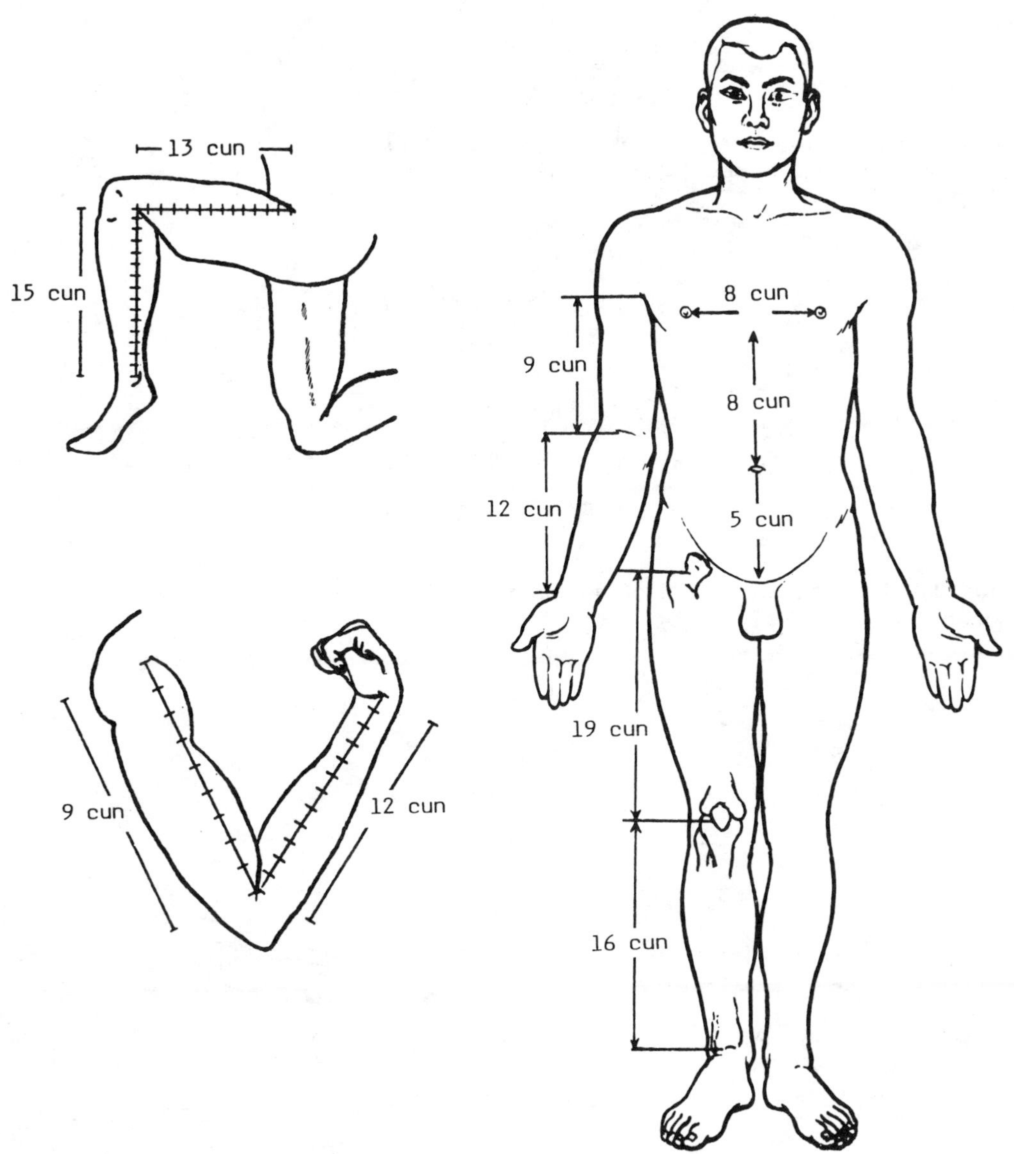

Figure 3.7. Examples of various proportional units in "human inches."

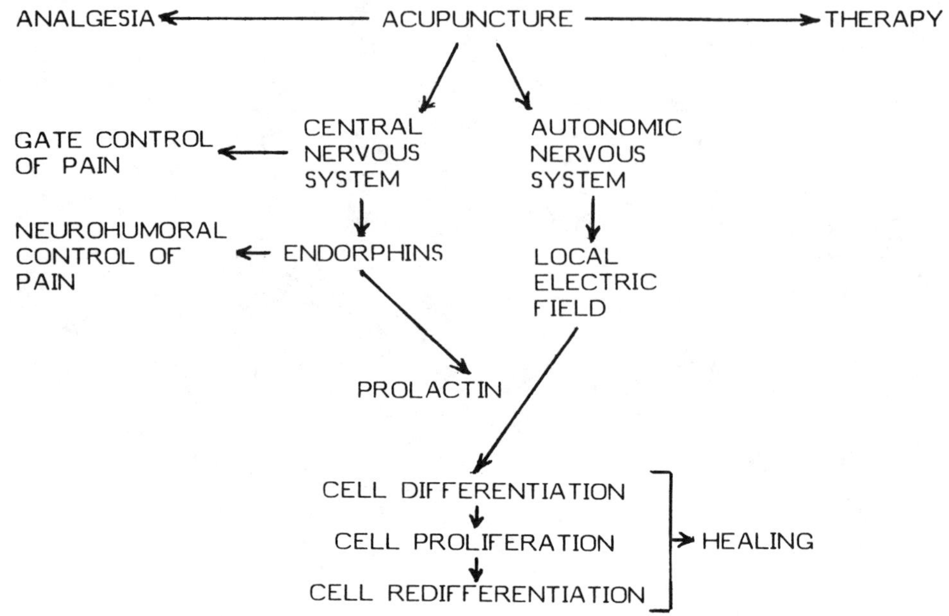

Figure 3.8. A schematic model of the primary effects of acupuncture, as depicted by Eckman.

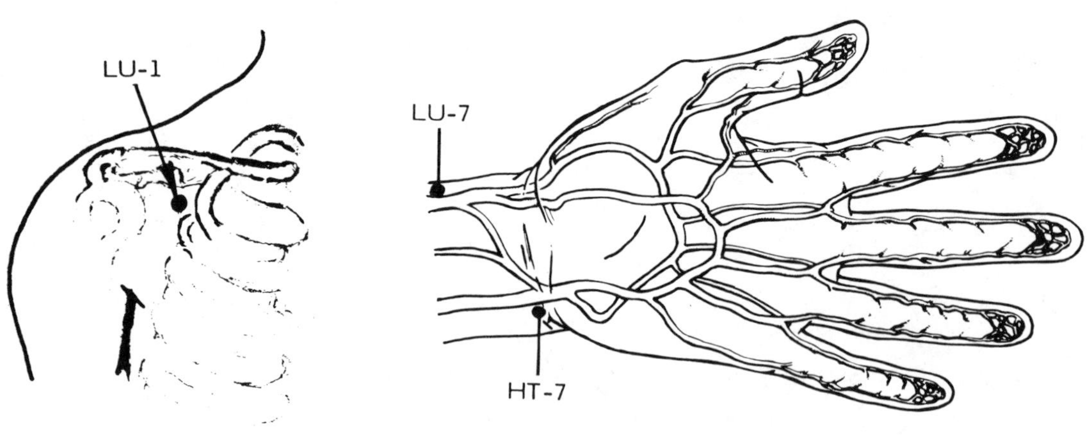

Figure 3.9. The major points on the lung meridian are LU-1 and LU-7. HT-7 is shown in the right diagram only for its relative position.

making a fist, this point is located at the highest spot on the domed muscle bulge between the thumb and index finger. More specifically, the point is located half way between the proximal and distal aspects of the 2nd metacarpal, just lateral to its radial side. See Figure 3.10.

Indications. This point (hoku or hegu) is another *master point.* Many authorities feel it is the most powerful acupoint of the upper body. It has been studied most extensively and is stimulated more often than any other site of the body. Extensive research has established a connection between stimulation of this site and alleviation of pain in the upper extremity and anterior neck or head. Stimulation of this site with electrodes attached to inserted needles is used to bring about anesthesia in the lower jaw or scalp prior to dental work or during certain surgical procedures. When it is used in combination with the most tender trigger point (Ahshi), pain in the upper extremity and anterior neck or head can be alleviated. We have also found that prolonged stimulation at this site (eg, over 15 minutes with needles) will trigger evacuation of the bowels and promote drainage of body fluids.

When used in combination with other sites, LI-4 may also influence other conditions. For example:

- LI-4 + LI-11 — dermatologic complaints
- LI-4 + ST-36 — gastrointestinal complaints
- LI-4 + SP-6 — gynecologic complaints.

Precautions. As this is a highly sensitive point, adverse reactions have been recorded with this site, the most frequent of which is syncope. Thus, if the patient complains of weakness, faintness, or nausea during therapy, the treatment should be discontinued. This site is also contraindicated during pregnancy, except to promote labor or medical abortion.

LI-11

Location. The location of this point (quchi) is located just distal to the lateral end of the transverse crease of the elbow joint when the arm is flexed on the forearm. See Figure 3.10. This point is frequently tender.

Indications. This point is treated for pains associated with lateral epicondylitis (eg, "ten-

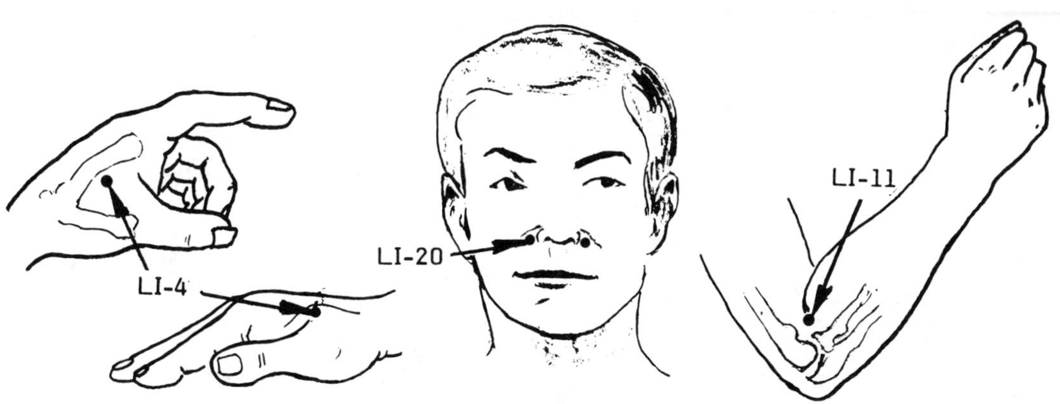

Figure 3.10. Major points on the large intestine meridian.

nis elbow'' syndrome) and is a special point used in the treatment of acute torticollis. Some studies have also indicated that, when stimulated bilaterally, it may lower blood pressure and affect the motor aspects of the nervous system. Used in conjunction with LI-4, it may be useful in the management of dermatologic and allergic nasorespiratory complaints.

LI-20

Location. This point (yingxiang) is found at the nasolabial groove on the side of the nasal ala. See Figure 3.10.

Indications. Stimulation of this site promotes drainage of the nasal sinuses and may be effective in combination with other focal sites in the treatment of facial paralysis.

Points on the Stomach Meridian

The major points on the stomach (ST) meridian are ST-2, ST-25, and ST-36.

ST-2

Location. This point (sibai) is found just below the orbit of the eye at the site of the infraorbital foramen. See Figure 3.11.

Indications. Stimulation at this site promotes drainage of the maxillary sinuses and is another site that may be utilized in patients with facial paralysis.

Precaution. Great care must be taken to avoid bruising the sensitive tissues in this area. Injury may readily lead to subcutaneous hemorrhage (ie, a ''black eye'').

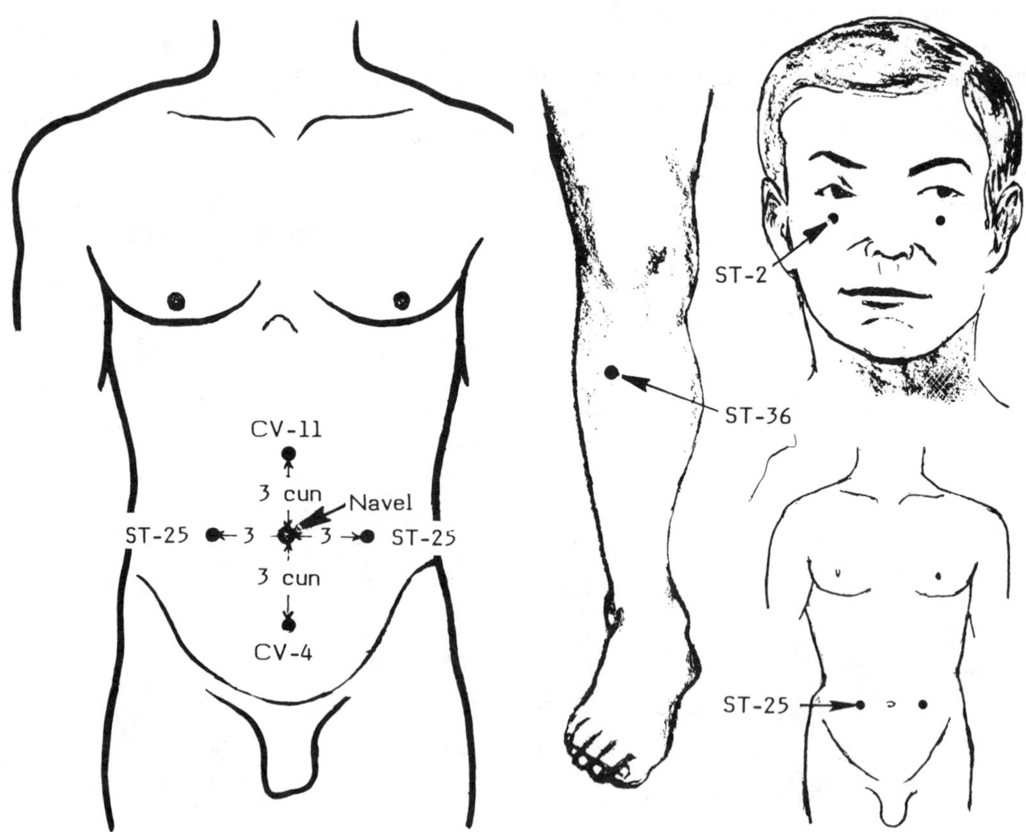

Figure 3.11. Major points on the stomach meridian.

ST-25

Location. The site of this point (tianshu) is located on a level with the umbilicus, 2—3 cun lateral to the midsagittal line, at the border of the rectus abdominis muscle. See Figure 3.11.

Indications. This site is often used in conjunction with CV-4 and CV-11 and appears most effective in treating gastrointestinal disorders, especially those of an acute nature. Note that this point is also the alarm point for the large intestine.

ST-36

Location. Have the seated patient flex a knee to a right angle and place the palm of the patient's ipsilateral hand over the patella. The tip of the index finger is slightly abducted. In this position, it should rest in a depression just below the heads of the proximal tibia and fibula. This depression is located about one finger's width lateral to the anterior crest of the tibia. See Figure 3.11.

Indications. This point (zusanli) is another of the seven *master points* of the body, and many authorities feel it is the most powerful acupoint of the lower body. It is thought to be the major body point for systemic tonification. Because of its location, it is also utilized in the treatment of conditions localized in the lateral aspect of the knee joint. Several studies have related this point to the cellular elements of the blood; thus, it has been indicated by some to be effective in the treatment of anemia and to increase the white cell count in patients with infections. Stimulation of this point is often used in conjunction with LI-4 (thought to be the most powerful acupoint of the upper body) in the treatment of chronic gastrointestinal complaints.

Points on the Spleen Meridian

The major points on the spleen (SP) meridian are SP-6 and SP-9.

SP-6

Location. This point (sanyinjiao) is found on the medial aspect of the ankle on the lower calf. It can be located by placing the lateral aspect of an ankle on the opposite flexed knee (as in the familiar male seated position) and placing the little finger of your hand (flexed knee side) on the medial malleolus of the exposed ankle so that the thumb points toward your flexed and rotated knee. The point is located 3 cun up the medial aspect of the calf, proximal to the medial malleolus. The point is located just posterior to the border of the tibia. See Figure 3.12.

Indications. This point is referred to as the *crossroads of the three Yin meridians* because the spleen, liver, and kidney meridians transverse each other at this site. Due to this fact, the point has multiple indications. As one of the seven master points, it is often used in the treatment of patients with gynecologic disorders, especially irregular or painful menstrual complaints and male sexual dysfunctions. It is also referred to as the *master of the circulatory system* as it affects various vascular conditions such as patients with cold extremities or those that bruise easily.

SP-9

Location. This point (yinlingquan) is located on the medial aspect of the knee joint, just below the lower border of the medial condyle of the proximal tibia. See Figure 3.12.

Indications. This point is primarily stimulated in the treatment of patients with osteoarthritis of the knee or sprains of the medial collateral ligaments.

Points on the Heart Meridian

There is one major point on the heart (HT) meridian, HT-7.

Location. This acupoint (shenmen) is located on the ulnar surface of the anterior wrist, just proximal to the pisiform bone. Exact lo-

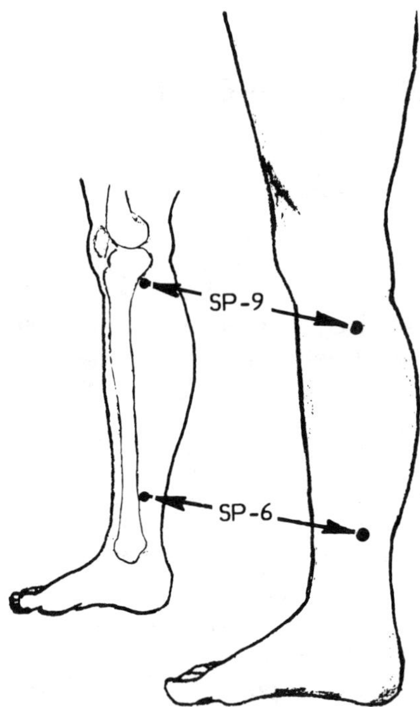

Figure 3.12. Major points on the spleen meridian.

calization places this point in a depression located just to the radial side of the flexor carpi ulnaris tendon, just medial to the ulnar artery. See Figure 3.13.

Indications. This specific point is stimulated in an attempt to relieve patients with symptoms of nervousness, irritability, anxiety, depression, hypertension, insomnia, and abnormal forgetfulness.

Points on the Small Intestine Meridian

The major points on the small intestine (SI) meridian are SI-3, SI-9, and SI-19.

SI-3

Location. To locate this point, make a tight fist and note the small triangular bulge on medial aspect of the supinated hand. The point is located at the end of the transverse crease just proximal to the head of the 5th metacarpal-phalangeal joint. See Figure 3.14.

Indications. This point (houxi) is treated when patients have pain in the contralateral lower back region and in patients suffering with various types of arthritis.

SI-9

Location. To locate the exact position of this point, have the patient hold their relaxed arm at the side. In this position, the point is located 1 cun above the top of the posterior axillary fold. See Figure 3.14.

Indications. This point (jianzhen) is stimulated whenever a patient complains of pain when flexing their arm behind their back (extension plus internal rotation) or when a patient exhibits signs of degenerative joint disease of the shoulder joint.

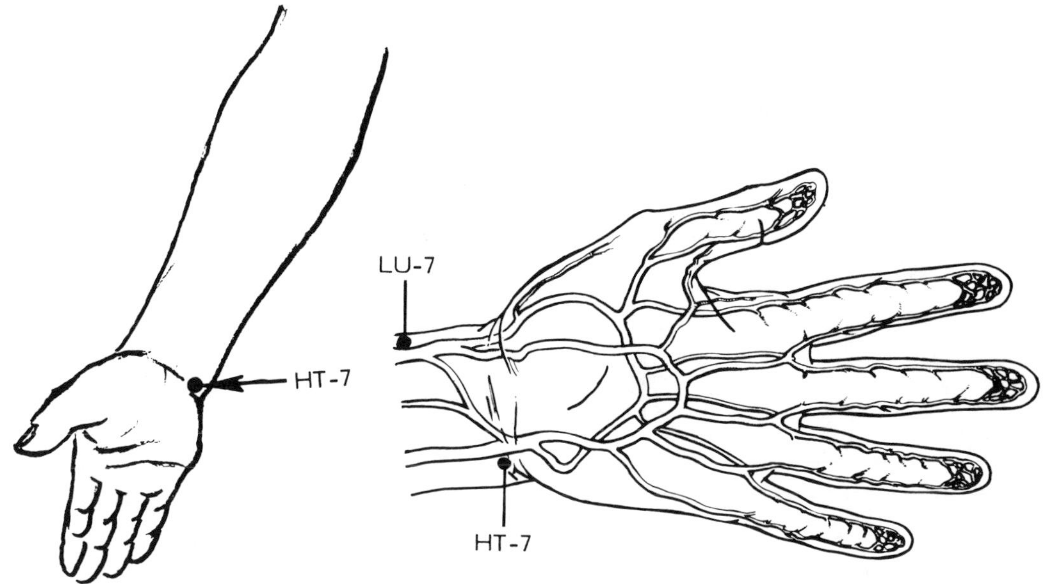

Figure 3.13. The major point on the heart meridian is HT-7. LU-7 is shown in the right diagram only for its relative position.

SI-19

Location. This point (tinggong) can be found by placing an index finger just anterior to the tragus of the ear and palpating between the tragus and the temporomandibular joint when the patient opens his or her mouth. See Figure 3.14.

Indications. This site is stimulated in various disorders of the ear such as earache, hearing loss, or tinnitus.

Precautions. Care must be taken when using a needling procedure to avoid major nerve and vascular structures in this area.

Points on the Urinary Bladder Meridian

The major points on the bladder (BL) meridian are BL-10, BL-23—25, BL-31, BL-51, BL-54, BL-57, and BL-60.

A large portion of the bladder meridian is made up of points referred to as association or associated points. These association points, which will be described later in this chapter, are located along the medial most aspect of this meridian (see Fig. 3.25). They appear to be related to various specific viscera in a manner similar to that of Meric Analysis where specific spinal segments are related to specific organs.

BL-10

Location. This point (tianzhu) is located two finger widths lateral to the midpoint between the spinous processes of C1 and C2, just lateral to the border of the trapezius muscle. See Figure 3.15.

Indications. This site is thought of as the atlas of acupuncture. Stimulation here is believed to have profound effects on the autonomic nervous system. Its stimulation may also relieve patients with thoracic outlet syndromes.

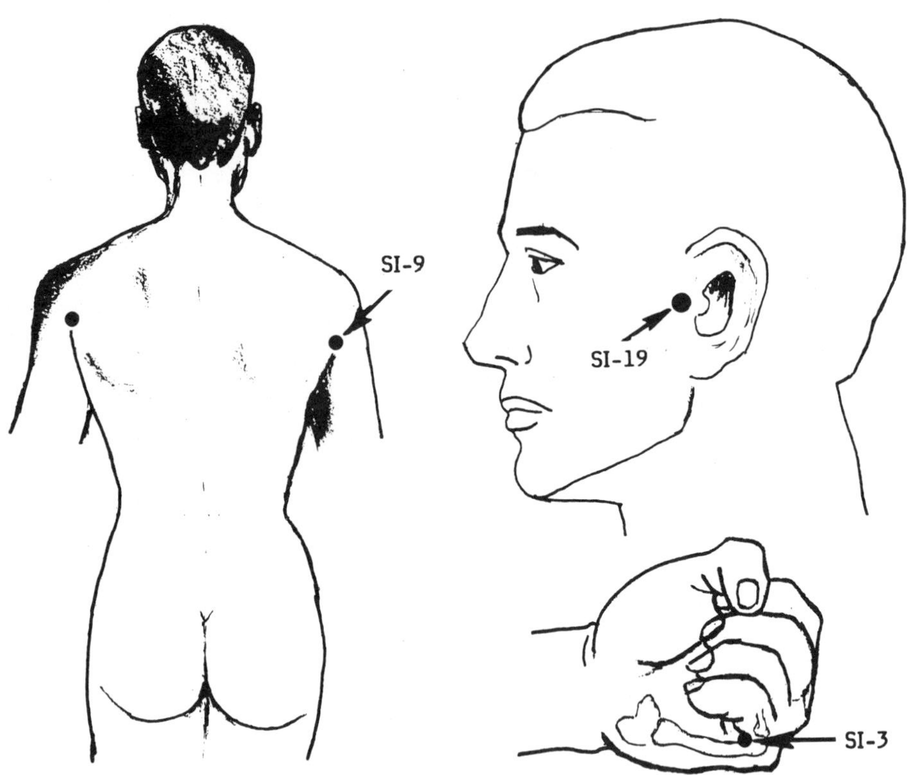

Figure 3.14. Major points on the small intestine meridian.

BL-23, BL-24, and BL-25

Location. These three points (shenshu, qihaishu, and dachangshu) are found two finger widths lateral to the midpoints of spinous processes of L2—L3, L3—L4, and L4—L5, respectively. See Figure 3.25.

Indications. Stimulation of these points is made in patients with low back pain, usually bilaterally, and sometimes combined with stimulation of GB-30 (see Fig. 3.15) and/or other points. The choice of specific stimulation in this area depends on the determined level of spinal involvement.

BL-31

Location. The site of this point (shangliao) is found in the depression of the first sacral foramen. See Figure 3.15.

Indications. This is an important point in the treatment of IVD syndromes, lumbar sprains and strains, and other afflictions of the lower back. Some reports of experiments with male animals have indicated that treatment of this point may elevate sperm count.

BL-51

Location. This point (yinmen) is found in the longitudinal midline of the posterior thigh, halfway between the gluteal and popliteal creases. See Figure 3.15.

Indications. This is an important point in the treatment of low back pain, especially when there is sciatic radiation to the thigh.

BL-54

Location. This posterior point (weizhong)

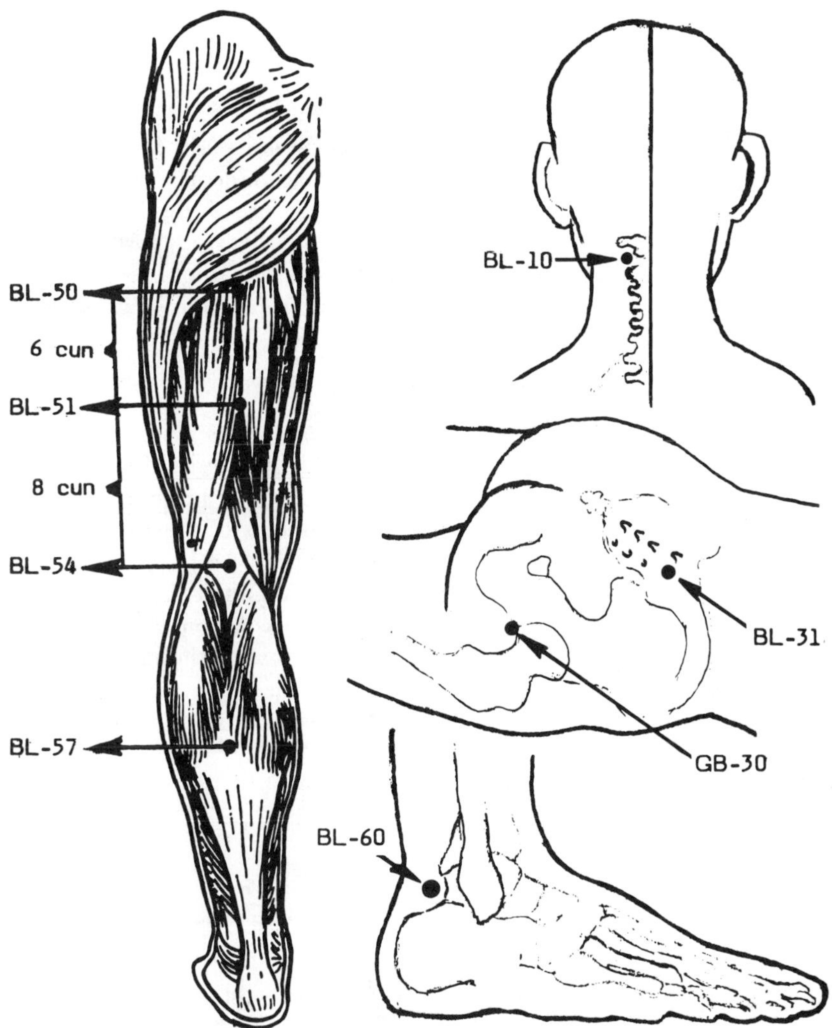

Figure 3.15. Some major points on the bladder meridian.

is located on the transverse crease of the posterior knee, just lateral to the center of the popliteal space. See Figure 3.15.

Indications. Stimulation of this point is made in patients with arthritis of the knee or sciatic pain that radiates to the knee.

Precautions. If needling is conducted, it is best to slightly flex the joint so that tension will be removed from the popliteal tissues. Care must be taken not to pierce one of the many vascular structures in this area.

BL-57

Location. This point (chengshan) is found halfway down the back of the calf, at the longitudinal midpoint between the knee and the ankle joint, where the split of the gastrocnemius muscle is located. See Figure 3.15.

Indications. Stimulation of this point is indicated in cases of sciatica that manifest pain radiating to the calf.

BL-60

Location. This point (kunlun) is found on the external side of the ankle, at a level of the midpoint of the lateral malleolus longitudinally and halfway between the Achilles tendon and the lateral malleolus transversely. See Figure 3.15.

Indications. This site has been found to be of value in patients with generalized body pain, foot problems, and sciatic-like pains that radiate from the lower back to the ankle.

Points on the Kidney Meridian

The major points of the kidney (KI) meridian are KI-1, KI-2, and KI-27.

KI-1

Location. This point (yongquan) is found on the plantar surface of the foot in a depression at the junction of the anterior and middle third of the sole, between the 2nd and 3rd metatarsophalangeal joints. See Figure 3.16.

Indications. Although one of the most tender acupuncture sites of the body, this point is one of the best sites to stimulate when a patient has problems related to the feet. It is also stimulated in patients with dry skin and complaints of impotency.

KI-2

Location. This point (rangu) is found anterior and inferior to the medial malleolus of the ankle. If an imaginary line is drawn from the midpoint of the foot (midpoint between the front and back), the point can be located in a depression at the anterior-inferior border of the navicular bone. See Figure 3.16.

Indications. Stimulation of this point is often made when patients show signs of excessively moist skin (ie, hyperhidrosis).

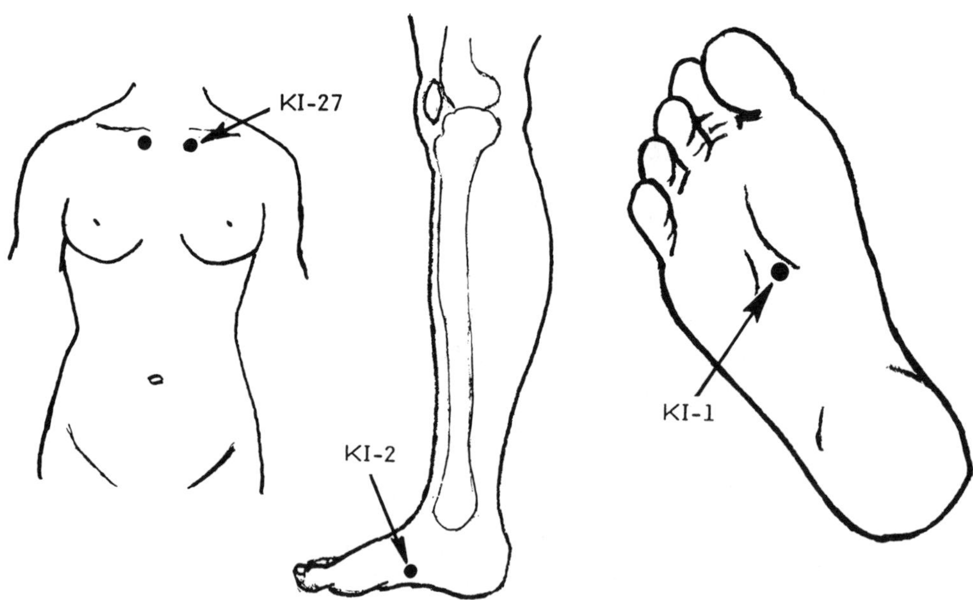

Figure 3.16. Major points on the kidney meridian.

KI-27

Location. The site of this point (shufu) is found in the depression between the 1st rib and the lower border of the clavicle, just lateral to the manubrium of the sternum. See Figure 3.16.

Indications. This point is often referred to as the "reset button" by kinesiologists. Manual stimulation of this site is thought to temporarily balance the meridians or to "reset" them prior to muscle testing or checking for overall energy balance in the meridians.

Points on the Heart Constrictor Meridian

There is only one major point of the heart constrictor (HC) meridian, HC-6. It should be noted that this meridian is also referred to just as frequently by many authorities as the pericardium (P) or circulation/sex (CS or CX) meridian.

Location. This point (neiguan) is found on the anterior surface of the forearm, directly in the midline, 2 cun from the largest transverse crease of the wrist. See Figure 3.17.

Indications. Stimulation of this point is indicated for patients presenting with thoracic pain (eg, rib pain, intercostal neuralgia, postherpetic neuralgia, thoracic strain/sprain, and painful disorders of the lungs). Some authorities have reported that stimulation of this site may stop singultus (hiccups), although we have yet to have our first success using this point for hiccups.

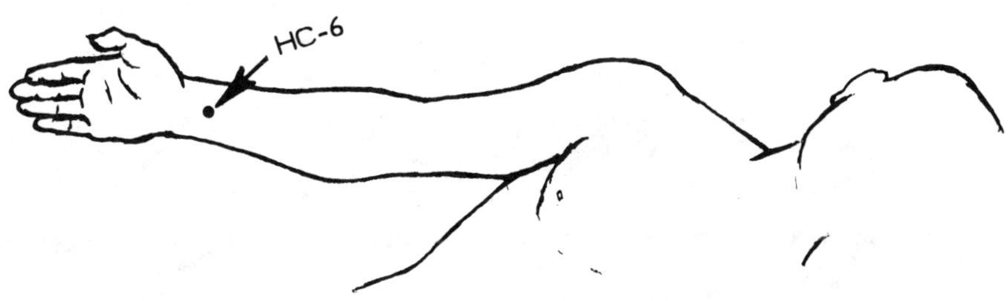

Figure 3.17. Major point on the heart constrictor meridian.

Points on the Triple Heater Meridian

The major points on the triple heater (TH) meridian are TH-5 and TH-17.

TH-5

Location. This point (waiguan) is positioned on the dorsum of the wrist, exactly in the center, at a point two cun proximal from the flexure crease of the wrist. It is located directly opposite to HC-6. See Figure 3.18.

Indications. This site is the major point of energy balance in the body. Stimulation of this point is thought to equalize the autonomic nervous system and balance unilateral problems in the body (eg, unilateral hearing loss, unilateral knee problems).

TH-17

Location. This point (yifeng) is found posterior to the earlobe in the depression located between the mastoid bone and the angle of the mandible. See Figure 3.18.

Indications. The indications for stimulating TH-17 are hearing loss, tinnitus, and earache.

Precautions. If needling is performed, insertion to a depth greater than 1½ cun is absolutely forbidden.

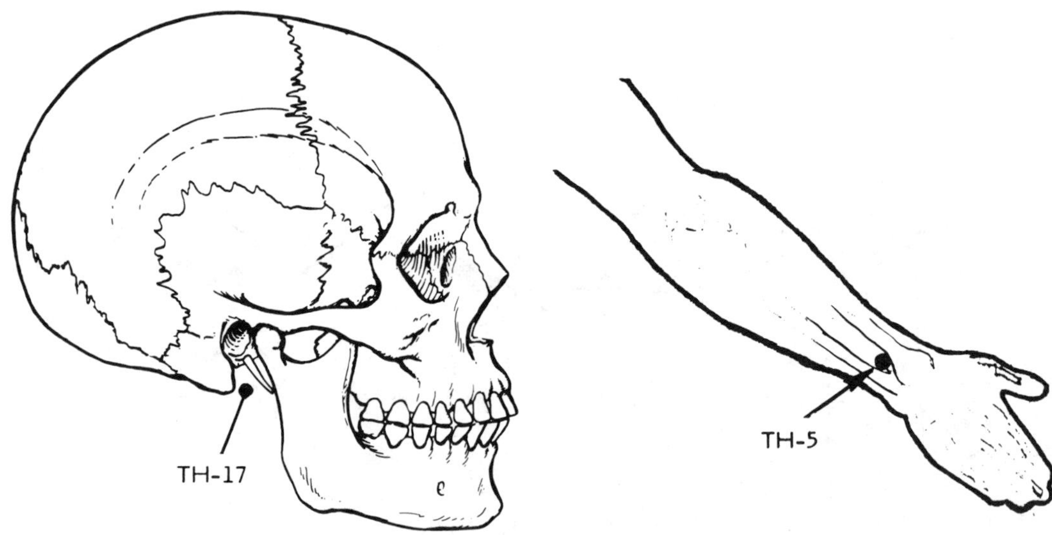

Figure 3.18. Major points on the triple heater meridian.

Points on the Gallbladder Meridian

The major points on the gallbladder (GB) meridian are GB-20, GB-21, and GB-34.

GB-20

Location. This point (fengchi) is found just inferior and medial to the mastoid process, in a depression (usually tender) that is located between the sternocleidomastoideus and the trapezius muscles. See Figure 3.19.

Indications. This site, one of the seven *master points,* influences the autonomic nervous system. It is also an excellent point to stimulate in patients with suboccipital headaches.

Precautions. When needling, the line of insertion is directed toward the opposite eye. Deep insertion of a needle greater than 1½ cun may trigger adverse effects; thus, such depth is forbidden.

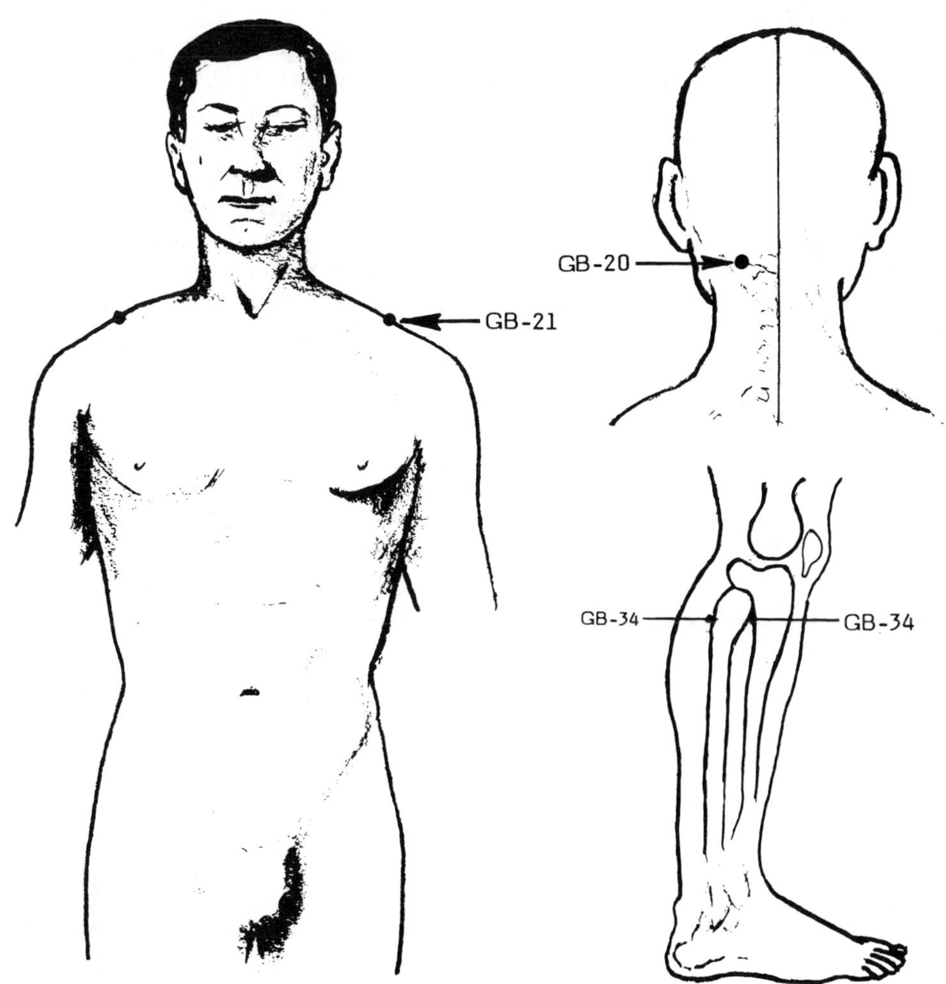

Figure 3.19. Major points on the gallbladder meridian. Note that some authorities place GB-34 anterior to the head of the fibula and others place it posterior.

GB-21

Location. The site of this point (jianjing) is located midway between the spine and the acromion of the shoulder. With the patient seated, hands folded in the lap, head forward, run your palpating finger from the tip of the acromion halfway up toward the spine, splitting the trapezius down the middle. The site will be found as a tender depression at the halfway point. See Figure 3.19.

Indications. This is probably the best point there is to stimulate patients with muscle spasm in the *upper* half of the body.

Precautions. Perpendicular needle insertions are discouraged. Insertion should be made at an angle directed toward the midline. Do not exceed a depth of 1 cun, as the apex of the lung might be punctured.

GB-34

Location. This point (yanglingquan) is found in a depression located anteroinferior or posteoinferior to the head of the fibula, depending on which authority is followed. Most likely, there are two sites: GB-34 anterior and GB-34 posterior that may be effective stimulation sites. Both sites are shown in Figure 3.19, bottom right.

Indications. These points are the best sites on the body used to influence patients with muscle spasm, especially in the *lower* half of the body. Either or both points may also be stimulated in patients with pain on the lateral aspect of the thigh and/or leg.

Points on the Liver Meridian

The major point on the liver (LV) meridian is LV-3.

Location. This point (taichong) is found on the dorsum of the foot between the 1st and 2nd metatarsals, approximately 2 cun from the margin of the web between the toes. See Figure 3.20.

Indications. This point is often stimulated in an attempt to detoxify the body and for the treatment of patients with neurologic complaints. Some evidence indicates that it is one of the best points on the body for treating patients with migraine.

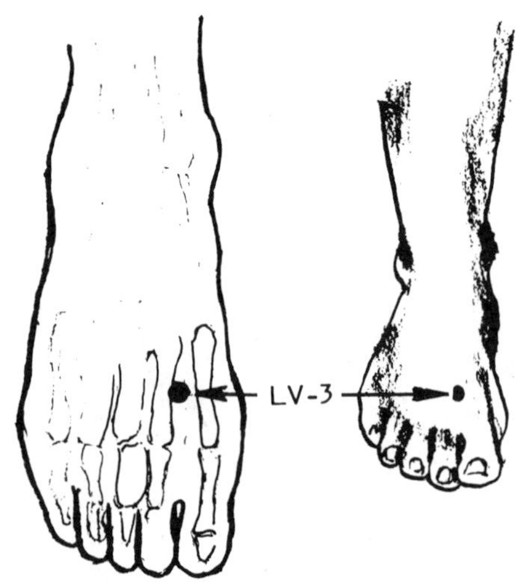

Figure 3.20. Major point on the liver meridian.

Points on the Conception Vessel Meridian

There are two unilateral meridians on the body: one on the anterior midline that bisects the chin, navel, and pubis (the conception vessel), and one on the posterior midline that cuts through the spinous processes (the governing vessel).

There are two major points on the conception vessel (CV), CV-4 and CV-8.

CV-4

Location. This point (guanyuan) is located in the anterior midline, 3 cun below the navel. See Figures 3.21 and 3.11.

Indications. Stimulation of this point is thought to affect patients with pelvic disorders (eg, menstrual pain, gastroenteritis, polyuria, etc). Treatment may also be given to this point to generally relax the patient.

CV-8

Location. This point (shenjue) is found in the center of the navel. It is a "forbidden" point and should never be treated. See Figure 3.21.

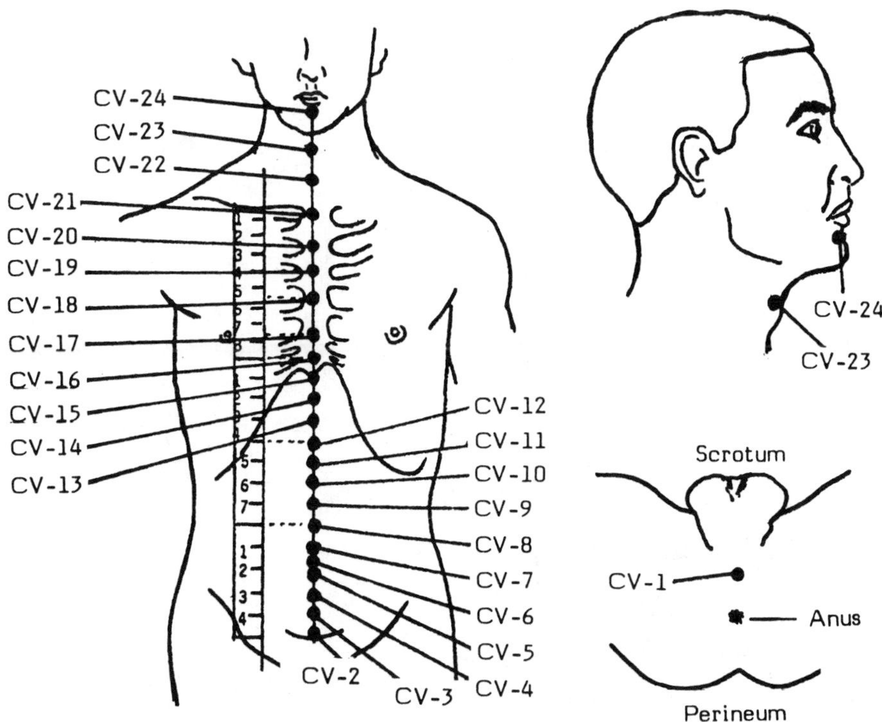

Figure 3.21. Points on the conception vessel meridian.

Points on the Governing Vessel Meridian

The major points on the governing vessel (GV) meridian are GV-3, GV-14, GV-16, GV-20, and GV-26.

GV-3

Location. The site of this point is found between the spinous processes of L4 and L5. See Figure 3.22.

Indications. This point is a good point to treat for low back pain.

GV-14

Location. This point is found between the spinous processes of C7 and T1. See Figure 3.22.

Indications. This point is used in the treatment of thoracic outlet syndromes, neck pain, and shoulder pain. It is referred to as a *reunion point* because it interconnects with other meridians and often takes on the functions of those meridians.

GV-16

Location. This site is found directly in the midline just below the external occipital protuberance, at the base of the occiput. See Figure 3.22.

Indications. Stimulation of this point is used in the treatment of suboccipital headaches. Some studies have indicated a relationship between this point and the endocrines.

GV-20

Location. This point is located in the midsagittal line of the scalp, on a line drawn between the apex of both ears. See Figure 3.22.

Indications. Relationships have been drawn between this point and treatment of patients with hemorrhoids or hypertension.

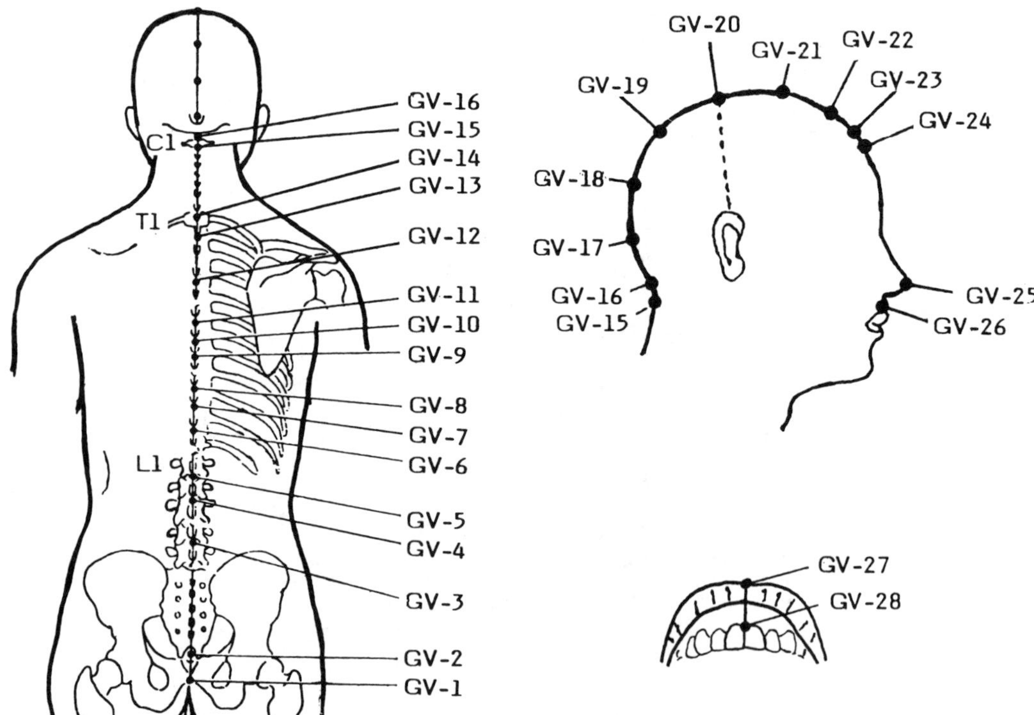

Figure 3.22. Points on the governing vessel meridian.

GV-26

Location. The site of this point is found at the philtrum, in the angle formed by the nose and the upper lip. See Figure 3.22.

Indications. Firm manual stimulation of this point is indicated in patients who feel faint.

Alarm Points

As previously described briefly, there are several reflex points for the meridians that are located on the anterior surface of the body. Spontaneous pain, pain on pressure, or excessive electropermeability at one of these points may indicate that some disorder is present in the associated meridian. For example, it is empirically claimed that spontaneous pain at LU-1 indicates a problem in the lung meridian, whose alarm point is LU-1.

All alarm (mo) points are located on the ventral surface of the thorax and the abdomen, and each point is associated with one of the 12 main meridians and its function. Six of the meridian alarm points are located on the conception vessel meridian, thus they are unilateral. The other six alarm points are bilateral, giving a total of 18 alarm points in all.

It is thought by Oriental physicians that tenderness or pain elicited by light pressure on or spontaneous pain at any of these points indicates that the meridian has excessive energy (Chi). Tenderness only on heavy pressure indicates that there is a deficiency of Chi. Generally, the alarm points are associated with the Yin types of diseases; viz, those diseases associated with cold, depression, and weakness.

Table 3.1 lists the alarm points for the 12 meridians and gives the anatomical location of each. These points are also depicted in Figure 3.23.

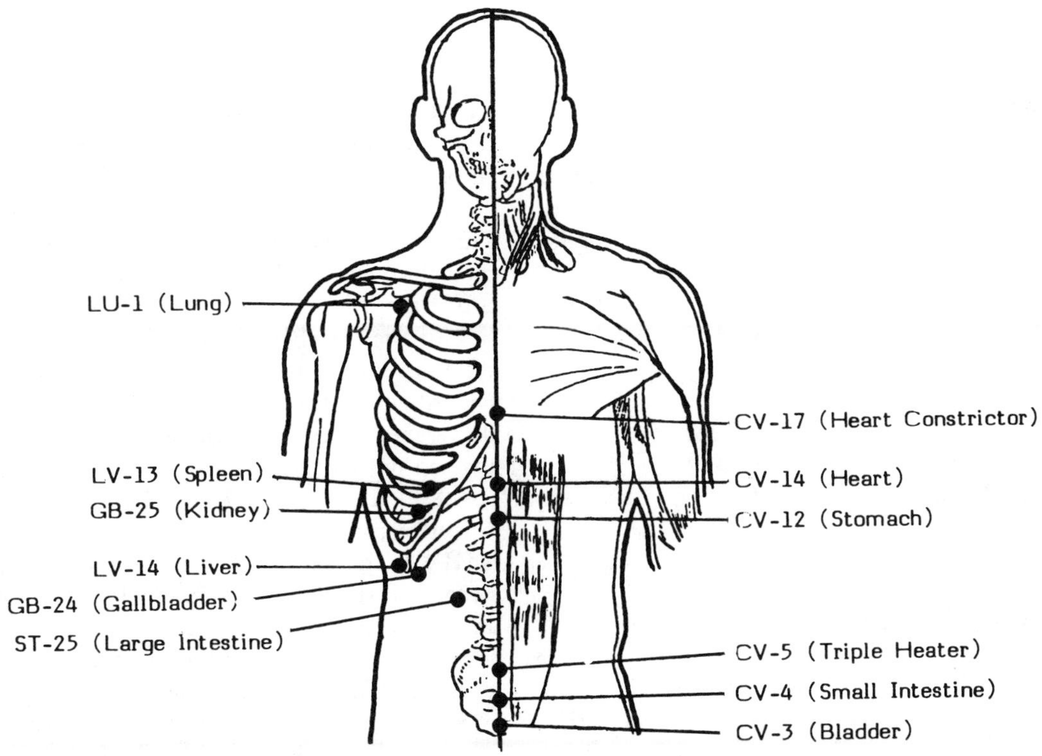

Figure 3.23. Alarm points.

Table 3.1. Alarm Points of the Body

Meridian	*Alarm Point*	*Location*
		BILATERAL POINTS
Lung	LU-1	1 cun below clavicle, lateral interspace 2nd—3rd ribs.
Liver	LV-14	On vertical nipple line, between 6th—7th ribs.
Gallbladder	GB-24	On vertical nipple line, between 8th—9th ribs.
Spleen	LV-13	Anterior tip of 11th rib.
Kidney	GB-25	Anterior tip of 12th rib.
Large intestine	ST-25	2 cun lateral to navel.
		MIDLINE POINTS
Heart constrictor	CV-17	Midsternal, nipple level, ¾ths down from episternal notch.
Heart	CV-14	6 cun above navel, just below xiphoid process.
Stomach	CV-12	4 cun above navel, epigastrium, midway between the sternum and navel.
Triple heater	CV-5	2 cun below navel.
Small intestine	CV-4	3 cun below navel.
Bladder	CV-3	4 cun below navel.

Master Points

The seven master points are the primary points of the body, and they are used more frequently than other points. See Figure 3.24. Generally, they will all be tender to the touch and the effects from stimulating them are usually pronounced. These points, in review, are:

- LI-4
- SP-6
- BL-54
- LU-7
- ST-36
- GB-20
- LV-3

Association Points

Associated points were briefly described with the bladder meridian. An association point (or associated point, as it is sometimes called) is a reflex site for an affiliated meridian. Generally, it allegedly becomes tender when the meridian's Chi is abnormally disturbed.

All meridians have an associated point. This point is located along the back on the medial course of the bladder meridian, 1½ cun from the spinous processes, on either side of the vertebral column. That is, all association points may be found approximately two finger widths lateral to the midline of the spine. There are also associated points that do not correspond with a specific meridian. See Table 3.2 and Figure 3.25.

In this context, a special point to be noted is KI-27. This point is located on the anterior surface of the body and supposedly acts as an associated point for the entire series. It is sometimes referred to as the "home of all associated points." Refer to Figure 3.16.

Some authorities contend that these association points, when tender, are the best points to treat for tonification or sedation of the affiliated meridian because of a lesser possibility of an adverse reaction or side effects.

The associated points have certain characteristics in contrast to the alarm points, according to Felix Mann:

1. Classically, they are points of sedation. Sedation of an association point in turn causes sedation of the meridian preceding it and the meridian which follows it. This is typically the reverse of what occurs when alarm points are stimulated.

2. These points, because of their general calming effect, are used in Yang diseases such as those associated with fever and/or overexcitation.

3. Association points also serve well as points of tonification.

4. Chinese osteopathy uses these points in the correction of minor displacements of the vertebrae.

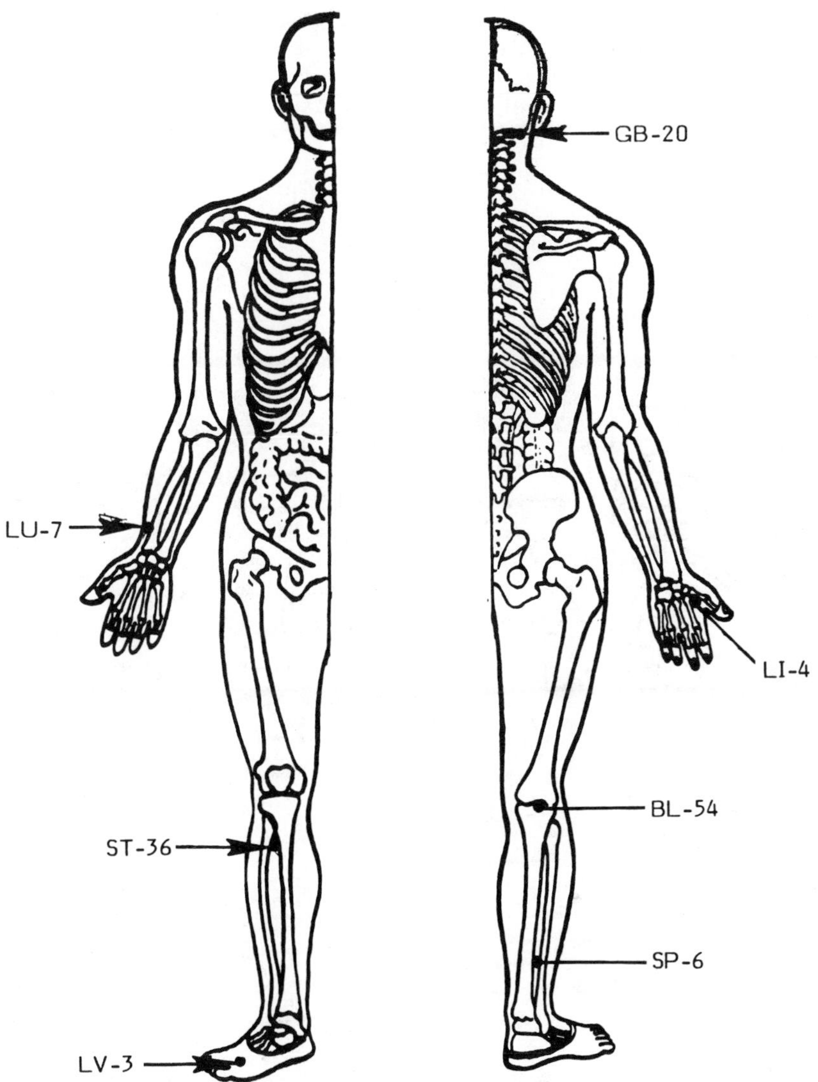

Figure 3.24. Master points.

Table 3.2. Associated Points

Meridian	*Assoc. Point*	*Location*
LU	BL 13	1½ cun lateral to spinous processes, between T3 and T4.
HC	BL 14	1½ cun lateral to spinous processes, between T4 and T5.
HT	BL 15	1½ cun lateral to spinous processes, between T5 and T6.
GV	BL 16	1½ cun lateral to spinous processes, between T6 and T7.
LV	BL 18	1½ cun lateral to spinous processes, between T9 and T10.
GB	BL 19	1½ cun lateral to spinous processes, between T10 and T11.
SP	BL 20	1½ cun lateral to spinous processes, between T11 and T12.
ST	BL 21	1½ cun lateral to spinous processes, between T12 and L1.
TH	BL 22	1½ cun lateral to spinous processes, between L1 and L2.
KI	BL 23	1½ cun lateral to spinous processes, between L2 and L3.
LI	BL 25	1½ cun lateral to spinous processes, between L4 and L5.
SI	BL 27	At the level of the S1 foramen.
BL	BL 28	At the level of the S2 foramen.

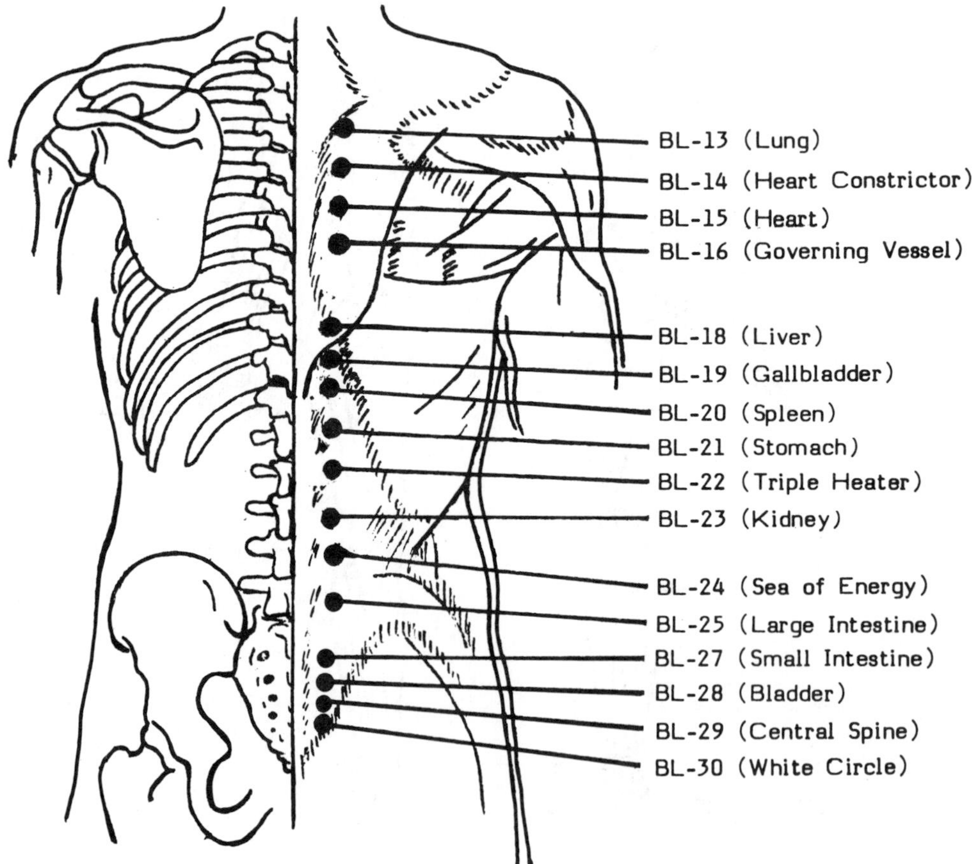

Figure 3.25. Association points.

CLOSING REMARKS

Although needling procedures are frequently mentioned in this chapter, the skillful use of such penetrating techniques require specialized instruction beyond the scope of this discourse. However, this information as presented will be of extreme value when nonneedling techniques (eg, electric stimulation) are utilized in adjunctive therapeutics.

REFERENCES

1. Jayasuriya A: Medicina alternativa strategy for the integration of healing methods. *International Journal of Chinese Medicine,* 2(1):7-14, March 1985.
2. Jaskoviak PA: *Manual of Meridian Therapy.* Lombard, IL, National College of Chiropractic, 1979, pp 10-15.
3. Han KB: *On the Kyungrak System.* Pyongyang, Korea, Foreign Language Publishing House, 1964.
4. Mann F: *Acupuncture, The Ancient Chinese Art of Healing and How It Works Scientifically.* New York, Vintage Books, 1971, p 5.
5. Mann F: Papers presented to the International Acupuncture Conference in Vienna and German Acupuncture Conference in Weisbaden.
6. Vannerson JF: A neurological explanation of acupuncture. *Digest of Chiropractic Economics,* March/April, pp 22-28, 1974.
7. Mann F: *Acupuncture, The Ancient Chinese Art of Healing and How It Works Scientifically.* New York, Vintage Books, 1971, p 5.
8. Takase K: Revolutionary new pain theory and acupuncture treatment procedure based on new theory of acupuncture mechanism. *American Journal of Acupuncture,* 11(4):305-328, October-December 1983.
9. Hu Y, Qi Y: The Phenomena of energy circulated in the meridian system. *International Journal of Chinese Medicine,* 1(4):7-14, December 1984.
10. Sato A: Spinal and medullary reflex components of the somato-sympathetic reflex discharges evoked by stimulation of the group IV somatic afferents. *Brain Research,* 51:307-318, 1973.
11. Kunert W: Functional disorders of internal organs due to vertebral lesions. *Ciba Symposium,* 13(3), 1965.
12. Coote JH, et al: Reflex discharges into thoracic white rami elicited by somatic and visceral afferent excitation. *Journal of Physiology,* 202:141-159, 1969.
13. Dittmar E: Cutaneo-visceral neural pathways. *Journal of Physical Medicine* (British), 15:208, 1952.
14. Kuntz A, Hazelwood LA: Circulatory reactions in the gastrointestinal tract elicited by local cutaneous stimulation. *American Heart Journal,* 20:743-749, 1940.
15. Kuntz A: Anatomic and physiologic properties of cutaneo-visceral vasomotor reflex arcs. *Journal of Neurophysiology,* 8:421-429, 1943.
16. Richins CA, Brizzee K: Effect of localized cutaneous stimulation on circulation in duodenal arterioles and capillary beds. *Journal of Neurophysiology,* 12:131-136, 1949.
17. Mann F: *Acupuncture, The Ancient Chinese Art of Healing and How It Works Scientifically.* New York, Vintage Books, 1971, p 7.
18. Travell J, Rinzler SH: Relief of cardiac pain by local block of somatic trigger areas. *Proceedings of the Society for Experimental Biology and Medicine,* 63:480-482, 1946.
19. Dale RA: The principles and systems of micro-acupuncture. *International Journal of Chinese Medicine,* 1(4):15-42, December 1984.
20. Mann F: *Acupuncture, The Ancient Chinese Art of Healing and How It Works Scientifically.* New York, Vintage Books, 1971, pp 8-9.
21. Ussher NT: The viscerospinal syndrome: a new concept of visceromotor and sensory changes in relation to deranged spinal structures. *Annals of Internal Medicine,* 1940, pp 427-432.
22. Weiss S, Davis D: The significance of the afferent impulses from the skin in the mechanism of visceral pain; skin infiltration as a useful therapeutic measure. *American Journal of Medical Science,* 176:517, 1928.
23. Gutstein R: A review of myodysneuria (fibrositis). *American Practitioner and Digest of Treatment,* 6: 570-577, 1955.
24. Mann F: *Acupuncture, The Ancient Chinese Art of Healing and How It Works Scientifically.* New York, Vintage Books, 1971, pp 8-9.
25. Matsumoto T: *Acupuncture for Physicians.* Springfield, IL, Charles C. Thomas, 1974, pp 19-20.
26. Pennell RJ, Heuser GD: *The "How to" Seminar of Acupuncture.* Independence, MO, IPCI, 1973, pp 25-30.
27. Mann F: *Acupuncture, The Ancient Chinese Art of Healing and How It Works Scientifically.* New York, Vintage Books, 1971, pp 8-9.
28. Ibid.
29. Keegan JJ, Garrett FD: The segmental distribution of the cutaneous nerves in the limbs of man. *Anatomical Record,* 102:409-439, 1948.
30. Sherrington CS: *The Integrative Action of the Nervous System.* New York, Scribner, 1906.
31. Downman CBB: Skeletal muscle reflexes of splanchnic and intercostal nerve origin in acute spinal and decerebrate cats. *Journal of Physiology,* 18:217-235, 1955.
32. Mann F: *Acupuncture, The Ancient Chinese Art*

of Healing and How It Works Scientifically. New York, Vintage Books, 1971, pp 8-9.
33. Downman CBB, McSwiney BA: Reflexes elicited by visceral stimulation in the acute spinal animal. *Journal of Physiology,* 105:80-94, 1946.
34. Kellgren JH: On the distribution of pain arising from deep somatic structures, with charts of segmental pain. *Clinical Science,* 4:35-46, 1942.
35. Travell J, Bigelow NH: Referred somatic pain does not follow a simple segmental pattern. *Federation Proceedings,* 5:106, 1946.
36. Koblank A: *Die Nase als Reflexorgan.* Haug, Ulm, Germany, 1958.
37. Melzack R, Wall PD: Pain mechanisms: a new theory. *Science,* 150:871-879, 1965.
38. Melzack R: Phantom limb pain. *Anesthesiology,* 35:409-419, 1971.
39. Casey KL: Pain: A current view of neural mechanisms. *American Scientist,* 61:194-200, 1973.
40. Hart FD (ed): *The Treatment of Chronic Pain.* Philadelphia, F.A. Davis, 1974, pp 4-5.
41. Melzack R: Phantom limb pain. *Anesthesiology,* 35:409-419, 1971.
42. Noordenbos W: *Pain: Problems Pertaining to the Transmission of Nerve Impulses Which Give Rise to Pain.* New York, Elsevier, 1959, pp 95-96, 182.
43. Fox JL: Neuropacemaker for relief of intractable pain. *Medical Annals of the District of Columbia,* 40:577-579, 1971.
44. Matsumoto T, Hayes MF: Acupuncture, electric phenomena of the skin, and postvagotomy gastrointestinal atony. *American Journal of Surgery,* 125:176-180, 1973.
45. Pennell RJ, Heuser GD: *The "How to" Seminar of Acupuncture.* Independence, MO, IPCI, 1973, pp 25-30.
46. Macheret EL: Some theoretical prerequisites for the use of acupuncture. *International Journal of Chinese Medicine,* 2(1):27-30, March 1985.
47. Fields A: Acupuncture and endorphins. *International Journal of Chinese Medicine,* 1(2):5-15, June 1984.
48. Slagoski JE: Resolution of acute dysmenorrhea with one-point therapy. *International Journal of Chinese Medicine,* 1(1):23-24, March 1984.
49. Tseung A: Some clinical cases responding to acupuncture in general practice. *International Journal of Chinese Medicine,* 1(1):49-51, March 1984.
50. Vazharov K: Observations on some conditions responsive to treatment with acupuncture. *International Journal of Chinese Medicine,* 2(1):31-32, March 1985.
51. Kitzinger E: Vertebragenic syndromes and nondrug treatment. *International Journal of Chinese Medicine,* 1(3):3-7, September 1984.
52. Shafshak TS: Electroacupuncture versus physiotherapy in the treatment of tension myositis. *International Journal of Chinese Medicine,* 1(1):35-38, March 1984.
53. Odell SW: Acupuncture as major tool in reprogramming therapy. *International Journal of Chinese Medicine,* 1(3):15-17, September 1984.
54. Hyodo M: *Ryodoraku Treatment: An Objective Approach to Acupuncture.* Japan Ryodoraku, Osaka, Japan, Autonomic Nerve Society, 1975.
55. Sin YM: Acupuncture and inflammation. *International Journal of Chinese Medicine,* 1(1):15-20, March 1984.
56. Academy of Traditional Chinese Medicine: *An Outline of Chinese Acupuncture.* Peking, China, Foreign Languages Press, 1975, pp 91-95.
57. Eckman P: Acupuncture and science. *International Journal of Chinese Medicine,* 1(1):3-7, March 1984.

Uncited References

Berman DA: Pain relief and acupuncture: the if, why and how. *American Journal of Acupuncture,* 7:31-41, 1979.

Bowers JZ: Reception of acupuncture by the scientific community: from scorn to a degree of interest. *Comparative Medicine East & West,* 6:89-96, 1978.

Ene EE, Odia GI. Effect of acupuncture on disorders of the musculoskeletal system in Nigerians. *American Journal of Chinese Medicine,* 11:106-111, 1983.

Hansen, PE, Hansen JH: Acupuncture treatment of chronic facial pain: a controlled cross-over trial. *Headache,* 23:66-69, 1983.

Lee Peng CH, Yang MMP, Kok SH, Woo YK: Endorphin release: a possible mechanism of acupuncture analgesia. *Comparative Medicine East & West,* 6:57-60, 1978.

Lenhard L, Waite PME: Acupuncture in the prophylactic treatment of migraine headache: pilot study. *The New Zealand Medical Journal,* 96:663-666, 1983.

Lewith GT, Turner G, Machin D: Effects of acupuncture on low back pain and sciatica. *American Journal of Acupuncture,* 12:21-32, 1984.

Pontinen PJ: Acupuncture in the treatment of low-back pain and sciatica. *Acupuncture and Electro-Therapeutics Research,* 4:53-57, 1979.

Rozeiu AM: Clinical decisions: a normative approach. *Journal of the Canadian Chiropractic Association,* 26:102-106, 1982.

Shibutani K, Kubal K: Similarities of prolonged pain relief produced by nerve block and acupuncture in patients with chronic pain. *Acupuncture and Electro-Therapeutics Research,* 4:9-16, 1979.

Wei LY: Scientific advance in acupuncture. *American Journal of Chinese Medicine,* 7:53-75, 1979.

Wyke B: Neurological mechanisms in the experience of pain. *Acupuncture and Electro-Therapeutics Research,* 4:27-35, 1979.

Yue, S: Acupuncture for chronic back and neck pain. *Acupuncture and Electro-Therapeutics Research,* 3: 323-324, 1979.

Chapter 4

Superficial Heat Therapies

This chapter describes the physiologic principles involved with the use of heat and reviews some of the more common types of superficial heat modalities.

INTRODUCTION

The use of heat in treating the body is almost as old as the history of mankind. From the time of the earliest bath houses, people have sought to relieve aches and pains by this method. The warmth of fire, hot coals, warm compresses, and similar modalities have come down through the ages as useful healing tools.

Historical Background

In 1666, Sir Isaac Newton demonstrated, by means of a prism, the various colors of the visible spectrum. Scientists were unaware of the fact that light travels at a fixed rate until 1673, when the Danish astronomer Olaus Romer reported his findings that proved this to be true.

Sir Oliver Lodge defined light as "an electromagnetic disturbance of ether." It was at first thought that this disturbance occurred in the form of extremely small oscillations, and light was described as "the propagation of energy in the form of waves" (wave theory).

James Clerk Maxwell enunciated his electromagnetic theory of light in 1768. Through his genius, the great mass of existing knowledge at that time was brought under a single "ether" theory. This theory, known as the electromagnetic principle, showed that, if we assume the existence of a single ether that is capable of bearing electric and magnetic strains, any movement of electricity or of a magnetized body entails changes in the electrical or magnetic forces throughout space. This led to the development of computing the initial concepts of the electromagnetic spectrum.

In 1800, Sir William Herschel found there was an area *beyond the red* end of the visible spectrum that caused a thermometer to register an even higher degree of heat than in the red area. Thus were discovered the *invisible heat* rays, which, because of their position beyond the red rays, were called *infrared* rays. A year later, Johann Ritter found that there were rays beyond the *violet* end of the spectrum, which darkened silver chloride. Thus were discovered the invisible "chemical" rays, which, because of their position beyond the violet end of the spectrum, were called *ultraviolet* rays.

Physiotherapeutic innovations took a giant leap forward about the same time as D. D. Palmer discovered contemporary chiropractic. A mercury vapor lamp enclosed in glass was invented by Arons in 1896, and first manufactured by Peter Cooper Hewitt in 1902. The quartz mercury vapor lamp, devised chiefly by Kromayer, was first made in 1904.

Niels Ryberg Finsen, who established a

"Light Institute" at Copenhagen in 1897 is generally recognized as "The Father of Light Therapy" because of his seemingly miraculous cures of lupus by using carbon-arc lights. Italians, however, claim that Sciascia of Sicily undertook experiments in "pyrophototherapy" as early as 1880 that included the successful treatment of lupus. However, it was the work of Finsen that aroused intercontinental interest in artificial light therapy.

Max Karl Ernst Ludwig Planck of Berlin devised the quantum theory of light radiation in 1900. A few years later, Rollier of Leysin introduced a systematic method in 1903 for the application of sun's rays to the whole body, especially in the treatment of extrapulmonary tuberculosis. He stimulated much interest in methods of natural and artificial light therapy.

It was not until 1924, by careful spectroscopy, that Millikan, who had photographed the ultraviolet spectrum, was able to span the distance between the shortest ultraviolet rays and the longest roentgen rays.

The Electromagnetic Spectrum

The electromagnetic spectrum is a graphic representation of the various energy waves in ascending order of wavelength and descending order of frequency. See Table 4.1. Among the energy forms available in general practice, the longer the wavelength, the deeper the penetration—with the exception of cosmic waves, of which we know relatively little at this time. The longest rays are the Hertzian waves, which are used in wireless telegraphy, that may have wavelengths of a mile or more.

Very broadly, the application of electromagnetic energy with wavelengths between 1850 Angstroms and 150 kilometers, approximately, can be applied in the form of longwave diathermy, shortwave diathermy, microwave diathermy, infrared therapy, heliotherapy, ultraviolet therapy, Grenz ray therapy, or medical deep x-ray and radium therapies.

Physiologic Effects of Local Heat

Heat (superficial and deep) is applied in a number of fashions such as:

- Electric pads
- Fluidotherapy
- Hot moist packs
- Hot water
- Hydrocollator packs
- Incandescent lamps
- Infrared rays
- Microwaves
- Paraffin dips
- Radiant heaters
- Sauna-like hot air
- Shortwave diathermy
- Steam baths
- Sunlight
- Ultrasound
- Ultraviolet lamps
- Warm sand and mud
- Whirlpools

The surface effects of heat on tissues are essentially the same, but deeper effects vary according to intensity, concentration of application, duration, wavelength, and the vascularity of the area.

The primary physical effect of the use of heat is thermal. As the modality of heat is placed over a treated part, that part increases in temperature. This increase in local temperature further increases the heating effects, which in turn precipitates three basic reactions: (1) an analgesic or calming effect, (2) a slight increase in local metabolism, and (3) some sedation of sensory nerves, which is most likely due to the triggering of enkephalin production.

Enkephalin, hypothesized to be an endogenous neurotransmitter, is a pentapeptide that is found in many parts of the brain. It binds to specific receptor sites, and many of these sites are considered to be pain-related opiate receptors.

As local metabolism increases, this further increases the local temperature and gives rise

Table 4.1. The Electromagnetic Spectrum

Approximate Frequency per second	*Approximate Wavelength*	*Application*	
		Therapeutic	*Technical*
0 cycle		Galvanism, electrocautery	Direct current
1 cycle		ECG, EEG, muscle stimulation, electrodiagnosis, Ryodoraku	Common alternating current
10 cycles			
10^2 cycles			
	1000 km		
10^3 cycles	100 km		Low frequency current
10^4 cycles			
	10 km		
10^5 cycles			Longwave radio
	1 km		
10^6 cycles	100 m	High frequency surgery (longwave diathermy)	Midwave radio
10^7 cycles			Shortwave radio
	10 m		
10^8 cycles		Shortwave diathermy	
	1 m		
10^9 cycles			
	10 cm	Microwave diathermy	Ultrashortwave radio
10^{10} cycles			
	1 cm		
10^{11} cycles			
	1 mm		
10^{12} cycles			
		Infrared therapy	
10^{13} cycles			Radiant heat
	0.01 mm	Heliotherapy	
10^{14} cycles			
	0.001 mm	Ultraviolet therapy, air sterilization	
10^{15} cycles			Light waves
	100 m mu		
10^{16} cycles			Ultraviolet radiation
	10 m mu		
10^{17} cycles			
	1 m mu		
10^{18} cycles			
	2 A	Grenz ray therapy	
	1 A		Fine-structure analysis
10^{19} cycles			
		Roentgenography	
	0.1 A	Deep x-ray therapy	
10^{20} cycles			
	0.01 A	Radium therapy and radioactive isotopes	Material testing
10^{21} cycles			
	0.001 A		

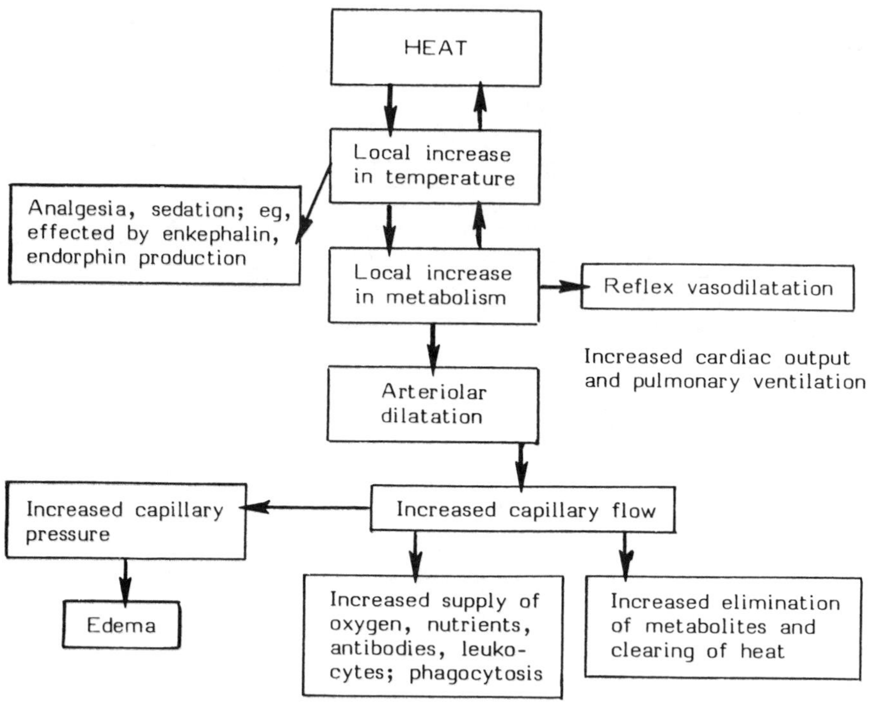

Figure 4.1. The physiologic effects of local heating.

to the release of histamine or histamine-like substances that bring about arteriolar dilatation. This dilation of arterioles increases capillary flow and pressure.

If heat is applied at too high a temperature or for too long a duration, edema may result. Such effects mimic the reaction following tissue tearing such as in a sprain.

The ideal situation occurs when the correct treatment time is utilized. Then, the beneficial healing effects of heat are obtained; viz, increased elimination of metabolites and an increased supply of oxygen, nutrients, antibodies, and leukocytes, which lead to increased phagocytosis.[1] The basic effects of heat are shown in Figure 4.1.

The body responds to the application of heat according to the temperature degree produced in the tissues and the duration that the temperature is elevated. Treatments for brief periods, where there is little or no heat buildup in the tissues, seem to have little, if any, therapeutic effect.

In recent years, there has been a tendency to avoid thermotherapy for many musculoskeletal complaints for which it was once frequently used. In fact, there is considerable evidence that indicates an overutilization of heat when pain and swelling are present. This is especially true with acute complaints, where heat tends to aggravate the complaint and prolong healing time by increasing local edema. Heat definitely has a beneficial effect therapeutically, but it must be used properly and only when indicated.

As with cold, the exact physiologic mechanisms by which heat achieves its effects are not completely understood. For example, paradoxical decreases in intra-articular temperatures have been recorded after superficial heat has been applied, and increases in intra-articular temperatures have been recorded with surface cold. However, these findings are not the general rule. The anticipated effects of superficial heat can be divided into two general categories: localized effects and remote reflex effects.

Localized Effects of Heating

Heat, when properly utilized, has several specific localized effects on the body. Heat brings about a transient vasoconstriction in the circulatory system that is followed by vasodilation and hyperemia. Heat increases the flow of blood to and from the area being treated, and it initially increases metabolism within the parts being treated. However, when heat is used too long, it may lead to local congestion, edema, and reduced metabolism.

One of the many effects of heat and one extremely important rationale for its use is the effect that it has on the skin and underlying fatty tissue. Heat promotes sweating, which helps to remove toxic wastes—keeping in mind that if the heat applied is beyond the tolerance of the patient, a burn may result.

Heat may also increase the threshold of cutaneous sensory receptors, and this effect may, in turn, trigger enkephalin production. This pain-control effect is generally minimal and certainly not sufficient to warrant its utilization as an ideal modality for pain control.

Heat is much more effective in its influence on the psyche. There is no question that heat tends to relax a patient, and herein arises a potential problem with heat when it is utilized for musculoskeletal complaints. Heat almost always feels good to the patient. To the typical patient's thinking, "If 5 minutes of heat feels good, then 20 minutes of heat should produce even better effects." It has been the authors' experience, however, that heat should rarely be used for acute musculoskeletal complaints, especially if pain and/or edema are present. The major reason for this is that when heat is used it is almost always overused—leading to increased edema, which prolongs the patient's recovery time.

The rule of thumb is that heat should never be applied to a body part until 48—72 hours after injury, or even longer if recurrent bleeding or swelling is a danger. When tissue is injured, the body establishes a defensive inflammatory mechanism that temporarily blocks circulation as white and red blood cells hasten to the affected part. After the acute stage has passed, fresh blood must be brought to the injured part to carry on the battle to enhance healing processes. Because lesion waste products are difficult to move through the small venous vessels, heat is then an aid.

Remote Reflex Effects of Heating

Heat may stimulate increased blood flow, metabolism, and healing far distant from the site of application. This is especially true when shortwave diathermy is used as the modality for heat production. An example of its use would be the application of shortwave diathermy over the low back region of patients with poor circulation in the lower extremities. Its use here may help to stimulate, albeit temporarily, an increase in peripheral circulation. This effect is undoubtedly a lumbosacral parasympathetic vasomotor response.

Systemic Effects of Heating

The clinical effects of heat on the body may be summarized as:

1. *Increased oxidation.* The law of van't Hoff states that for every temperature rise of 10 °C (18 °F), the velocity of chemical reactions in the body (eg, rate of oxidation) is increased 2—3 times. This means that even slight increases in temperature can have a profound effect on cellular oxidates and, of course, on systemic physiology. For example, when ultrasound is used in the forearm or thigh, temperature increases are typically 1.8 °—3.6 °F. At the extreme, when fluido-

therapy is utilized, a temperature increase of about 8 °F can be noted, which substantially affects membrane permeability, oxidation, and hence, metabolic activity.[2,3]

2. *Tachycardia.* Increased circulation has an effect on pulse rate. For every 1 °F of temperature increase, there is a correspondingly rise in the pulse rate of about 10 beats.

3. *Hypotension.* As heat is utilized over a body part, blood pressure gradually lowers as more blood flows from the central venous system toward the part being treated.

4. *Tachypnea.* The respiratory rate increases in response to the factors listed above.

5. *Polyuria.* Heat triggers an increase in urine formation, with its constituent water, salts, urea, and nitrogenous wastes.

6. *Alkalemia.* Heat has been noted to slightly increase alkalinity in the blood of the area being treated.

7. *Increased plasma blood volume and oxygen consumption.* These states occur frequently when the patient is treated within heated water because there is no fluid loss due to perspiration evaporation.

Methods of Therapeutic Heating

Heat is transferred superficially by means of three primary methods: conduction, convection, and radiation.

CONDUCTION

Conduction occurs when two or more adjacent objects (media) of unlike temperature are placed in contact and a state of energy exchange affects successive portions of each. Heat is transferred (conducted) from the warmer to the cooler body by the process of conduction. See Figure 4.2.

The *rate of heat exchange* depends essentially on (1) the difference in temperature of the adjacent bodies, (2) the different properties in heat conductivity, and (3) the length of time the process is allowed to continue. Numerically, conductivity is the reciprocal of unit resistance (resistivity).

Certain objects conduct heat better than others. Metals such as gold, silver, and copper are some of the best conductors of heat because they offer relatively little resistance to thermal energy. Generally, substances that are good conductors of heat are good conductors of electricity (eg, tissue water).

Almost any solid, liquid, or gas can be used in conducting heat to a patient. What determines the choice are such factors as what part of the body is to be treated, what end-effects are desired, and whether or not it is preferred that the patient be in motion during therapy.

The major disadvantages of any conductive heating modality (eg, heating pad, hot pack) is that the part being treated cannot be visualized during therapy and it is often difficult to apply evenly to irregularly shaped parts such as an extremity joint. Due to the pressure involved, it is unsuitable for open wounds, draining fistulas, or ulcerations.

CONVECTION

Convection involves the exchange of heat between a surface and a fluid (liquid or gas) moving over that surface. Hubbard tanks, whirlpool baths, and fluidotherapy are good examples of applications of convection heat. An air current moving across or through heated coils (eg, an electric room heater) is another example.

RADIATION

In radiation, the objects between which the transfer of heat energy occurs are separated by an intervening medium that does not become warmer as a result of the heat being transmitted through it. The heat transferred generally travels through the air to the patient from a source of radiation that is in the infrared portion of the spectrum.

Table 4.2 summarizes the forms of therapeutic heating commonly used.

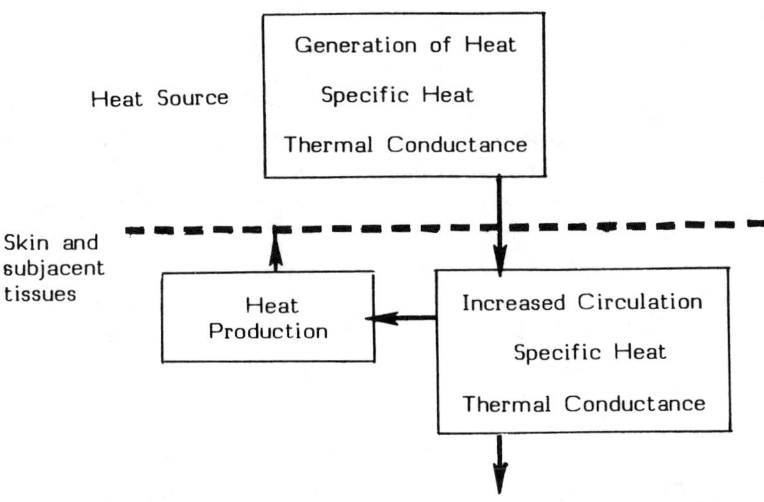

Figure 4.2. Heat exchange by conduction.[4]

Table 4.2. Sources of Superficial Heat

Method of Transmission	*Source of Heat*	*Form of Energy*
Conduction*	Electric heating pad Hot water bottle Hydrocollator pack Kenny pack Heated paraffin	By motion of the involved molecules
Convection	Agitated water baths Moist air baths Hot air baths Fluidotherapy Whirlpool**	By movement of the involved molecules

Radiation	Infrared lamp
	  Luminous
	  Nonluminous
	Sunlight
	Ultraviolet rays
		By means of radiation

* Partly by convection.
** Partly by conduction.

CONVERSION

Heat can also be transferred deep within the body by the process of conversion. Conversion is that process whereby a high frequency electric current or vibrations passing through a part converts the oscillations into heat energy. The heat buildup in this instance is due primarily to friction and molecular bombardment as the current meets cellular resistance. Typical examples are witnessed in the use of shortwave, microwave, and ultrasound diathermy, which are described in a future chapter.

Physical Effects of Heating

Regardless of the type of modality utilized, the immediate effect on the body is purely a physical one; ie, a rise in temperature (hyperthermia) in the tissues to which the heat is directed. The degree, and somewhat the extent, of the effects of this thermal effect vary in proportion to (1) the degree of heat, (2) the speed in which the thermal effects are dispersed, (3) the duration the heat is applied, and (4) to a greater extent, the particular source of the heat.

It takes time for heat to penetrate. For example, when hot water bags whose water temperature is 133 °F are continually placed on an extremity, the outside of the towel covering the bag will be about 122 °F. It takes about 30 minutes for the skin temperature to rise from 90 °F to 110 °F, about 40 minutes for subcutaneous tissue to rise from 91.2 °F to 105.5 °F, and about 50 minutes for intramuscular temperature to rise from 94.2 °F to 99.6 °F.[5]

Heat should never be applied above patient tolerance or in situations where the patient doesn't have the ability to discriminate how hot the modality is. As a general rule, the average maximum tolerance of the skin to radiant heating has been shown to be 113.9 °F for the surface and 117.8 °F for the undersurface.

As heat is applied, the patient should feel warmth between 92 °F and 98 °F, hot between 98 °F and 104 °F, and increasingly uncomfortably hot at 104 °F and over. The usual therapeutic range for heat modalities is from 100° to 115 °F, depending on an individual patient's tolerance. It should be noted, however, that temperatures as low as 107.6 °F can cause thermal damage if left on for several hours.[6] The rule of thumb when applying heat is that 113 °F at close contact for a 30-minute duration is the maximum safe exposure time.

General Indications and Contraindications

Local heat relieves muscle spasm, dilates superficial blood and lymph vessels, increases phagocytosis and perspiration, and sedates the nervous system. It also reflexly dilates blood and lymph vessels in deeper tissues in various degrees depending upon the application site.

General heat applied to the body increases circulation, heart rate, perspiration, respiration, and urine formation. The blood tends to become more alkaline while the tissues become more acidic.

Some authorities have shown that variations of temperature applications to various parts of the body will produce vascular shifts and also have a toning effect upon the blood vessels, thus explaining the benefits of alternate hot and cold applications.

Local heat is usually contraindicated in acute inflammations, suppuration, hemorrhagic tendencies, impaired or hypersensitive thermal sense, or over encapsulated swellings where vasodilation may result in rupture or dispersion. Heat should never be applied to an acute injury where extravasated blood and fluids occur as great damage can be done by increasing localized edema and bleeding from ruptured capillaries. Great care must be used in applying local heat to the diabetic.

The general indications and contraindication of local heat are listed in Table 4.3.

Table 4.3. General Indications and Contraindications of Local Heat

GENERAL INDICATIONS	
Relaxation of spasticity	Enhance the absorption of exudates
Decrease myospindle response to stress	Enhance local nutrition
Increase the suppurative processes	Enhance local blood alkalinity and tissue acidity
Increase hyperemia, vasodilation	Produce general sedation and local analgesia
Increase threshold of pain receptors	Promote sweating
Increase local circulatory and metabolic rates	Increase blood volume
Decrease vascular stasis	Increase pulse rate and cardiac volume
Decrease diastolic blood pressure	Increase lymph flow
Increase urinary output	
GENERAL CONTRAINDICATIONS	
Deficient vascularity due to organic disease of the blood vessels	Over acute skin conditions such as rashes, sunburn, gangrene, etc
Anesthetic areas or areas of diminished sensation (eg, scars)	In infants, the elderly, or severely debilitated patients
Malignant neoplasm in the body area being treated	After counterirritant ointments or lotions have been applied
With patients receiving roentgen therapy	Over recently formed scars
Bleeding tendency	Over extremely fair skin
Active cases of tuberculosis	Over metal such as rings, bracelets, underwater clips, implants, etc
Over the pregnant uterus	To the eyes
Over deep acute inflammatory processes, especially suppurating lesions	To contact lenses; they should be removed when treating near the face
Over localized edema	To patients with a high fever

Note: Avoid exposure that is too intense or prolonged; overheating skin can result in mottling or even blisters. When applying heat to the face, the eyes should be protected by pieces of absorbent cotton that have been moistened with water and then flattened against the eyelids. As always, the final determination as to use depends on the clinical impressions derived from the examination and case history.

Basic Rules of Application of Heat

Six general rules should be recognized when heat is utilized:

1. Test the heated object on yourself before you apply it to the patient.
2. When the heat to the patient is increased (eg, with an infrared lamp), discontinue the therapy if the patient complains of excessive warmth.
3. Be sure that the patient's skin is dry.
4. When applying heat directly to a bony prominence or over sensitive areas, pad or drape the area.
5. Do not apply heat for too long a duration.
6. Check the patient every 3—5 minutes after starting the treatment.

HOT MOIST PACKS

Perhaps the most commonly used heat modality is the hot pack such as a hydrocollator pack. Such packs transfer heat to the patient primarily by conduction, but some convection may be involved when contact is not firm. A typical heating unit is shown in Figure 4.3.

Application

When any type of hot pack is used, the part to be treated should be uncovered and checked for scar tissue, areas of decreased circulation, and diminished sensation. Explain the therapy to the patient and that it will take a few minutes before they feel the buildup of warmth.

The patient should feel comfortably warm, but not hot. Place an alarm bell next to the patient so that if the packs get uncomfortable from either the heat or weight, the patient can call for assistance.

The packs should be completely wrapped, using either:

1. A "four towel wrap," where four Turkish towels are folded in half lengthwise so there are eight layers between the skin and the hot pack. See Figure 4.4.

2. A "three towel wrap," where three Turkish towels are folded in half so that there are six layers between the hot pack and the patient. See Figure 4.5.

Once they have been wrapped in towels, the packs should be placed on the patient. The wrapping towels should always be dry, never damp or wet, and the patient should never be allowed to lie over the hot pack or let the pack directly touch the skin.

It takes approximately 5—10 minutes before maximum heat will reach the patient;

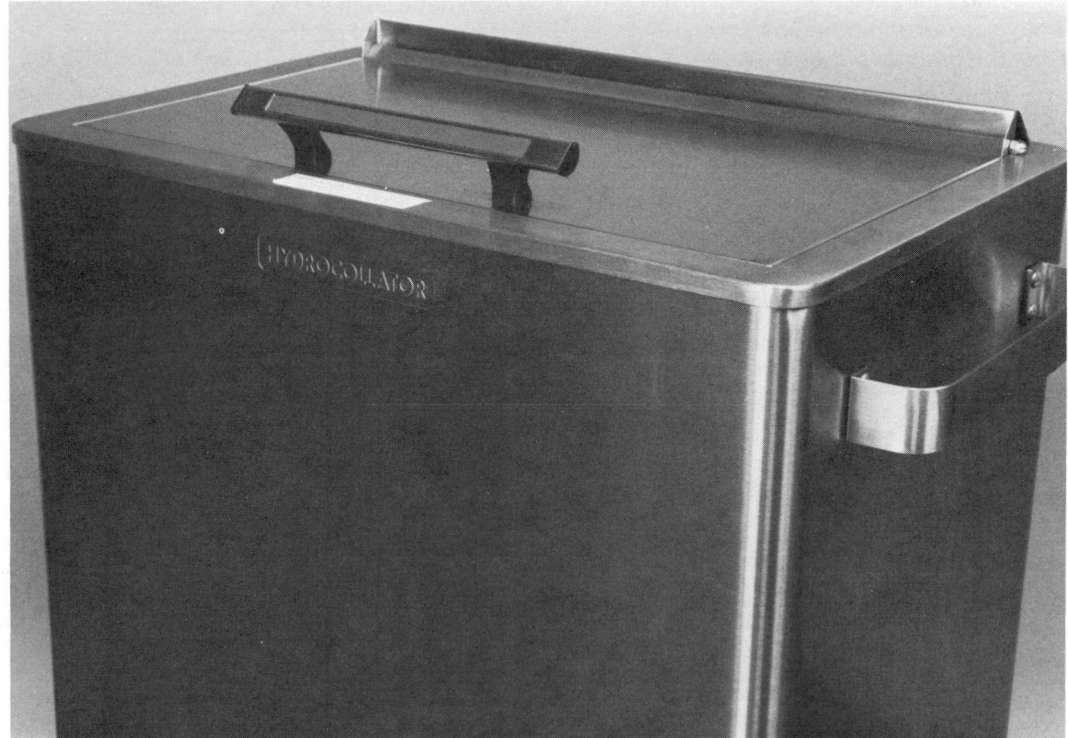

Figure 4.3. A standard hydrocollator unit. The water temperature should be maintained from 150° to 170°F.

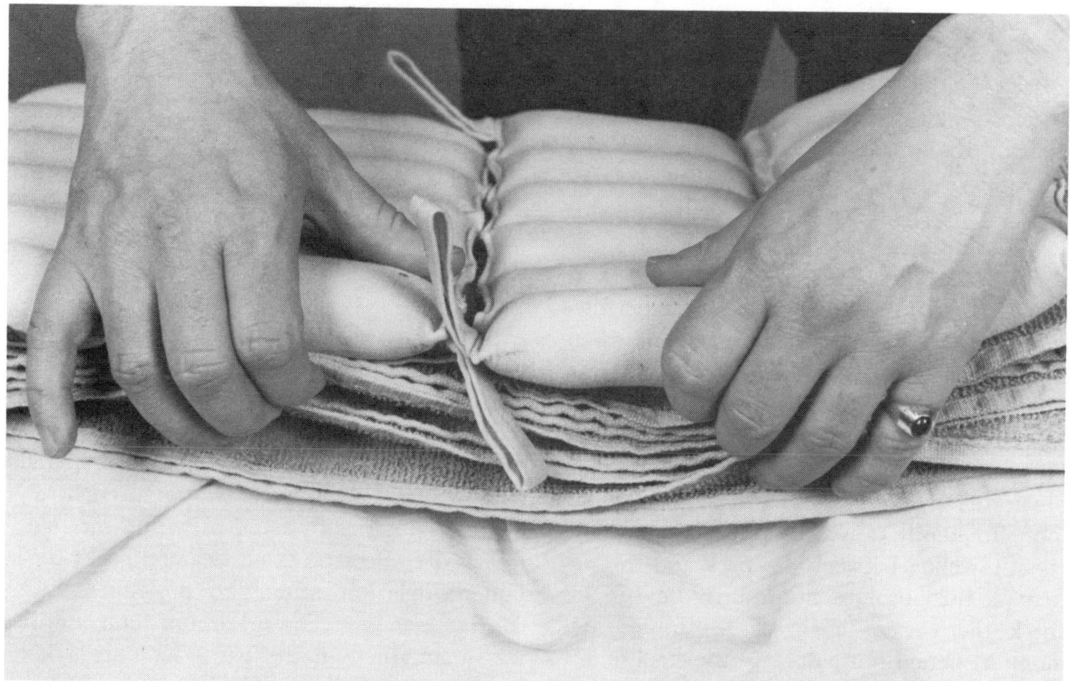

Figure 4.4. In using a "four towel" wrap, eight layers of toweling are placed between the patient and the hot pack.

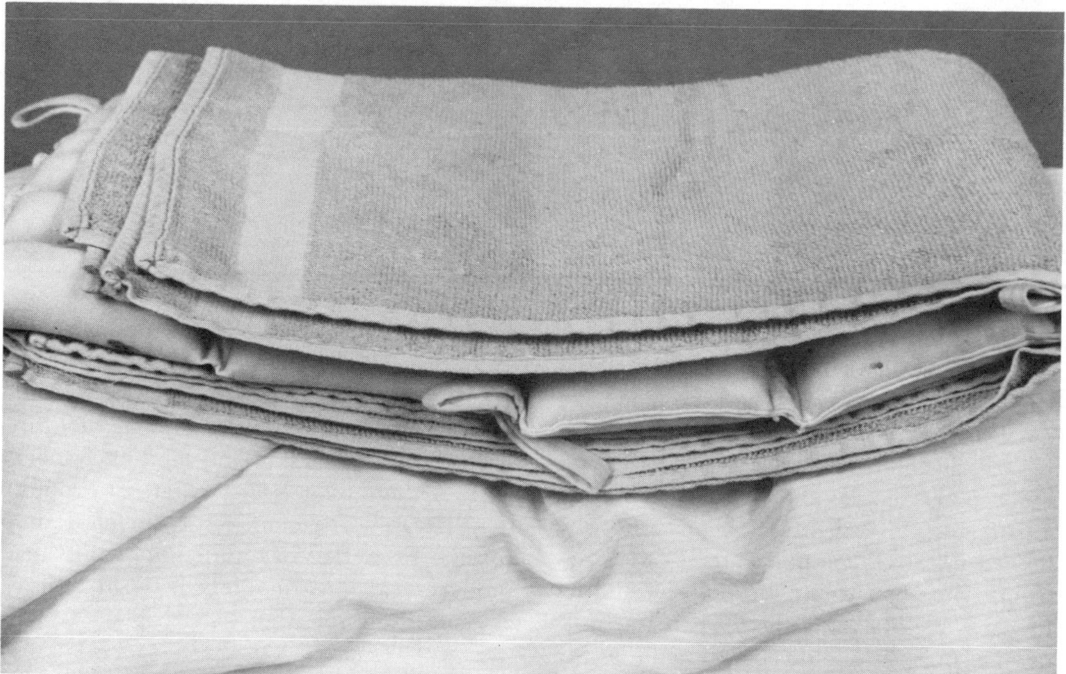

Figure 4.5. A modified "three towel" wrap, with six layers of toweling between the patient and the hot pack.

however, the patient should be checked every 3—5 minutes after the treatment has started to see if the heat from the packs is becoming uncomfortable. Check the patient's skin for signs of abnormal hyperemia such as *erythema ab igne* (localized erythema due to exposure to heat). Typical treatment time is 20—30 minutes.

At the end of the therapy, the packs should be returned to the tank and the towels placed in a storage container to await cleaning. This will avoid cross-contamination from patient to patient.

A special caution should be noted here. The most common cause for malpractice in physiotherapy today is burns, and they are most frequently caused by hot packs. Six layers of toweling between the pack and the patient is the absolute minimum. Be sure to check the patient after 3—5 minutes and monitor periodically during the treatment. Do not just ask the patient how they feel, for the area may have become desensitized. Remove the hot pack, and visually observe the patient's skin.

Types of Packs

HYDROCOLLATOR PACKS

Commercially purchased hot packs should be kept in a tank whose temperature is maintained from 150°—170°F. See Figure 4.6. The packs should be totally submerged in water for a minimum of 30—40 minutes between use to regain the correct temperature. Hydrocollator packs retain their therapeutic temperature for a long time (about 20 minutes) because they contain a silica gel that readily absorbs water.

Hot packs should not be allowed to dry out because this will cause them to become dry and brittle. If the packs are not used frequently, it is best to unplug the unit and let the packs soak in the water. When reactivating the unit, it should be turned on the night before because it takes about 12 hours to build up the proper temperature. Assure that the unit is grounded.

A unit should be drained and cleaned at least once each month, using a mild disinfectant and a nonabrasive soap. Some doctors feel that it is good policy to tag the unit to be sure this procedure is completed. Routinely date and initial the tag after each cleaning.

KENNY HOT PACKS

A therapy that was once popular in the treatment of poliomyelitis utilized the Sister Kenny hot pack, which originated in Australia. These hot moist packs were made of soaked wool or wool-like blanket material from which the hot water was removed by repeated wringings by hand or with a mechanical device. Because these steamed packs contained little moisture, the prolonged heat content was low. The maximum temperature was maintained in the packs for only a few seconds; thus, they could be used at much higher temperatures—up to 140°F at the time of initial application. The packs were left in place from 10 to 20 minutes, and then replaced once or twice. The entire treatment lasted about 1 hour. It was felt that the intense short-term temperature stimulus had a strong effect on the involved nerves and muscles. However, their use today has fallen out of vogue.

THERMAPHORE PACKS

These units are either electrically or chemically controlled hot packs. The electric type is really a dry heat pack (similar to a common heating pad) that develops its moisture from the patient's skin and inhibits evaporation. A thermostat is incorporated to control temperature. The nonelectric chemical unit consists of a flat bag containing salts that produce heat when moistened. It can be used as a substitute for a hot water bag.

Indications and Contraindications

Since heat promotes sweating, it is desir-

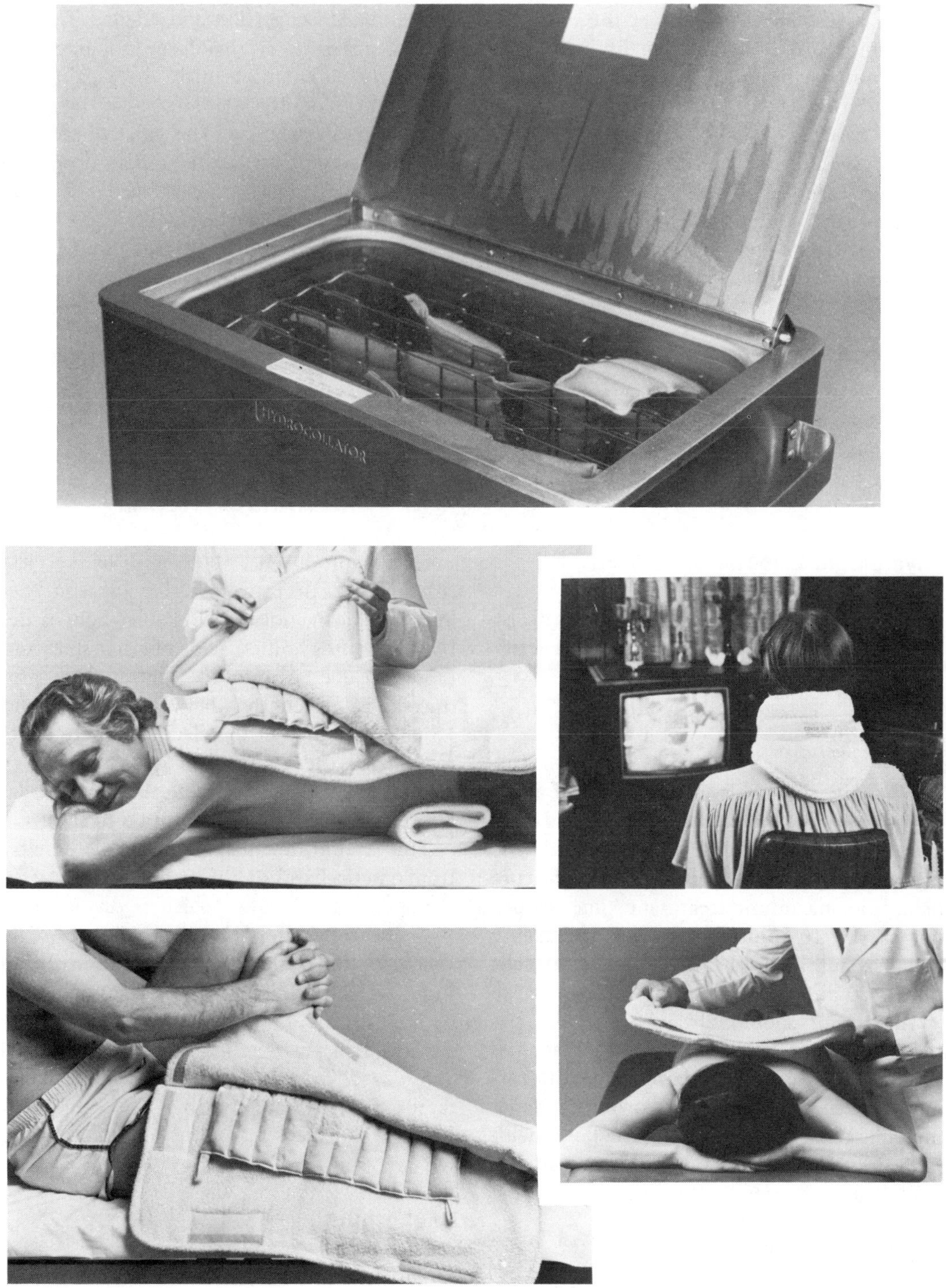

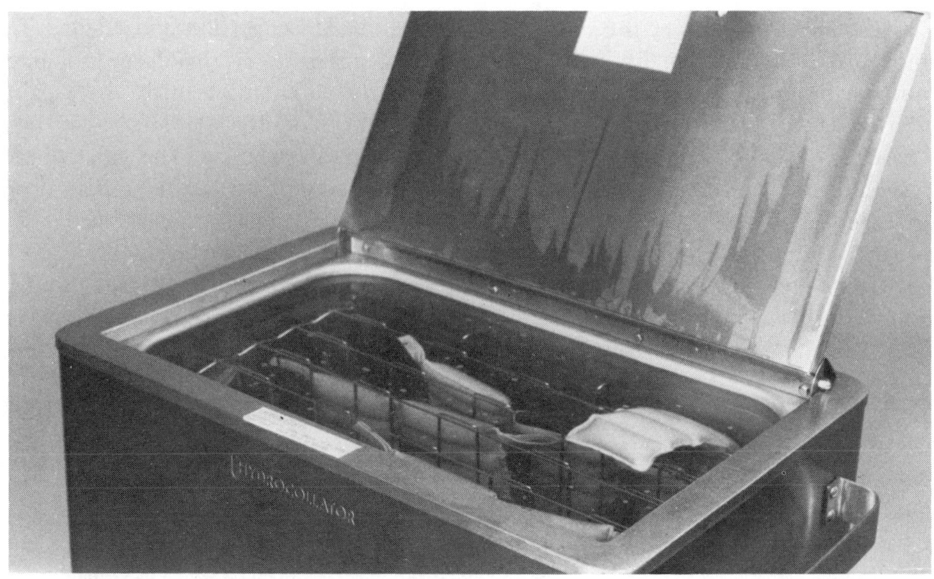

Figure 4.6. *Top photograph,* hot packs should be completely immersed in the water in order to regain their therapeutic temperature after each use. *Bottom photographs,* hydrocollator packs in use (courtesy of the Chatanooga Corporation).

able to use hot packs whenever the objective is to remove toxic wastes from the body. Another primary indication would be whenever the objective is to localize heating on a specific part.

Heat should not be used in any acute strain or sprain, as this will increase swelling, aggravate the complaint, and prolong healing time. Other areas of contraindication or precaution were shown in Table 4.3.

HEATING PADS

Heating pads receive little use in the office of the practitioner or therapist. The use of a heating pad is much more common in a patient's home.

Physiologic Effects

Heating pads transfer dry heat mainly by conduction and less by convection. Penetration is far less than that of moist heat.

Application

When heating pads are used, the following rules should be kept in mind: (1) Never allow a patient to lie on a heating pad. See Figure 4.7. (2) If used during times of acute pain, the maximum treatment time should not exceed 10 minutes. If used after acute pain has subsided, the maximum treatment time is 20 minutes.

The doctor should always advise the patient *not* to use heat until after the pain has subsided. Many authorities feel that the earliest heat should be used following an acute musculoskeletal insult is after 36 hours with professional supervision; 72 hours for "at home" use.

Contraindications

Most patients have the tendency to lie on a heating pad. This has the effect of drying tissues, which later produces or enhances the formation of congestion and edema. The patient's suffering is therefore prolonged, as the increased edema leads to more pain. Unfortunately for the patient, heat tends to produce a vicious cycle. The sedative effect of heat feels good, and this initial deception encourages further use that leads to more pain and stiffness. See Table 4.3.

One way that a heating pad can be used without causing a dehydration effect is to use moistened towels between the heating pad and the skin. If this procedure is used, it must be made certain that the heating pad has been manufactured for this purpose and that there are no exposed wires.

INFRARED THERAPY

Heat is produced at both ends of the electromagnetic spectrum. At the low end (below 4,000 Angstroms), ultraviolet light is derived. At the other end of the spectrum (above 7,000 Angstroms), infrared is produced. Wavelengths between 4,000 and 7,000 Angstroms in the electromagnetic spectrum have the appropriate quantum energy to trigger those photochemical reactions that are responsible for the perception of light.

This section describes that part of the electromagnetic band at the red end of the visible spectrum of light, which is divided into the "near infrared" band that is closer to visible light (7,500—93,097 Angstroms) and the "far infrared" band that extends from 93,097 to 100,000 Angstroms. Heat energy produced in this band is referred to as *radiant heat* or *infrared radiation.* Far infrared is rarely used therapeutically. The units that produce infrared radiation contain glowing red wire coils. See Figure 4.8.

Background

Various units have been developed that direct radiant energy toward the patient. Depending on the exact wavelength that comes from the source, the body reflects the rays,

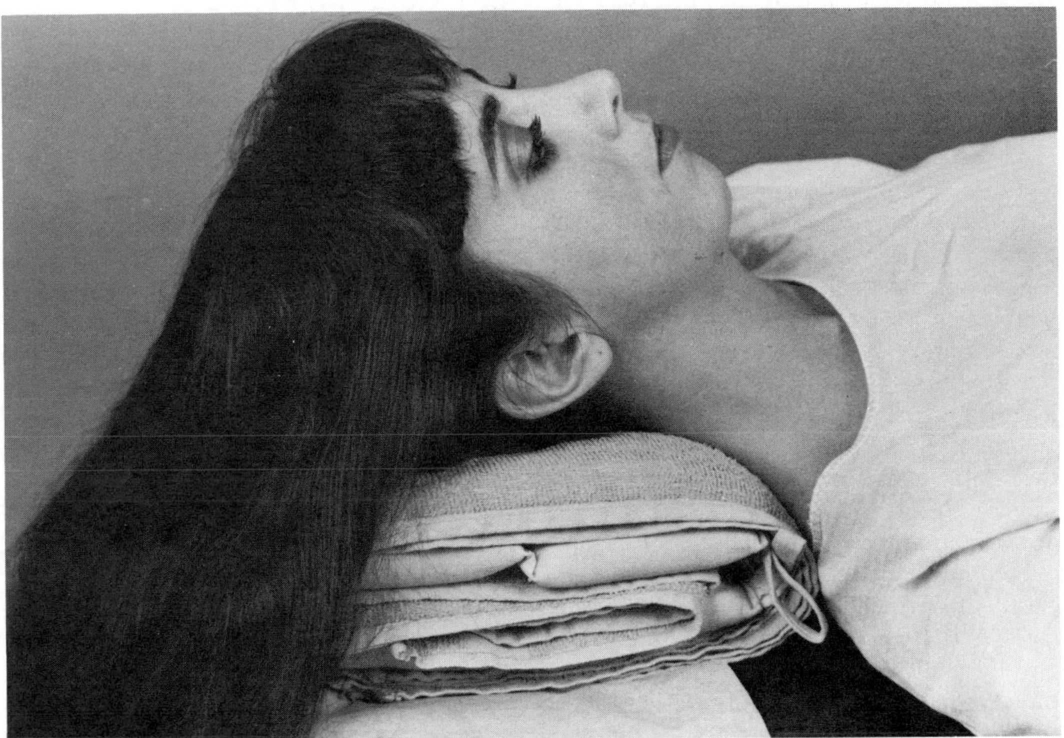

Figure 4.7. Although this patient appears quite comfortable, an electric heating pad or a hot pack (shown) should not be used under the patient.

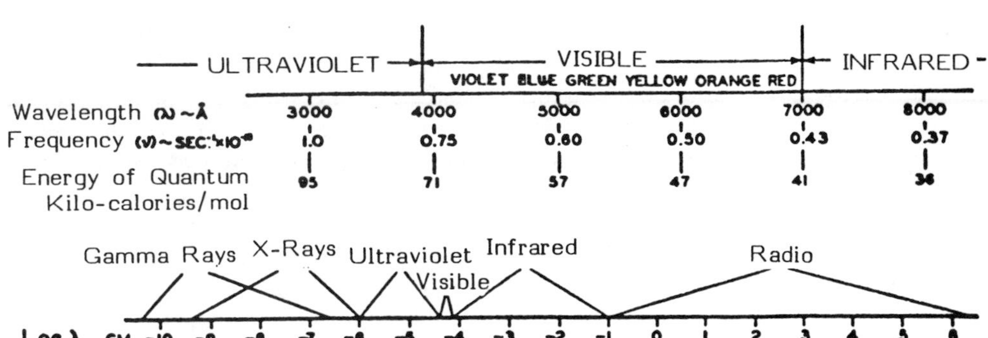

Figure 4.8. The electromagnetic spectrum, showing the relationship of quantum energy to wavelength. The spectral ranges are mapped on two different scales: in Angstrom units on the upper scale, centimeters on the lower scale.[7]

absorbs the rays, or transmits the radiation through the skin. In the infrared region, human skin will absorb the vast majority of the energy, with minimal reflection and transmission. The maximum penetration that can occur with the various types of heat lamps and luminous bulbs in common use is about 3 mm at 12,000 Angstroms, and only a small part of the energy penetrates that deep.

Near infrared wavelengths penetrate less than those of far infrared. The energy of near infrared is almost totally absorbed in the superficial 0.1 mm of the skin. Wavelengths longer than 30,000 Angstroms can be absorbed by the moisture on the surface of the skin. Wavelengths of 100,000 Angstroms, however, may penetrate to a depth of several centimeters.

Common infrared units and relatively enclosed "bakers" have some significant advantages over several other heat modalities. They provide the patient with constant heat for the set treatment time without ever dropping to or below body temperature. They also have a lessened danger of burning the patient because there is no pressure and the area can be viewed during therapy. Because the heat is constant, the operator is better able to control the treatment—hence, the therapeutic results will be more predictable.

Infrared Treating Units

Infrared radiations can also be given off (with varying degrees of efficiency) by any hot object (eg, household electric heaters, hot water bottles, heating pads, stoves, etc). The major difference in a household heater is that the reflector is designed to widely disperse the heat throughout a room, while the more concave reflector of a therapeutic unit is designed to converge the radiations upon a small area.

Infrared treatments are generally administered by units falling into one of two general classifications: (1) luminous and (2) nonluminous.

LUMINOUS INFRARED

Luminous units are also called near, short, or high-temperature-operating (3000 °C) infrared units. Short infrared rays are emitted to some degree by all heated objects (eg, hot water bottle, heating pad). The wavelengths are typically in the range of 1,500—1,200 millimicrons, and the heat penetration depth is about 5—10 millimeters.

The luminous (referring to the associated bright light) infrared generators in use today transfer superficial heat to the body from a tungsten or calcium filament that is heated to high incandescence either in a conical bulb or a clear or red glass, with the reflecting mirror built into the inside of the funnel-shaped part or in a glass bulb (with widely varying wattages) mounted at the focal point of a concave reflecting mirror. The heat source is usually attached to a floorstand apparatus.

Studies have shown that, of the total radiation at a short infrared wavelength, about 30% of the radiation can penetrate deeply into the skin (up to 10 mm). See Figure 4.9.

Such sources of radiation are valuable because they furnish a more penetrating heat and will therefore be quite effective (after the acute stage of an injury has passed) in treating musculoskeletal complaints when such superficial heating is desirable.

An outdated procedure once utilized a "baking" unit, which consisted of a polished reflector shaped like a tunnel that was supported on four or more legs. It was essentially used for treating extremities. The patient was treated for 30—45 minutes. Then, after a 15—30 minute rest period, the limb was massaged. This therapy was thought to be especially effective when pain and stiffness of an extremity was the outstanding feature of a disorder.

The chief source of luminous heat radiation in the professional office are heat lamps. See Figure 4.10. Unfortunately, their utilization in clinical practice has too often been to

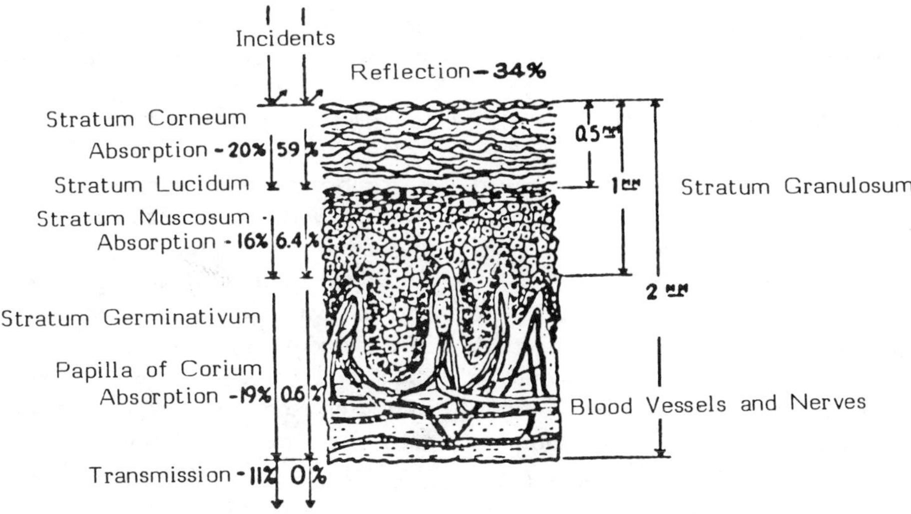

Figure 4.9. The percentage difference of the absorption of infrared by skin in an adult Caucasian, with radiation from tungsten at 2970°K (A) and from iron at 1000°K (B).[8]

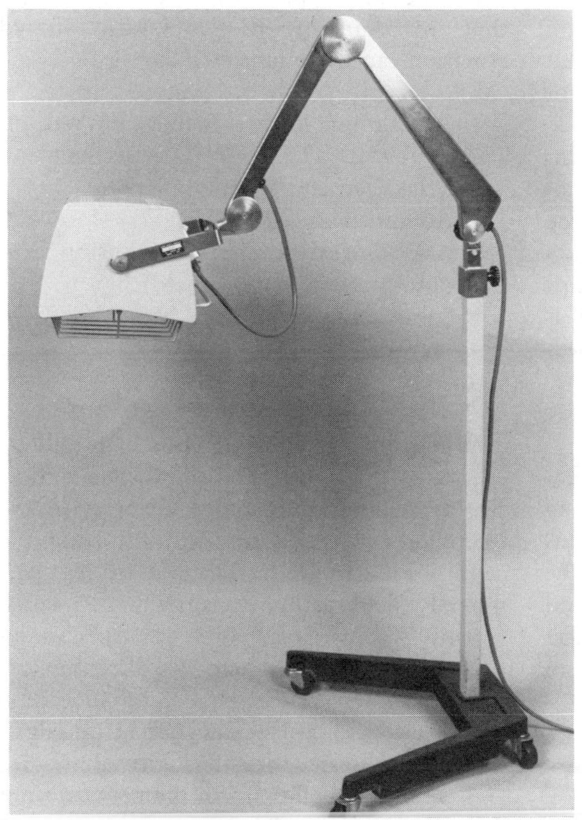

Figure 4.10. A Burdick infrared heating lamp.

"babysit" the patient until the doctor was ready to provide other therapy.

NONLUMINOUS INFRARED

Nonluminous units are sometimes called far, long, or low-temperature-operating (500°—600°C) infrared units. Such rays are emitted by all incandescent bodies.

Units utilizing nonluminous infrared are more often used in the clinical setting than the luminous modalities. The light is not as bright as short infrared, hence the terminology *nonluminous.* This type of lamp is sometimes preferred because it has no glare. The radiations produced are typically between 15,000 and 40,000 millimicrons, and the depth of penetration is about 0.1—0.2 mm.

The commercial generator consists of heating elements that are constructed of resistant materials placed in a suitable reflector. The heating element is often made of coils of resistant metal wires that are wound around a cylindrical or cone-shaped piece of porcelain or similar material that has the property of efficiently reflecting infrared radiation.

In contrast, penetration with luminous infrared is deeper than that for longwave modalities, with the maximum effects of the shortwaves being in a layer of tissue that lies 5—10 mm below the surface of the skin. Hence, longwave nonluminous radiation is more effective when the objective is to influence the peripheral blood vessels, nerve receptors, lymphatics, and other subcutaneous structures.

Individual patients often favor one heat source over another. Some patients seem to be bothered by the bright light of the luminous variety. However, in choosing the modality, the condition of the patient and the objectives the doctor wishes to effect should always be the determining factors in arriving at the clinical decision.

Physiologic Effects

Infrared radiation brings about those physiologic changes commonly associated with superficial heating modalities, with the depth of penetration being predicated on the source of the infrared rays.

The primary effect of infrared (as with any heat modality) is the stimulation of local circulation, with an ensuing hyperemia. Within and a short time after the application of infrared radiation, the skin begins to turn red and the patient perceives a sense of warmth. The erythema, appearing as reddish lines or spots, will generally persist for 15—45 minutes after exposure. However, repeated exposures or a prolonged exposure to infrared rays may lead to permanent pigmentation of the skin. Whereas ultraviolet waves lead to tanning, infrared rays may lead to mottling of the skin. This mottled appearance of the skin due to exposure to heat radiation is referred to as *erythema ab igne.*

As a vasodilator, radiant heat locally increases circulatory and metabolic rates. However, the major physiologic effects of heat that are commonly associated with infrared radiation can be summarized as:

- An almost instant feeling of warmth and erythema
- Relaxation and general sedation
- An antispasmodic effect
- A decongestant effect, enhancing exudate absorption (if not overused)
- Some analgesic effect

Therapeutic Indications

When these physiologic effects are indicated, radiant heat has been shown to be effective as an adjunct to other therapies in the treatment of nonacute arthritis, catarrhal conditions, chronic backache, fractures, peripheral neuropathy, posttraumatic stasis, spasms, sprains, stiff joints, strains, and superficial infections (where hot dressings are indicated). It can also be helpful in certain peripheral vascular diseases such as causalgia, Raynaud's disease, thromboangitis obliterans, and thrombophlebitis, with temperatures not exceeding 85°—90°F, when great care is used to avoid burns because of the poor circulation involved in these disorders.

The depth effects of various heat-therapy modalities are shown in Figure 4.11.

Contraindications and Precautions

Several contraindications and precautions should always be considered when infrared radiation is utilized. Refer to Table 4.3.

Technic of Use

The typical treatment time with standard luminous or nonluminous units is from 20 to 30 minutes, which should always be followed by a rest period and then massage of the area to aid the dispersion of residual heat.

The source of radiation should be placed at a distance of 18—20 inches from the part being treated and at a 90° angle to the surface being treated to avoid overheating at the interface. A dry or sometimes a moistened towel may be placed on the patient's skin below the light, either to protect the patient or prevent drying of tissues. See Figure 4.12.

Caution should be observed in positioning the lamp so that it does not fall on the pa-

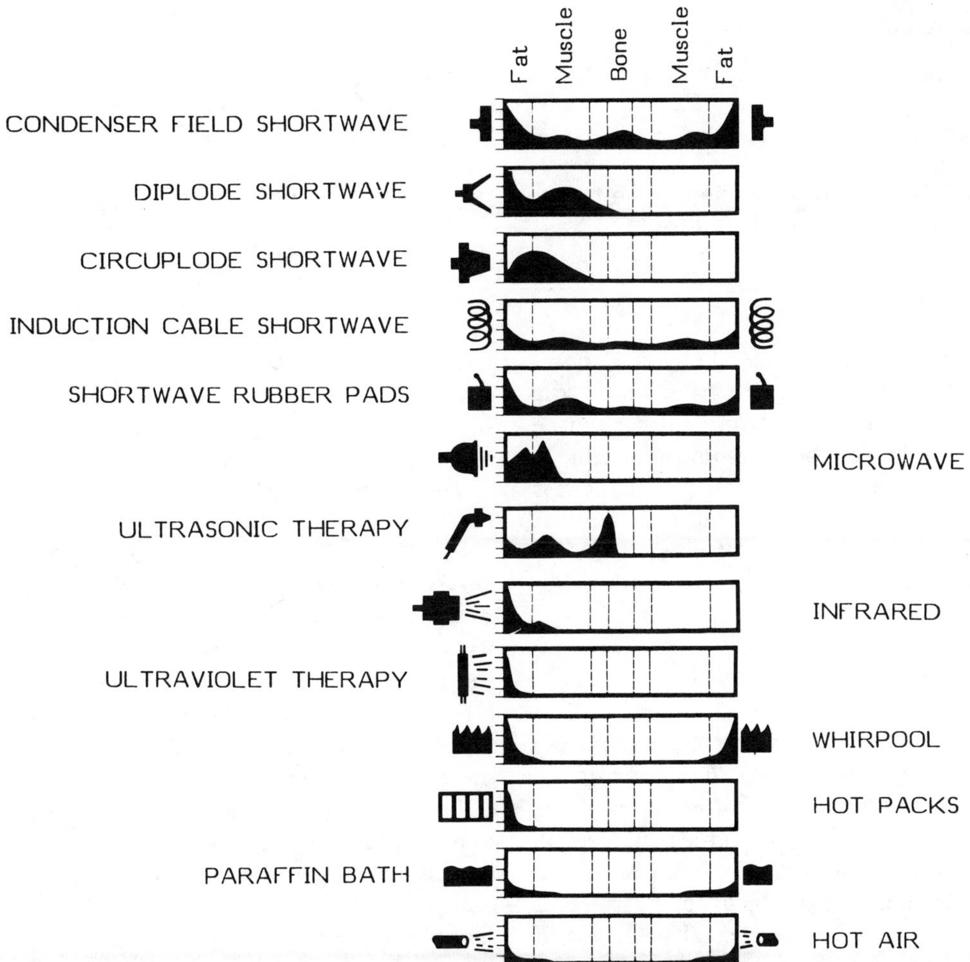

Figure 4.11. Depth effects of various heat therapy modalities.[9]

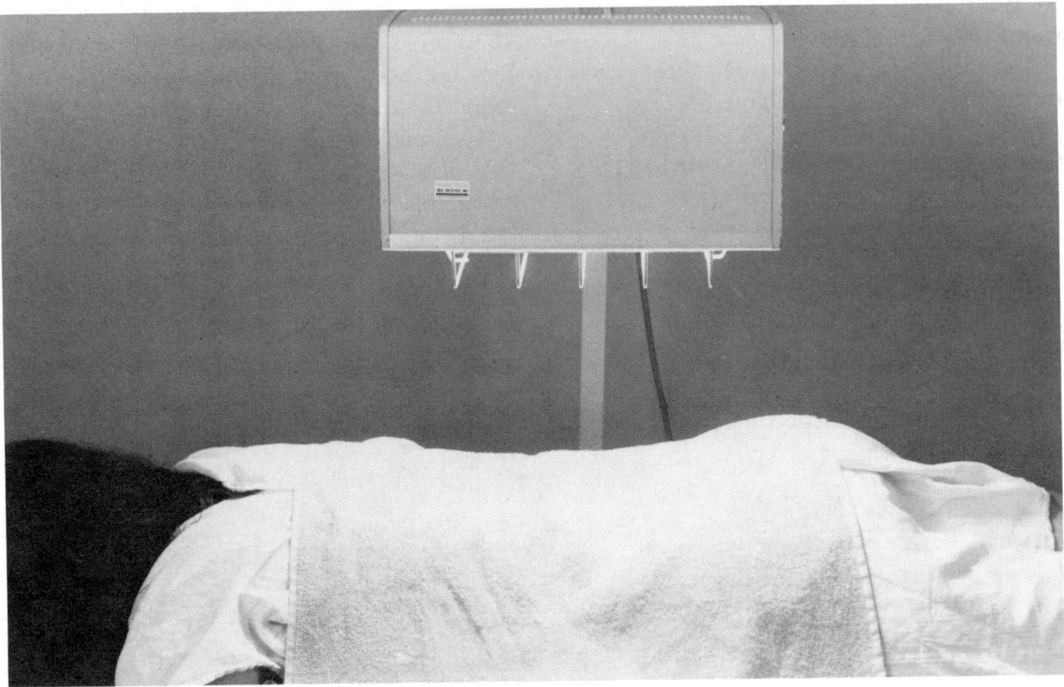

Figure 4.12. The infrared therapy unit should be positioned parallel to the skin, and the skin should be covered by a towel.

tient. If the patient cannot be closely monitored, it is a good idea to have within the patient's easy reach an alarm bell that can be rung if the therapy becomes uncomfortable.

To apply any type of therapeutic light rays intelligently, the physician must be familiar with three basic principles of physics: the inverse square law, the cosine law, and reflector absorption.

INVERSE SQUARE LAW

The intensity of radiation from any light source varies inversely with the square of the distance from the source. For example, if the distance between a lamp and a patient is 36 inches and this distance is reduced in half to 18 inches, the intensity will not be twice as great, but *four times* as great. Knowledge of this law is vital if one is to prevent overdosage when shortening the distance between an energy source and the patient.

COSINE LAW

The energy per square centimeter is proportional to a constant times the cosine of the angle made by a line connecting the energy source and the patient, and a line perpendicular to the patient's body. That constant is the light per square centimeter when the patient is perpendicular to the line joining the light and the patient. Thus, this law states that light rays are most intense when the part to be irradiated is at right angles to a line joining the patient and the light source, and that there is a gradual diminution in intensity as the patient becomes more oblique to this line. At an inclination of 30° (one-third of a right angle), twice the exposure is necessary to produce the same radiation as at 90° (a right angle).

This law indicates that, to obtain the maximum intensity from a light source, the part to be treated should be at right angles to a line joining this part and the light source. See Figure 4.13.

In the application of a light source that is enclosed in a reflector, these laws still apply. However, curved surfaces reflect the rays at so many angles that the reflected rays proceed at a right angle to many portions of the surface area being treated.

REFLECTOR ABSORPTION

It should also be kept in mind that reflected rays are never as intense as direct rays. Some of the rays are sure to be absorbed by the reflector. There is always a considerable loss of energy if the reflector feels hot during use. Thus, it is wise to have the line joining the patient and the light as near to a right angle to the treated part as is possible.

Because all substances absorb light rays to some extent, chemical and biological phenomena result such as fluorescence, phosphorescence, ionization, photoelectric effects, and chemical catalysis.

ULTRAVIOLET LAMPS

Ultraviolet radiation is that portion of the electromagnetic spectrum between visible light and x-radiation. Because of its particular place in the spectrum, it possesses powerful actinic properties, especially at certain bands within the ultraviolet area.

Within the spectrum, ultraviolet rays are divided further into near ultraviolet (320—420 millimicrons); midultraviolet (290—320 millimicrons) where germicidal effects take place; and far ultraviolet (180—290 millimicrons), such as that filtered through window glass. See Figure 4.14.

To utilize ultraviolet radiation therapeutically, the radiating substance producing the ultraviolet rays must be heated to an extremely high temperature (5,400 °F or higher). The major sources of therapeutic ultraviolet radiation are electric arcs, which are produced between electrodes of metal, carbon, or mercury in quartz.

The major characteristics of ultraviolet and infrared rays are compared in Table 4.4.

Physiologic Effects

The primary effect of ultraviolet radiation is photochemical. Whether emitting directly from the sun or from an artificial source, ultraviolet rays have many physiologic effects. The most obvious of these are witnessed in the erythema and tanning effects of sunlight.

Many people go to great length to benefit from the sun's tanning effects. It's amusing, in a way, to think that at the turn of the century a tanned skin was considered to be a sign of a common laborer, while now it is associated with the "in" people—reflecting images of leisurely resorts, tropical beaches, or a pool-side life-style. This is further evidenced by the growing popularity of neighborhood tanning salons.

The best spectral band at which tanning occurs is between 290 and 320 Angstroms. No tanning is produced by wavelengths that are longer than 3,300 Angstroms. The chief mechanism by which tanning occurs is thought to be by means of absorption of the specific quanta by proteins within the melanin granules that are found around the prickle cells of the stratum spinosum. As tanning occurs, the cells are destroyed and this triggers a releasing of a vasodilator substance that is sensitive to temperature changes. This substance then diffuses to the subdermal level where vasodilation is produced. This process occurs over a period of several hours. As the reddening occurs, the stratum corneum thickens in an attempt to provide some protection against further exposure to the sun's rays.

A normal sequel to the reddening process is a migration of granules of melanin toward the surface from the deeper layers of the

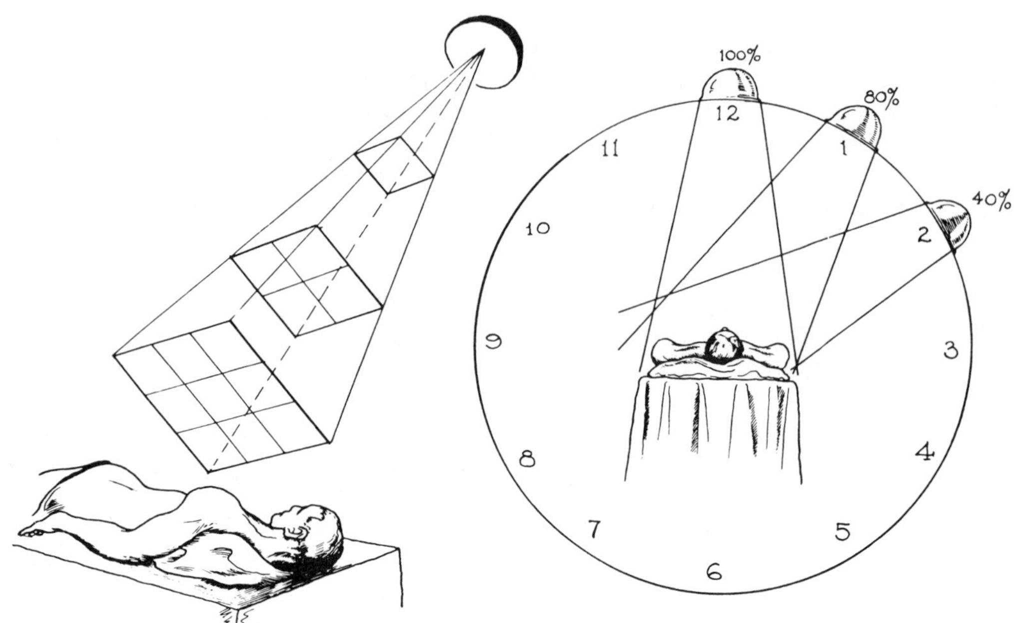

Figure 4.13. *Left,* depicting the Inverse Square Law. *Right,* graphic representation of Lambert's Cosine Law. This law may be visualized by imagining the face of a clock and picturing the patient as being at the center of the clock's face, with the light source at 12 o'clock. In this position, the light rays would be at right angles to the patient and maximum intensity would be obtained. If the light source is moved either to 1 o'clock or 11 o'clock, the rays will fall upon the patient at an angle, and there will be only 80% of maximum intensity. If the light source is moved further to 10 o'clock or 2 o'clock, the inclination of the rays will be even greater, and only 40% of the maximum intensity of radiation will be obtained.

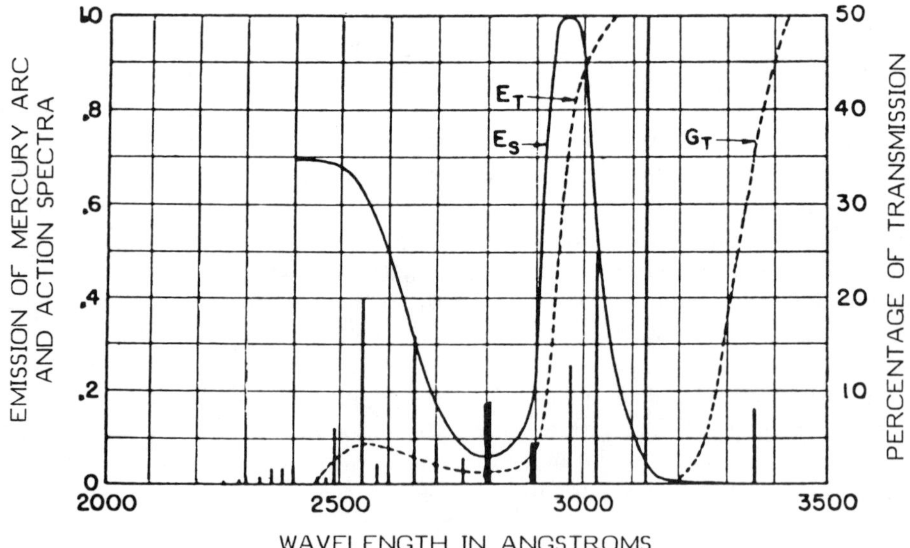

Figure 4.14. Various phenomena in the ultraviolet portion of the electromagnetic spectrum. The vertical lines at the bottom of the graph indicate the position and relative intensity of "hot quartz" mercury vapor lamps.[10]

Table 4.4. Comparison of Ultraviolet and Infrared Radiations

	Long Ultraviolet	*Short Ultraviolet*	*Long Infrared*	*Short Infrared*
Wavelength (millimicrons).	400—200	200—180	150,000—15,000	15,000—7,200
Penetration	0.3—0.5 mm	0.1—0.3 mm	0.1—0.3 mm	10—30 mm

	Ultraviolet	*Infrared*
Appearance of erythema..	Lighter red, sharp borders	Dark red spots or pattern
Development of erythema.	After several hours	Immediate
Duration of erythema.....	Several hours/days	Less than 1 hour
Pigmentation............	Diffuse tanning	Mottled
Tolerance...............	Constantly increases	Occasionally develops

skin. This tanning process occurs without oxygen. A second type of tanning may occur; but it requires oxygen and it is reversible. It consists of a deeper darkening of preformed pigment and occurs from prolonged exposure to radiations with wavelengths of 3,000—4,400 Angstroms (eg, sunlight, carbon-arc source).

Other effects, some well documented and some debatable, are summarized below:

1. Chemical or antirachitic effects occur. When ultraviolet rays with wavelengths below 320 millimicrons are absorbed in the corneum, upper layers of the skin, hair follicles, sebaceous glands, and sweat glands, vitamin D forms as a by-product. Calcium absorption and calcium-phosphorus metabolism are also enhanced.
2. Serum globulin, reticulocytes, and red blood cells are increased.
3. Skin tone, color, elasticity, and secretory functions are improved.
4. Muscular tone is improved.
5. Bactericidal and related actions occur. Several studies indicate that some bacteria, fungi, and viruses are destroyed at about 2,652 Angstroms, with a lethal rate of 90% at 2,537 Angstroms.
6. Biologic effects occur. Ultraviolet tends to increase circulatory and metabolic rates, which, in turn, accelerate cellular growth and activity.

Mercury-Vapor Arcs

These types of artificial ultraviolet production are the result of a mercury vapor that is encased in a quartz envelope and then activated by an electric current.

HOT QUARTZ LAMPS

This category of artificial ultraviolet has a high vapor pressure in the order of 1 to 10 atmospheres. Such units are the most common type used for applying therapeutic ultraviolet radiation. See Figure 4.15. The larger of these lamps produce minimal erythema, using a 15-second exposure with an arc—skin distance of 30 inches.

The Kromayer type is water cooled; thus, it has the advantage of being able to be used close to the patient's skin without danger of burning the patient by radiant heat. There is also a small orificial unit that can be safely used for about 5 seconds at 2 inches.

COLD QUARTZ LAMPS

This category of ultraviolet has a low vapor pressure of about 0.001 atmosphere. Because both the current and pressure are low, the glow of the tube is minimal and the tube is maintained at a relatively cool temperature.

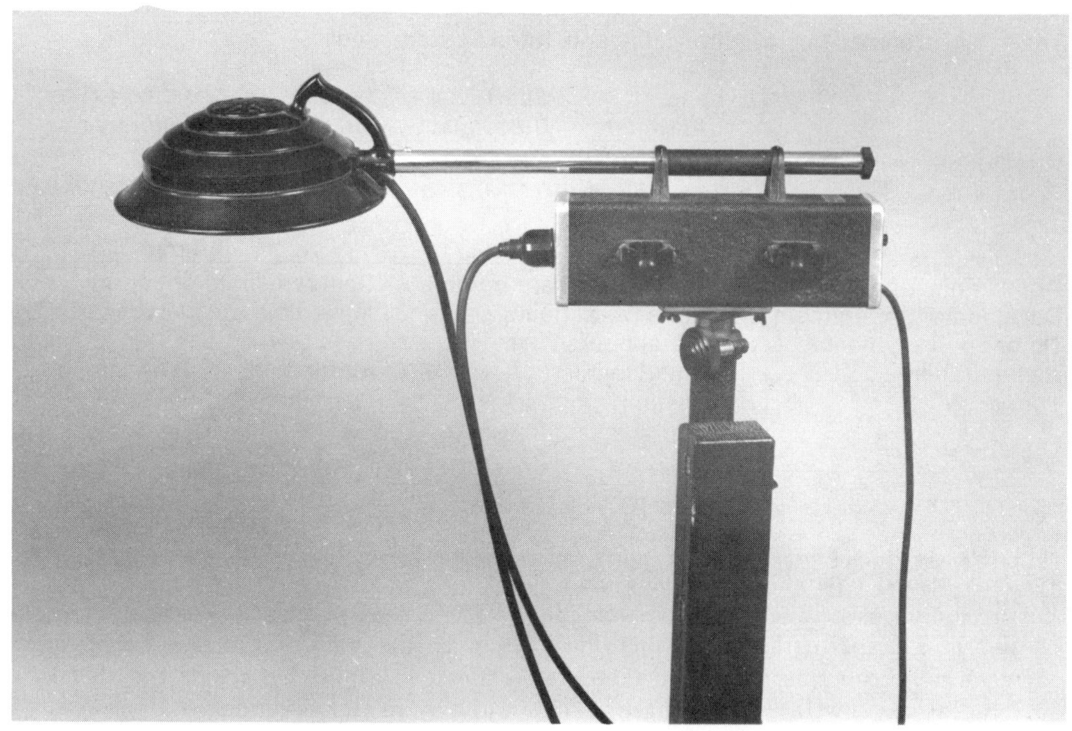

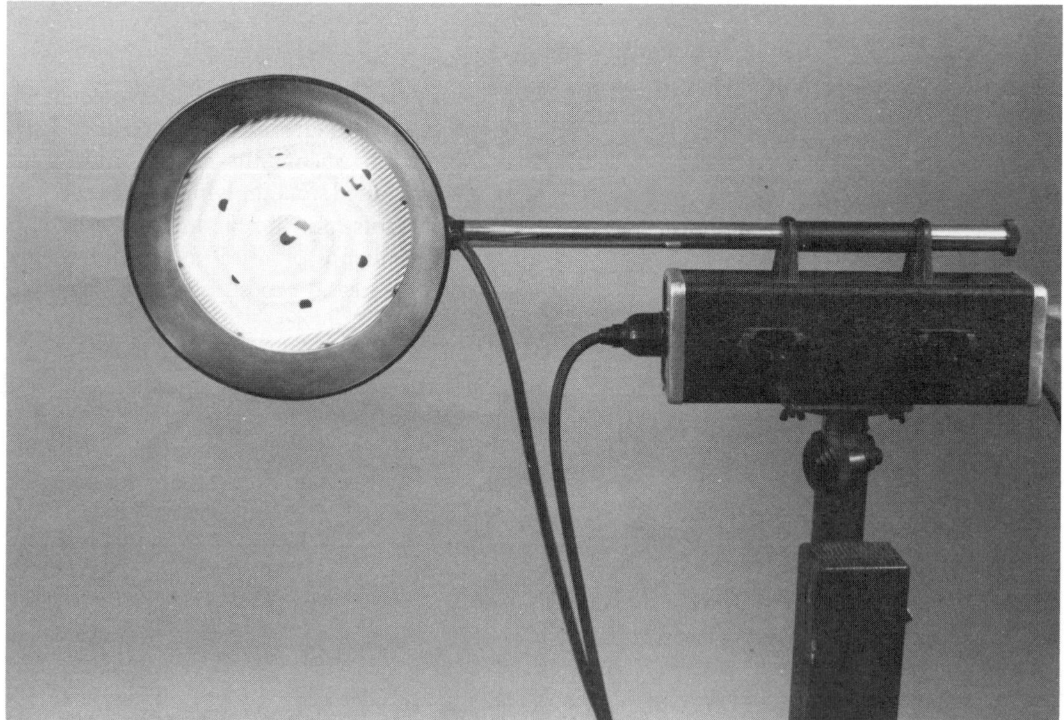

Figure 4.15. A hot quartz ultraviolet unit.

This allows the lamp to be placed near the body or inserted into a body orifice (eg, external ear, throat). See Figure 4.16.

At 253 millimicrons, the ultraviolet band has enough penetrating power to (1) stimulate biologic and therapeutic effects, (2) stimulate erythema without considerable pigmentation; and (3) bring forth the antirachitic effect. The primary effect is bactericidal, and because of this, such units tend to be used almost exclusively in air disinfection (eg, germicidal lamps).

SUN LAMPS

The various sunlamps available have a medium pressure of about 0.1 atmosphere. The two major types are fluorescent sunlamps and reflector sunlamps (RS lamps), both of which can produce an erythema within a few minutes.

Carbon Arcs

Carbon-arc lamps are rarely used therapeutically. Their wavelengths range from infrared to far ultraviolet. They were once used chiefly because of their antirachitic effect; however, modern nutritional practices have made their use obsolete. Today, they are primarily used in the printing industry to expose light-sensitive lithography plates or films.

Black Light Lamps

Blacklight "Wood's rays" are used diagnostically because of their ability to detect fluorescent materials in the skin and hair in certain diseases (eg, tinea capitis). The terms "Wood's light" and "Wood's lamps" are frequently used synonymously for Wood's rays, even though they are technically misnomers.[11]

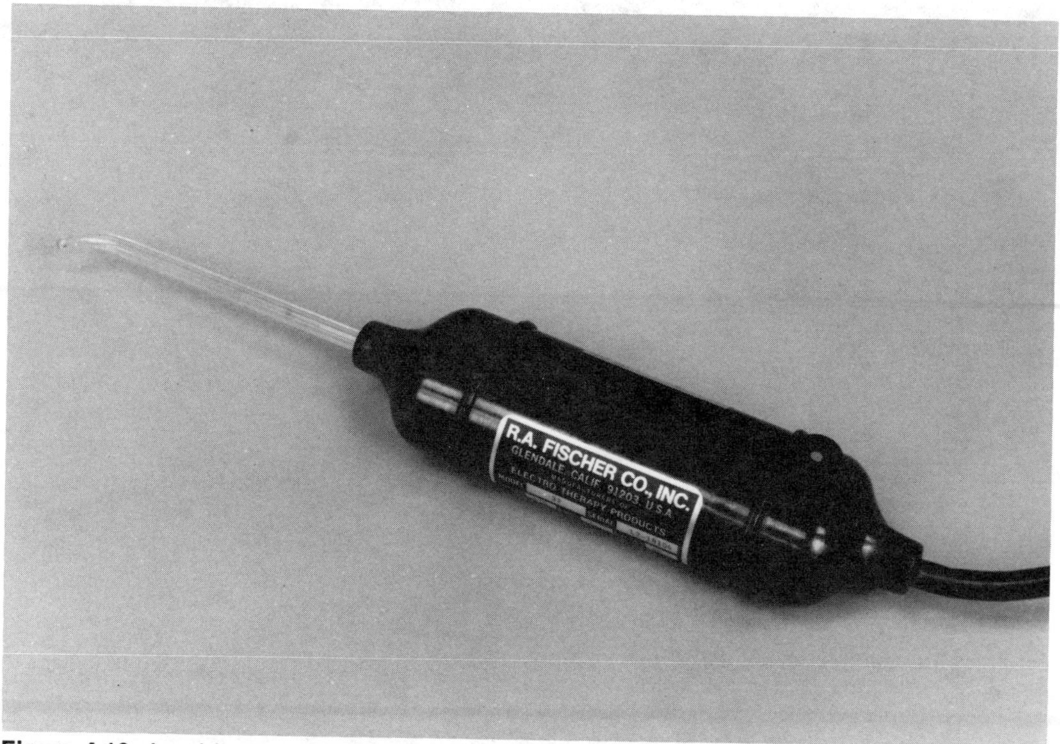

Figure 4.16. A cold quartz ultraviolet unit with an orificial applicator.

Application and Dosage

Because of the danger of severe sunburn, care must be taken in the application of ultraviolet (UV) radiation. Both the patient and the operator must be careful not to receive excessive exposure. Careful screening or draping will assure that only the part to be treated will be exposed. See Figure 4.17. As the eyes are especially sensitive to ultraviolet rays, both the patient and the operator must wear special goggles during the time of application.

ESTABLISHING THE MINIMAL ERYTHEMAL DOSE

As the ultraviolet dosage must be carefully regulated, a minimal dose should be established prior to the first treatment. This is arrived at by establishing the minimum quantity of ultraviolet radiation that can be used at a specific distance over a set period of time. That is, because the most quickly evident reaction to ultraviolet radiation is erythema, the exact exposure necessary to develop erythema determines an individual's degree of intrinsic (reactive) sensitivity.

Sleeve Test. The typical testing procedure is to drape the patient so that a small area on the abdomen, inner thigh, or volar surface of the forearm is exposed. Areas of new skin, scar tissue, sunburn, abrasions, or with thick hair should be avoided. The exposed area is covered with a cloth or piece of flexible cardboard that has five or six 1-inch square openings (cut-outs), separated approximately 1 inch apart. The UV lamp is then placed 30 inches from the skin if it is a hot quartz lamp, 1 inch from the skin if it is a cold quartz lamp, or in slight contact with the skin if it is an orificial lamp.

If a new hot quartz lamp is being used, the openings are exposed at 5-second inter-

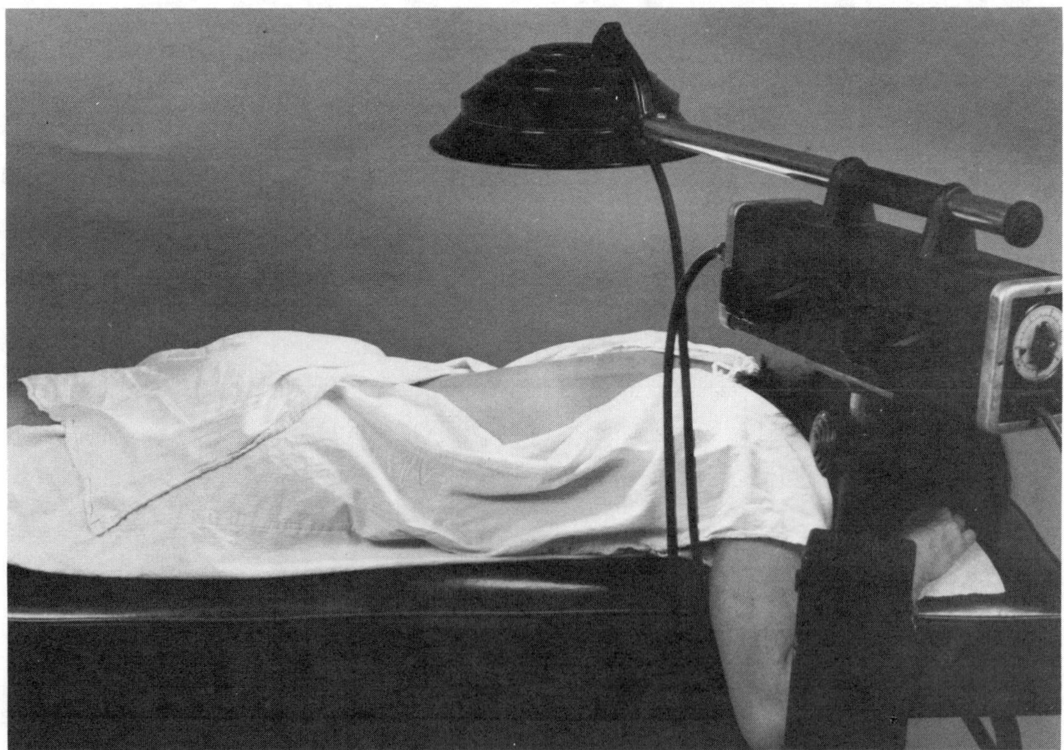

Figure 4.17. Treating with a hot quartz ultraviolet unit.

vals and then covered. That is, opening #1 is covered at the end of 5 seconds, opening #2 at the end of 10 seconds, opening #3 at the end of 15 seconds, etc. If a cold quartz lamp is used, the same technique is used at 1-second intervals.

The minimal erythemal dose is that patch area where the erythema is first perceptible after about an 8-hour period and then disappears after 24 hours. If that area had been treated at a distance of 30 inches for 5 seconds, this would be the MED (minimal erythemal dose) for that particular patient.

As a general rule once the MED has been established, the patient can then be safely exposed an additional 15 seconds each succeeding treatment.

Some therapists establish an MED initially for their ultraviolet units and use this dosage on each patient. However, we recommend that an MED be established for *each* patient to avoid the danger of producing severe itching or sunburn from an overdose. A new MED should be established for a patient that has not been treated with ultraviolet rays in 3 months.

Experience has shown that individuals with fair or light complexions are considerably more sensitive to UV rays than are individuals with darker skin tones, and females are about 20% more sensitive than males. Such reasons add to the importance of establishing an MED for each patient.

In applying ultraviolet radiation, it is well to be aware that any extrinsic or intrinsic factor which might enhance increased skin circulation will increase an individual's sensitivity to ultraviolet rays. Different areas of the skin (eg, those rarely exposed to the sun) and certain applied or ingested substances (eg, photosensitive drugs) may also make one part of the body more sensitive than another.

DOSAGE REACTIONS

The degrees of erythema can be classified into four groups of severity:

- *First degree.* This is the MED. There is slight reddening of the skin, without desquamation, and possibly a slight itching may be produced. This result follows after what is often called a *tonic dose.* A reaction below this level is referred to as being the result of a *suberythemal dose.*
- *Second degree.* This resembles a mild sunburn. A definite reddening of the skin occurs, followed by slight desquamation, with some associated sensation of itching or burning. The erythema typically becomes visible in about 6 hours and usually fades within 2 days.
- *Third degree.* A marked reddening of the skin occurs after 3 hours, some edema and blisters develop, and this stage is followed by obvious desquamation, which is exhibited by epithelial scales and epidermal peeling or shedding in sheets that is similar to that following a severe sunburn. The associated pruritus and hyperesthesia can be quite uncomfortable.
- *Fourth degree.* Intense reddening occurs after a couple of hours, which is followed by blistering and peeling that persists for several days. Exudation and deep pigmentation often occur. This condition is sometimes called a reaction to a *bactericidal* or *destructive dose.*

TREATING WITH HOT QUARTZ

Hot quartz is used primarily in the management of dermatologic complaints (eg, psoriasis, acne).

The operator should preheat the lamp for about 5 minutes before application and be certain that any ointments, lotions, medications, or cosmetics have been removed from the skin before an exposure is made. The lamp should be centered over the draped patient and placed parallel to the surface of the body to be treated. The distance from the light source to the skin should be carefully measured, and the exposure time should be exactly set on a timer.

Since a gradual tolerance to ultraviolet rays will increase with each treatment up to a point, the dosage can be increased at each therapy session. If treatments are applied each day, the dosage is normally increased by one-half the MED each day. Although tolerance is accumulative to a great extent, the maximum dosage to the patient should not exceed 10 MEDs. If treatments are administered less frequently than daily, then the rate of increase should be relatively less.

TREATING WITH COLD QUARTZ

Spot and Grid Exposures. These techniques are generally used over open wounds or ulcerated areas of the skin (eg, decubitus or varicose ulcers). As with hot quartz applications, foreign materials should be removed from the skin prior to exposure. No prewarming time is necessary, but the exposure time should be exact. The lamp should be held parallel to the skin at a distance of 1 inch. It should be noted that mercurochrome enhances the effects of UV rays.

Orificial Exposures. The sanitary applicator should be sterilized by being prewarmed for about 15 seconds prior to use. The patient and the operator must be shielded from the UV rays during both this warmup and the actual therapy. If the throat is to be treated, for example, the applicator is then inserted into the oropharyngeal orifice and held about half an inch from the mucous membranes. See Figure 4.18. The applicator is turned on, and an exposure is made (usually for 10—15 seconds). Following the therapy, the applicator should be cleaned with alcohol, sterilized, and stored according to the manufacturer's instructions.

Indications, Contraindications, and Precautions

The use of ultraviolet radiation is indicated when its physiologic, antirachitic, bactericidal, biologic, or chemical effects would be considered beneficial to the disorder at hand. See Table 4.5.

PARAFFIN

Paraffin is a white, tasteless, wax-like substance that is often used for sealing jars and in making candles. It may be used for therapy in the office or at home by the trained patient. While not widely used in out-care services, it has been found to be of considerable value, especially with arthritic pain and disability.

Background

Paraffin therapy is essentially hot wax that consists of seven parts paraffin and one part mineral oil, according to most authorities. Some authorities, however, recommend a 4:1 ratio. Regardless, the purpose of the mineral oil is to lower the melting temperature of the wax. Without it, the melted wax would be far too hot for therapeutic purposes.

The wax is melted in a double boiler, which is usually the 1½ quart size. Professional tubs are available commercially that typically have a preset temperature of 125°—130°F after warmup, which is near the typical melting point of 125.6°F. See Figure 4.19.

Because the paraffin-oil mixture has a low specific heat, it can be applied directly to the skin if the circulation to the part is normal. Before application, the part to be treated should be cleaned and dried, the thermesthetic sense should be ascertained to be normal, and all jewelry on the part to be treated should be removed.[12]

The temperature of the melted wax should be checked with a thermometer, but a finger pretest by the doctor or therapist will even more assure the apprehensive patient that the mixture is not too hot.

Physiologic Effects

Paraffin offers the same physiologic effects and advantages as any other form of superficial heat that is transferred by conduction. Some long infrared rays of brief duration

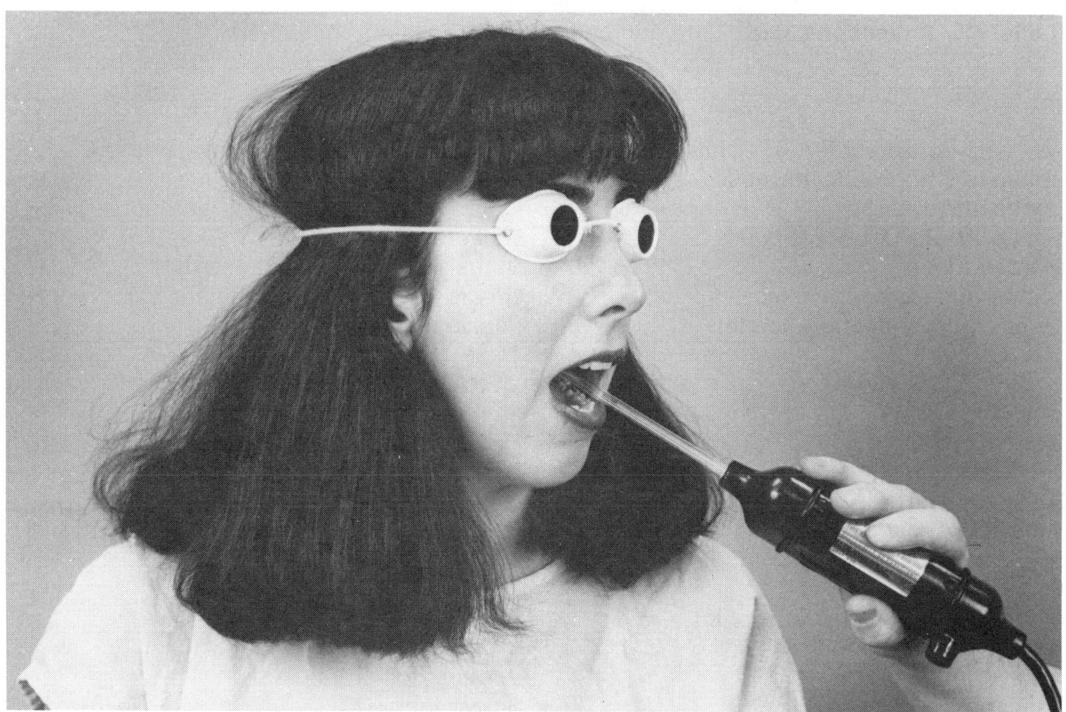

Figure 4.18. Note the use of protective goggles when ultraviolet rays are used. Both the patient and the operator, or anyone else in attendance, should wear protective goggles.

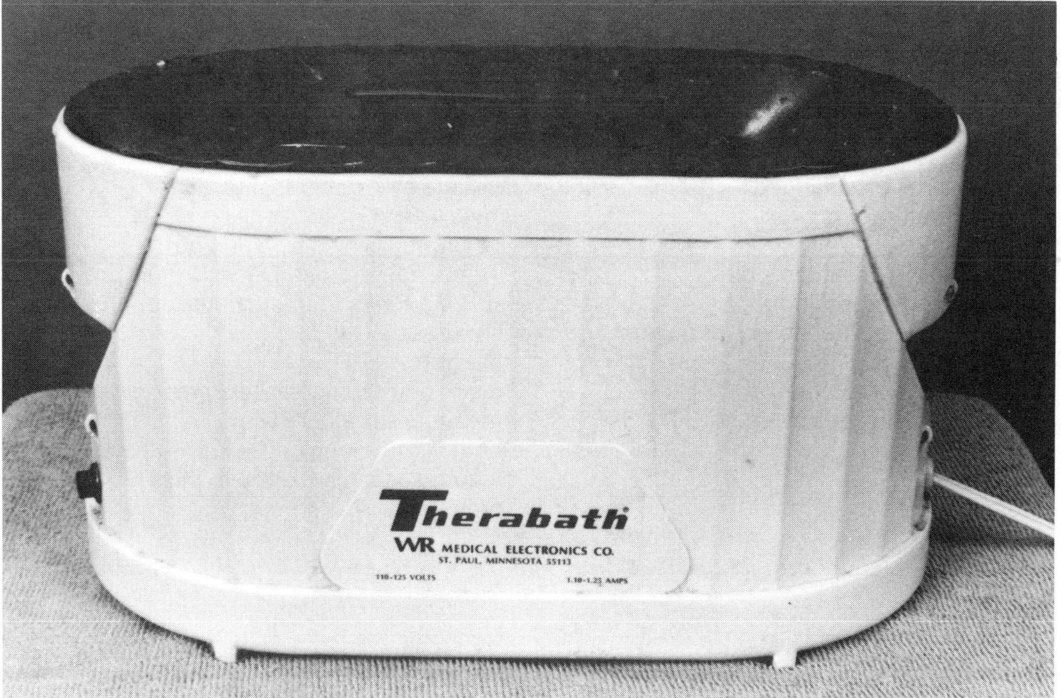

Figure 4.19. A paraffin wax unit.

Table 4.5. Indications and Contraindications of Ultraviolet Radiation

PRIMARY INDICATIONS

Dermatologic disorders (eg, chronic psoriasis, acne vulgaris, abscess, boils, tinea, etc)
For antibacterial effects
Herpes zoster
Lupus vulgaris
Open wounds (septic, aseptic)
Oropharyngitis (except for beta-streptococcal infections)
Osteomalacia (pregnancy, lactation)
Rickets
Sinusitis (eyes well protected)
Ulcers (eg, decubitus, indolent, varicose)

OTHER CONSIDERATIONS

Acne conglobata
Acne rosacia
Acne varioliformis
Adenoma sebaceum
Alopecia areata
Alopecia prematuria
Arthritis (atrophic, hypertrophic)
Asthma (bronchial)
Bone/joint tuberculosis
Bronchitis
Burns (mild)
Chilblains
Chlorosis
Delayed fracture union
Dermatitis herpetiformis
Dermatophytosis
Erysipelas
Erythema induratum
Impetigo contagiosa
Pityriasis rosea
Pruritus (secondary)
Pustular folliculitis
Scleroderma
Scrofuloderma
Sinusitis
Spasmophilia

GENERAL CONTRAINDICATIONS

Active and progressive pulmonary tuberculosis
Adrenal insufficiency
Arteriosclerosis (advanced)
Diabetes mellitus
Eczema (acute)
Exanthema (eg, measles, pox)
Heart disease (advanced)
Hemophilia and other hemorrhagic disorders
Hepatic insufficiency
Herpes simplex (controversial)
Hyperthyroidism
Keratosis
Keloids
Lupus erythematosus
Malignancy
New skin (eg, posttraumatic)
Over the eye, genitals, buttocks, female breast
Over sunburn or x-radiation burns
Patients on photosensitive drugs (eg, sulfonamides, tetracyclines, quinine, green soap)
Pellegra
Poison plant toxicosis (eg, poison ivy)
Precancerous skin lesions
Renal insufficiency
Weeping eczema (controversial)
Xeroderma

Note: Extreme caution must be used with infants, the elderly, or severely debilitated patients.

may also be involved because the heat is quite penetrating. In addition, warm paraffin tends to soften indurated or calloused skin.

Application

The melted paraffin-oil mixture can be applied by brush, but the most common method used is to slowly dip the involved part (eg, a hand or foot) into the wax and then remove it from the pot. See Figure 4.20. The part is repeatedly reimmersed from 7 to 10 times or more to build up a thick coat of wax (eg, a white glove-like appearance). Upon each reimmersion, the sensation of heat will be greatly diminished.

After the wax cools somewhat to a semisolid state (ie, a degree of palpable firmness), it should be covered with a paper towel or wax paper, wrapped in a heavy towel, and left to rest for 15—20 minutes. The wax is then removed. It easily peels from the skin because of the mineral oil content. See Figure 4.21. The part should appear quite reddish, moist, and soft. Next, an important part of the therapy, the part should be massaged and passively exercised (mobilized). The entire treatment usually takes about 25—30 minutes.

A variation of paraffin dipping is called paraffin immersion. After the part has been dipped 7—10 times, the part is removed and the paraffin is allowed to solidify. The part is then returned to the tub (which should have a padded edge) and allowed to remain there from 20 to 30 minutes, or until the paraffin melts.

Paraffin can also be painted on with a brush or poured on from a cup to a body part. The tub temperature for these procedures is about 160°F. Either procedure is messy and of questionable value because of the heat lost between applications to large areas of the body.

Hot paraffin wraps were once commonly used. The part is dipped once or twice and then covered with one thickness of gauze. This procedure is repeated about 7—10 times, and the final dip is covered with wax paper or paper towels. It is a wasteful procedure because it is difficult to save the wax, and few, if any, benefits over the regular dipping procedure have been noted.

HOME THERAPY

Many practitioners provide their arthritic patients with a commercial heating unit (Therabath) for home use after the patient has been properly trained in the technique. While contraindicated in acute rheumatoid or septic arthritis, this therapy is an excellent method of applying heat to painful, stiff, and deformed extremity joints after the acute stage has passed.

The typical routine is to have the patient use the paraffin coating twice a day for about a month and then once a day thereafter if necessary. Chronic cases may be benefited by using this method for months or years. To achieve maximum benefit, the patient must be instructed to follow each dipping session with massage and exercise of the involved part(s). For example, each digit should be passively moved throughout the range of motions up to but not exceeding the threshold of discomfort. This is followed by a few minutes of active exercise. If, for example, the hand is being treated, an attempt should be made to have the thumb touch each finger. See Figure 4.22. The patient can also be instructed to squeeze a moderately soft rubber ball. Similar exercises can be devised for the feet.

Indications, Contraindications, and Precautions

Paraffin therapy is primarily indicated for nonacute arthritic joints, especially where there is limited mobility. Several authorities also recommend it for bursitis, postfracture stiffness, strains and sprains, tenosynovitis, and indurated scar tissue or contractures that limit motion. Paraffin should not be used

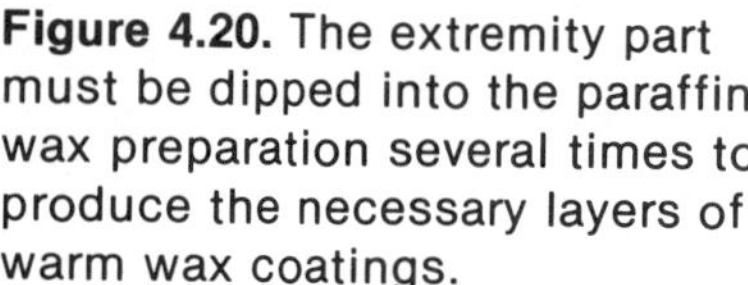

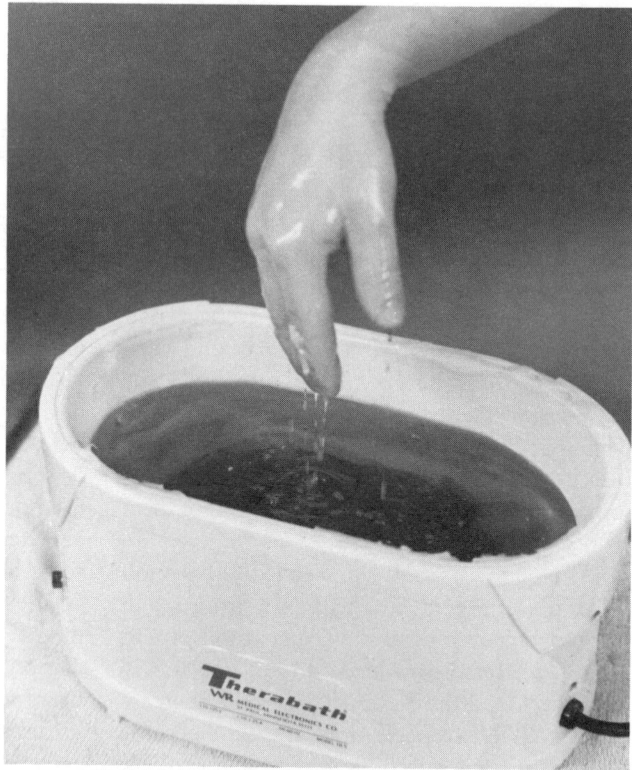

Figure 4.20. The extremity part must be dipped into the paraffin wax preparation several times to produce the necessary layers of warm wax coatings.

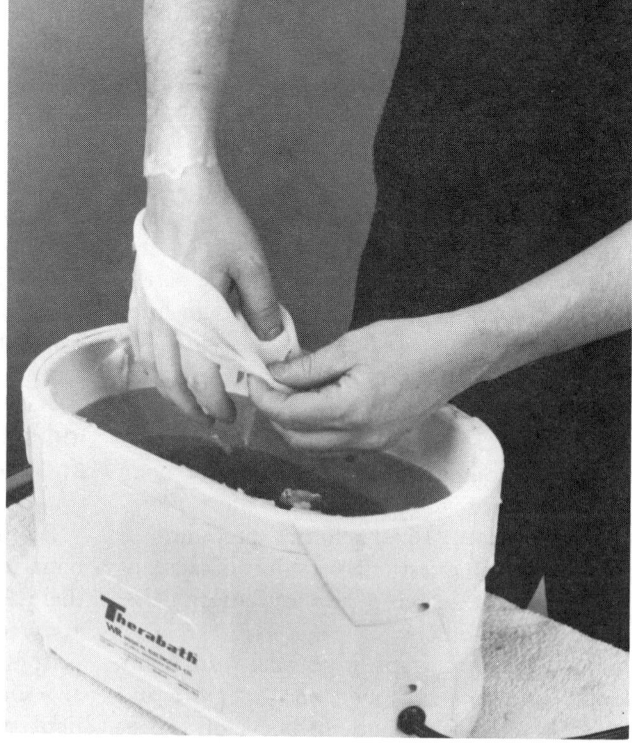

Figure 4.21. Used paraffin peels off readily. It may then be returned to the tank.

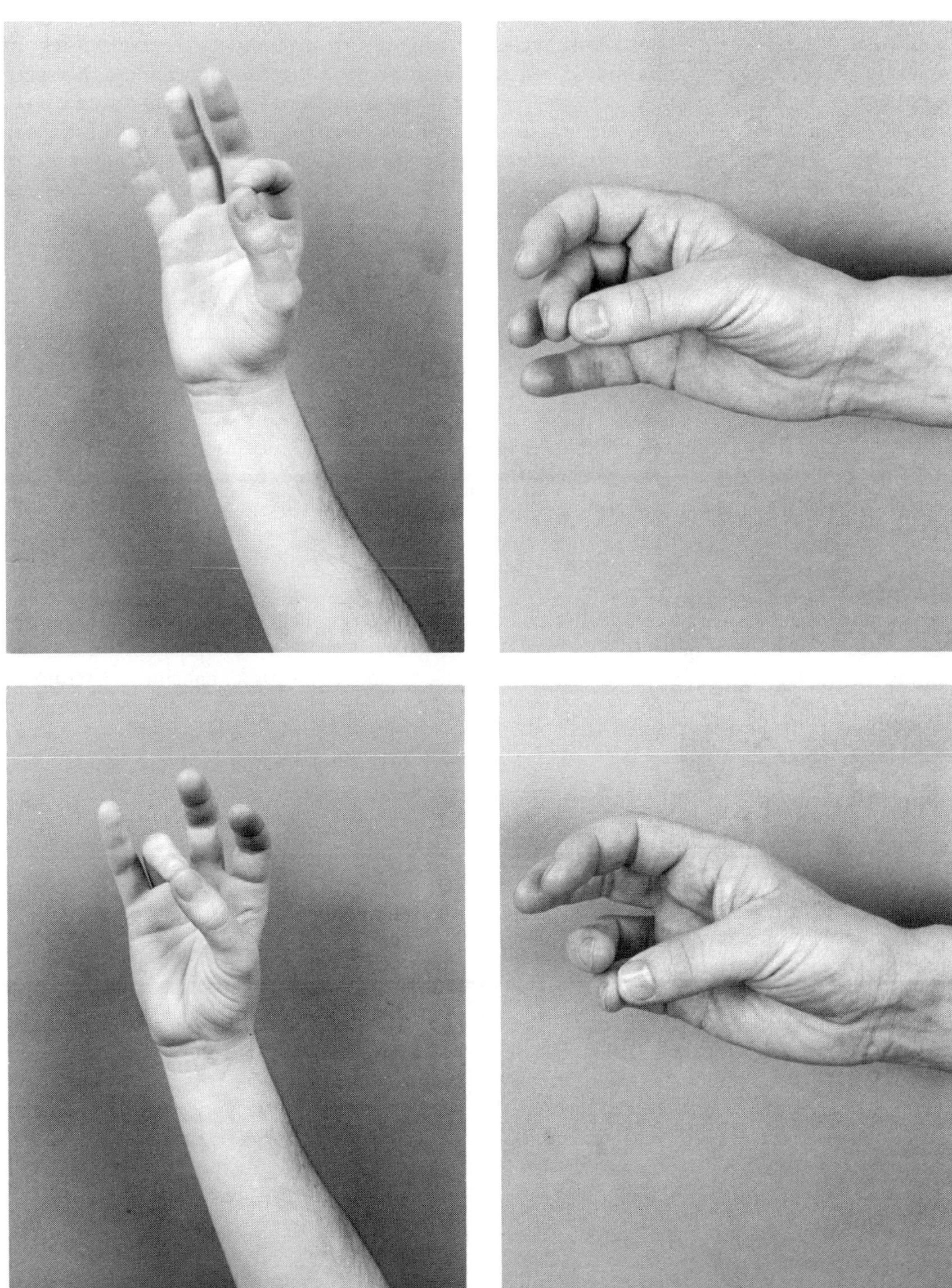

Figure 4.22. After the paraffin has been removed, massage and exercise should be performed to enhance joint mobility and tissue elasticity. Photographs show posttherapy active thumb-to-finger exercises.

over open wounds, abrasions, acute skin disorders, or where there is diminished sensation.

Following use, the wax can be returned to the melting pot. Used wax will again become sterile after it remains at the melting point for about an hour. A small amount of wintergreen can be added to used paraffin to disguise the odor of accumulating skin debris.

The heating unit should be cleaned at least every other month and the wax-oil mixture replaced. Most units have a disposable container that holds the wax. The tank can be cleaned with soap and water, and hardened areas of wax drippings can be removed by scrubbing with a rough cloth soaked in alcohol.

Common paraffin is quite flammable. Thus, caution must be taken to keep it away from an open flame. A double boiler must be used to heat the wax and oil.

FLUIDOTHERAPY

In the earlier parts of this chapter, several different types of heat modalities were described. An explanation was given of those modalities that transfer either wet or dry heat primarily by conduction (eg, hot moist packs, electric heating pads, paraffin) or by radiation (eg, infrared and ultraviolet units). In subsequent chapters, the deep heating diathermies and units that transfer heat through water (hydrotherapy) will be described. In the concluding section of this chapter, attention will be focused on one of the newest modalities on the market today—Fluidotherapy. See Figures 4.23 and 4.24.

Background

Fluidotherapy is a relatively economical multifunctional modality that simultaneously applies heat, micromassage, levitation, stimulation, and pressure oscillations. This modern innovation was first developed by Ernst Henley to treat lesions of the extremities. Its main purpose is to develop intense therapeutic heat as it swirls a mixture of air and small cellulose particles around a submerged part. The patient's extremity is inserted into an enclosed port located either at the side or top of the unit; then the unit's timer, temperature regulator, and blower intensity controls are set and activated. See Figure 4.25.

Fluidotherapy units are essentially dry whirlpools. A unit encases solid particles of fine cellulose (Cellex) that are actually finely ground corn cobs, which are rapidly whirled in the air by means of an extremely high-powered blower. Because of the rapid movement of the fine particles against the skin, combined with the movement of the extremity that occurs passively, high intensities of heat and micromassage can be produced without the danger of burning the patient.

The bed of Cellex is heated by a stream of pressurized air that flows upward through an electric heater, thus enhancing its temperature. As the velocity of the air is increased to a point where the pressure drop of the air becomes equal to the weight of the Cellex, the bed begins to expand. Thus, the air/Cellex mixture begins to take on the characteristics of a heterogeneous fluid of an extremely low viscosity. This phenomenon is reflected in the term—*fluidization.*

Because the unit transfers dry heat in motion, the patient is able to tolerate much higher temperatures without discomfort, as contrasted with comparable heat levels in paraffin baths or hydrotherapy—in fact, some studies have shown that the amount of heat absorbed by the patient is from four to six times greater.[13] See Figure 4.26.

Fluidotherapy temperatures can be tolerated by the average patient up to 120°—125°F. When heat production was compared for Fluidotherapy, paraffin, and hydrotherapy, the maximum skin temperature rise was 16.7°F for Fluidotherapy, which is considerably greater than for either paraffin or hydrotherapy. See Table 4.6.[14] In addition, the initial thermal shock experienced in paraffin

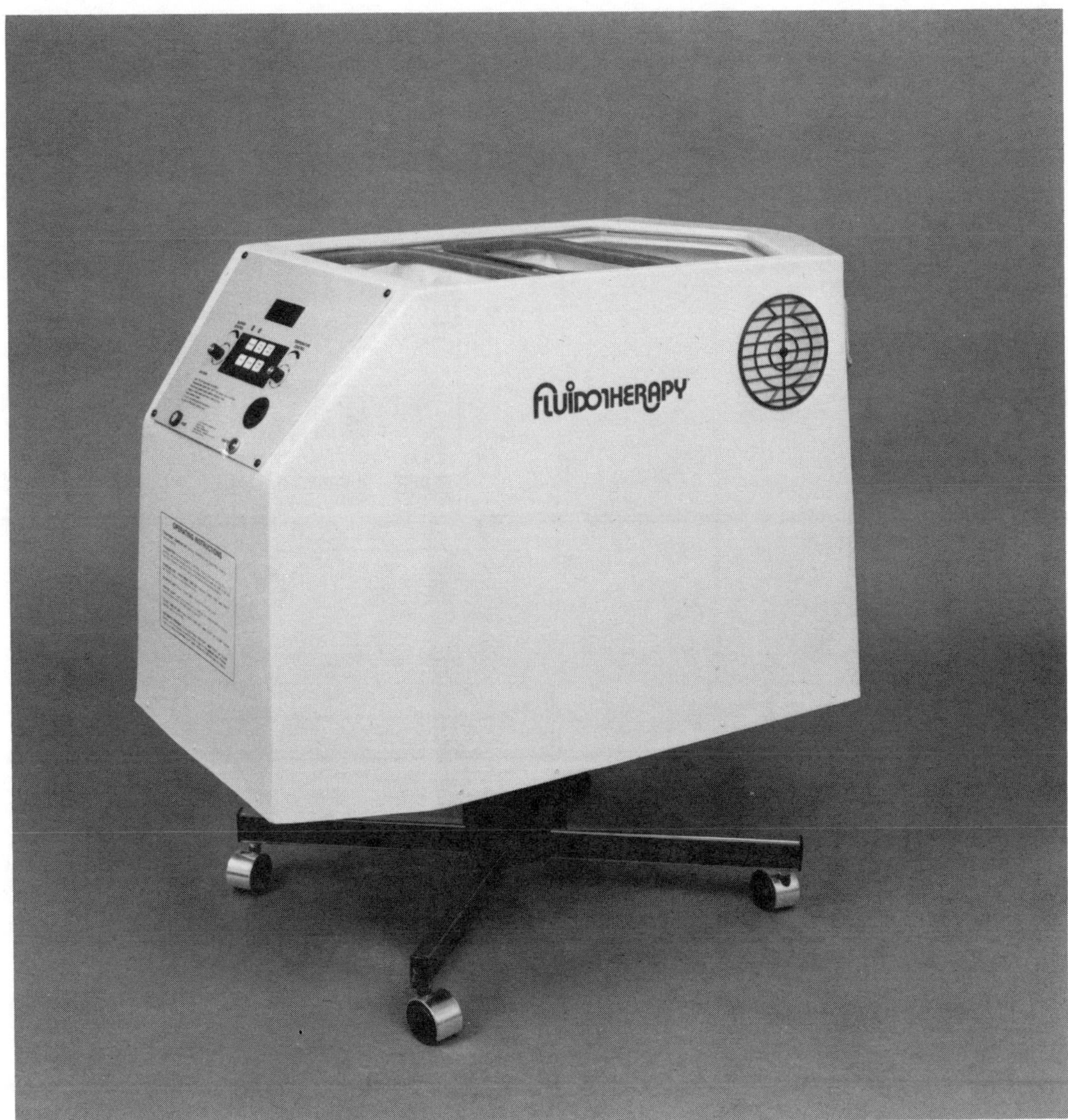

Figure 4.23. Diagonal side view of a typical Fluidotherapy unit.

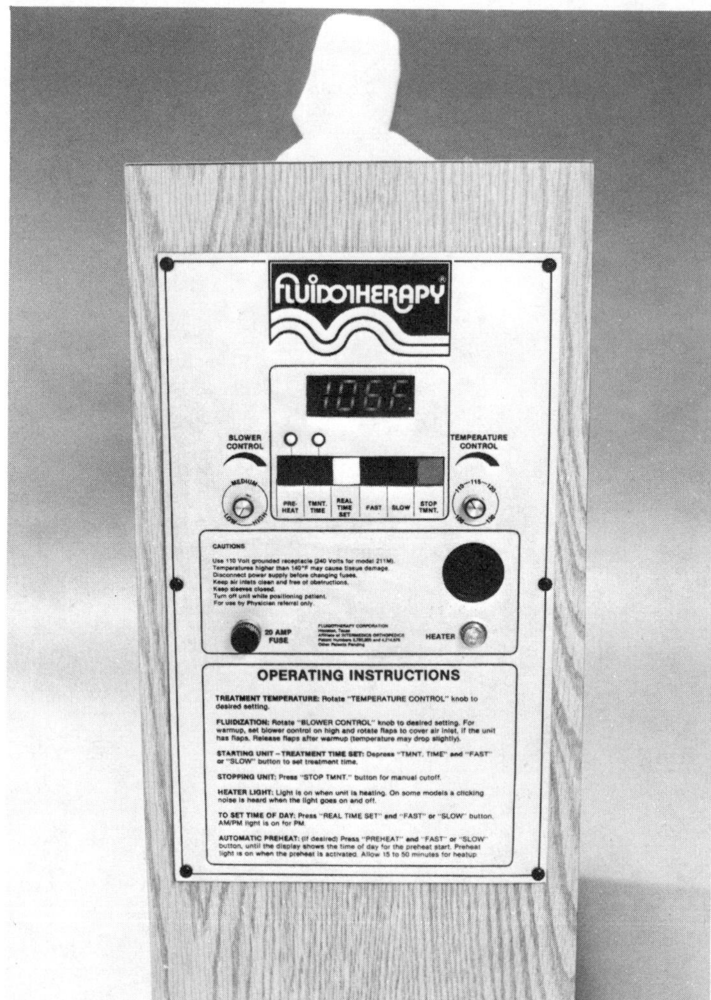

Figure 4.24. View of the control panel of a Fluidotherapy unit.

Table 4.6. Comparison of In Vivo Temperatures Produced by Fluidotherapy, Hydrotherapy, and Paraffin Wax Treatments

Modality	*Application Temperature*	*Maximum Joint Capsule Temperature Rise (0.5 cm depth)*	*Maximum Joint Muscle Temperature Rise (0.5 cm depth)*
Fluidotherapy.	118°F	16.2°F	9.5°F
Hydrotherapy	102°—104°F	10.8°F	7.7°F
Paraffin therapy (9-dip)	126°F	13.5°F	8.1°

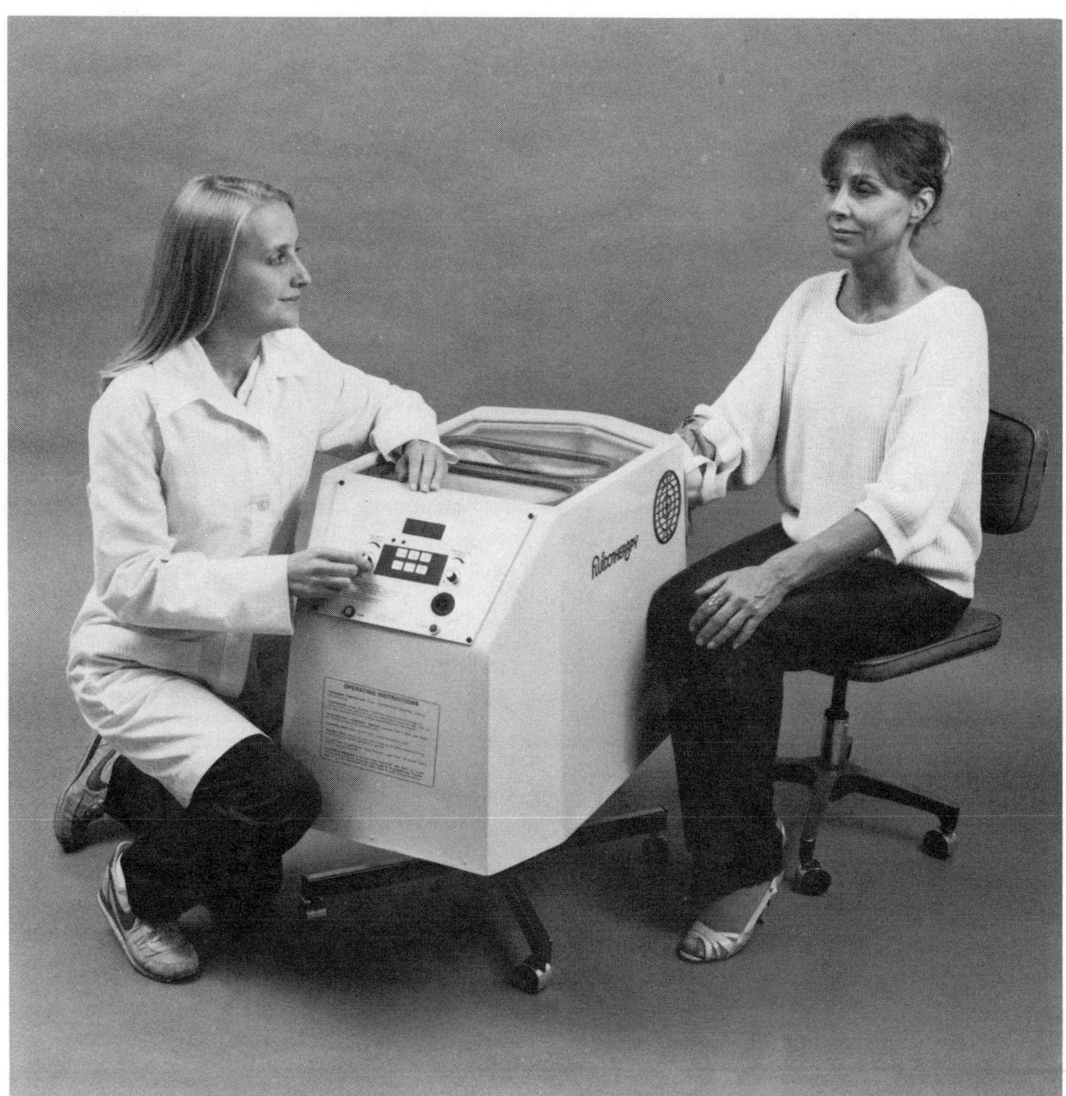

Figure 4.25. After an extremity is placed in the unit, the therapist sets the control dials. With the front-loaded unit shown, the patient may be seated on a chair during the treatment.

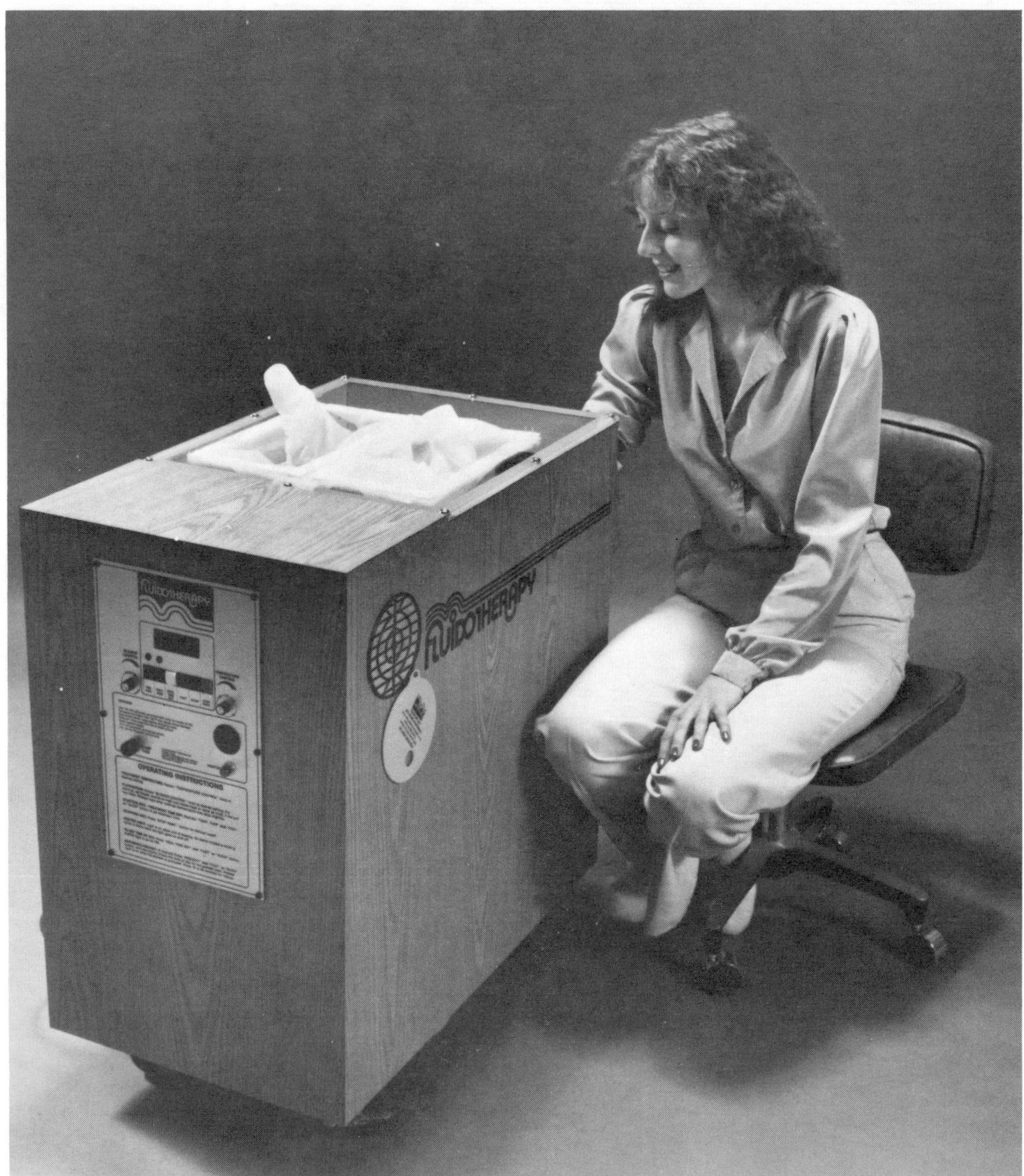

Figure 4.26. Applying Fluidotherapy to the right hand and wrist.

therapy is avoided because the hot air/solid fluidized mixture has a lower thermal conductivity than either water or paraffin.

Tests have shown that the Cellex does not need to be routinely changed. It appears that the high temperatures created during use and the aerobic atmosphere inherent within the system destroy any pathognomonic organisms that might be introduced by a patient or from the environment.

Physiologic Effects

The unit's powerful blower transfers high degrees of kinetic energy by way of the whirling Cellex for micromassage and stimulation of both mechanoreceptors and thermoreceptors. The rapid pressure fluctuations (1.5—3.0 Hz) of short duration (0.1—0.3 seconds) contribute to the reduction of edema/swelling. In addition, the fluidized air/solid medium has properties that gives it the advantages of a fluid without the disadvantages of a wet medium. As with any heat modality, it produces systemic relaxation and a sedative effect.

The major physiologic effects of Fluidotherapy are:

1. *Increased temperature of the treated part.* Treatments can increase internal temperatures considerably. At a unit setting of 118 °F, foot capsule temperatures as high as 114 °F have been recorded. See Table 4.6.

2. *Increased pulse rate.* The average pulse increase has been measured to be 5—6 additional pulses/minute.[15]

3. *A slight rise in total body temperature.* Several patients studied have indicated an oral temperature gain of 0.213 °F.

4. *A slight decrease in systemic blood pressure.* The average reduction is 2.21 systolic, 3.45 diastolic.

Safety Aspects

During the use of most types of thermotherapy, the patient's safety is compromised if the individual is subjected to the possibility of a burn from high temperatures, an electric shock, or infection from contamination. The design of the Fluidotherapy system is such that these factors have been greatly minimized, inasmuch as equipment error and human error must occur simultaneously for an accident to occur.

To prevent a patient from receiving an accidental burn, a high-temperature cut-off is incorporated in the system, duplicate temperature measuring devices (thermistors) have been installed, and a circuit breaker will open the circuit if the control circuit fails. The danger of a dust explosion or of the pulverized corn cobs catching on fire is almost nil because of the particle sizes used and the fact that corn cob particles are self-extinguishing. Thus, an inflammatory hazard does not exist.

To avoid the possibility of an accidental shock, all electrical switches and devices adhere strictly to UL codes, an automatic cut-off is provided in the event of a voltage drop to the motor or the motor fails, and there is separate fusing on the heater and motor circuits.

Cross-contamination from patient to patient is always a safety concern in a health-care facility. Repeated studies have shown that when bacterial and mycotic contaminants (eg, Eschericia coli, Pseudomonas aeruginosa, Staphylococcus aureus, Candida albicans) were injected into the inflow of the unit, no viable pathogens could be found in the outflow after 15 minutes had passed.[16] However, to assure additional safety, it is recommended that if there is any danger of cross-infection between patients, the bed of the unit should be purged for 15 minutes between treatments.

One might think that there would be danger of a contact dermatitis because of the pulverized corn cobs used as a medium. This has not been reported to be true, even after thousands of patients had been treated.

Indications

Fluidotherapy may be utilized whenever there is desire to increase the temperature of an extremity part. It is an excellent modality when a physician wishes to increase local temperature and simultaneously exercise the part. Thus, patients with musculoskeletal injuries or arthritis of the extremities can benefit tremendously after the acute stage has passed, especially when stiffness and restricted joint movement are present. See Figure 4.27. Many patients report that they prefer the sensation of Fluidotherapy over that of other superficial heat modalities.

A considerable amount of study has been done with Fluidotherapy in the treatment of acute injuries (eg, compound fractures, burns), especially open wounds. In the cases of open wounds studied, a plastic glove or bag is placed over the extremity part that has been injured to prevent the whirling particles becoming embedded in the wound or dressing.

The primary indications for Fluidotherapy are the treatment of pain, range of motion restriction, blood flow insufficiency, certain types of edema, and open or closed wound healing enhancement:

1. *Pain.* The mechanical and thermal stimulation of the skin produces counterirritation that tends to modulate sensory input, thus blocking pain perception and response.[17,18,19]

2. *Restricted range of motion.* The high tissue temperatures that can be produced by Fluidotherapy acts upon such tissue components as structural fibers, synovia, and exudates to lower their viscosity, improve the elasticity, and alter their biomechanical deformation (rheologic) properties—thus improving the joints range of motion in a physiomechanical manner.[20,21,22] See Figure 4.28.

3. *Blood flow insufficiency.* The blood vessel dilation resulting from the high treatment temperature dramatically increases blood flow.[23,24,25]

4. *Wounds.* The high tissue temperatures produced by Fluidotherapy accelerate the biochemical reactions involved in cell division and regeneration to new healthy tissues.[26,27,28]

A unit that treats the low back has been recently developed. See Figures 4.29 and 4.30. Studies of its clinical efficacy are in their infancy, but the early data indicate extremely beneficial results in enhancing healing of various musculoskeletal injuries.

Application

Treatment temperature protocols:

Back	-	123°—126°F
Foot/feet	-	114°—118°F
Hands/arms	-	116°—120°F
Knee(s)	-	118°—120°F
Leg (one)	-	116°F
Legs (both)	-	114°F

Treatment duration generally varies from 15 to 20 minutes per session. When in doubt, Borrell recommends 110°F for 20 minutes.[29] The typical length of therapy varies from 2 to 6 weeks, depending upon the extent and chronicity of the disorder.

Contraindications and Precautions

As with almost any thermotherapy, care should be taken not to treat the acute inflammatory types of arthropathies such as early rheumatic, psoriatic, gonorrheal, or suppurative arthritis. Special precautions should be used in treating the very young, aged, or debilitated patient. See Table 4.7. Treatment should always be terminated in any case where unusual erythema or swelling is observed.

The total amount of energy absorbed by the patient in Fluidotherapy is at least 100 times greater than that of ultrasound. However, ultrasound would be the preferable modality where deep penetration into a small isolated area is desired (eg, a heel or shoulder spur).

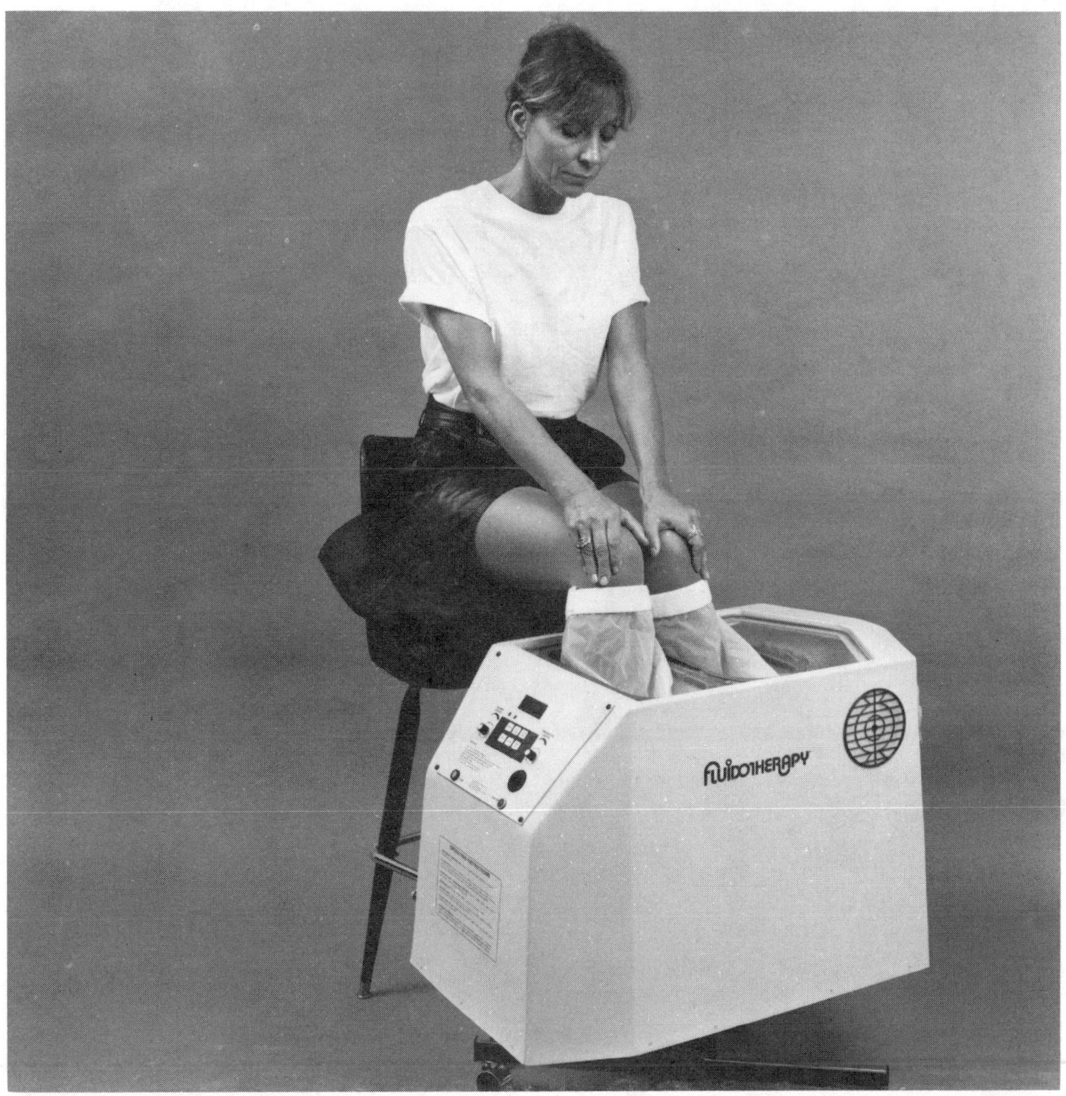

Figure 4.27. A fairly high stool should be provided to the patient if the lower extremities are being treated.

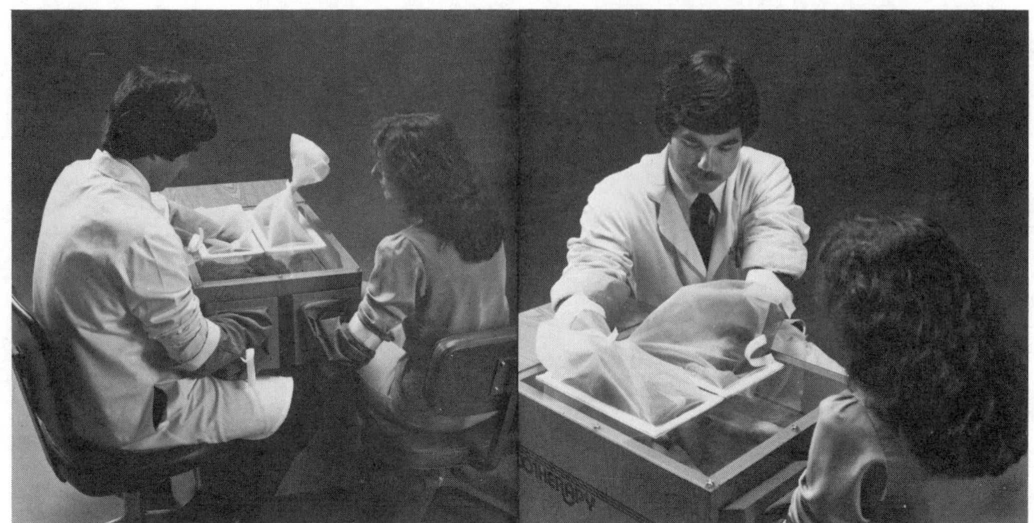

Figure 4.28. The doctor or therapist may sometimes wish to provide manipulation, massage, or passive exercise to the patient during the therapy.

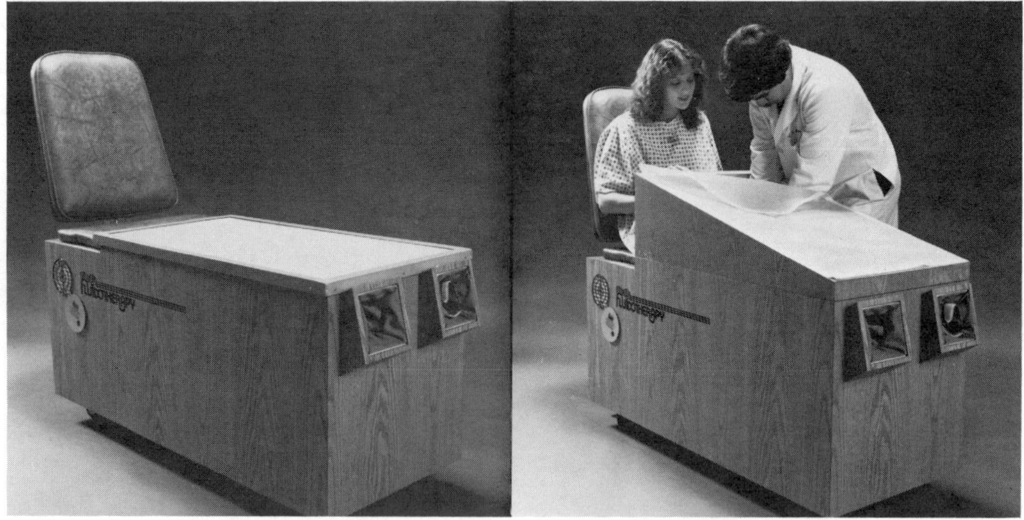

Figure 4.29. *Left,* a Fluidotherapy unit design for treating the back. *Right,* a back unit being adapted for treatment of the lower extremities.

Table 4.7. General Indications and Contraindications of Fluidotherapy

GENERAL INDICATIONS

Pain:	Range of motion:
Dislocation	Arthritis
Epicondylitis	Dermatogenous contractures
IVD syndrome	Following immobilization
Low back pain	Myogenous contractures
Overstrains	Neurogenous contractures
Rheumatic tissue alterations	Postfracture restrictions
Soft-tissue trauma	Postsurgical restrictions
Spinal sprains	Posttraumatic inflammation
Subluxation	Posttraumatic innervation
Sudeck's dystrophy	Posttraumatic ischemia
Tenosynovitis	Sports injuries
	Tendogenous contractures
Wounds and swellings:	Blood flow insufficiency:
Closed wounds	Raynaud's syndrome
Contusions	Reflex sympathicotonia
Dislocations	Stasis ulcers
Open wounds	Sympathetic dysfunction
Sprains	Carpal/tarsal tunnel syndromes
Subluxations	Vegetative dystonia
Surgical wounds	

GENERAL CONTRAINDICATIONS

Acute cardiorenal edema	Acute inflammatory processes
Chronic venous insufficiency	Suppurating lesions
Vascular disease	Infants or the elderly
Hypesthesia	Severe debilitation
Malignancy	Over metal such as rings, bracelets, underwear clips, implants, etc.
Pyrexia	
Active cases of tuberculosis	

CLOSING REMARKS

Inasmuch as some professional papers concerning thermotherapy are written with temperature values in Fahrenheit and other in Celsius, equivalents are shown in Table 4.8.

This chapter has generally described the basic concepts underlying the physiologic effects of local heat, localized heating, and reflex heating. The systemic effects of heat, the methods of therapeutic heating, and the common sources of superficial heat have been portrayed. In addition, the physical effects of heating, the general indications and contraindications of superficial heat, and the basic rules of applying therapeutic heat have been depicted. An understanding of these basic factors is necessary to apply modalities producing superficial heat in a professional manner. Depth and temperature effects are compared for several superficial heat modalities in Figure 4.31.

Specifically, the physiologic effects, indications, application, and contraindications have

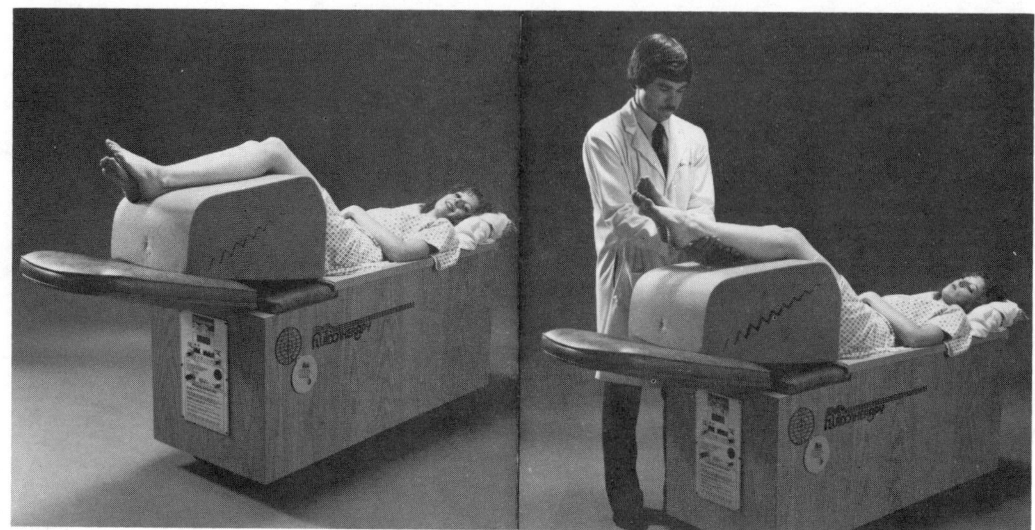

Figure 4.30. Treatment of the lower back with Fluidotherapy.

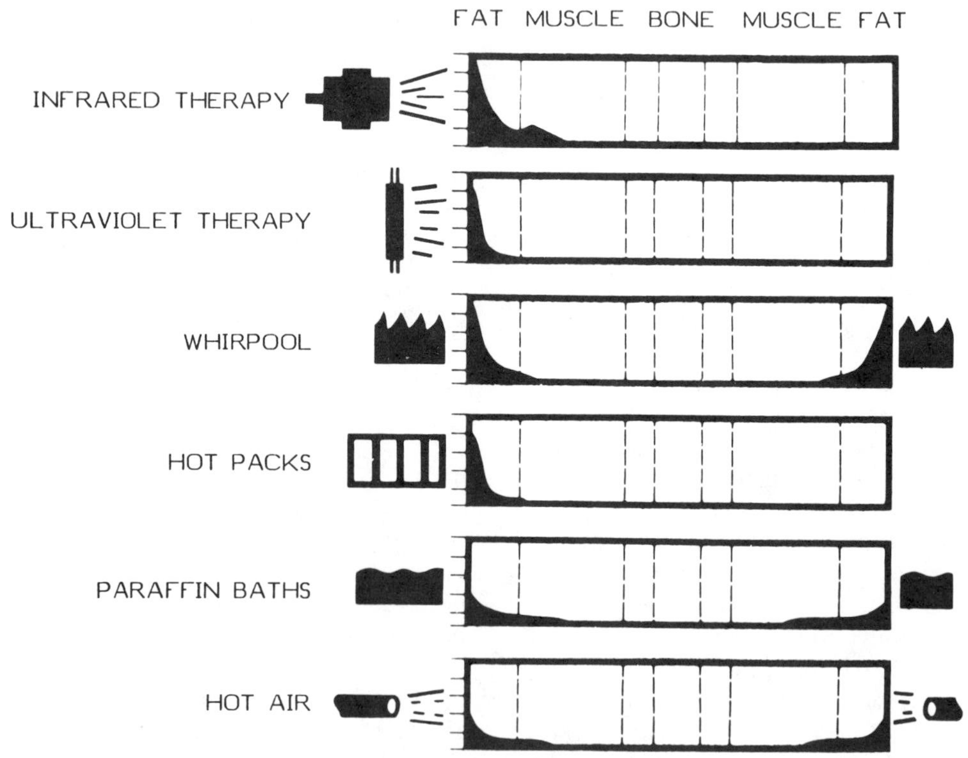

Figure 4.31. Comparison of depth/temperature relationships for various types of superficial heating modalities.

Table 4.8. Celsius and Fahrenheit Thermometric Equivalents

C°	F°	C°	F°	C°	F°	C°	F°
0	32	26	78.8	52	125.6	78	172.4
1	33.8	27	80.6	53	127.4	79	174.2
2	35.6	28	82.4	54	129.2	80	176
3	37.4	29	84.2	55	131	81	177.8
4	39.2	30	86	56	132.8	82	179.6
5	41	31	87.8	57	134.6	83	181.4
6	42.8	32	89.6	58	136.4	84	183.2
7	44.6	33	91.4	59	138.2	85	185
8	46.4	34	93.2	60	140	86	186.8
9	48.2	35	95	61	141.8	87	188.6
10	50	36	96.8	62	143.6	88	190.4
11	51.8	37	98.6	63	145.4	89	192.2
12	53.6	38	100.4	64	147.2	90	194
13	55.4	39	102.2	65	149	91	195.8
14	57.2	40	104	66	150.8	92	197.6
15	59	41	105.8	67	152.6	93	199.4
16	60.8	42	107.6	68	154.4	94	201.2
17	62.6	43	109.4	69	156.2	95	203
18	64.4	44	111.2	70	158	96	204.8
19	66.2	45	113	71	159.8	97	206.6
20	68	46	114.8	72	161.6	98	208.4
21	69.8	47	116.6	73	163.4	99	210.2
22	71.6	48	118.4	74	165.2	100	212
23	73.4	49	120.2	75	167	101	213.8
24	75.2	50	122	76	168.8	102	215.6
25	77	51	123.8	77	170.6	103	217.4

Note: Given a temperature on the Celsius (Centigrade) scale, it can be converted to Fahrenheit by multiplying by $9/5$ and adding 32. Given a temperature on the Fahrenheit scale, convert to Celsius by subtracting 32 and multiplying by $5/9$.

been described for hot moist packs, heating pads, infrared units, ultraviolet lamps, paraffin and Fluidotherapy. These factors should be frequently reviewed by all health-care personnel involved.

REFERENCES

1. Stillwell GK: The use of physical medicine in office practice with particular emphasis on the aftercare of fractures. *Journal of the Iowa Medical Society,* 53:12-18, 1963.
2. Abramson DI, et al: Effect of paraffin bath and hot fomentations on local tissue temperatures. *Archives of Physical Medicine and Rehabilitation,* 45: 87-94, 1964.
3. Abramsom DI, et al: Changes in blood flow, oxygen uptake, and tissue temperatures produced by the topical application of wet heat. *Archives of Physical Medicine and Rehabilitation,* 42:305-318, 1961.
4. Krusen FH, et al: *Handbook of Physical Medicine and Rehabilitation,* ed 2. Philadelphia, W.B. Saunders 1971, p 262.
5. Schafer RC: *Chiropractic Management of Sports and Recreational Injuries.* Baltimore, Williams & Wilkins, 1982, p 199.
6. Krusen FH, et al: *Handbook of Physical Medicine and Rehabilitation,* ed 2. Philadelphia, W.B. Saunders 1971, p 262.
7. Blum HF: *Photodynamic Action and Diseases*

Caused by Light. New York, Reinhold Publishing, 1941.

8. Anderson WT Jr: in *Archives of Physical Therapy, X-Ray and Radium,* 18:699, 1937.
9. Hill LL: *Parameters of Physiotherapy Modalities.* Lombard, IL, National Chiropractic College, class notes, date not shown, pp 3-4.
10. Glasser O: *Medical Physics.* Chicago, Year Book Publishers, 1944, pp 1145-1157.
11. Thomas CL (ed): *Taber's Cyclopedic Medical Dictionary,* ed 14. Philadelphia, F.A. Davis, 1981, p 1577.
12. Hill LL: *Parameters of Physiotherapy Modalities.* Lombard, IL, National Chiropractic College, class notes, date not shown, p 40.
13. Valenza J, et al: A clinical study of a new heat modality: fluidotherapy. *Journal of the American Podiatry Association,* 69(7):440-442, July 1979.
14. Borrell RM, et al: Comparison of in vivo temperatures produced by hydrotherapy, paraffin wax, and fluidotherapy. *Journal of the American Physical Therapy Association,* 60(10):1273-1276, October 1980.
15. Valenza J, et al: A clinical study of a new heat modality: fluidotherapy. *Journal of the American Podiatry Association,* 69(7):440-442, July 1979.
16. Sharbough RJ, Hargest BA: The effect of air-fluidized systems on microbial growth. In Artz CT, Hargest BS (eds): *Air Fluidized Beds, Clinical and Research Symposium.* University of South Carolina, 1975.
17. Borrell RM, Henley EJ: Fluidotherapy in a hand clinic. *Archives of Physical Medicine and Rehabilitation,* 60:536, 1979.
18. Brown DM, Ellis RA: A physiological basis for desensitization of the hypersensitive upper extremity. Paper presented to the American Society of Hand Therapists, Las Vegas, 1980.
19. Fuentes LF, Lopez DA: An evaluation of a new heat modality: fluidotherapy. Paper presented to the National Physical Therapy Association, Atlanta, 1979.
20. Borrell RM, Henley EJ: Fluidotherapy in a hand clinic. *Archives of Physical Medicine and Rehabilitation,* 60:536, 1979.
21. Fuentes LF, Lopez DA: An evaluation of a new heat modality: fluidotherapy. Paper presented to the National Physical Therapy Association, Atlanta, 1979.
22. Henley EJ: A novel fluidized-bed application: fluidotherapy. *CHEMTECH,* accepted for publication, 1982.
23. Borrell RM, et al: Comparison of in vivo temperatures produced by hydrotherapy, paraffin wax, and fluidotherapy, op cit.
24. Henley EJ: A novel fluidized-bed application: fluidotherapy. *CHEMTECH,* accepted for publication, 1982.
25. Lober S: Quantitative analysis of fluidotherapy heat treatment on the human hand. Houston, TX, University of Houston, 1980. Thesis.
26. Borrell RM, Henley EJ: Fluidotherapy in a hand clinic. *Archives of Physical Medicine and Rehabilitation,* 60:536, 1979.
27. Lober S: Quantitative analysis of fluidotherapy heat treatment on the human hand. Houston, TX, University of Houston, 1980. Thesis.
28. Valenza J, et al: A clinical study of a new heat modality: fluidotherapy. *Journal of the American Podiatry Association,* 69(7):440-442, July 1979.
29. Borrell RM, Eastburn J: Treatment protocol for fluidotherapy in hand rehabilitation. Paper presented to the Annual Meeting of the American Congress of Rehabilitative Medicine, Honolulu, American Academy of Physical Medicine and Rehabilitation, November 1979.

Chapter 5

Deep Heat Therapies

This chapter describes the therapeutic applications of high frequency currents; namely, the shortwave, microwave, and ultrasonic diathermies.

HISTORY OF HIGH FREQUENCY CURRENTS

Electric currents with high frequencies were first analyzed therapeutically in 1890 by a French physiologist, D'Arsenval. The method he used consisted essentially of damped oscillations of an extremely short duration with a high frequency current. The impulses were interrupted by pauses that lasted about 500 times as long as the oscillations themselves. The heat generated by body resistance during treatment with high frequency currents was used for the first time by von Zeynek and, independently, by Nagelschmidt who was the first to call the process *diathermy*.

In the 1920s at the University of Jena, physicist Esau discovered that flies exhibited a peculiar behavior when they were brought into a high frequency electrical field. This led to his development of a powerful generator to produce such a field. He also called the process *diathermy*.

In Germany during the early 1930s, Schliephake and others further investigated the phenomena, recognized its therapeutic value, and established the physical and biological functions associated with its use. These and other studies led to the development of classical shortwave therapy. The rapid advance of decimetric-wave and centimetric-wave techniques in the field of RADAR, made especially after World War II, led to the introduction of microwave diathermy.

ALTERNATING HIGH FREQUENCY CURRENT

In contrast to a direct current of moderate intensity where a flow occurs from one pole to another and produces the transfer of electrically charged particles (iontophoresis), an ionic transfer does not take place when the polarity is changed rhythmically (eg, alternating current) because there is an equal flow of positive and negative current. When extremely high frequency alternating currents are employed such as in millions of cycles per second (eg, at 27 MHz for shortwave diathermy or 2,450 MHz for microwave diathermy), direct contact of the electrodes with the skin is not necessary as the energy can pass through the air, an insulated pad, or an insulated cable and then through the body. Thus, firm contact on irregular surfaces is not a concern.

For practical purposes, clinical applications of high frequency currents can be classified as follows:

1. Shortwave diathermy
   A. Induction or coil field
   B. Condenser field
2. Microwave diathermy
3. Ultrasonic diathermy.

The term "diathermy" means deep heating; a procedure by which body heat is elevated by passage of a high frequency current through tissues (ie, transthermia, thermopenetration). The heat that develops in the tissues results from the resistance offered by tissue constituents to the passage of the electrical current.

High frequency currents utilize electromagnetic oscillations with frequencies higher than 300,000 Hz. Electromagnetic oscillations at these frequencies do not cause depolarization of nerve fibers.

SHORTWAVE DIATHERMY

Shortwave therapy is a form of high frequency electrotherapy, which has become one of the most common therapeutic forms of deep-heat therapy during the past several decades. It is far superior to longwave therapy, and midwaves have no heating effect. See Figure 5.1. Shortwave diathermy is broadly defined as an oscillating electric current of extremely high frequency (10—100 million Hz) and short wavelength (3—30 meters).[1]

Physics

Therapeutic shortwave modalities generally use oscillations with a frequency of 27.12×10^6 Hz, which corresponds to a wavelength of 11.06 meters when produced in a vacuum. This frequency of oscillations was established by international agreement in order to prevent disturbance of other transmitting devices. In fact, all shortwave units are regulated by the Federal Communications Commission (FCC) in this country to prevent their interference with radio waves.

It has been shown in recent years that wavelength in itself is not a primary factor in tissue heating. There is no optimum wavelength for heating specific body tissues. The major factors are the energy delivered to the patient and the equipment and technique being used.

The major physical effect of high frequency treatment is thermal; ie, the buildup of heat in human tissues. However, any electrical current will heat tissues in accordance

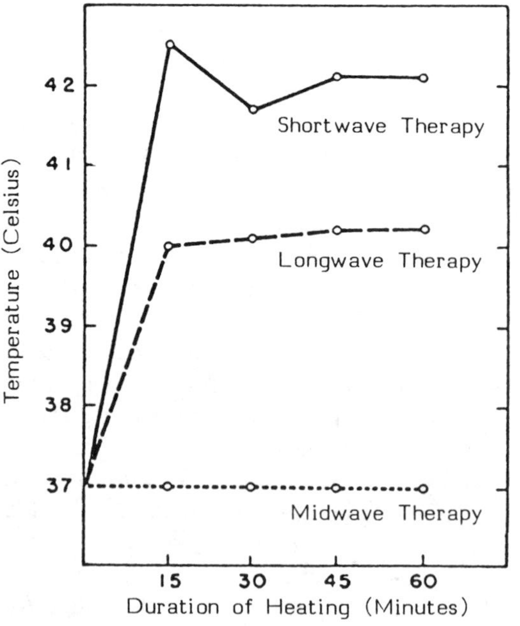

Figure 5.1. Mean rectal temperature charted during intrapelvic heating, comparing the effects of shortwave, longwave, and midwave diathermy.

with Joule's laws: (1) heat is produced in direct proportion to the square of current strength; (2) heat produced by a given amount of current is directly proportional to the resistance of the conductor, and (3) the heat produced is directly proportional to the duration of current flow.

Superficial heat applied at an intensity sufficient to affect deep tissues would undoubtedly burn the skin. Low frequency currents are not as suitable for triggering heat production in tissues because, if they were utilized at an intensity that would produce tissue heating, the corresponding effects on polarity would trigger tissue destruction. This later effect would only be logical as used in surgical diathermy (high frequency electrocautery), which destroys tissue to seal blood vessels and arrest bleeding.

DEMONSTRATION OF EFFECTS

Three classical experiments are described below that demonstrate the primary physical effects of high frequency currents on conductors.

The Light Bulb Experiment. In this experiment, a participant holds a cylindrical electrode in each hand. Attached to the base of one terminal is a light bulb. The other terminal is attached to the diathermy unit. As soon as the shortwave machine is turned on, the electric bulb lights, yet the patient does not experience any physical sensation or muscular reaction even though the current is passing through the patient. This demonstrates that *a high frequency current can exert an electrothermic effect on the body without triggering a perceptive or neuromuscular reaction.*

The Wrist Experiment. The subject in this experiment is asked to grasp a shortwave cable or cylindrical electrode in each hand while holding the wrists straight. When the current of shortwave unit is turned on, the subject will feel more heat in the wrists than in the hands or forearms. This draws the conclusion that *the greatest heating effect occurs along that path of the high frequency current which is shortest and where the tissue density is greatest.*

The Water Experiment. The conducting coils from the terminals of the diathermy unit in this experiment are placed 2 inches apart in a container filled with tap water. The meter will indicate passage of the current when the unit is activated to a fair amount, yet bubbles do not form at the electrodes in the water. Neither does the addition of some salt to the water bring about bubble formation, indicating that *shortwave diathermy does not exhibit electrolytic or electrochemical properties.*

ELECTROMECHANICAL CRITERIA

Short wavelengths range between 7 and 100 meters; ie, between medium radio waves and those for television. There are three specific frequencies that are permitted and regulated by the FCC for shortwave units: 13.66, 27.33, and 40.98 megacycles. The wavelengths corresponding to these frequencies are 22, 11, and 7.5 meters, respectively. Most units commercially available have a frequency of 27.33 megacycles and a wavelength of 11 meters.

The shortwave diathermy units in use today have three basic components in their circuitry that are common to all; ie, (1) the power supply, (2) the oscillating circuit, and the (3) patient circuit. Typical units are shown in Figures 5.2, 5.3, 5.4, and 5.5.

To absorb the generation of the oscillating circuit, a condenser is necessary. See Figure 5.6. The basic unit consists of two separated plates. When the plates are supplied with a constant voltage, one plate becomes charged positively and the other negatively. Thus, an electric field is created between the two plates. When an insulator is placed between the two plates, it is called a *dielectric.*

The energy course with an electric oscillating unit starts when the condenser begins to discharge over the coil and the oscillating energy is converted into magnetic energy. See

Figure 5.7. In the second sequence, the condenser voltage drops to zero as the magnetic field in the coil reaches its peak, and this recharges the condenser with a different polarity (third sequence). In the final sequence, the condenser discharges and the magnetic field of the coil develops again.

Because the patient is an integral part of the shortwave circuit, the patient's skin resistance must be a consideration during applications because the patient's electrical impedance is an integral part of the impedance of the shortwave circuit. Thus, it is necessary to retune the variable patient circuit to resonance during any given therapeutic application. In older units, this impedance factor is corrected by means of a knob that manually makes adjustments so that the patient circuit is tuned into resonance.

Tuning of the patient circuit should always be made at a low output level to prevent a surge that may cause excessive heating. Failure to properly tune the patient can lead to a burn because small movements by the patient may change circuit impedance that would alter current flow. After tuning is accomplished, the unit's output can be adjusted to the desired level. In modern units, tuning is effected by a variable capacitor that automatically tunes the patient into resonance.

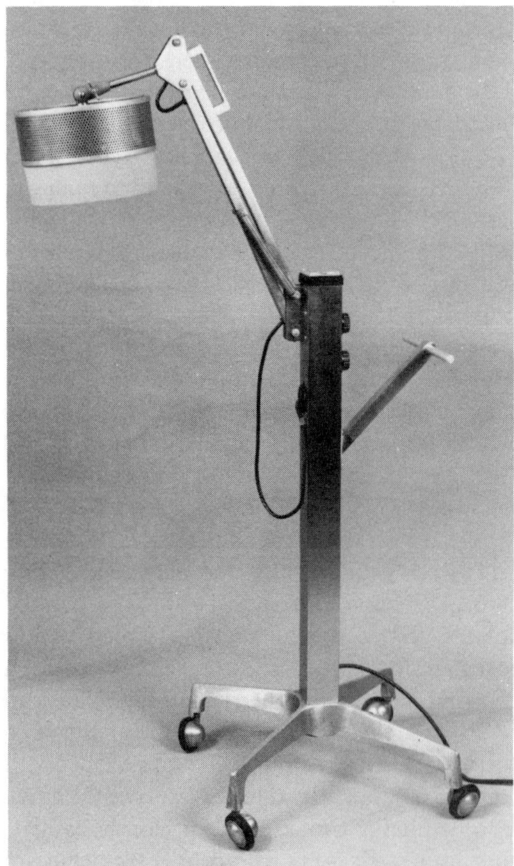

Figure 5.2. An Authotherm induction field diathermy unit.

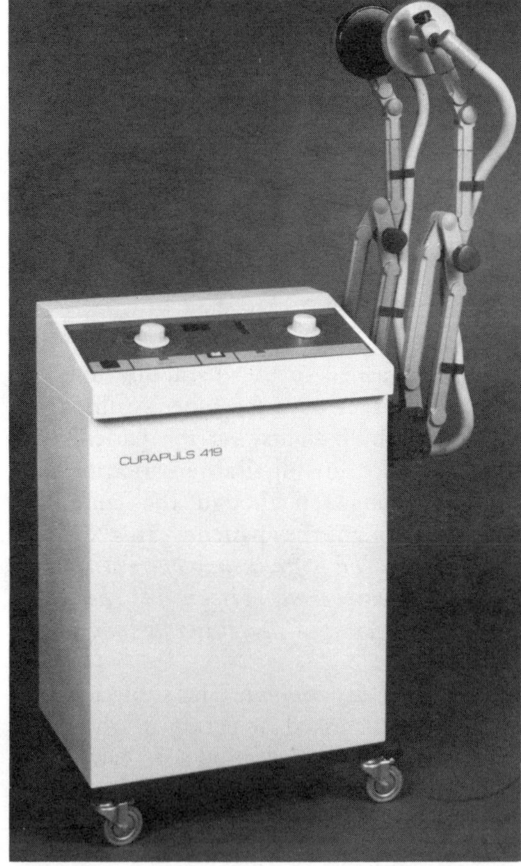

Figure 5.3. The Curaplus 419 space-plate condenser-field diathermy unit.

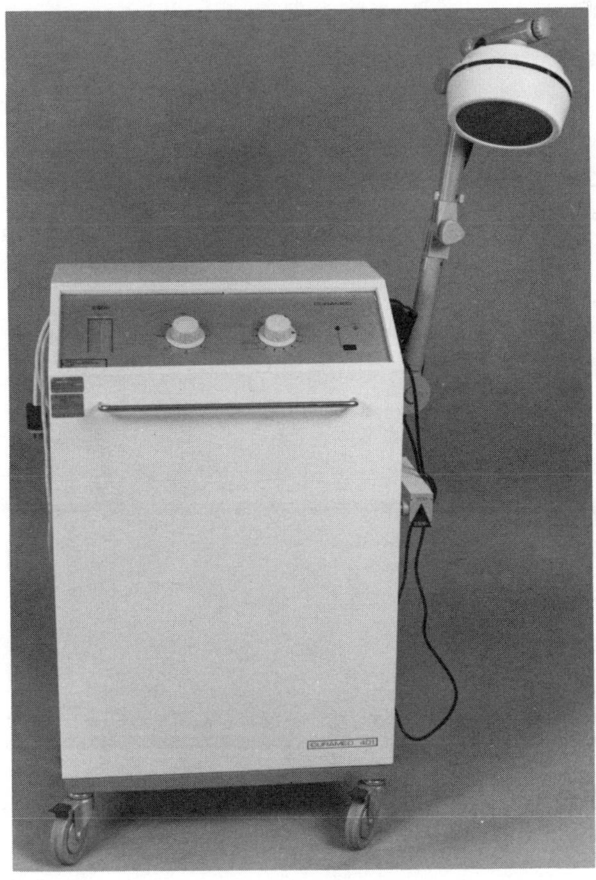

Figure 5.4. A Curamed 401 induction field shortwave unit.

Physiologic Effects

A definitive understanding of how high frequency energies affect the body has yet to be reached. It is known, however, that the application of high frequency electromagnetic energy causes ions in the cells to vibrate. This vibration, in turn, causes tissue heating to occur, depending on the intensity of the energy applied and the body's ability to dissipate the heat produced. The process is the simple result of the conversion of electrical energy into friction-created thermal energy within the tissues involved. The stimulation effect, with or without a buildup of heat, is a significant factor.

When used therapeutically, a high frequency current is an expandable kinetic (not static) energy field that is exhibited by the formation of heat. Emphasis in the past was placed primarily on the heating effects of diathermy. As a result, authors began to recommend longer and longer treatment times, stressing only the buildup of heat. However, our clinical observations have indicated that the longer treatment times utilized in diathermy to build tissue heat is actually counterproductive. This point cannot be stressed too strongly.

Some therapists have used shortwave therapy with heat buildup as their primary objective. They treat all patients by creating fairly

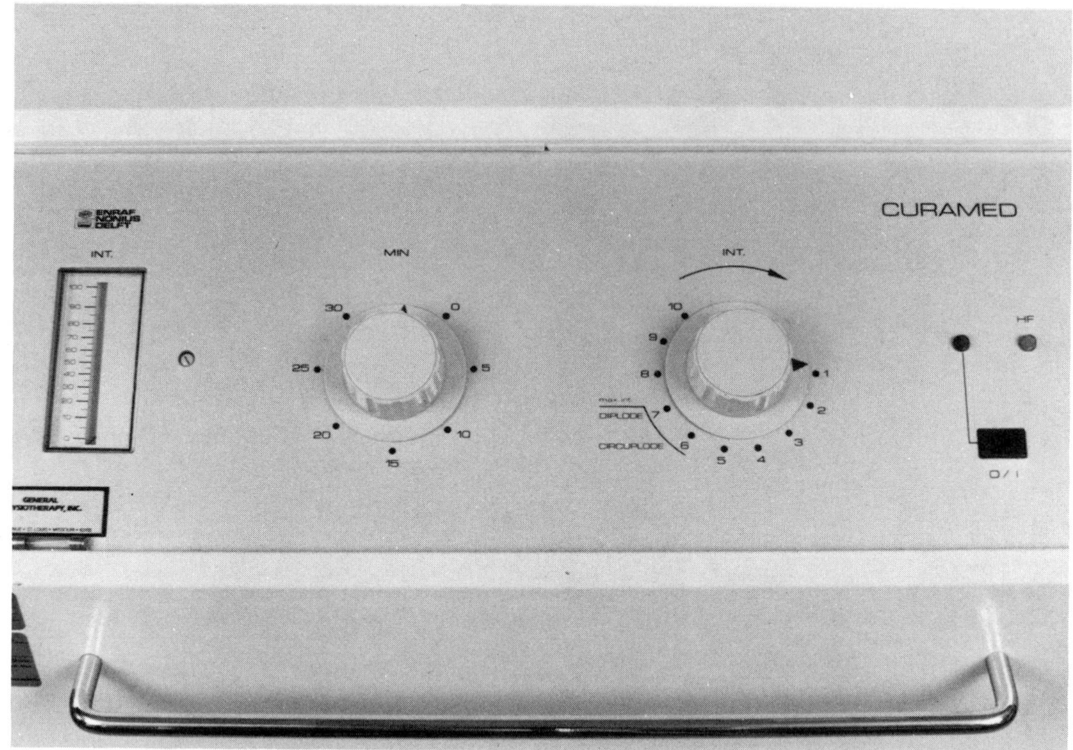

Figure 5.5. View of the control panel of a Curamed 401 induction field shortwave unit.

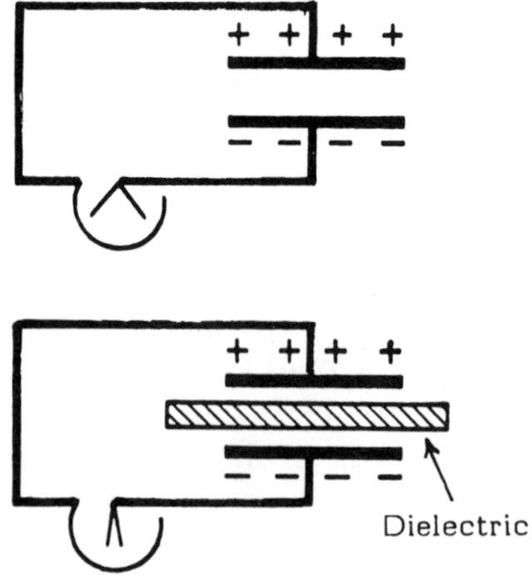

Figure 5.6. *Top,* schematic of a condenser without a dielectric. *Bottom,* condenser with a dielectric.

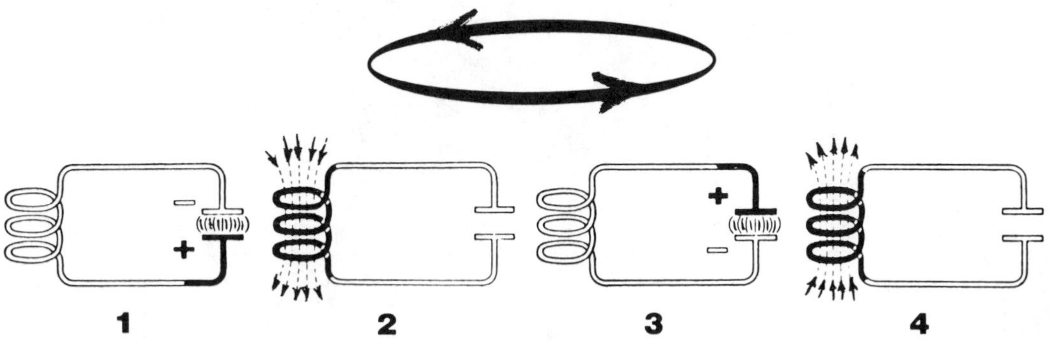

Figure 5.7. The energy course within an electric oscillating unit.

high tissue temperatures, and then wonder why the patients are not responding as anticipated or are getting worse. What happens is that the body is unable to dissipate the thermal energy rapidly enough, and excessive tissue heat is produced. Thus, the primary objective should not be to create heat; it should be to trigger energy expenditure that produces the desired results in the tissues. The heat that is produced and the corresponding tissue temperature rise are not the therapeutic factors. They are merely the measuring devices used to determine the rate at which the energy is expended.

It should also be noted that inasmuch as the temperature of the inflowing blood is likely to be lower than that of the heated tissues, the blood can be considered to be a cooling agent. When energy is produced in tissues faster than the cooling mechanisms of the body can dissipate, there will be a temperature increase that produces unpleasant reactions. Again, heat is not the therapeutic factor—it is only a clinical "yardstick." The energy expenditure is what produces the desired results in the tissues. Thus, the energy and the rate of its expenditure should be the determining factor in calculating proper dosage.

Many studies have been conducted on the specific physiologic effects of shortwave therapy. In essence, almost all physiologic reactions that have been attributed to shortwave diathermy applications are due to stimulating the movement of molecules and heating. A typical application is shown in Figure 5.8. Ten major effects are briefly summarized below:

1. *Thermal.* The primary undisputed physical effect of shortwave diathermy is the production of heat. In addition to its local effects, homeostatic heat-regulating vasomotor mechanisms are activated to dissipate the excessive temperature whenever external heat is applied to the body. This is manifested in general circulatory readjustments via cardiovascular mechanisms, along with vasoconstriction of the renal and splanchnic vascular beds, which tend to compensate for the effects of local heating.

2. *Stimulation.* The stimulation of tissue by means of high frequency current has been found to trigger the release of histamine. In turn, histamine (a vasodilator) produces further capillary dilatation both qualitatively and quantitatively. In addition, the thermal stimulation of cutaneous sensory receptors produces vasodilation via the axon reflex.

3. *Capillary pressure.* The effected increase in tissue temperature tends to considerably elevate capillary pressure.

4. *Blood flow.* Because of the factors enumerated above, the circulatory rate is increased. It should also be noted that while

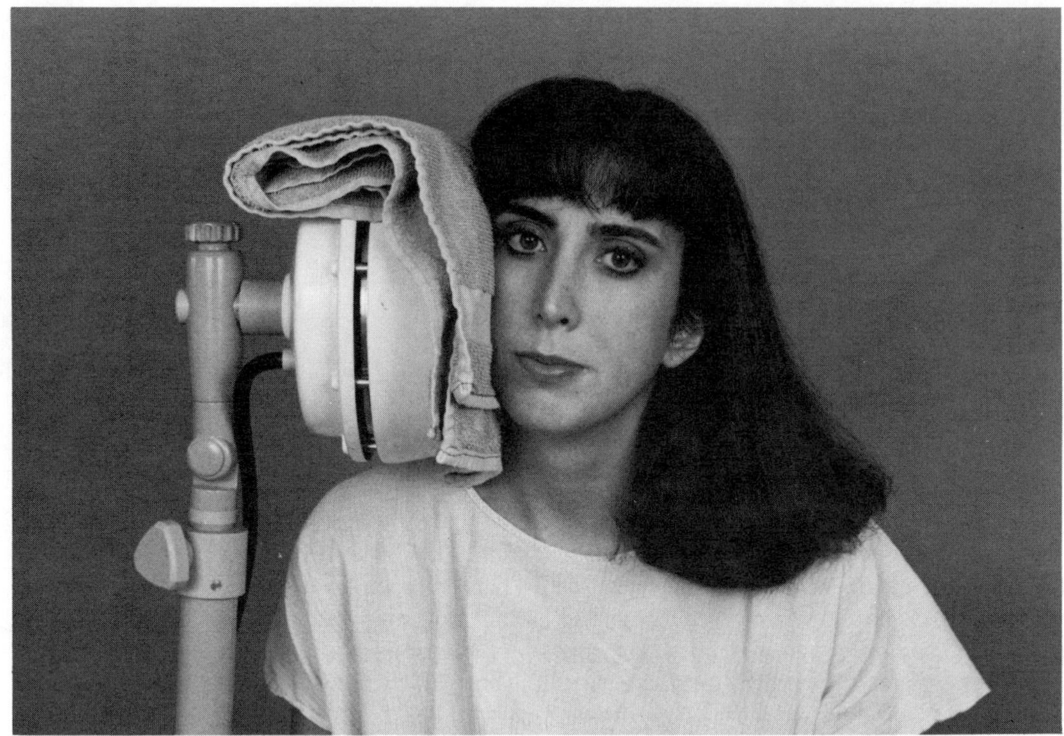

Figure 5.8. Monode application of induction-coil diathermy to the right TMJ area.

superficial heat produces dilatation in the subcutaneous capillaries, shortwave diathermy has a much greater effect on arteriolar and arterial dilatation. Such factors tend to increase the outflow of lymph and hormones, improve cellular nourishment and water balance, and enhance the absorption of infiltrates and exudates. The combined deep hyperemia and lymphedema tends to temporarily increase the volume of the part affected, and the associated tissue stretch undoubtedly stimulates involved autonomic receptors when viscera are treated.

5. *Oxidation.* In accord with the *law of van't Hoff,* for every rise of 10 °C, the rate of oxidation is increased 2½ times. The rate of cellular oxidation throughout the body is influenced by changes of temperature, even when it is less than 1 °C. This stimulating factor is important in affecting the physiologic processes of the internal organs. In other words, a slight rise in temperature greatly increases the oxygen-carrying capacity of erythrocytes and, in turn, this slight increase in oxygen supply to cells has a pronounced stimulating effect on the metabolic rate of the involved cells. In addition to the dilatory effects of other factors, the liberated metabolites (via autonomic mechanisms) expand the lumen of the blood vessels and increase the quantity of patent vessels so that vascular channels are opened widely.

6. *Phagocytosis.* High frequency fields have been found to stimulate increased white blood cell ingestion and digestion of solid substances (eg, other cells, bacteria, bits of necrosed tissue, foreign particles). For an unexplained reason, this effect has been shown to be due to the energy's influence on blood serum rather than on the leukocytes themselves. Obviously, this can be an important factor in activating body defense mechanisms. Initial-

ly, there is a leukopenia but it is quickly followed by a distinct leukocytosis, especially of the lymphocytes, that persists for about 24 hours.[2]

7. *Detoxification.* Studies have shown that the dilating effect of high frequency currents on the capillary system (both venous and arterial sides) enhances the resorption of toxic substances (eg, inflammatory exudates, metabolic by-products) that interfere with optimum cellular anabolism and catabolism.

8. *Hypotonicity.* High-frequency currents build tissue heat that leads to relaxation of spastic muscles and softening of other tissues (eg, ligaments, adhesions). It has been shown repeatedly that heated tendons, joint capsules, and scars yield more readily to stretch—indicating a distinct change in the physical properties of the tissues affected.[3,4]

9. *Endocrine changes.* Experiments by Schliephake and Weissenberg have shown that the activity of the endocrine glands can be increased by shortwave diathermy. They demonstrated changes in blood sugar level, cholesterol level, eosinophil count, and water balance. For example, it was shown that blood sugar levels rise in hyperthyroidism and certain forms of diabetes after the pituitary gland is irradiated; in Cushing's syndrome, a lowered blood sugar level is produced. On the other hand, irradiation of the upper abdomen increases the level of blood sugar in diabetics, and the secretion of ketosteroids is enhanced.[5] See Figure 5.9.

10. *Visceral circulation.* Shortwave diathermy, utilizing the condenser field, increases circulation within the internal organs under the electrodes by over 20%.[6] Superficial heat tends to decrease visceral circulation, via compensating homeostatic vasomotor mechanisms, while deep heat tends to increase visceral circulation. For example, when an increase in liver circulation is desired, shortwave or interferential current should be the therapy of choice. The findings of Pabst on this subject are summarized in Table 5.1.

Indications, Contraindications, and Precautions

Like most any form of physiotherapy, shortwave diathermy is considered an adjunct to be employed with other therapeutic measures, and certain indicative situations, contraindications, and areas of precaution have been established by sophisticated research and extensive empirical findings. See Table 5.2.

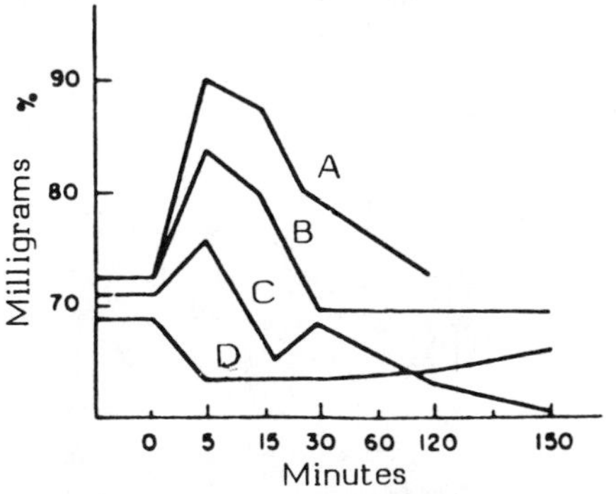

Figure 5.9. Analysis of shortwave therapy on the endocrine system. In the above chart, *Curve A* shows the effects of treating the pituitary gland by placing the patient's head within a condenser field, producing the greatest increase in the patient's blood sugar level. Note that the most change occurs after 5 minutes of a 10-minute therapy, then sharply declines within an hour. *Curve B* exhibits the effects of treating the adrenals by placing condenser field applicators over the patient's lateral abdomen. *Curve C* depicts the effects of treating the gonads by locating two condenser plates over the testes or ovaries. *Curve D,* where the blood sugar level is hardly altered, represents the effects of treating the arm musculature in a condenser field.

Table 5.1. Changes in Blood Circulation in the Liver After Physical Therapy

Modality		*Effect on Hepatic Circulation*
Hot water bath	(-)	Decreased circulation 27%
Moist heat	(-)	Decreased circulation 11%
Infrared radiation	(0)	No uniform reaction
Interferential current	(+)	Increased circulation 12%
Shortwave condenser field	(+)	Increased circulation 21.9%

DEEP HEAT

In a capacitor arrangement where connective tissue is placed between two electrodes emitting an extremely high frequency current, some of the current passes as a conduction current and some as a capacitative component. The higher the current frequency during application, the smaller the conduction current and the greater the capacitative current. A typical application is shown in Figure 5.10.

Because of the dielectric property of some tissues that are normally poor conductors, high frequency currents can be effectively utilized to heat regions that would be unac-

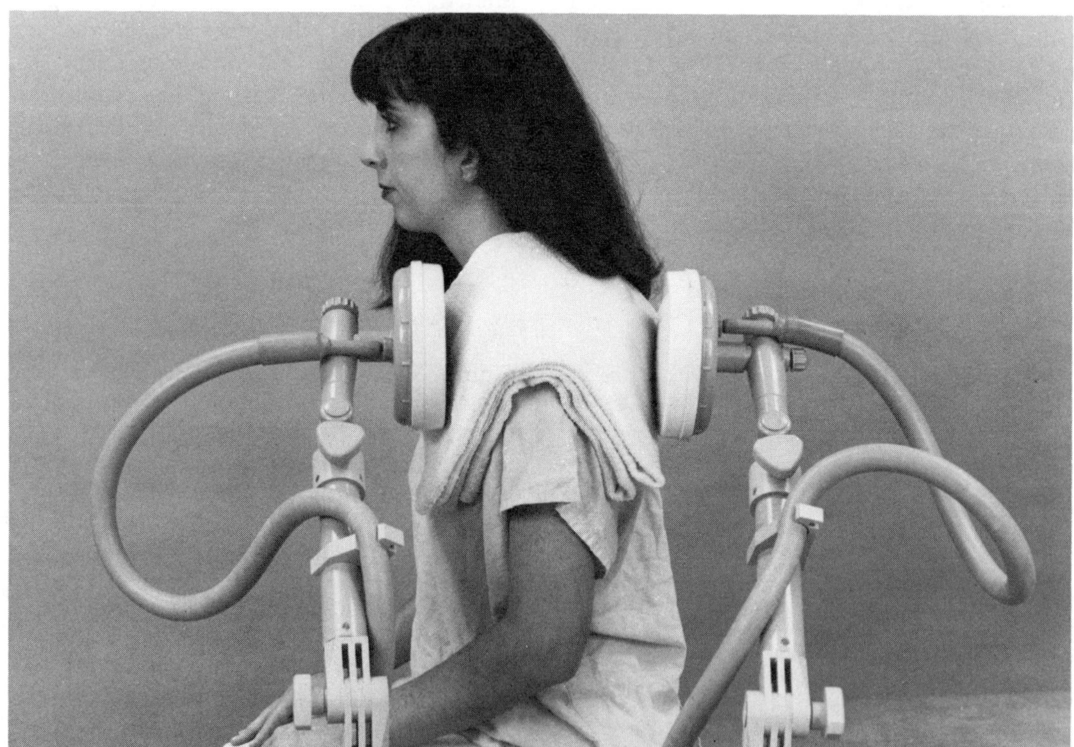

Figure 5.10. Space-plate application of condenser-field diathermy through the left shoulder area.

Table 5.2. General Indications and Contraindications of Shortwave Diathermy

GENERAL INDICATIONS

Adnexitis	Myalgia
Amenorrhea	Myositis
Brachial plexus neuritis	Neuritis
Bronchiectasis	Osteoarthritis (chronic)
Bronchitis	Otitis externa, media (extreme caution)
Bursitis (subacute, chronic)	Parametritis
Colic	Pelvic inflammatory disease (subacute, chronic)
Contusions	Periostitis
Dislocations	Peripheral vascular disease (remote application only, to cause a reflex vasodilation)
Diverticulitis	Pleurisy
Dysmenorrhea	Prostatitis
Epicondylitis	Pyelitis (subacute, chronic)
Facet syndrome	Rheumatoid monoarthritis (subacute, chronic)
Fibrositis	Sprains (with posttherapy massage and exercise)
Fibrous fixation/ankylosis (eg, post-traumatic)	Strains (with posttherapy massage and exercise)
Furuncle/carbuncle (superficial)	Subluxations
Gastrointestinal neurosis	Tenosynovitis
Hypertonia	Vasomotor headaches
Intercostal neuralgia	
Ischialgia (chronic)	
IVD syndrome (eg, sciatica)	
Lumbago	
Mastitis	

ABSOLUTE CONTRAINDICATIONS

Attached hearing aid	Over contact lenses
Fractures (recent) in the young	Over moist dressings
Hemoptysis, epitaxis, melena, and other hemorrhagic tendencies	Over pregnant uterus
Malignancy (diagnosed, suspected)	Over wet skin
Menstruation (profuse period)	Patients with pacemaker
Metallic dental appliances	Peptic ulcers (bleeding)
On a metal table	Pyretic states
Over adhesive strapping	Rheumatoid arthritis (acute)
Over casts	Septic arthritis (acute)
	Tuberculosis (pulmonary or joint)

RELATIVE CONTRAINDICATIONS

Areas of decreased vascularity	Osteoporosis (advanced)
Arteriosclerosis (advanced)	Over growing epiphyseal plate
Arthritis deformans	Patients on anticoagulant therapy (authorities differ)
Decompensating heart condition	Patients on cortisone therapy
Hypothermesthesia (extreme caution)	Patients on gold therapy
Infants and the debilitated elderly	Peripheral vascular disease (occlusive)
Intrauterine device (metallic)	Poliomyelitis (acute stage)
Metallic buttons, zippers, hairpins, buckels, clasps, keys, knives, etc	Polyneuritis with impaired circulation
Metallic implant	Suppurating inflammatory processes
Metallic jewelry, watches	Thrombosis
Nondraining cellulitis	Transcerebral applications (deep)
Osteomyelitis	Varicose veins

Note: This table is only a guide. Extreme caution must be used when any inflammatory condition is being treated. Each patient must be treated as an individual and in accord with high standards of professional judgment as directed by the diagnosis.

cessible to a purely conductive current. Thus, shortwave diathermy is an excellent modality to locally increase temperatures within thick muscle, viscera, and para-articular structures. See Figure 5.11. The general effect of diathermy is rapid peripheral vessel dilatation that is accompanied by a rise in body temperature, which in turn, stimulates the hypothalamic thermostat to increase pulse rate, respiration, and general metabolism.

ANALGESIA

A chemical substance, most likely a metabolic by-product, found in normal tissue that is similar to lactic acid may irritate nociceptors and produce pain if it is not continually removed by an adequate blood flow (eg, as in ischemia, stasis). The application of high frequency energy such as that of shortwave diathermy tends to produce local dilatation and an increased circulatory rate, thus reducing the tissue concentration of this chemical below the threshold of the nociceptors.

SEDATION

Although the mechanism is not completely understood, diathermy has shown to produce a marked sedative effect on irritated motor nerves (eg, hypertonia, cramps, spasms of both striated and smooth muscle) and sensory nerves (pain, hyperesthesia, deep tenderness). A typical application is shown in Figure 5.12.

TRANSCEREBRAL CONDUCTION

Transcerebral applications are generally discouraged. Extreme caution must be used in treating the ears, sinuses, eyes, face, mouth, neck, cervical muscles, or cranium (eg, for headaches) even with induction-field therapy. Early adverse signs consist of headache, nausea, and vertigo. Such conditions as hordeolum, iritis, otitis, facial palsy, gingivitis, stomatitis, mastoiditis, laryngitis, parotitis, or sinusitis can usually be treated physiotherapeutically with less liability by applications of

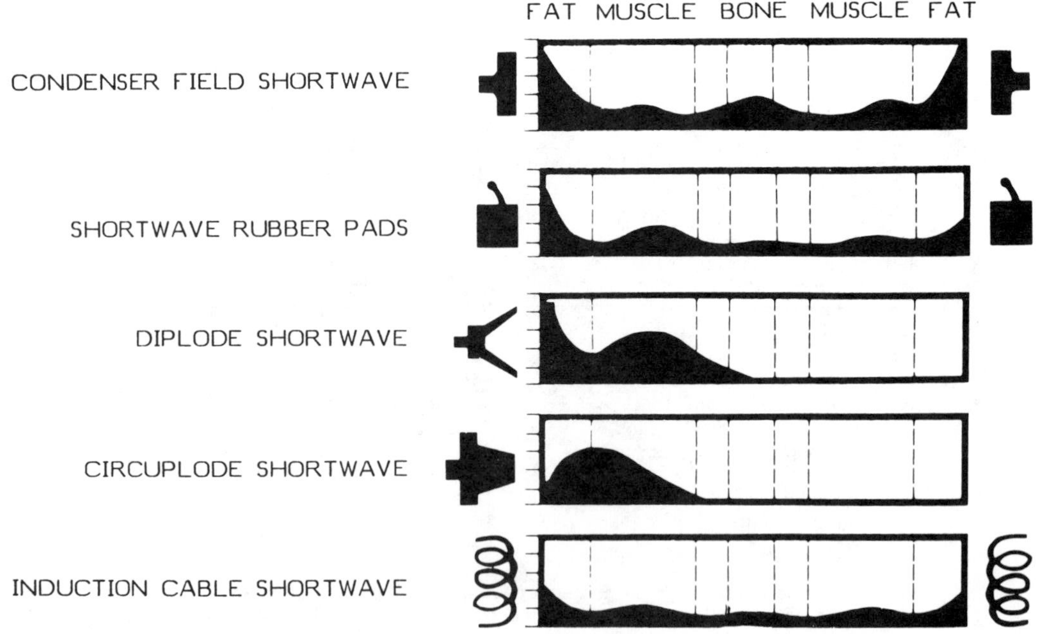

Figure 5.11. Comparison of depth/temperature relationships for various types of shortwave diathermy modalities.

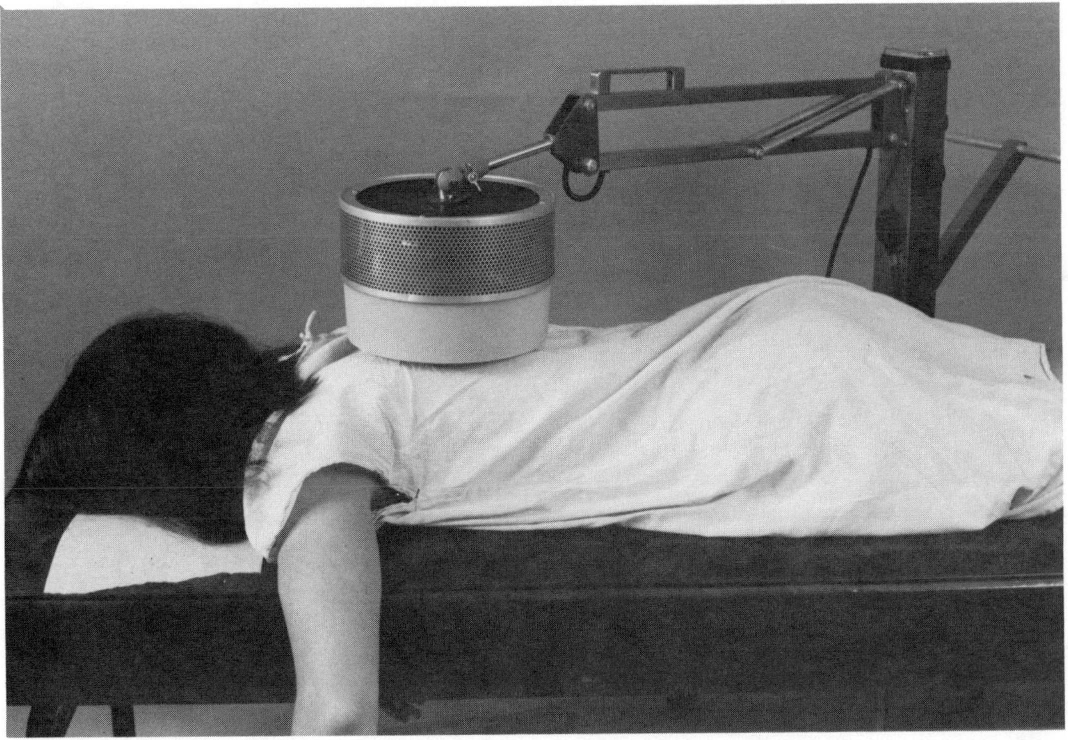

Figure 5.12. The application of induction-field shortwave diathermy for treatment of the thoracic area.

superficial heat or cold, or with diathermy by a remote reflex therapy.

While not considered an inflexible standard, some authorities feel that deep heat is contraindicated in any disease process that will respond to the simpler methods of superficial heat which give satisfactory results.

SAFETY PRECAUTIONS

The general rules for applying therapeutic heat should always be followed. Check for frayed wires or loose connection on the equipment. As with all forms of therapeutic heat, diathermy should be applied to an unclothed body part only. See Figure 5.13. Inspect the patient's skin for scars or broken skin, and ascertain the quality of heat perception.

Advise the patient of what to expect, and administer therapy by gradually increasing the current to the desired level. The patient should be warned not to touch cords, the machine, or any metal during therapy. Make sure that the equipment is grounded. During therapy, it is a good safety procedure to allow the patient to have control of the "off" switch. See Figure 5.14.

Several other precautions should be considered:

1. While metallic dental fillings are not usually contraindications, plates, bridges, and other dental appliances containing metal must be removed prior to therapy. Hearing aids must be placed at least 4 feet from the treatment field.

2. Shortwave diathermy should not be applied simultaneously with another form of

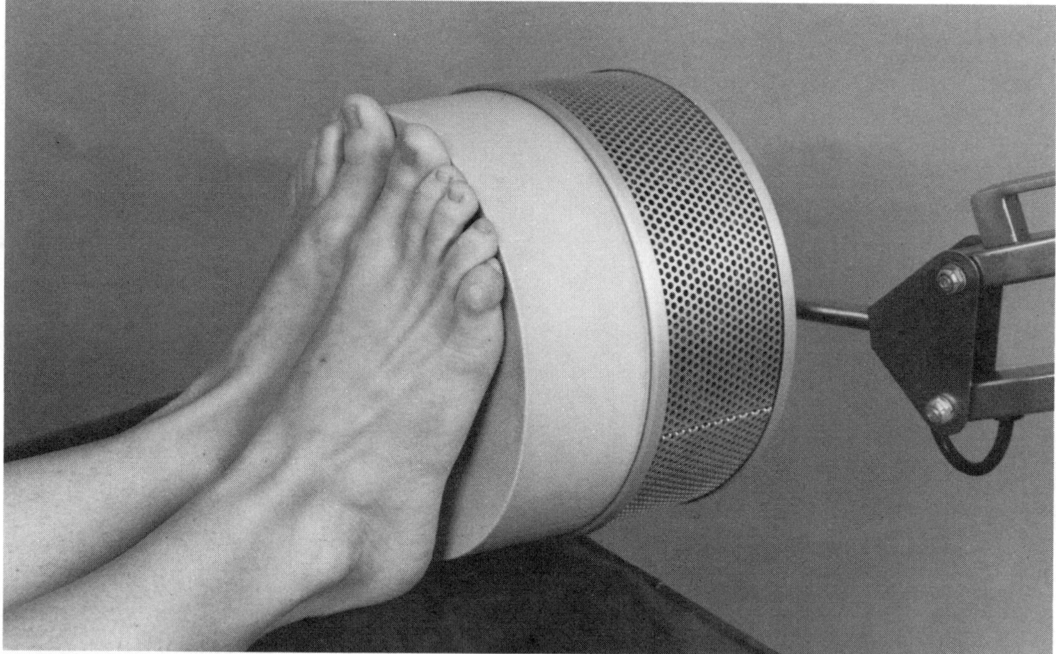

Figure 5.13. Although toweling is not necessary for spacing with induction field diathermy (as shown in the above photograph), care must be taken to assure that buildup of perspiration does not occur at the applicator—skin interface.

electrotherapy, nor should more than one shortwave unit be used on the same patient at the same time.

3. When two appendages are being treated at the same time (eg, both knees, feet, hands), several layers of toweling should be placed between them. See Figure 5.15.

4. Care must be taken to assure that the applicator is parallel to the surface of the skin. If an applicator is angled, heat will be excessively concentrated at the edge of the applicator nearest the skin.

5. When electrodes must be inspected, adjusted, or relocated, the current must be turned off during the process and then gradually increased again after the site of application has been examined and been found to be satisfactory.

6. Periodically review the contraindications listed in Table 5.2.

Dosage

For the most part, the regulation of dosage with shortwave diathermy is presently empirical, depending on the patient's perception of warmth and communicative ability. Patient tolerance should always be the prime consideration. To date, this subjective measure is our primary guideline and is based on normal heat perception by the patient. Only with an orificial electrode in which a thermometer can be incorporated will truly objective data be available. If a patient does not have normal innervation, the use of shortwave therapy should only be applied with extreme caution. With these thoughts in mind, the following dosages are recommended.

Dosage Level I. For patients who have no appreciable specific pain or in the treatment of visceral conditions, gradually increase tem-

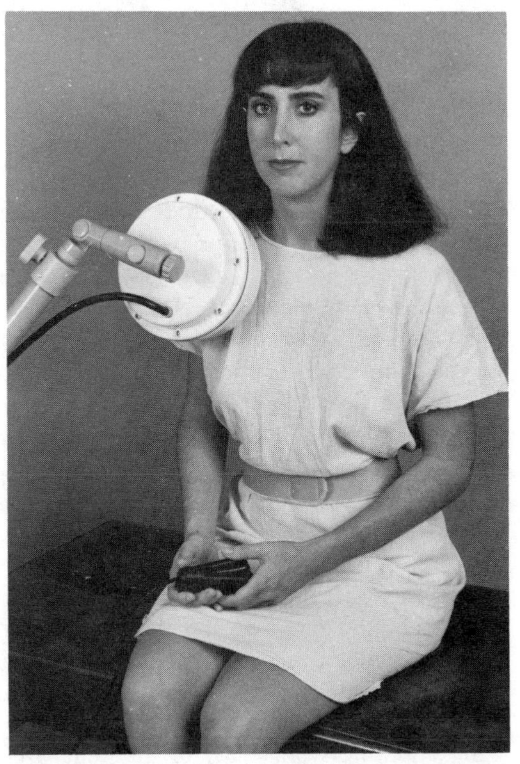

Figure 5.14. A patient holding the "off" switch during the application of induction-field shortwave diathermy to the right shoulder area.

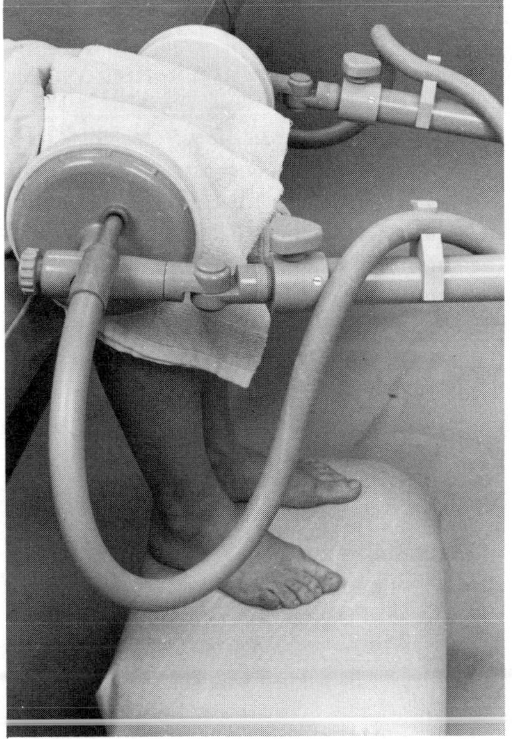

Figure 5.15. Space-plate application of condenser-field diathermy through both knees.

perature to where the patient just perceives a comfortable yet distinct (but never intense or painful) sensation of "velvety" warmth. Keep in mind that heat sensors are located only in the skin, not in deeper tissues.

Dosage Level II. For patients who have pain, the temperature is increased to a point just below the level of Dosage I. Likewise in acute inflammatory conditions, no detectable sensation of warmth should be perceived by the patient.

The general rule is that the more acute the condition to be treated, the less temperature elevation and the shorter the treatment duration. Weaker currents applied to the hands and feet and to trophic lesions are also generally indicated.

Treatment Time

A rapid buildup of heat that might surpass homeostatic safety measures should always be avoided. It takes time for the tissues to reach the desired and fairly constant temperature level. Normally, from 3 to 5 minutes elapse before maximum current reaches its peak effect.

Each unit contains a timing device that can be preset for the duration of the treatment. A maximum treatment time of 10 minutes is recommended for most situations. While some authorities recommend longer durations, various studies have shown that little added effect is achieved after 10 minutes. Acutely painful/tender and inflammatory processes usually require a duration of 5—10 minutes at Dosage II. Durations in excess of 10 minutes at Dosage I, but not exceeding 20 minutes, are generally reserved for deep, chronic, noninflammatory joint lesions; eg, in the treatment of osteoarthritis of the shoulder, hip, or knee where buildup is desirable.

Initially, typical sessions are usually conducted daily or on alternate days, depending on the physician's clinical judgment of the situation at hand. As the problem begins to resolve, the interval between applications may be extended but widely spaced intervals (eg, 4—5 days or more) are difficult to justify.

Positioning of Capacitor Electrodes

The three common electrode positions are (1) transverse, (2) longitudinal, and (3) coplanar.

Transverse (Horizontal) Applications. In this common application technique, the tissues are located in perpendicular layers relative to the field lines (ie, connected in series). Because energy absorption increases in tissue quadratically with the current's field-line density, care must be taken to localize the highest field density accurately to obtain the most efficient results. See Figure 5.16.

If it is desirable to produce greater heat superficially on one side and deeper heat on the other side, this can be accomplished by using a bilaterally variable electrode—skin distance. The same effect can be achieved by using applicators bilaterally of different size; ie, the energy concentration will be greater at the side of the smaller electrode. Thus, electrode—skin spacing and electrode diameter can be varied to achieve optimal effects. See Figure 5.17.

Longitudinal Applications. In this technique, the subcutaneous tissue layers are approximately in line with the direction of the field lines (ie, connected in parallel) between the condenser plates. See Figure 5.18.

Co-planar Applications. The electrodes are placed in the same plane in this technique (ie, on the same side of the body part to be treated). Because of this placement, the energy absorption in deep tissues is quite low, especially if the applicators are separated 1½ times their diameter or more. See Figure 5.19.

Therefore, with these three different types of electrode positions, the following factors will affect the site of the highest field-line density:

1. Electrode—skin distance.
2. Location of electrodes, in relation to

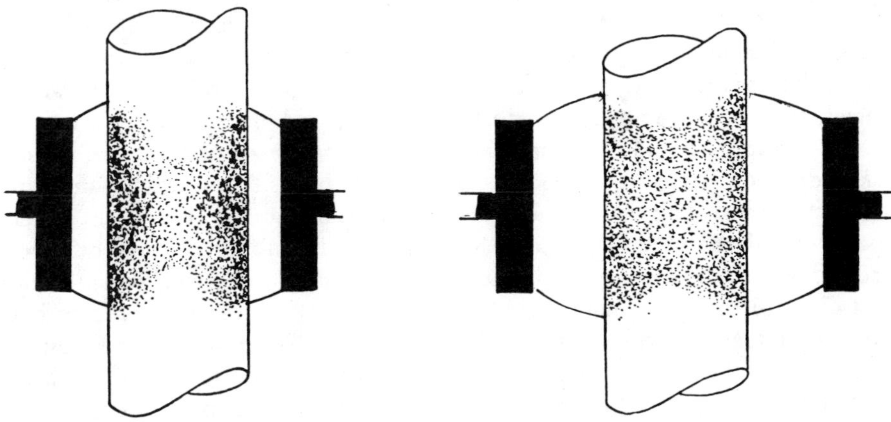

Figure 5.16. Extent of transverse condenser field depth effect. The drawing on the left depicts fairly close spacing, where a greater increase in superficial heat is produced. When the placement offers a greater electrode—skin distance, as shown in the drawing on the right, the temperature is increased in deep tissues almost as much as it is superficially.

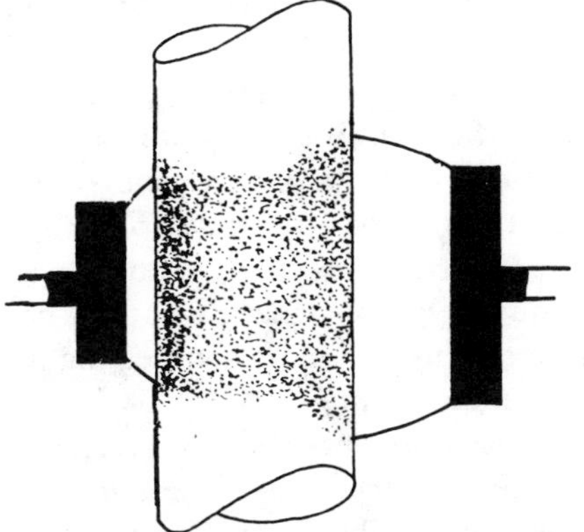

Figure 5.17. Schematic of transverse condenser field effect where the applicator diameters and electrode—skin spaces have been varied. Superficial heat will be greatest at the side with the smaller diameter applicator and the shorter electrode—skin distance.

each other and to the body part being treated.

3. Size of electrodes, in relation to each other and to the body part being treated.

In general, the thicker the body part to be treated, the greater should be the electrode—skin distance, which is provided by air spacing or towels. This is true whether plates, pads, or coils are used. The reason for such spacing, when excessive superficial heat is to be avoided, is that the most rapid decrease in field intensity occurs close to the applicator.[7] Most manufacturers offer specific instructions for correct spacing in relation to the power output of their equipment.

CONDENSER FIELD APPLICATIONS

Shortwave diathermy applications involve the application of either condenser field heating or electromagnetic field heating, and both methods require tuning of the patient circuit to resonance. In the condenser field technique, the part to be treated is placed between two condenser plates, pads, or cuffs that give rise to a high frequency alternating voltage. The peak current is inversely proportional to the resistance offered by the conducting tissues, which, in turn, is determined by the involved tissue's resistivity. Because of this, strong conduction currents can readily be established in tissues with a relatively high fluid content.

Modified applications of this standard technique are made with:

1. *Space plates.* An air-spaced plate is a condenser applicator that is enclosed in a rigid plastic material. The plastic ring surrounding each plate is attached to a self-retaining adjustable arm to provide for proper spacing between the condenser plate and the surface of the body part to be treated. All condenser-field units have their greatest effect near the skin, but, as penetration must cross from electrode to electrode, secondary effects are produced in muscle and bone.

2. *Glass envelopes.* In this design, each condenser plate is enclosed in a glass envelope. The position of the condenser plate within the envelope is usually adjustable, and the distance between the condenser plate and body part surface can be varied by positioning.

3. *Condenser pads.* These pads consist of pliable plates that readily conform to the surface being treated. The plates are enclosed in a flexible rubber or plastic material, with electrode—skin spacing provided by dry toweling (1—2-inch layer) or heavy moisture-free felt (½—1-inch layer). This absorbent spacing material also reduces the risk of a superficial burn resulting from the accumulation of perspiration. The applicators can be fixed in position by sandbags or rubber straps.

4. *Internal metal electrodes.* These electrodes have been specially designed for use in the rectum or vagina. When utilized, a large belt-like electrode is applied over the abdomen, which produces a higher current density around the smaller internal electrode. Shortwave diathermy internal electrodes are an efficient deep heating agent for application to pelvic organs.[8] See Figure 5.20. The largest internal electrode that will fit the orifice should be used because poor contact can produce a severe burn. Thus, a variety of sizes should be available in the office.

INDUCTION COIL APPLICATIONS

Whereas an electric field current is formed between the two condenser electrodes, a magnetic field is generated by a coil-field in induction therapy. In this type of electromagnetic field heating, a drum, a monode, an insulated cable loop, or a pancake coil (an encircled continuous coil, resembling a coiled rope) is generally utilized. In the latter two techniques, electromagnetic coil-field heating (inductothermy) is used when heating a large part or an entire limb.

1. *Drum technique.* In this technique, the coil is enclosed in a plastic container, which is sometimes flexible at the hinges (eg, Diplode) so that it can be angled to conform to the body part being treated. A plastic hous-

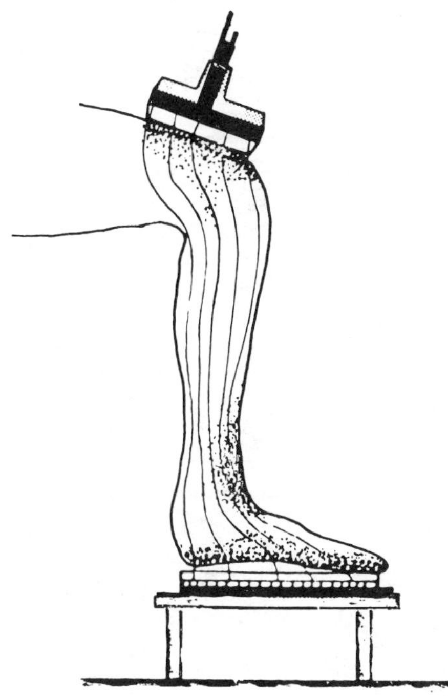

Figure 5.18. Diagram of longitudinal condenser field application in the leg. In longitudinal applications, the voltage through the tissues is relatively the same and the current density will follow the path of least resistance (ie, tissues with the highest water content).

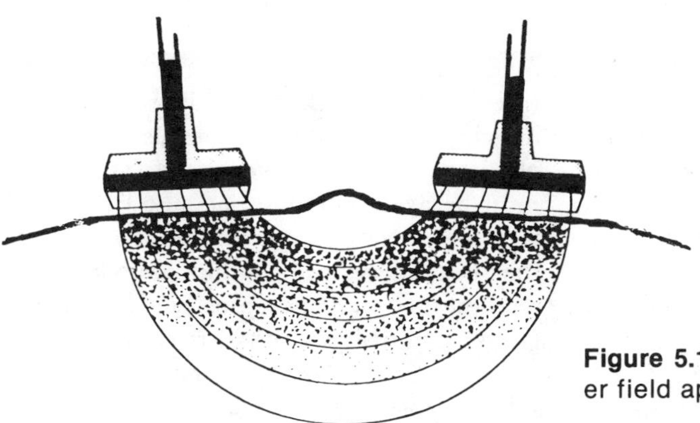

Figure 5.19. Diagram of co-planar condenser field application to the back.

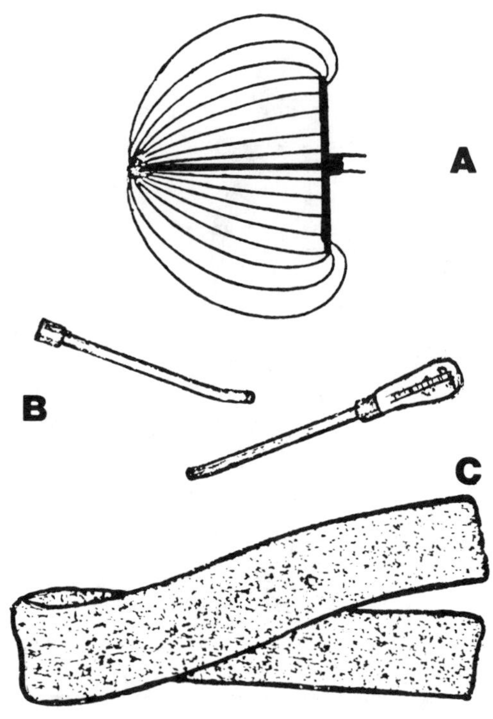

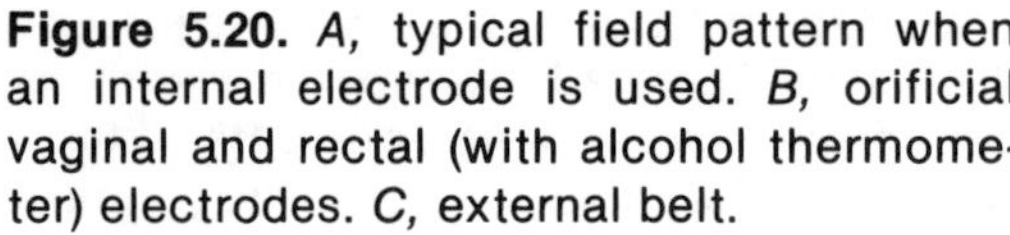

Figure 5.20. *A*, typical field pattern when an internal electrode is used. *B*, orificial vaginal and rectal (with alcohol thermometer) electrodes. *C*, external belt.

ing provides some spacing between the loops of the cable and the surface of the body part. The primary field density of a drum is in muscle tissue, a moderate effect is produced in subcutaneous fat, and only a negligible amount reaches deep bone.

2. *Monode technique.* A conventional monode is a helical induction coil applicator that operates on principles and has heat-producing effects that are similar to those of a drum, except that the applicator itself is not flexible. See Figure 5.21. Peak temperatures of a monode will penetrate to a depth of 1—2 centimeters in muscle tissue.[9]

A special type of unit is called a Circuplode. The applicator incorporates a special screen that is placed in front of a coil electrode. See Figure 5.22. Its function is to stop the electric field but allow the magnetic field to pass. This offers a distinct advantage in that it decreases the heat in the subcutaneous fatty tissue to a minimum, allows a greater thermal effect to be produced within muscle tissue, yet its effect on bone is almost nil. The reason for this is that muscle is a better conductor than fat or bone. Thus, it is an efficient modality when the desire is to heat muscle but not the subcutaneous layer of fat or deeper bone. However, its application must be made cautiously because the patient will not perceive any sensation of heat until the heat developed within muscle tissue reaches the thermoreceptors in the surface layers, essentially via conduction.

3. *Insulated cable technique.* A heavily insulated cable of 2—4 circles can be shaped to almost any desirable form of application; eg, "pancake" coil, spaced about 1-inch apart, "hair pin" loop, or coil for wrapping around an extremity. See Figure 5.23. Wooden

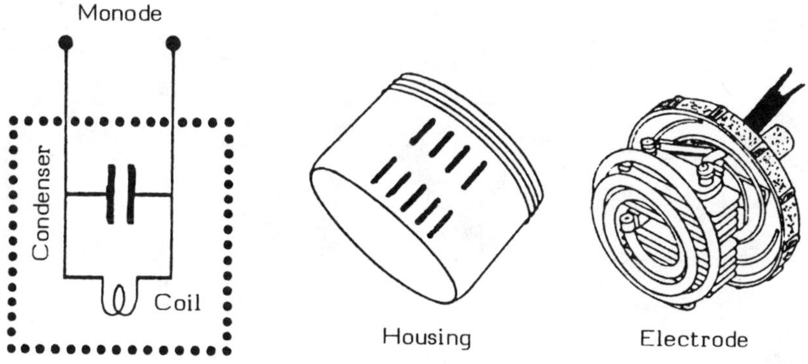

Figure 5.21. Wiring diagram (left) of a typical monode applicator (right).

"spacers" are available to assure a symmetrical design. The cable ends should never be crossed, and the two ends leading to the diathermy unit should be of equal length and separated by at least the distance the outlets on the control unit are separated. Whenever coil—skin spacing is required, towels can be used. Typical thickness is 1—2 inches.

The high frequency current flowing through a looped or coiled cable creates a magnetic field that induces *eddy currents* in the body part located within the field. Eddy currents within the limb flow in opposite directions to those of the coil current and generate heat within the tissues (inductothermy). It is an efficient method for heating an entire extremity.

The major factors relating to electromagnetic field heating are:

1. The distance between the coil and the skin, the distance between coil windings, and the magnitude of the insulating material's dielectric contents—all of which determine coil capacity.

2. The length and shape of the coil, which determine the magnitude of coil inductance.

3. The frequency of oscillation. If the frequency of the electrical energy is large compared with the natural frequency of the coil, then the coil will function capacitatively by capacitor field heating. On the other hand, if the electrical frequency is small relative to the frequency of the coil, then the coil will function inductively by eddy current heating.

Induction current is greatest where the magnetic field is strongest. When an induction coil is used, the current density is greatest close to the cable and at the fat—muscle, interface. See Figures 5.24 and 5.25.

ENERGY TRANSFER

Regardless of the type of shortwave therapy used, the intensity of the heat produced will be determined by the strength of the current, current density, and conductivity of the tissues involved. According to *Kirchhoff's law,* the greatest level of heat will be produced in the area of greatest current density.[10] It is this *area of current density* that differs among the various techniques.

For all practical purposes, tissue conductivity is proportional to its water content; ie, the higher the water content, the better the conductivity because the greatest current flow will occur in tissues with the least resistance.[11] For example, edematous tissue will be selectively heated to a higher temperature than muscle tissue, and muscle tissue will be selectively heated to a greater level than bone under the same conditions.

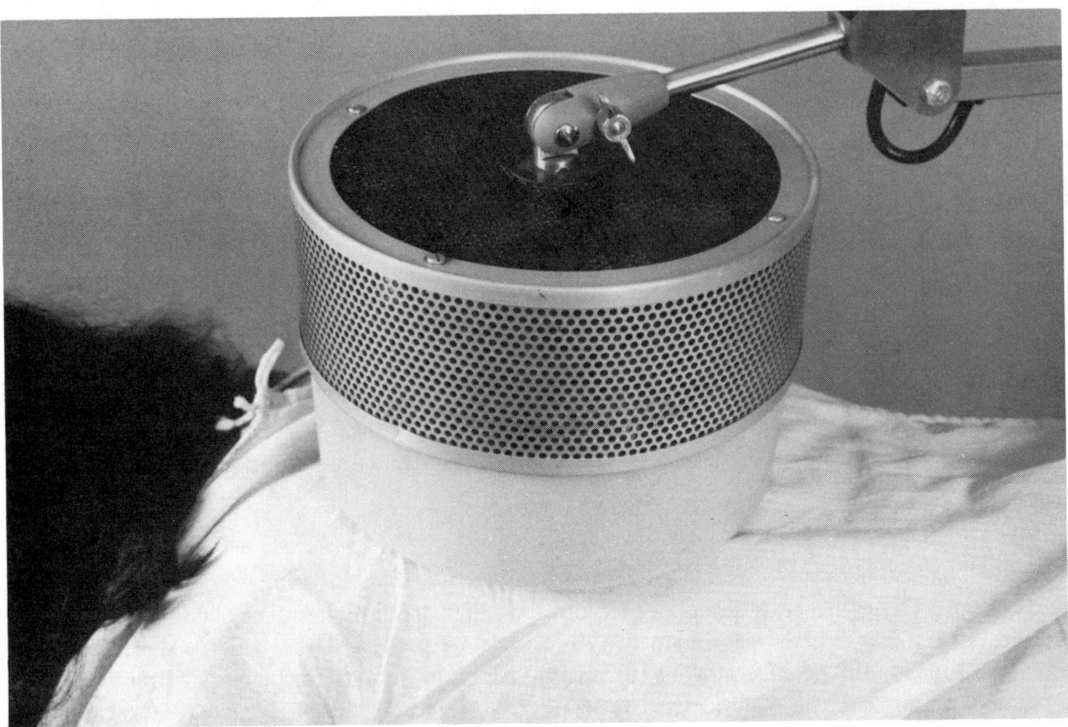

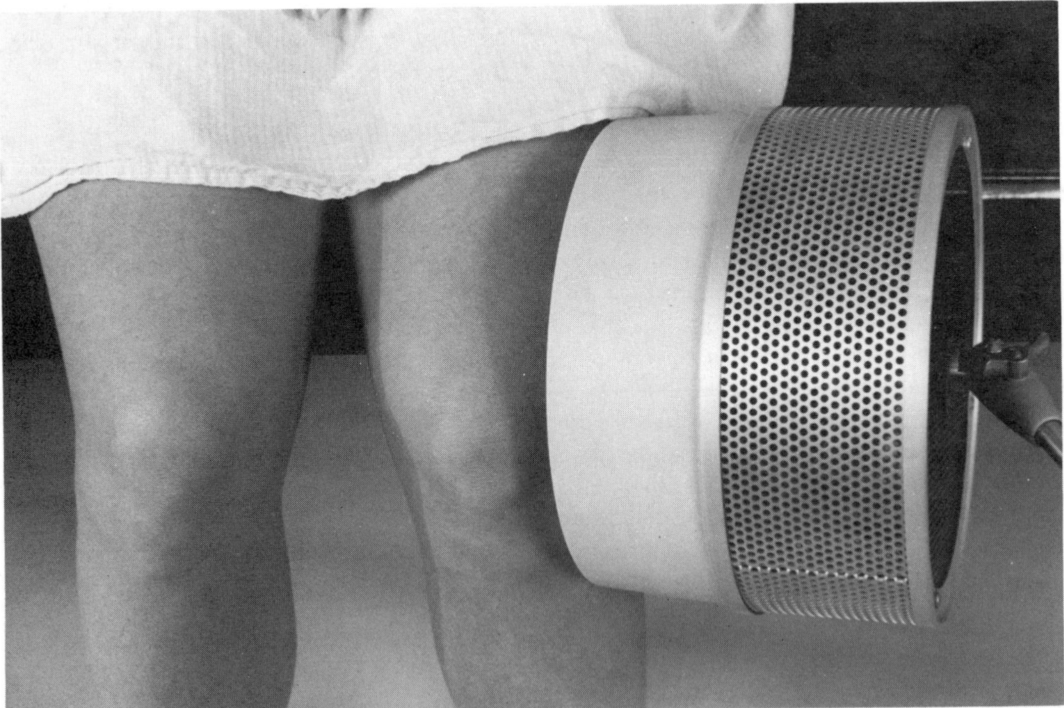

Figure 5.22. *Top,* Circuplode application of induction-coil diathermy to the thoracic area; *bottom,* to the lateral aspect of the left knee.

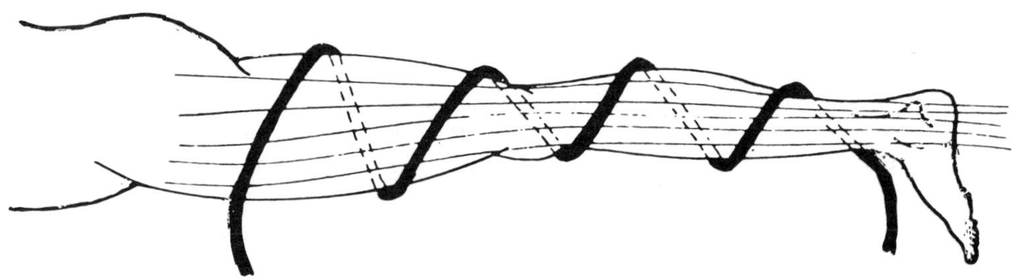

Figure 5.23. Schematic of a wraparound induction coil applied to a lower extremity.

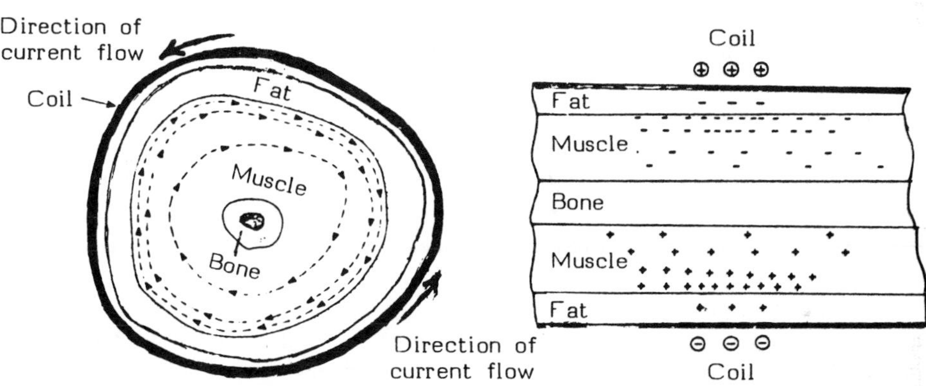

Figure 5.24. Wraparound induction coil electromagnetic field. In the left diagram, depicting a transverse section of a limb that has been enclosed in a wraparound induction coil, note that the tissue current density is greatest at the fat—muscle interface. The diagram on the right portrays this process in a schematic longitudinal section.

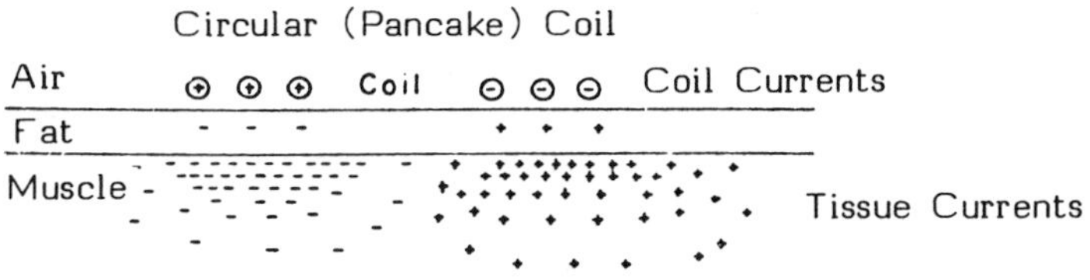

Circular (Pancake) Coil

Air ⊕ ⊕ ⊕ Coil ⊖ ⊖ ⊖ Coil Currents

Fat

Muscle Tissue Currents

Figure 5.25. Circular (pancake) induction coil electromagnetic field. As with a wraparound coil, the tissue current density with a pancake coil is greatest at the fat—muscle interface.

Some examples of tissue water content are:

Tissue	Water Content
Bone	5—16%
Brain	68%
Fat	14—15%
Muscle	72—75%
Skin	5—16%

The importance of these percentage figures can be better appreciated when it is realized that the ratio of temperature increase in muscle as compared with that of fat is 1:10 with the condenser method and 1:1 with the induction cable technique.[12]

Due to its high density and conductivity, a metallic implant and the adjacent tissues will be heated selectively far beyond that of other tissues in the field when induction currents are used. With the condenser method, the metal itself is not heated but the surrounding tissues become excessively hot.

Specific Applications

As previously described, effective therapeutic heating essentially depends on apparatus capabilities, proper dosage, treatment duration, and electrode position. Another important factor is the selection of the proper method of treatment among the alternatives available. In general, all forms of intelligently applied diathermy will produce satisfactory results. However, certain techniques offer specific conveniences or safety benefits in specific situations. One example is shown in Figure 5.26.

The shortwave condenser field is the method of choice when treating internal organs. The energy of the electromagnetic field will not penetrate deep enough to create the stimulation effect desired when induction applicators are used (eg, drum, cables).[13]

Typical applicator utilization for various parts of the body is shown in Table 5.3.

Pulsed Shortwave Diathermy

In recent years, the application of pulsed high frequency currents have been preferred over currents with a continuous frequency. It has been the authors' experience that, except in the treatment of osteoarthritis, it is generally preferable to use a pulsed shortwave current whenever possible. A typical unit is shown in Figures 5.27 and 5.28.

When pulsed shortwaves are used, a primary objective is to select the highest possible pulse power while producing as little heat as possible. Hardly any perceptive heat is generated during pulsed shortwave diathermy; thus, it is particularly indicated when perceptible heat is to be avoided (submitis dose) but the stimulation effect would be of benefit.

Most units that employ a pulsed current operate at a frequency of 27.12 megacycles, with a pulse duration of 65 microseconds and an adjustable pulse rate of 80—600 Hz. The current is applied via an induction coil (eg, drum) or a condensor field.

Some authorities claim that a pulsed current achieves deeper penetration than a continuous current, but this claim is widely disputed. Nevertheless, various benefits have been established. Studies have shown that collagen formation, fat activity, fibroblastic alignment, hematoma canalization, histocytic activity, phagocytosis, and white cell infiltration were enhanced by pulsed shortwaves when wounds were treated.[14] Research has also shown that the larvae of Drosophila were killed more effectively by pulsed diathermy than by continuous applications.[15] Various other papers have reported excellent results in the treatment of arthritis, the stimulation of the body's defensive mechanisms, the resolution of calcific bursitis, sinusitis, lymphadenitis, and recurrent otitis media with the use of pulsed diathermy.[16,17] In addition to these benefits, reports have been made of rapid pain reduction, rapid absorption of hematoma and edema, rapid fracture healing, and powerful stimulation to peripheral circulation.[18]

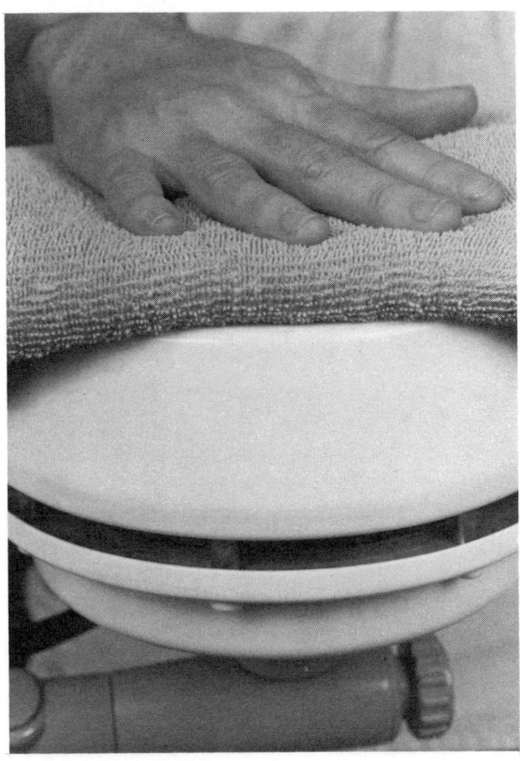

Figure 5.26. The use of shortwave diathermy in the treatment of a hand.

Table 5.3. Application Techniques of Shortwave Diathermy

Body Part(s)	*Common Techniques*
Abdominal organs	Condenser pads or plates
Back	Condenser pads or plates, pancake coil (patient prone), or drum
Coccyx	Pancake coil (patient prone) or drum
Elbow	Condenser pads, plates, or wraparound coils
Eyes	Condenser pads with spacing by gauze and terrycloth
Foot	Condenser pads
Hands/wrists	Condenser spaced plates or pads, rarely a pancake coil
Head/sinuses	Condenser plates with spacing provided by space plates
Hip/thigh	Condenser pads, drum, pancake coil, or coil and pad
Knees/ankles	Condenser plates, pads, wraparound coil, or circular cuff
Neck	Condenser pads, spaced plates, wraparound coil, or pancake coil
Pelvic organs	An internal electrode is the method of choice. Raise the temperature reading of the alcohol thermometer mounted within the electrode to 113°F (45°C) for 5—15 minutes.
Perineal area	Drum placed under a wooden chair of the sitting patient
Shoulder	Condenser plates, pads, or flexible drum

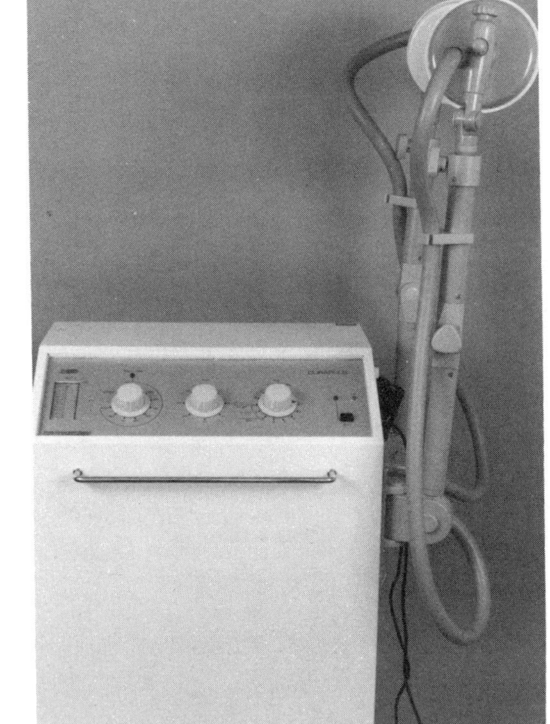

Figure 5.27. A Curapuls space-plate condenser-field diathermy unit.

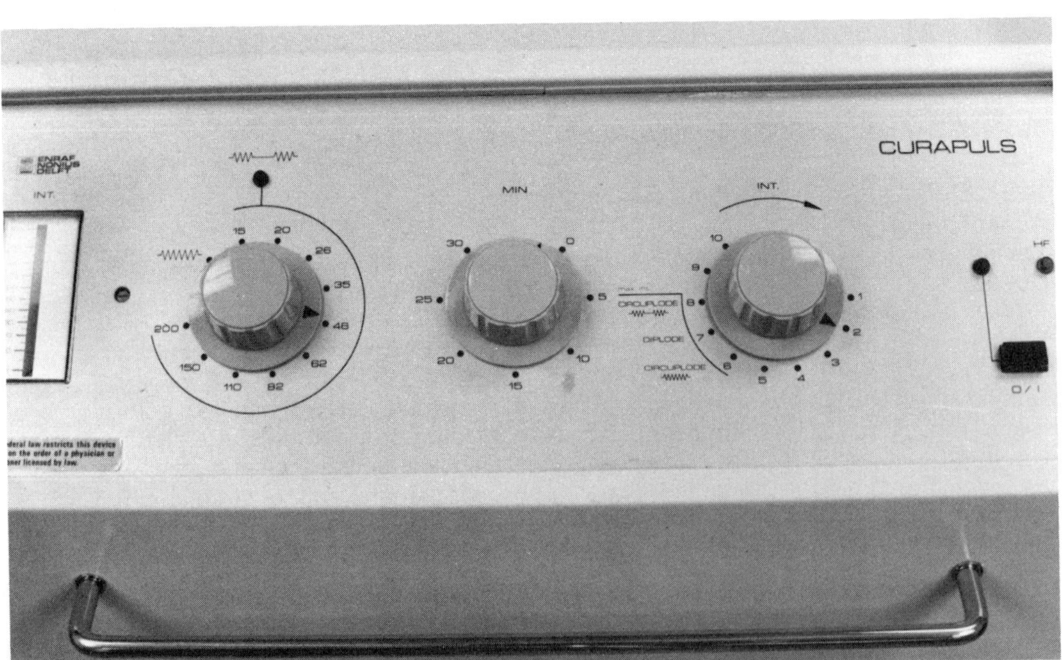

Figure 5.28. Close-up view of the instrument panel of a Curapuls space-plate condenser-field diathermy unit.

MICROWAVE DIATHERMY

Microwave diathermy was born out of research conducted during and after World War II. In 1946, Dr. Frank H. Krusen developed a water-cooled multicavity magnetism device that generated a frequency of 2450 megacycles at a wavelength of only 12.2 centimeters. These electromagnetic radar waves are in a band between radio waves and the visual spectrum—almost 90 times higher in frequency than shortwaves and about 300 times lower than infrared waves.

Physics

As do other electromagnetic waves, high frequency microwaves travel at the speed of light. The energy that is produced by a microwave device is made possible by a two-element generator called a magnetron, which generates an oscillating, highly stabilized, continuous, high frequency wave. The power input provides the rectified high voltage that is applied on the magnetron's anode and the current necessary for the various relays and filaments. The maximum output is about 100 watts. The energy is finally beamed from an antenna or radiator, called a director, that serves as the applicator. As with shortwave diathermy, no direct contact of the energy source with the skin is necessary. See Figure 5.29.

The particular frequency produced by the magnetron is made possible by a series of cavities linked together that contain the necessary capacitance and inductance, and one cavity contains a coupling loop. The field of the magnet causes the electrons leaving the cathode, located in the center, to make a circular path. As the velocity of the electrons increases, the cavities begin to resonate and electromagnetic radiation is generated. The coupling loop picks up the energy and carries it from the magnetron to a director (radiating element) via a coaxial cable. The director transmits the energy in a specific predetermined pattern toward the patient. Thus, it can be said that the electromagnetic radiation is "directed" to a specific site on the patient like a reflected beam of light. See Figure 5.30.

The degree of microwave-ray absorption by a patient depends on (1) the characteristics of the tissues that are exposed, (2) the frequency of the unit, and (3) the power density of the field produced.

Various types of microwave directors can be used in clinical practice, and each is unique in its characteristic heating pattern. The configuration of a pattern is determined and controlled by the distance that it is placed from the patient and the shape of the reflector incorporated into the unit. The power output of the microwave unit is adjusted in accordance with the size and shape of the body part being treated.

Physiologic Effects

The physiologic effects of microwaves are similar to those of the more powerful high frequency shortwaves, but the extent of reaction is different:

1. The smaller heat output of a microwave unit warms tissues in a much more local area. The heat in this smaller area can be much more readily dissipated by the area's vascular circulation.

2. There is little penetration into deeper organs—and this may be an advantage in some cases. Most of the microwave energy is used in heating the subcutaneous fat and the fat—muscle interface. Penetration into deep muscle tissue is only about a third as strong as that with shortwave diathermy.[19,20]

3. There is also a difference in the general cardiovascular adjustments. It has been shown that the distinct changes in blood flow after shortwave diathermy (eg, vasoconstriction of the renal and splanchnic vascular beds) are comparatively absent after microwave therapy. Thus, with microwave therapy, counteracting systemic homeostatic mechanisms are not put into play.

Most of the physiologic effects of micro-

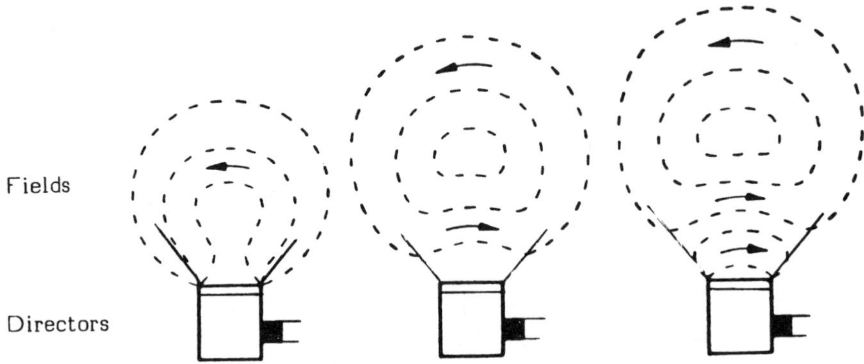

Figure 5.29. Diagrams showing the formation of the electric field emitted from a microwave director.

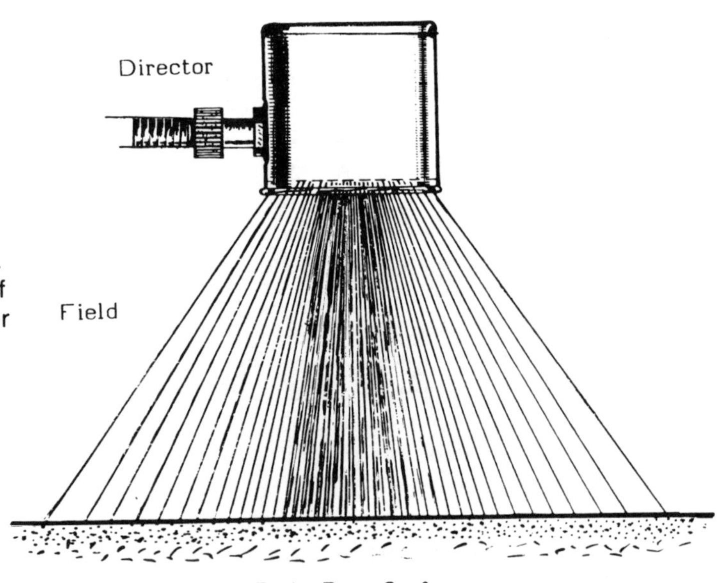

Figure 5.30. Schematic of a circular field microwave director, showing the conical radiations being beamed to a patient. Note that the lines of force are denser at the center and decrease in density toward the sides.

wave radiation are due to heating of tissues by conversion. The heat buildup occurs mainly because of the resistance offered by tissue constituents to the high frequency current, and a specific temperature distribution results within body tissues. This temperature distribution depends on the specific propagation and absorption characteristics of the tissues that are being treated.[21] Those tissues with a high water content (ie, good conductors) are the most likely to absorb the microwaves.

Some studies have indicated that, in addition to the thermal effects of microwave radiation, there may be some nonthermal changes. Commonly noted is a "pearl chain" formation, which is also seen as a by-product of pulsed shortwave diathermy, where serum blood cells and fat globules become aligned like a necklace. However, the clinical significance of this unusual pattern has not been determined. In addition to this effect, some investigators have reported blood coagulation changes—either increased or decreased, depending on dosage.[22] Other nonthermal effects of therapeutic microwaves such as the effect on bone growth and vasodilator responses have only been established in animal studies.

Indications

Whenever mild heat buildup or associated reflexes are desired in a specific site (eg, the deltoid insertion) that is localized and not too deep, microwave irradiation is the treatment of choice. See Figure 5.31. Microwave therapy has many of the advantages of certain types of superficial and deep heat. Contact is not necessary, and smaller, confined areas can often be treated more effectively. Orificial heating, however, cannot be applied by microwave irradiation, and the field that can be heated at any one time is relatively small. Microwave therapy has little, if any, effect on deep joints or viscera.

A large number of papers report good results with the use of microwave therapy in the treatment of many disorders of the eye. Iridocyclitis, scleritis, and keratitis are just three examples. However, because of the danger involved and the specialized skills necessary, such applications are usually best left to the experienced ophthalmologist than to the general practitioner.

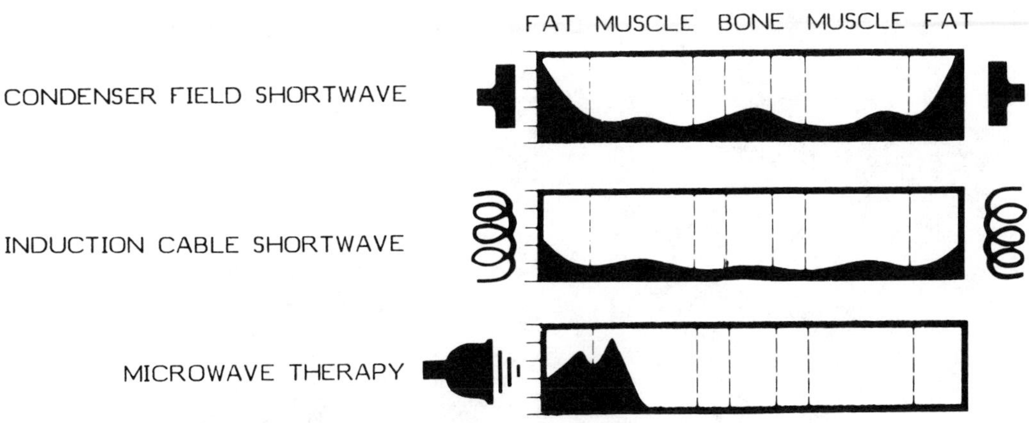

Figure 5.31. Comparison of depth/temperature effects of condenser field, induction field, and microwave diathermy.

Precautions During Use

If vigorous heating effects are desired, the applicator must be brought close to the surface of the skin (ie, within 1 inch). This is especially true when treatment is to be directed to a specific site. The applicator should not be brought into contact with the skin, as this may cause the development of intensely heated areas that are close to the antenna rod or director. This is invariably true when an "A Type" director is used. See Figure 5.32.

Precautions must be taken to avoid the formation of sweat droplets forming on the skin that can be selectively heated, leading to a superficial burn. This can be avoided by placing a towel between the applicator and the skin, but this procedure is not recommended by several authorities. It is better to keep the area open to inspection and wipe the area dry as is necessary.

Microwaves are known to cause lenticular opacities several days following direct exposure, but this is usually an accumulative effect. During treatment near the head, the eyes of the patient should be shielded with special goggles that incorporate a fine mesh of copper wire padded with felt. See Figure 5.33.

Watches must be kept away from the high frequency field or they might become magnetized. Hearing aids must be placed at least 4 feet from the treatment field. Take care never to cover the vent holes on the unit and that the equipment is well grounded.

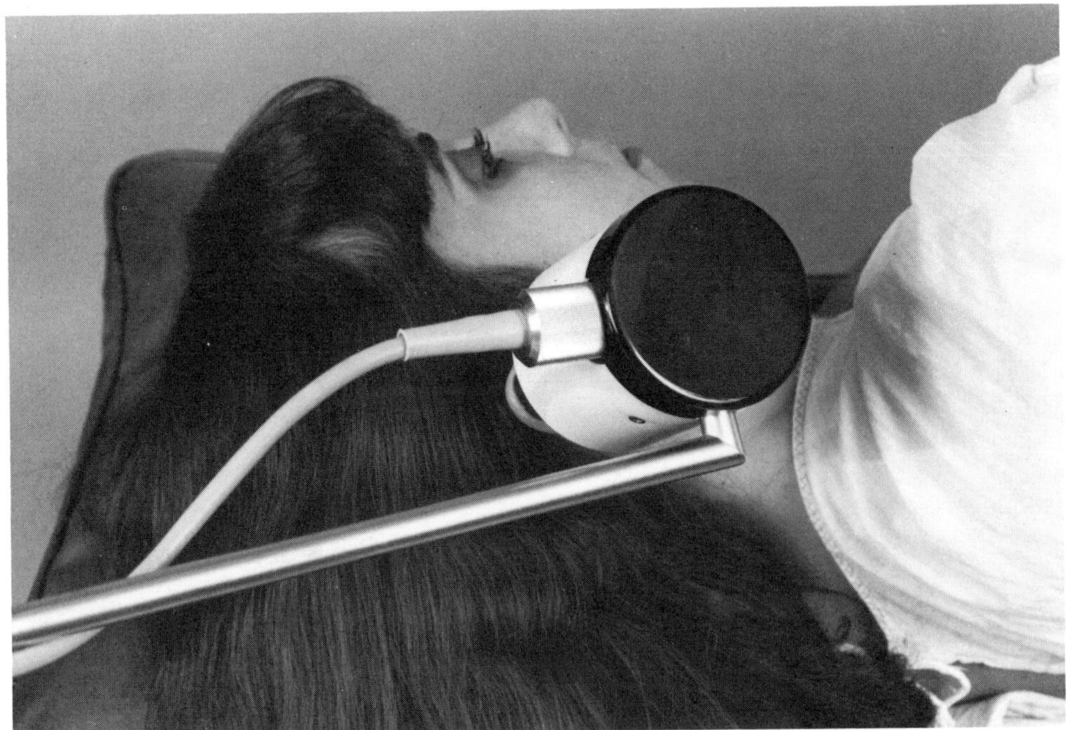

Figure 5.32. Microwave therapy to the right ear.

Contraindications

All the general contraindications to therapeutic heat should be considered. Applications to the very young or old should be conducted with great care. In addition, extreme caution should be used when applications are made to bony prominences. Current concentration on high spots will encourage the development of painful blebs. Also see Table 5.4.

The use of any high frequency current is usually contraindicated over ischemic tissue (eg, that associated with peripheral vascular diseases). However, Gersten found no difference in heating ischemic and normal tissue after radiations of 5 and 10 minutes. It was not until microwave exposures of the same intensity were increased to 15 and 20 minutes that damage to ischemic areas occurred. It is interesting that the average temperatures recorded in the damaged tissues were no higher than those registered in the uninjured tissues that had normal circulation.[23]

Specific Applications

The clinical effectiveness of a microwave unit's energy output essentially depends on (1) the type of unit used, (2) the electrode—skin distance, and (3) the amount of surface area to be treated. Generally, when the surface area is increased, the electrode—skin distance must be increased, and more power output is necessary. A typical unit is shown in Figure 5.34.

Various types of simply controlled directors can be used. The director should be spaced from 1—7 inches from the patient, depend-

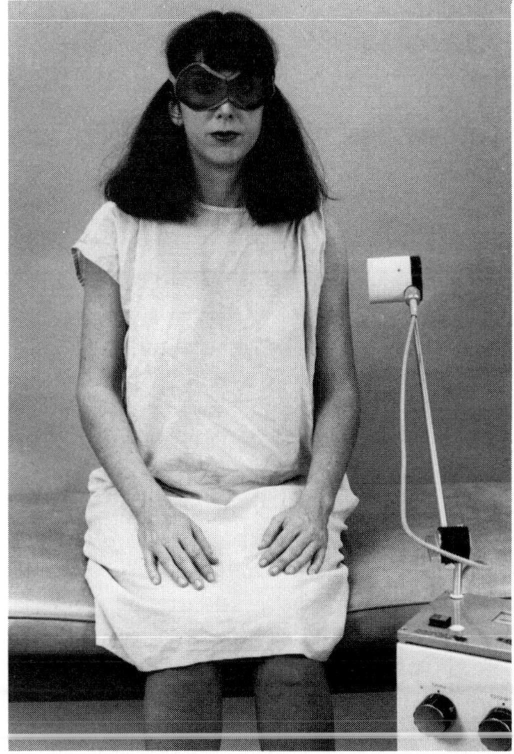

Figure 5.33. Microwave therapy to the left deltoid insertion. Note the use of special goggles.

Table 5.4. General Indications and Contraindications of Microwave Diathermy

GENERAL INDICATIONS	
Bursitis (subacute, chronic)	Radiculitis
Fibrositis	Rheumatoid arthritis (subacute, chronic)
Hematoma (aged)	Sinusitis
Myositis	Spondylosis
Neuritis	Sprains (subacute, chronic)
Osteoarthritis	Strains (subacute, chronic)
Pelvic inflammatory disease (chronic)	Subluxations
Pleurisy	Tenosynovitis
Otitis externa	
GENERAL CONTRAINDICATIONS	
Area of hypothermoesthesia	Over metallic implants
Attached hearing aid	Over moist dressings
Edematous areas	Over pregnant uterus
Hemorrhagic tendencies	Over scars
Into the brain	Over the eye
Metastatic carcinoma	Over the scrotum (authorities differ)
Osteomyelitis	Over wet skin
Over adhesive tape	Patient with a pacemaker
Over casts	Peripheral vascular disease (occlusive)
Over lumbar or abdominal regions during profuse menstruation	To patient in a metal bed or chair
	Tuberculosis

Note: This table is only a guide. Each patient must be treated as an individual and in accord with high standards of professional judgment as directed by the diagnosis.

ing on the type that is used. The size and shape of each pattern depends on the electrode—skin distance and the shape of the director's reflector. Keep in mind that as the electrode—skin distance is increased, the amount of radiation per surface unit decreases but the area of the surface irradiated increases. See Figure 5.35.

Common types of directors are described in Table 5.5. These general guidelines should be considered during the application of microwave diathermy. It should also be noted that the power output meter of a microwave unit is calibrated in percentages of power rather than in milliamperes, with maximum power being set at 100%.

The smaller types of directors incorporate an antenna and a hemisphere reflector. They produce a beam that has a ring-shaped cross-sectional field pattern, with a diameter of several inches. Thus, they produce circular patterns, some with maximum heating occurring at the periphery to help equal skin temperatures when irregular surfaces are irradiated. The larger corner-reflector-type directors produce an oval or nearly rectangular pattern, with the maximum intensity found in the center, that can be positioned to cover a much larger area (eg, a large part of the back or of a thigh).

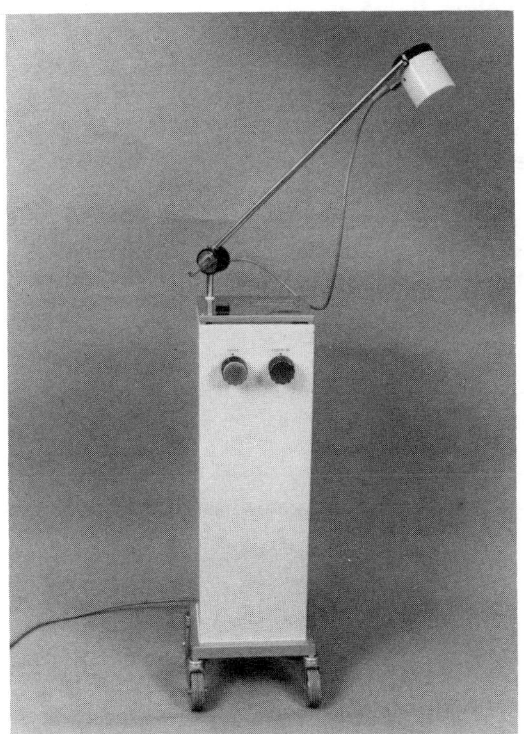

Figure 5.34. An Elmed microwave diathermy unit.

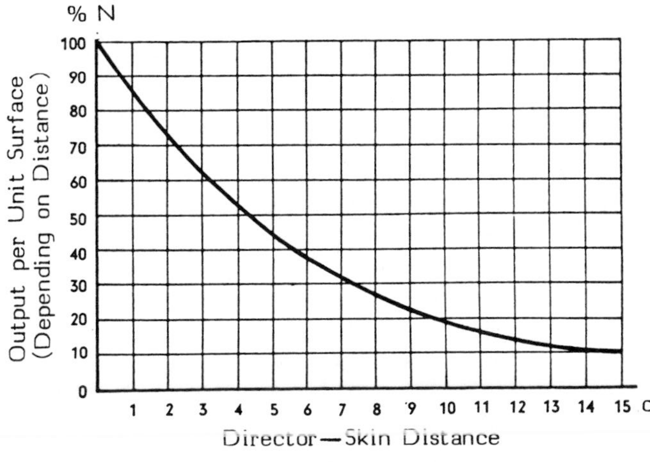

Figure 5.35. Graph showing how various applicator—skin distances influence output per surface unit in microwave therapy.

Table 5.5. Microwave Director General Application Data*

Type	*Description*	*Approximate Size of Heating Pattern*	*Spacing*	*Suggested % of Power*
A	Small hemisphere	4-inch diameter	1 inch	30—40
		6-inch diameter	2 inches	50—60
B	Large hemisphere	7-inch diameter	2 inches	40—50
		9-inch diameter	3 inches	50—80
		10—12-inch diameter	4 inches	50—80
C	Small rectangular reflector	6 square inches	1 inch	15—20
		8 square inches	2 inches	20—30
		21 square inches	3 inches	60—70
		37 square inches	4 inches	70—80
		57 square inches	5 inches	90—100
D	Intermediate-size rectangular reflector	Back: C7—Coccyx	5 inches	90
			7 inches	100
E	Large rectangular reflector		1 inch	20—40
			2 inches	60—80
			3 inches	80—90
			4 inches	80—100
		6 x 15 inches	5 inches	90—100

* Based on Burdick Unit.

Dosage and Treatment Time

Microwave therapy is one of the easiest modalities to use for the application of subcutaneous heat, and dosage is quickly measured and controlled. See Figure 5.36. As with other forms of electromagnetic energy, dosage is the product of applied energy times duration of exposure.

Proper dosage and treatment time, as with shortwave diathermy, are essentially based on subjective perception of heat if the patient's thermoesthetic faculties are normal. However, even a healthy perception of heat should be modified downward by the practitioner's experience when necessary. Keep in mind that the skin of different patients may have different absorptive and reflective characteristics.

Some general guidelines are shown in Table 5.6. It is well to keep in mind that these guidelines and those supplied by a manufacturer are average instructions. They cannot take unusual situations into consideration, and only with experience and caution should the physician exceed the recommended limits of power percentage and/or reduce the suggested spacing distance.

A treatment duration exceeding 20 minutes is inadvisable. Studies conducted by Worden and his associates found tissues temperatures to be lower after an exposure of 30 minutes than at 20 minutes.[24] See Figure 5.37.

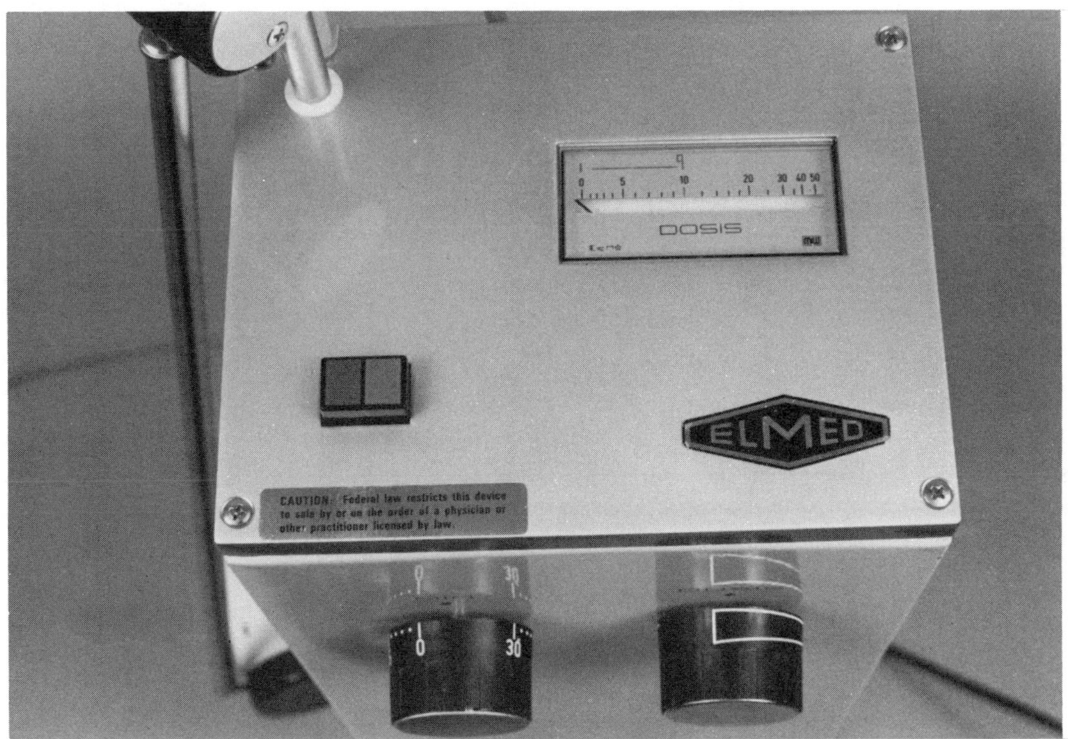

Figure 5.36. Top diagonal view of an Elmed microwave unit showing meter and controls.

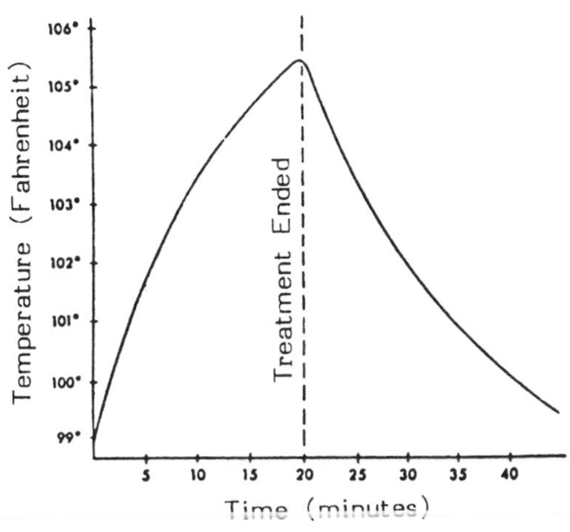

Figure 5.37. Time/temperature effects during microwave irradiation. Note that, during the 50-minute exposure, the maximum temperature peak is reached at 20 minutes and then rapidly decreases.

Table 5.6. Microwave Dosage and Treatment Duration*

Dose Level	Subjective Sensation	Typical Indications	Treatment Time (minutes)	Intensity
I	No detectable warmth	Acute, inflammatory processes	5—10	Low
II	Barely detectable warmth	Subacute inflammatory conditions	5—10	Low
III	Distinct, pleasant warmth	Nonspecific pain syndromes	10—20	High
IV	Intense warmth	Chronic disorders	10—20	High

* Based on Elmed Microwave 150

ULTRASOUND DIATHERMY

The term *ultrasound* or *ultrasonics* refers to acoustic vibrations above those frequencies, which are not available to the human ear, that penetrate into the deeper layers of tissue. Therapy with this deep heating modality is generally referred to as *ultrasound* or *ultrasound diathermy*.

Historical Background

The biologic effects of ultrasound were first noted by Langevin when he watched fish as they died after swimming into a beam of ultrasonic waves in 1917. Others expanded upon his studies, particularly Wood and Loomis who, in 1927, set down most of the basic principles on which present day ultrasound units operate. Their conclusions were first published in a paper titled, "Physical and Biological Effects of High-Frequency Sound Waves of Great Intensity."

In 1944, Horrath experimented with the use of inaudible sound waves in treating superficial malignant growths. His apparent success in the treatment of cutaneous sarcomas surprised the medical community, and it gave great impetus to the utilization of ultrasound therapy throughout the health-care field.

During the late 1940s, further studies and usage spread rapidly in Europe, especially in Germany, and to a lesser extent in this country. However, it wasn't until 1952, when the Council on Physical Medicine and Rehabilitation presented its first report on ultrasound therapy, that the therapy really came of age in the United States.

Today, the number of technical papers and articles relative to ultrasound diathermy number in the thousands, with some of the current research being directed toward its possible role as a cancer therapy; thus returning to Horrath's original interest 4 decades later.

Physics

Ultrasound equipment consists essentially of a high frequency generator (similar to that of a diathermy generator) and an applicator (sound head). See Figure 5.38. Electric oscillations (about 0.8—1 megacycle) produced by the generator cause a transducer in the applicator to vibrate and generate the ultrasonic waves. The generator itself is composed of three electrical components: a power input, an oscillating circuit to produce the high frequency current, and a transducer circuit.

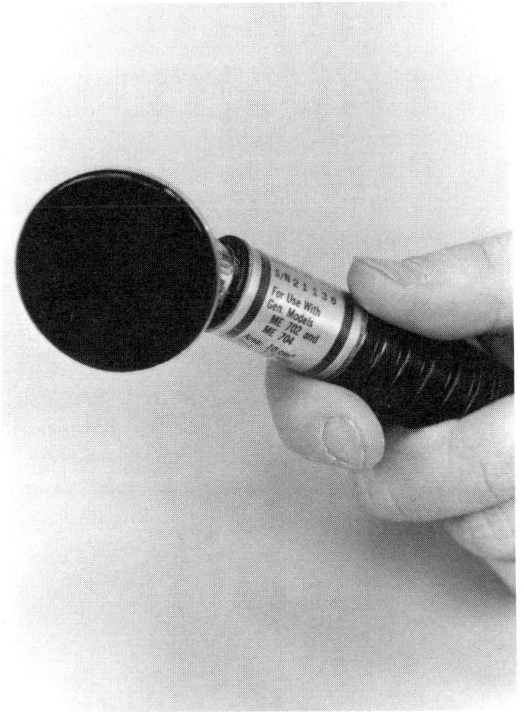

Figure 5.38. An ultrasound applicator (sound head).

Ultrasonic vibrations are produced when a crystal or crystals located between two electrodes are subjected to high voltages of electrical energy. When this occurs, the crystals rapidly contract and expand. The higher the wattage, the greater the expansion. The rapidly alternating expansion and contraction, in turn, initiates the formation of the longitudinal compression waves that travel at speeds up to millions of cycles per second. Thus, the process is one of transforming electrical energy into mechanical energy due to surface pressure—thus a *piezoelectric* effect.

As previously described, the ultrasound emission is a high frequency acoustic vibration that is imperceptible to the human ear. Except for the higher frequency range, however, an ultrasonic wave is a mechanical vibration (a longitudinal compression wave) that is identical to that of an audible sound wave.

Vibrations of frequencies above 17,000 cycles/second or more are usually above the range normally perceptible by the adult auditory mechanism. In the equipment in use today, the frequencies that are produced far exceed this level, ranging from 30,000 to 1 million cycles/second (1 MHz).[25]

Ultrasonic waves travel at a velocity of approximately 330 meters/second in air. In comparison, electromagnetic waves travel at 3×10^8 meters/second. The velocity of sound in a fluid at room temperature is about 1,450 meters/second.

As the ultrasonic waves are propagated into human tissue, tissue molecules are set into vibration at a frequency that is near that of the ultrasound unit's output. It is well known that the high frequency pitch of a forceful singer can cause a glass to shatter. So too, the high frequencies of ultrasound, when specifically directed into human tissue, may cause certain tissue substances to disintegrate at the molecular level.

CRYSTALS

The crystals utilized in ultrasound today are of three types: barium titanate ($BaTiO_3$), quartz sulfate (SiO_2), and lithium sulfate ($LiSO_4$). Barium titanate, a manufactured ceramic-like substance, is the most popular as it requires relatively little voltage (about 100 volts) to activate. Quartz sulfate is very stable but requires extremely high voltage (eg, 2000 volts). Lithium sulfate is of medium impedance, requiring about 500 volts. It is man-made, ie, "seeded" in the laboratory.

A single crystal may be the entire transducer, as with the Mettler ultrasound unit, or located within the sound head, as is common in most units. Multiple crystals may also be used, as with the Lindquist unit.

COUPLING MEDIA

In order for ultrasound to effectively penetrate human tissue, an appropriate conducting medium must be utilized. See Figure 5.39. This medium should prevent an air gap between the applicator and the skin, remove all gas bubbles clinging to the skin, and afford an easy glide for the sound head during direct application.

Several studies have emphasized the importance of the media used. Although there has been conflicting data reported, this issue bears some special consideration. For example, Beid and Cummings found a thixotropic gel in 1973 that conducted over 70% of the transducer's energy output. In studying other coupling media in use at that time, they

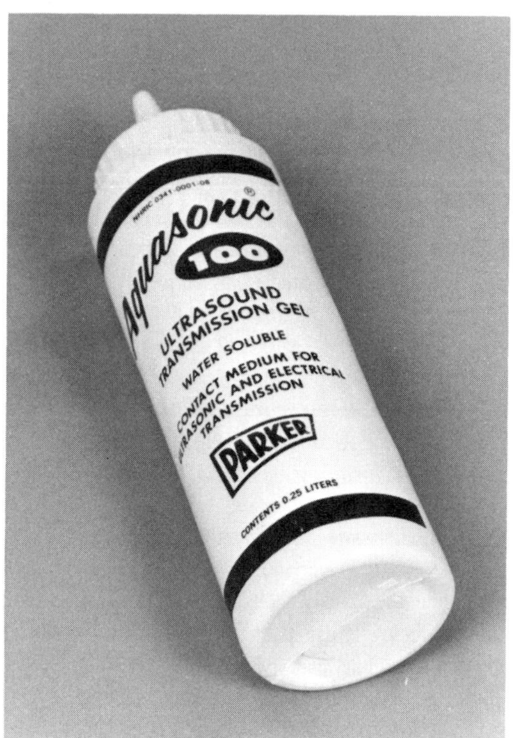

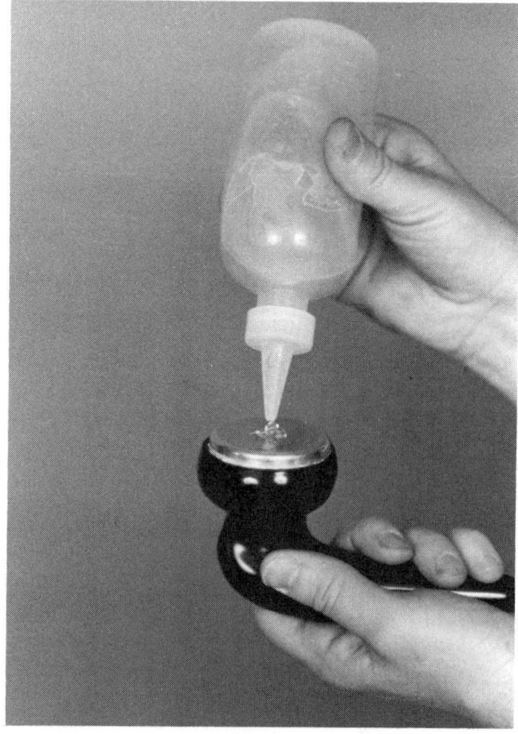

Figure 5.39. *Left,* Aquasonic, a commercially prepared coupling medium. *Right,* Application of coupling gel to the sound head.

found that glycerol (a vegetable oil) transmitted an average of 67.75%, ECG creams and body lotions about 26%, and mineral oil only about 20%. Air was not found to transmit any appreciable quantity of therapeutic ultrasound, and it is for this reason that a relatively air-free medium must be used.

In 1976, however, Warren published data that seemed to refute these earlier studies. He found that, among the gels studied, there was no significant difference in transmitted waves when the direct contact method to administer ultrasound was used.

A review of Griffin's data, published in 1980, is summarized in Figure 5.40. This more recent study seems to suggest that, although questions may be raised as to specific percentages, there appears to be a definite difference when the relative transmissivity of water, glycerine, and mineral oil is compared. When ultrasound treatment is considered relative to tissue temperature changes, transmissivity was greatest when glycerine was used; but, as intensity increased, the relative temperature change invariably increased. Thus, certain conclusions might be drawn from these and other studies:

1. There is a significant difference in transmissiveness among water, glycerine, and mineral oil, with the greatest transmissiveness in tap water.

2. Transmissiveness is the reciprocal of temperature rise.

3. The superiority of water as a coupling agent is supported by the relatively small temperature change associated. See Figure 5.41.

4. If the intention is to increase the temperature within the part to be treated, immersion in a nonaqueous coupling medium apparently produces an *infrared* effect (especially with glycerine). If the goal is to produce both an infrared and ultrasonic effect, preheated water or a nonaqueous coupling medium should be used.

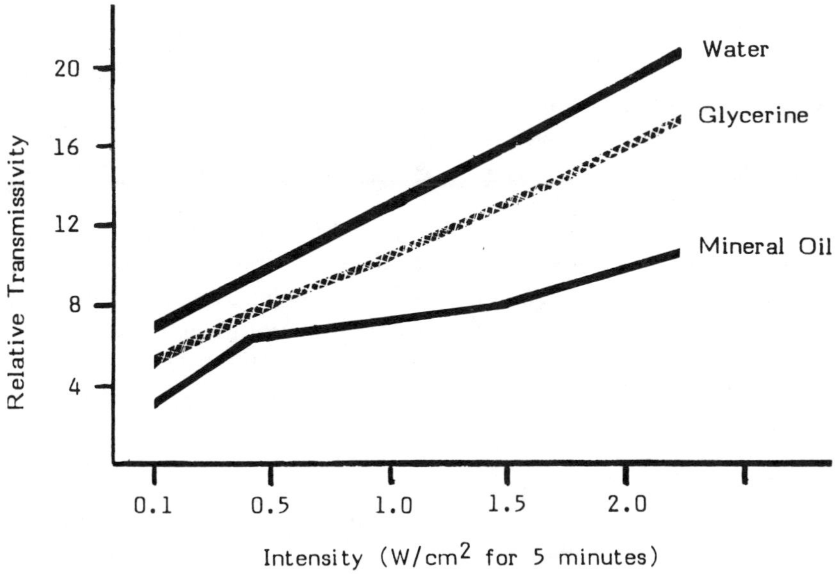

Figure 5.40. Relative transmissivity of three coupling media (water, glycerine, mineral oil) when subjected to various intensities of ultrasound.

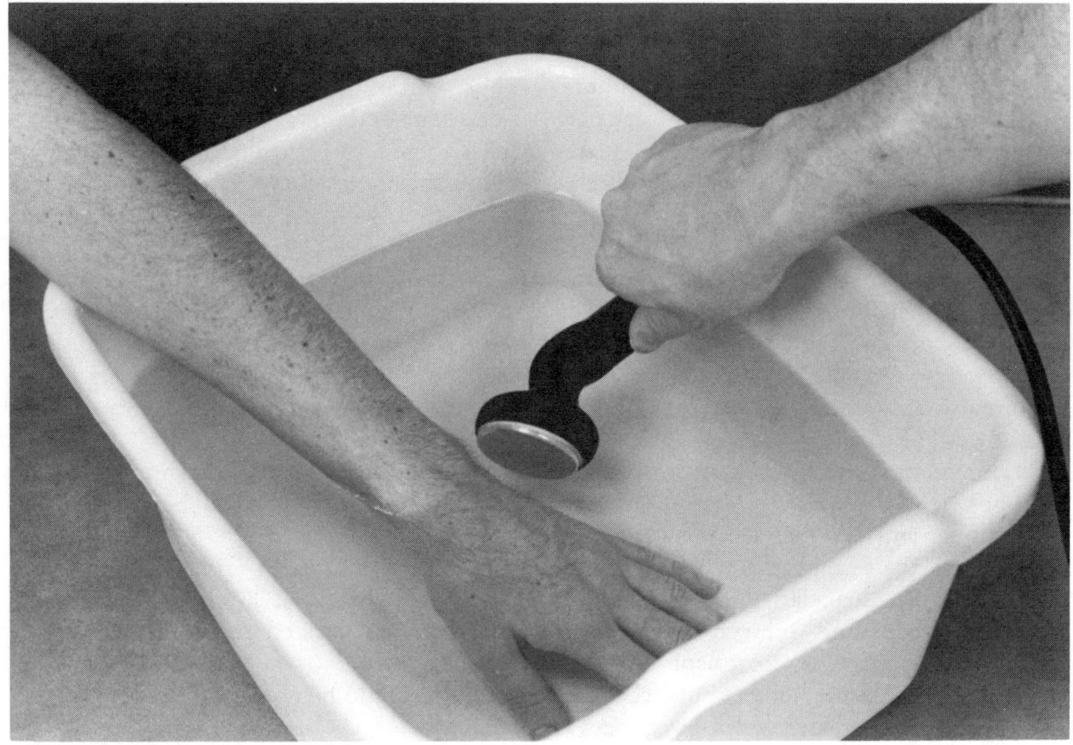

Figure 5.41. Ultrasonic therapy to a wrist using water as the coupling medium.

POWER

When averaged over a period of time, the amount of ultrasonic energy that is produced at the surface of the crystal(s) in the transducer head is known as the *average power* (measured in watts). This power is an important parameter because it, along with exposure time, determines the amount of energy delivered to the tissues being treated. In therapeutic applications, the peak intensity should not exceed about three times the average intensity if undesirable side effects are to be avoided. See Figure 5.42.

Another important parameter is that power is measured per unit area. This is generally expressed in watts per square centimeter (W/cm^2). This value is obtained by dividing the total power by the area affected by the ultrasonic beam radiating from the applicator. For example, 10 watts delivered to 5 square centimeters has an average power of 2 $watts/cm^2$. The same average power would be found if 20 watts were delivered to 10 square centimeters by using a larger sound head.

Some units show both total watts and W/cm^2. It is more common, however, to see only the latter registered. Power levels in commercial units rarely exceed 2.5 W/cm^2. A typical control panel is shown in Figure 5.43.

CAVITATION

In animal studies, cavitation has been seen to occur in tissues when excessive dosage is used, but it rarely occurs in clinical practice. As the sound wave enters body tissue, it is possible to quantitatively assess the ampli-

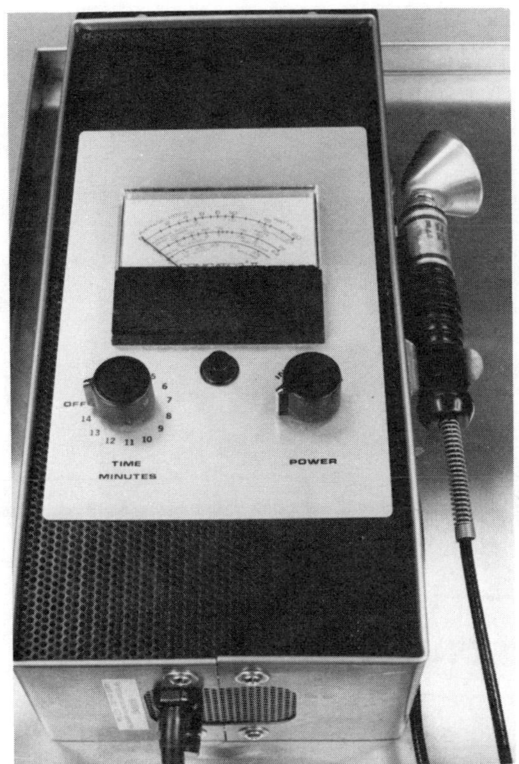

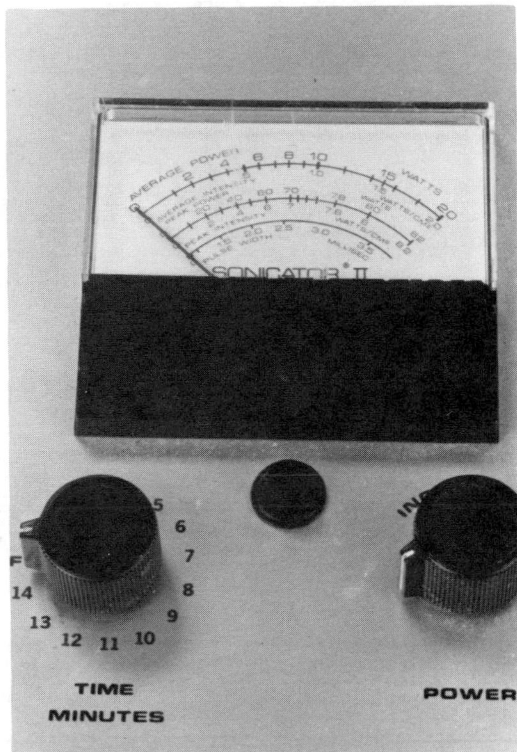

Figure 5.42. *Left,* a Sonicator II ultrasound unit. Right, close-up view of the average-power dial.

tude of displacement of specific cellular molecules by rarefaction and compression processes. Powerful ultrasonic forces may trigger secondary reactions in body tissues and, because dissolved gases are always present in body tissues, gaseous cavitation may develop.

During the phase of rarefaction, as the tissues become less dense, it is possible to produce gas-filled cavities. During the following compression phase, these cavities might collapse and bring about a high energy concentration in the form of shock waves. As the gas bubbles are alternately compressed (and some gas moves out of the bubbles into surrounding fluid) and rarefacted (the bubbles expand), there is a net gain of tissue gas moving into bubbles.

Associated electrical and chemical phenomena have been described as being the result of this cavitation process. Mechanical destruction may also be produced when the cavities collapse or when the gas bubbles grow large enough to vibrate in resonance with the sound waves. The occurrence of such gaseous cavitation can be prevented by an application of external pressure of sufficient force.

ABSORPTION AND REFLECTION

The heat generated is usually dissipated by conduction and convection, while the propagation of ultrasonic energy in tissues depends mainly on two factors: (1) the absorption characteristics of the biologic media and (2) the amount of reflected ultrasonic energy at tissue interfaces.

As ultrasound is transmitted through tis-

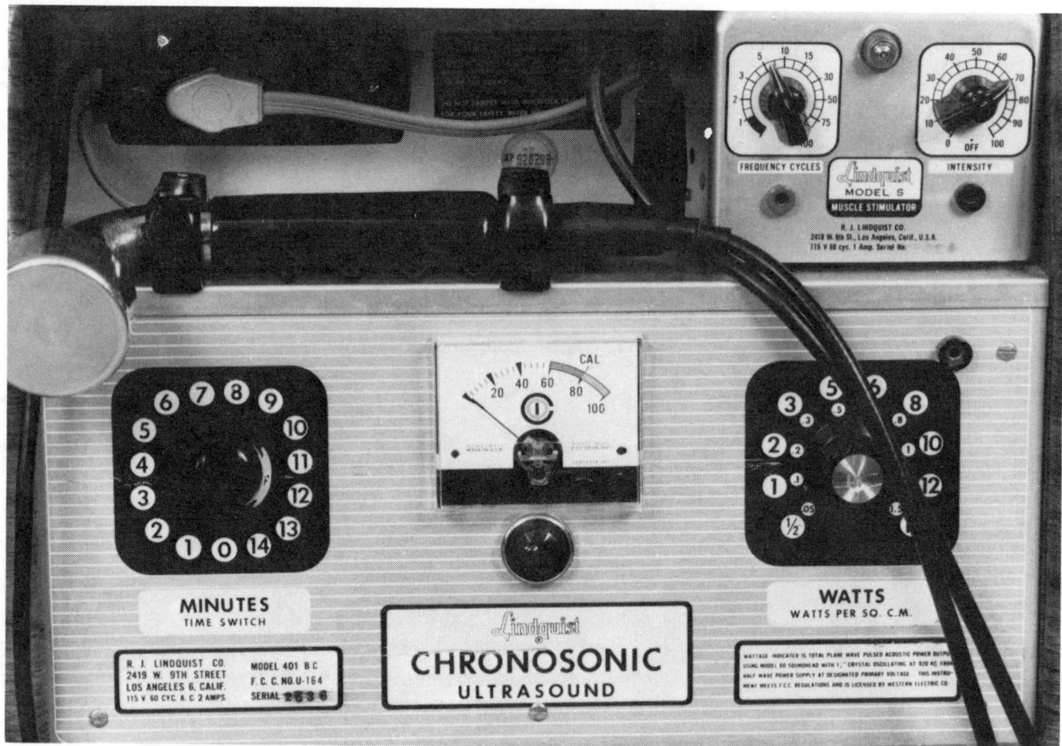

Figure 5.43. View of the control panel of a Lindquist ultrasound unit.

sue, it is gradually absorbed and converted into heat. Carstenson and Piersol, and their associates, separately demonstrated that ultrasound absorption occurs primarily in tissue proteins.[26,27] It is definitely a process of selective absorption. Attenuation of ultrasound in muscle tissue depends on whether or not the ultrasonic beam is perpendicular (sound head parallel) to the myofascial interfaces.

Depths of heat penetration into human tissue have been measured up to 5 centimeters, and the distribution within homogeneous tissues is fairly uniform (volume heating). The temperature buildup at the surface will be gradually attenuated in an exponential fashion.

When sound waves hit dense tissue, the waves tend to bounce back toward adjoining softer tissues, hence the greatest stimulating effect is closest and exterior to osseous tissue. The wavelength of ultrasound is small, 0.15 centimeter, and this allows ultrasound to scatter at interfaces and structures where sonic waves would be transparent.

Reflection readily occurs at interfaces between tissues of different acoustic impedance, and this may amount up to 30%. All unlike structures (eg, a metallic implant within bone) reflect and frequently focus ultrasound, further creating heat buildup in selective areas (structural heating). It is thought that the selective absorption of ultrasound which occurs at tissue interfaces may be related to scattering of ultrasonic energy as the result of reflection as well as to the production of transverse waves that are quickly attenuated. This localized heating at interfaces is unique to ultrasound; it is not associated with other forms of thermotherapy.

Physiologic Effects

Research conducted during the last 4 decades has shown that sound waves have extremely specific properties. At the high frequency and intensity levels used during therapy, animal studies conducted at the Uropathology Laboratories of Columbia-Presbyterian Medical Center in New York showed that ultrasonic therapy produced growth inhibition of implanted tumors. The effect appears to be triggered by altering the internal structure of cells and changing DNA synthesis. Although there did not appear to be any enhanced immunologic effect, the tumors also lost their ability to induce new tumors when injected into susceptible host animals.[28] However, ultrasound has not been proved to be an effective cancer treatment in itself because focal islets may still remain.

As previously described when ultrasound enters body tissue, it has been shown that the greatest buildup of heat occurs where two dissimilar structures are congruent. Note in Figure 5.44 that the greatest temperature increase occurs near the fat—muscle interface and the muscle—bone interface.

The primary physical effects of ultrasound can be considered to be a mechanothermochemical product; ie, producing physical, thermal, chemical, colloid chemical, and biologic effects. These effects may be summarized as follows:

1. *Heat.* Heat is generated within tissues, especially at the surface boundaries, by means of ultrasonic energy being converted into heat as the waves meet intra- and intercellular resistance (friction). This heat, along with other nonthermal biologic effects, increases peripheral arterial blood flow, increases the local metabolic rate, increases membrane permeability, temporarily blocks peripheral nerve impulses (especially small C fibers), alters spinal reflexes, and relaxes muscle spasms.[29-39]. Because of the neurologic effects, many authorities feel that it is important to treat the spinal root level and known areas of referred or reflex neurologic phenomenon, as well as the local site of involvement.[40]

2. *Specific Mechanical Action.* A specific mechanical action takes place that is attributed to the high alternating pressure forces at high accelerations and other physical phenomena.

3. *Micromassage.* A deeply penetrating, high frequency, fine vibratory action is intensely produced within tissue by ultrasonic waves.

4. *Tissue Alteration.* Ultrasound tends to break down the collagen fibrils of scar tissue by a specific action on the interstitial cement. When properly used over normal body tissue, however, it only tends to softens the tissue by decreasing its tonicity.

5. *Chemical Effects.* The chemical effects induced by ultrasound are products of an increased gaseous exchange, liquifaction of certain cellular gels, and increased oxidation.

6. *Clearing Agent.* Ultrasonic waves cause exudates and precipitates to be absorbed. Pulsed ultrasound, especially, tends to be effective is reducing edema.

7. *Microdestruction.* Ultrasound tends to disrupt tissue deposits (eg, spurs, calcified hematomas), but proof that spurs and deposits are dissolved is not conclusive.

8. *Analgesia.* Ultrasound slightly triggers enkephalin formation, producing a mild sedative effect.

Application

Ultrasound may be used on a continuous or pulsed setting and applied either underwater or directly to the skin using a contact medium. When used on the continuous setting, the major value of ultrasound is summarized with the phrase: "The greatest effects of treatment occur where two unlike structures interface."

Although many coupling agents are available, it seems that the greatest effects of ultrasound and the best transmissivity occur when a specially prepared ultrasound gel, cream, or immersion in water is used. During direct applications, it is better to use too much coupling medium than too little. As the medium tends to spread during application, a towel should be placed under the part to catch drips of gel or cream.

When ultrasound is applied directly upon the skin, it should be made with circular or oval movements while maintaining firm contact. The surface of the sound head should be held parallel to the surface being treated throughout the treatment. See Figure 5.45. The strokes are made at a moderate rate, about 1 inch/second. Firm light pressure should be used over areas where the tissue is thin, with firm heavier pressure used over thick muscle and fatty areas. When the part to be treated is placed within water, as should be the case when treating the extremities, the transducer head should be held in the water about an inch from the skin and moved in a somewhat circular pattern during the application.

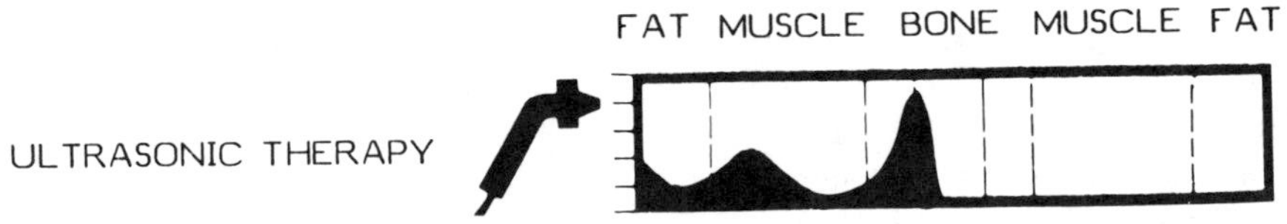

Figure 5.44. Depth/temperature effects of ultrasonic therapy.

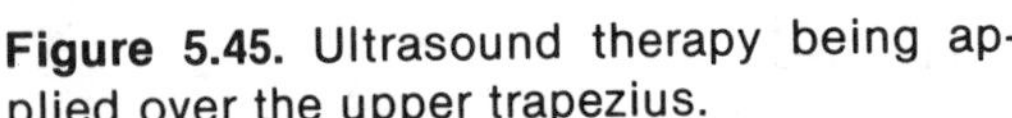

Figure 5.45. Ultrasound therapy being applied over the upper trapezius.

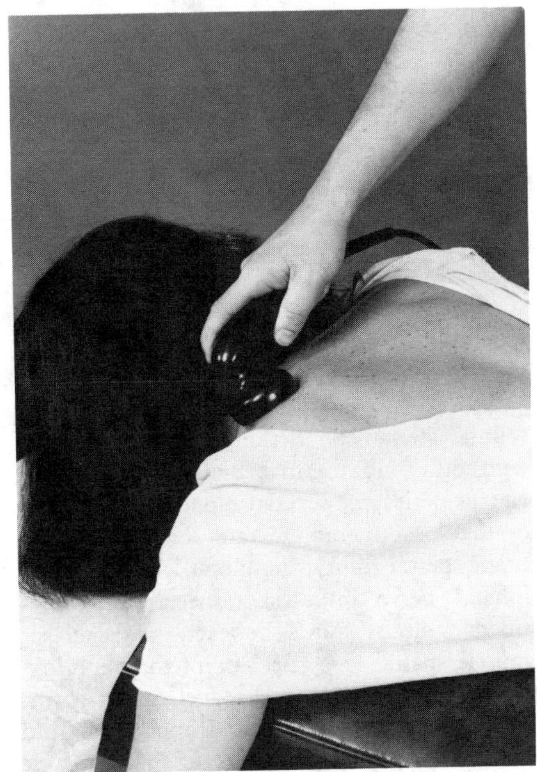

PULSED ULTRASOUND

All the biologic effects described may occur when ultrasound is applied on the pulsed setting, but the major effect of the pulsed waves is the reduction of edema. Many authorities, however, feel that pulsed ultrasound has an extremely limited therapeutic value over that of continuous ultrasound in that patients who would typically have edema (eg, acute sprain) also have pain, and ultrasound has a limited usefulness in pain control (ie, in endorphin/enkephalin production). In addition, pulsed ultrasound is only a process of rhythmically interrupting continuous ultrasound, thus fractionalizing the process and reducing the effect. Its major use is found in conditions where the micromassage effect is desired without the production of heat. Some typical units that have this function are shown in Figures 5.46 and 5.47.

STATIONARY TRANSDUCERS

A stationary transducer that does not need to be moved during therapy can be used with pulsed ultrasound utilizing 7—13 cm^2 transducers, or continuous or pulsed ultrasound may be used with 50 cm^2 transducers. As only a few areas will comfortably allow these large sound heads, the technique is not as popular as that for the mobile transducer.

COUPLING CUSHION TECHNIQUE

This technique is used when treating an irregular surface that cannot be submerged in water. A thin air-free rubber or plastic bag or condom is usually used as the cushion. A coupling gel is used between the cushion and the skin and between the cushion and the sound head. The moving technique is recommended when small transducers or continuous ultrasound are applied.

TRIGGER POINT AND MOTOR POINT THERAPY

A few papers report effective results when treating trigger and motor points with ultrasound; however, extensive comparisons with the more popular muscle stimulating alternating current have not been made at this writing. Pulsed oscillations are usually used because the intermittent cooling cycle gives the opportunity of holding the sound head stationary for 15—20 seconds when applying the therapy.

PHONOPHORESIS

Phonophoresis is in the early stages of investigation. The substance to be introduced into the skin is incorporated into the coupling medium. Polarity is not a concern in phonophoresis as it is in iontophoresis because it is administered mechanically rather than electrically.

COMBINED ULTRASOUND AND ELECTRICAL STIMULATION

Some units (eg, Medco-sonalator) offer combined ultrasound and electrical stimulation. The therapy may be applied directly or with the part to be treated immersed in water. However, authorities differ in their viewpoints whether this combined therapy is any more beneficial than singular therapy or therapy applied separately.

Dosage and Treatment Time

It has been found that different dosages (watt-minutes) of ultrasound can have different and sometimes opposite effects, yet dosage levels, while limited, are made strictly on an empirical basis. When using the proper conducting medium and a unit that is properly calibrated, the suggestions described in

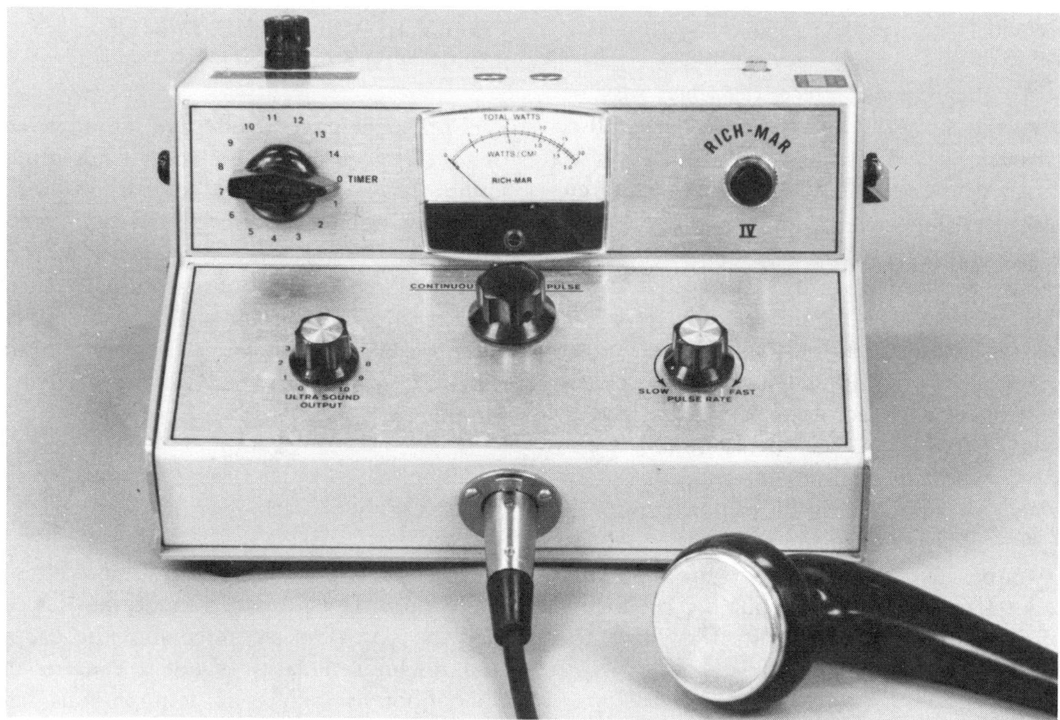

Figure 5.46. The Rich-Mar IV pulsed ultrasound unit.

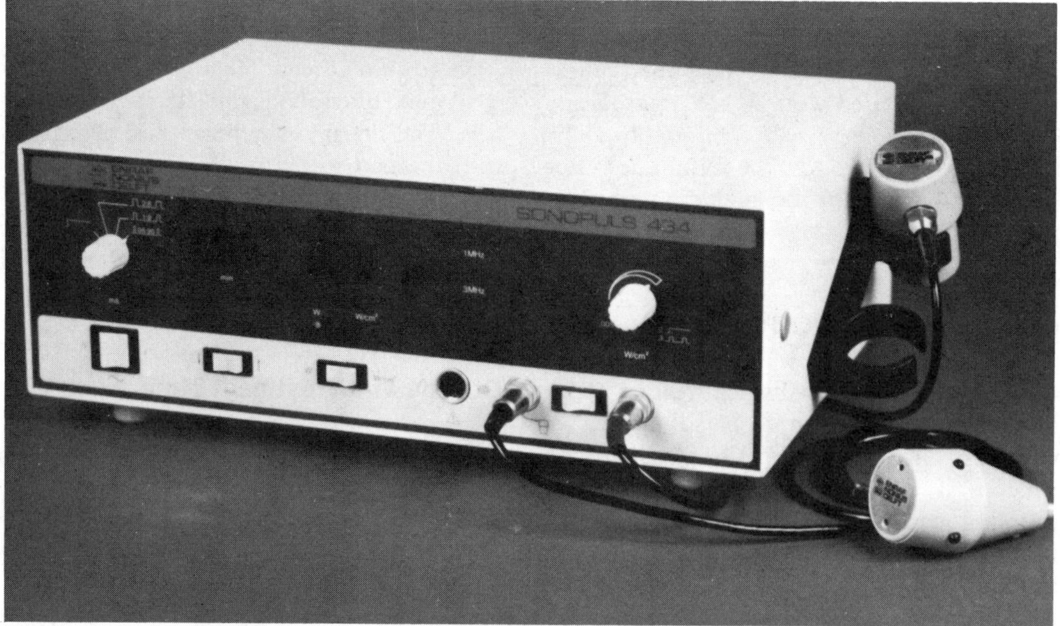

Figure 5.47. The Sonoplus 434 ultrasound unit.

Table 5.7 should be considered. As with most types of electrotherapy, acute conditions mandate a low intensity and stubbornly chronic disorders require a higher intensity—keeping in mind that different patients and different pathophysiologic processes will respond to the stimulation with varying tolerances.

The duration of treatment with ultrasound is typically from 4 to 8 minutes for each area treated in order for the patient to obtain maximum effects. If, for example, the spine is to be treated bilaterally, then 4—8 minutes of application should be given to each side; ie, first one side and then the other.

Indications, Contraindications, and Precautions

Ultrasound has the specific effect of building heat and producing a high intensity micromassage where muscles, tendons, and ligaments attach to bone. The "beaming" characteristic of ultrasonic therapy and its deep penetration make it an ideal therapy for localized therapy. Ultrasound, therefore, is an efficient therapy when used on the continuous setting for relaxing muscles in situations where the patient is not in acute pain. When used on the pulsed setting, ultrasound will be most effective over areas of chronic inflammation to remove edema or stasis.

The tissue softening effects of ultrasound have been demonstrated in a number of studies, especially when it was used in conjunction with other therapies. However, even when utilized alone, it has proved to be superior to microwave therapy in cases of periarthritis according to studies conducted by Lehmann and his associates.[41,42] Their findings are summarized in Table 5.8.

Ultrasound is contraindicated in a number of conditions and over certain areas. In addition to observing the general contraindications for heat, see Table 5.9. Large autonomic centers such as the stellate, celiac, and mesenteric ganglions should always be avoided. Extreme caution must be used when treating patients with advanced heart or vascular disease.

When patients complain of severe tingling, discomfort, or burning sensations during a treatment, they may be experiencing periosteal irritation. The fault is usually a failure to keep the sound head moving, moving the head too slow, moving the head in a circle with too small a diameter so that there is a continuous stroke overlap, or having the intensity setting too high. If treatment is continued in such a situation without correcting the fault, there is great danger in creating a severe periosteal burn.

Table 5.7. Dosage Considerations in Ultrasonic Therapy

Type of Case	*Type of Tissue*	*Contact Method of Application Dosage, W/cn²*	*Underwater Method of Application Dosage, W/cn²*
Acute	Thin	0.5—1.0	1.0—1.5
Acute	Thick	1.0—1.5	1.5—2.0
Chronic	Thin	1.0—1.5	1.5—2.0
Chronic	Thick	1.5—2.0	2.0—2.5

Note: In underwater applications, 0.5 W/cn² has been added to the figures for contact applications to compensate for the energy absorption between the applicator and the skin surface being treated.

Table 5.8. Range of Motion Increase After Ultrasonic and Microwave Therapy

Motion	*Average Range of Motion Gain from Ultrasound*	*Average Range of Motion Gain from Microwaves*
Abduction	32.6°	21.2°
Flexion	27.4°	16.1°
Rotation	45.4°	17.3°

Table 5.9. General Indications and Contraindications of Ultrasound Diathermy

GENERAL INDICATIONS

Bursitis (subacute, chronic)
Calcific bursitis
Causalgia
Decubital ulcers
Fibrositis (subacute, chronic)
Fibrotic polymyositis
Herpes zoster
Joint contractures
Myalgia
Neuralgia
Neuromas
Osteoarthritis
Painful neuroma
Periarthritis (nonseptic)
Radiculitis (subacute, chronic)
Raynaud's phenomenon
Rheumatoid arthritis (subacute, chronic)
Scars
Shoulder-hand syndrome
Spondylitis
Sprains (subacute, chronic)
Spurs
Strains (subacute, chronic)
Sudeck's atrophy
Tendinitis (subacute, chronic)
Trigger points
Varicose ulcers (chronic, with caution)

GENERAL CONTRAINDICATIONS

Acute infection
Areas of thermohypoesthesia (authorities differ)
Near hearing aid
Near malignant lesions
Near metallic implants
Near pacemaker
Occlusive vascular disease
Over bony prominences (eg, spinous processes)
Over epiphyseal plates of growing children
Over nerve plexuses
Over suspected embolus
Over the eye
Over the heart
Over the pregnant uterus (authorities differ)
Over the reproductive organs
Over the spinal cord after laminectomy
Radiculitis (acute)
Tendency to hemorrhage
Through the brain

Note: This table is only a guide. Extreme caution must be used when any inflammatory condition is being treated. Each patient must be treated as an individual and in accord with high standards of professional judgment as directed by the diagnosis.

CLOSING REMARKS

Since their original development, great strides have been made in the refinement of therapeutic shortwave, microwave, and ultrasonic diathermy equipment. It is now possible to elevate the temperature at the site of a pathologic lesion at most any level of depth.

However, while their physiologic effects overlap somewhat, shortwave, microwave, and ultrasound are not interchangeable in meeting a specific therapeutic goal. Each modality should be selected for a specific purpose, and each has its peak temperature distribution pattern. See Figure 5.48 and Table 5.10.

Likewise, each modality has specific contraindications and those that overlap with other deep-heating modalities. Proper utilization requires knowledge of the biophysics, pathophysiologic processes, and unique patient tolerances involved to apply each type of unit expertly and safely.

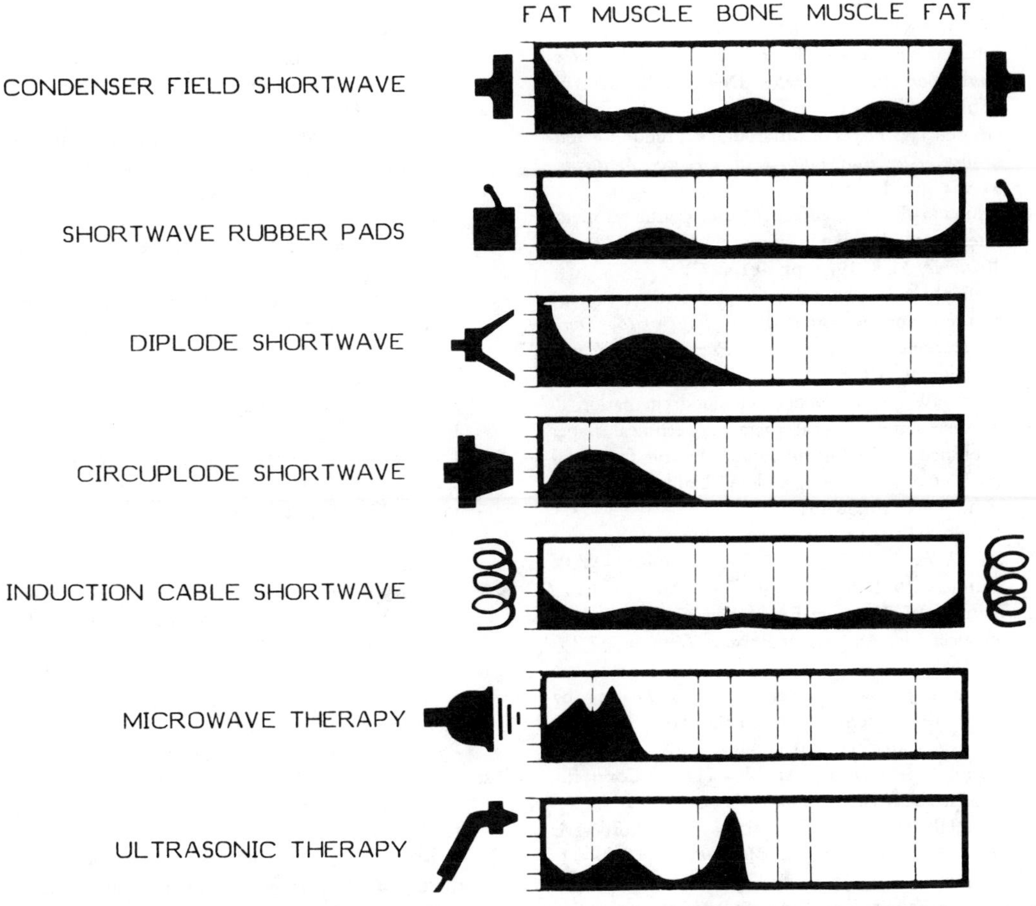

Figure 5.48. Comparative depth/temperature effects of shortwave, microwave, and ultrasonic therapy.

Table 5.10. Comparative Effects of High Frequency Current Modalities

Type	*Area of Major Effect*	*Area of Least Effect*
Microwave diathermy	Superficial muscle	Deep muscle, bone
Shortwave circuplode	Fat—muscle interface	Bone
Shortwave condenser field	Fat, muscle, viscera	Muscle—bone interface
Shortwave diplode	Fat, muscle	Bone
Shortwave induction field	Fat, muscle	Deep muscle, bone
Shortwave rubber pads	Fat, muscle	Bone
Ultrasound diathermy	Muscle—bone interface	Center of homogenous tissue

REFERENCES

1. *Stedman's Medical Dictionary,* ed 24. Baltimore, Williams &Wilkins, 1984, p 391.
2. van den Bouwhuijsen F, et al: *Pulsed and Continuous Short-Wave Therapy.* Delft, Holland, B.V. Enhaf-Nonius, p 15.
3. Gersten JW: Effect of ultrasound on tendon extensibility. *American Journal of Physical Medicine,* 34:362-369, 1955.
4. Lehmann JF, et al: Effects of therapeutic temperatures on tendon extensibility. *Archives of Physical Medicine,* 51:8, 1970, pp 481-487.
5. Schliephake E: The influence of shortwave therapy on the endocrine system. *Proceedings of the Third International Congress of Physical Medicine,* Washington, DC.
6. Pabst HW, et al: Changes in blood circulation in the liver after physical therapy. Technical paper published by the Institute and Polyclinic for Physical Therapy and Roentgenology, University of Munich, 40(62, 10):505-512.
7. Krusen FH, et al: *Handbook of Physical Medicine and Rehabilitation,* ed 2. Philadelphia, W.B. Saunders, 1971, pp 288-289.
8. Bierman W, Horowitz EA: A new vaginal diathermy electrode. *Archives of Physical Therapy,* 17:15-16, 1956.
9. Lehmann JR, et al: Selective muscle heating by shortwave diathermy with a helical coil. *Archives of Physical Medicine,* 50:117-132, 1969.
10. Licht S: *Therapeutic Heat.* New Haven, Connecticut, Elizabeth Licht, 1958, pp 55-115.
11. Scott HP: Heating of fatty tissues in a short-wave field. *Annals of Physical Medicine,* 2(48):48-52, 1954.
12. van den Bouwhuijsen F, et al: *Pulsed and Continuous Short-Wave Therapy.* Delft, Holland, B.V. Enhaf-Nonius, p 7.
13. Schliephake E: The influence of shortwave therapy on the endocrine system. *Proceedings of the Third International Congress of Physical Medicine,* Washington, DC.
14. Cameron BM: Experimental acceleration of wound healing. *American Journal of Orthopaedics,* 3: 336-343, 1961.
15. Witte E: Impulsdiathermie mit extremen feldstarken und ihre spezifischen biologischen effekte. *Strahlentherapie,* 97:146-148, 1955.
16. Ginsberg AJ: Pulsed short wave in the treatment of bursitis with calcification. *International Record,* 174:71-75, 1961.
17. Levy H: Pulsed shortwaves in sinus and allied conditions in childhood. *Western Medicine,* 2:246, 1961.
18. van den Bouwhuijsen F, et al: *Pulsed and Continuous Short-Wave Therapy.* Delft, Holland, B.V. Enhaf-Nonius, p 17.
19. Lehmann JR, et al: Heating patterns produced in specimens by microwaves of a frequency of 2456 megacycles when applied with "A," "B," and "C" directors. *Archives of Physical Medicine and Rehabilitation,* 43:538, November 1962.
20. Schwan HP, et al: Advantages and limitations of ultrasonics in medicine. *Journal of the AMA,* 149:125, May 10, 1952.
21. Ho HD, et al: Microwave heating of simulated human limbs by aperture sources. Special IEEE issue of *Microwave Theory and Techniques, Biological Effects of Microwaves,* February 1971.
22. Richardson AW: Blood coagulation changes due to electromagnetic microwave irradiation. *Blood,* 14: 1237-1243, 1959.
23. Gersten JW, et al: The effect of microwave diathermy on the peripheral circulation and on tissue temperature in man. *Archives of Physical Medicine,* 30:7-25, 1949.
24. Worden RE, et al: The heating effects of micro-

waves with and without ischemia. *Archives of Physical Medicine,* 29:751-758, 1948.

25. Wells PNT: *Biomechanical Ultrasonics.* New York, Academic Press, 1977.
26. Carstenson EL, et al: Determination of acoustic properties of the blood and its components. *Journal of the Acoustical Society of America,* 25: 286-289, 1953.
27. Piersol GM, et al: Mechanism of absorption of ultrasonic energy in blood. *Archives of Physical Medicine,* 33:327-332, 1952.
28. Longo F: Ultrasound therapy inhibits tumors in experiments. Research report presented to the annual meeting of the AUA. *Literature Review,* E 6-294, Elmed, Inc, Addison, IL.
29. Lehmann JF: The biophysical basis of biologic ultrasonic reactions with special reference to ultrasonic therapy. *Archives of Physical Medicine,* 34: 139-152, 1953.
30. Lehmann JF: Biophysical mode of action of biologic and therapeutic ultrasonic reactions. *Journal of the Acoustical Society of America,* 25:17-25, 1953.
31. Lehmann JF, Biegler R: Changes of potentials and temperature gradients in membranes caused by ultrasound. *Archives of Physical Medicine,* 35: 287-295, 1954.
32. Madsen PW Jr, Gersten JW: The effect of ultrasound on conduction velocity of peripheral nerve. *Archives of Physical Medicine,* 42:645-649, 1961.
33. Shealey CN, Henneman E: Reversible effects of ultrasound on spinal reflexes. *Archives of Neurology,* 6:374-386, 1962.
34. Gersten J: Changes in spinal cord thresholds following application of ultrasound, American Institute of Ultrasonics in Medicine. Detroit, *Proceedings of the 4th Annual Conference on Ultrasonic Therapy,* 1955, pp 31-39.
35. Lehmann JF, et al: Pain threshold measurements after therapeutic application of ultrasound microwaves and infrared. *Archives of Physical Medicine,* 39:560-565, 1958.
36. Stillwell DM, Gersten JW: Effect of ultrasound on spasticity. *Proceedings of the 4th Annual Conference on Ultrasonic Therapy,* Detroit, American Institute of Ultrasonics in Medicine, 1955, pp 124-131.
37. Fountain FP, et al: Decrease in muscle spasm produced by ultrasound, hot packs, and infrared radiation. *Archives of Physical Medicine,* 41:293-298, 1960.
38. Schroeder KP: Effect of ultrasound on the lumbar sympathetic nerves. *Archives of Physical Medicine,* 43:182-185, 1962.
39. Stuhfauth K: Neural effects of ultrasonic waves. *Journal of Physical Medicine* (British), 15:10-14, 1952.
40. ACA Council on Physiological Therapeutics: Physiotherapy guidelines for the chiropractic profession. *ACA Journal of Chiropractic,* IX:S-71-72, June 1975.
41. Lehmann JF, et al: Comparison of ultrasonic and microwave diathermy in the physical treatment of periarthritis of the shoulder. *Archives of Physical Medicine,* 35:627-634, 1954.
42. Lehmann JF, et al: The present value of ultrasonic diathermy. *Journal of the American Medical Association,* 147:996-999, 1955.

Chapter 6

Cryotherapies

This chapter describes the major physiologic principles and methodology associated with the therapeutic use of cold, together with related indications and contraindications. Specific ways in which cold therapy may be applied are also described; viz, by means of ice, cold packs and compresses, cryotherapy units, immersion, whirlpools, and vapocoolant sprays.

INTRODUCTION

One of the most effective modalities for the treatment of acute musculoskeletal injuries involves the therapeutic use of cold.[1] In years past, the heating pad was often used as a self-treatment by the layman at the first signs of back or extremity pain. In recent years, however, and at an increasing rate, clinicians have recommended applications of ice or cold to the area of insult. In fact, when a patient with a musculoskeletal injury is not responding to proper standards of care, it has often been found that a heating pad or some other form of heat has been applied at home.

Background

The use of cold as a therapy is not new. Peoples of the Scandinavian countries have recommended contrast baths for centuries, even to the extent of swimming in icy water after a sauna. The use of cold therapy has also been reported in the ancient writings or drawings of the Tibetan lamas, Mongolians, Germans, and American Indians. Cold wet bandages were first utilized in Prussia during the early 1800s by a Silesian farmer, Priessnitz Vincent, who is credited with their invention.

PHYSIOLOGIC EFFECTS

As a general rule, cold can trigger localized physiologic changes (as do other therapies). It can produce remote and/or referred effects.

Contrary to popular belief, it is not accurate to state that the effects of cold are exactly opposite to those involved with heat. In fact, several responses are quite similar.

General and Local Effects

It is obvious that the initial primary physical characteristic of cold is that it cools body tissues. Its basic effect is therefore hypothermal. The cooling of tissues then leads to a decrease in local tissue metabolism. Arterioles begin to constrict because there is a corresponding decrease in the formation of metabolites. The body then acts reflexively by sending blood to the skin and musculature, which produces a secondary hyperemia. As most circulatory activities are reduced, there is a decrease in the delivery to and utilization of nutrients in the involved tissues, a decrease in phagocytic activity, and a decrease in the production of lymph.[2] See Figure 6.1.

The general physiologic effects of cold include increased heart rate, respiratory rate,

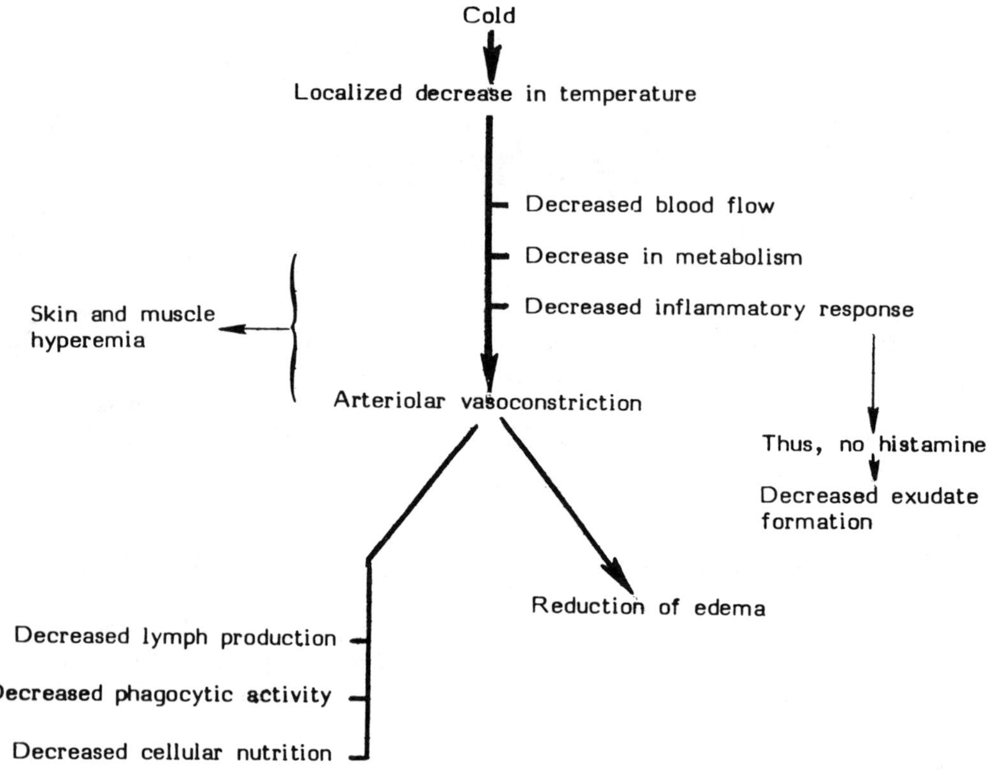

Figure 6.1. Physiologic effects of cold.

leukocytosis, and decreased fatigue. Skin color, occurring first as blanched skin, changes to red or blue-red in prolonged cold and is the result of a histamine release associated paradoxically with an increase in utilization of oxygen by local tissue. When cold is removed, the demand for tissue oxygen is increased and the vessels dilate in compensation to produce hyperemia.

When cooling is extreme (eg, immersion into ice water, ice massage), the body responds with regular "bursts" of vasodilation. These periodic reactions have come to be called the *hunting reaction* and are thought to occur in the area of arteriovenous anastomosis. This is a normal response, and failure of body tissues to react by vasodilation, via an autonomic reflex, may lead to injury to the local tissues from cryotherapy.[3,4]

Studies have shown that human body temperature can be repeatedly and successfully reduced to about 80°F (rectal) and the patient observed up to 8 days without subsequent abnormal effects.[5] The loss of function due to exposure to cold progressively goes from diminished light touch, then motor power, overt vasoconstriction, pain, and finally, loss of gross pressure perception.[6] The major physiologic effects of cold therapy are summarized in Table 6.1.

Effects of Prolonged Application

Prolonged applications of cold therapies may trigger paradoxical reactions in which the following may be noted:

1. Local vasodilation
2. Reflex internal vasodilation

Table 6.1. The Physiologic Effects of Cryotherapy

1. ***Localized Effects***
   A. Reduced nerve conduction velocities in both motor and sensory fibers (conduction can be eliminated when temperature decreases to 50°—59°F).
   B. Analgesia effected by a reduction of excitability of muscle afferents.
   C. Reduction of cell metabolism.
   D. Localized vasoconstriction.
   E. Decrease in exudates.
   F. Reduction in spasticity by way of a reduction of excitability of muscle afferents.
   G. Decreased capillary blood pressure, followed in 5—8 minutes by increased pressure and a slowed pulse.
   H. Increased musculature tone.

2. ***Reflex Effects***
   A. Reflex vasoconstriction of internal organs.
   B. Decreased perspiration and glandular activity.
   C. Anesthesia of the peripheral nervous system.
   D. Mild sedation of the CNS.

3. ***General Effects***
   A. Decreased muscle fatigue.
   B. Increased respiratory rate (hyperpnea).
   C. Increased heart rate (tachycardia).
   D. Increased leukocytosis.

3. Decreased heart and respiratory rates
4. Increased blood pressure.

Overcoming the Insulation Factor

The efficiency in which externally applied cold will depress tissue temperature depends essentially on the thickness of the overlying soft tissues, especially adipose tissues. The insulating property of fat significantly devalues the ability of a cold modality to lower deep muscle temperatures.[7,8] It has usually been found that the lowering of deep-tissue temperatures occurs only after applications that have a duration of 60 minutes or more.[9]

Penetration

The exposure of an extensive region of skin to cold will penetrate much more than modalities of heat. The effect will even result in body core temperatures lowering below normal.

Studies in ice massage show that the temperature drops 18°F at a depth of 1 cm with effects lasting up to 3 hours.[10] Ice massage can reduce surface skin temperature to 60°—58°F, and no ill effects to normal skin is seen until skin temperature is reduced below 50°F. But it takes time for the cold to penetrate. For example, when icebags whose water temperature is 32°F are continually placed on an extremity, the outside of the towel covering the bag will be about 40°F. It takes about 15 minutes for the skin temperature to drop from 84°F to 43°F, about 60 minutes for subcutaneous tissue to drop from 94°F to 70°F, and about 2 hours for intramuscular temperature to drop from 98°F to 79°F.

Comparative Effects of Heat and Cold

A comparison of the effects of heat and cold in the treatment of various complaints and conditions is shown in Table 6.2.[11,12]

METHODS OF COOLING

Regardless of the procedure used, a heat absorber must be placed in contact or near the tissue to be treated to subtract heat from the body. If this basic requirement is met, there are several ways that the tissues of the body may be cooled to lower their temperature:

1. The most commonly used method of therapeutic cooling is by means of *conduction,* where a solid, liquid, or gas is applied whose temperature is lower than that of the skin. This is usually effected by using cold packs or ice.

2. Another means to transmit coolness is by *evaporation,* where highly volatile liquids are sprayed onto the skin. In this method, a pressurized container of a volatile fluid is fitted with a calibrated nozzle that is capable of delivering a fine jet stream or mist to the skin. Typical examples are seen in the use of ethyl chloride and Fluori-methane.

3. A third method of therapeutic cooling is by *convection,* where a fluid medium is utilized. During World War II, for example, it was suggested that patients suffering the effects of cold immersion of the lower extremities might have their feet exposed to currents of cool air generated by an electric fan so that the return to normal temperature would be gradual. Likewise, cooling by convection might also serve some purpose in patients who have suffered a heat stroke.

It should always be kept in mind that the body is a large, relatively efficient, source of heat that has the capacity to compensate for temperature loss by modifying patterns of blood circulation via autonomic vasomotor responses. Thus, if vigorous cooling is to be produced, the medium to apply therapeutic cold must have a substantial heat-absorbing capacity. If not, the effect of the cooling medium will be overcome by the body's innate defensive mechanisms.

APPLICATIONS

Several different forms of cryotherapy exist. The more typical applications include cold packs, Priessnitz compresses, ice, cold therapy machines, vapocoolant sprays, humid-cold boric alcohol or aluminum acetate compresses, and clay packs.

McMaster compared the cooling effects of several modalities. His findings are shown in Table 6.3.[13]

Ice Massage

One of the easiest and undoubtedly the most economical ways to apply cold is by using ice massage. An ice cube may be grasped with a cloth or water may be frozen in a paper cup that serves as an insulated holder. See Figure 6.2.

In ice massage, the ice is applied directly to a patient's skin by using a circular or back-and-forth motion on the site to be treated.[14] Begin the massage about 12 inches from the exact focus of injury, and then slowly move centrally toward the lesion so that the massage is concentrated in an area that is approximately 6 inches in diameter.

STAGES OF RESPONSE DURING ICE MASSAGE

As the patient is treated, the reaction will usually go through four predictable stages in response to the cooling by ice massage:

1. *Coolness.* The first sensation that the patient perceives is that of coolness, which is felt almost immediately, evolving to an uncomfortable cold sensation that gradually progresses to Stage 2.

2. *Burning.* The uncomfortable coolness turns into a burning-type of feeling. This

Table 6.2. Comparative Effects of Heat and Cold

Symptom/Sign	*Heat*	*Cold*
Cellular metabolism		
Enzyme activity	Increases	Decreases
Membrane diffusion	Increases	Decreases
Oxygen consumption	Increases	Decreases
Inflammatory reaction	Increases	Decreases
Muscle spasm		
Spindle activity	Increases	Decreases
Fiber contractility	Increases	Decreases
Involuntary (reflex) contractions	Decreases	Decreases
Afferent activity		Decreases
Efferent activity		Decreases
Pain		
Nerve conduction velocity	Increases	Decreases
Enkephalins	Produced	Produced
Placebo effect	Positive	Highly variable
Psychic effect	Relaxation	May irritate
Joint response		
Connective tissue distensibility	Increases	Decreases
Contractures/adhesions	Softening	Less pain on stretching
Range of joint motion	Increases	Decreases
Synovial fluid viscosity	Decreases	Increases
Skin tissue	Local vasodilation	Local vasoconstriction
Vascular response		
Consensual	Vasodilation	Vasoconstriction
Local	Vasodilation	Vasoconstriction
Capillary permeability	Increases edema	Decreases edema
Vascular wall tone	Decreases	Increases

Table 6.3. Comparative Effects of Various Cooling Modalities

Modality	*Therapy Duration*	*Temperature Point of Depression*
Plastic bag of ice chips	60 minutes	51.8°F
Frozen flexible gel pack	60 minutes	46.4°F
Chemical cooling pack	60 minutes	37.4°F
Continuous cryotherapy unit	60 minutes	35.1°F

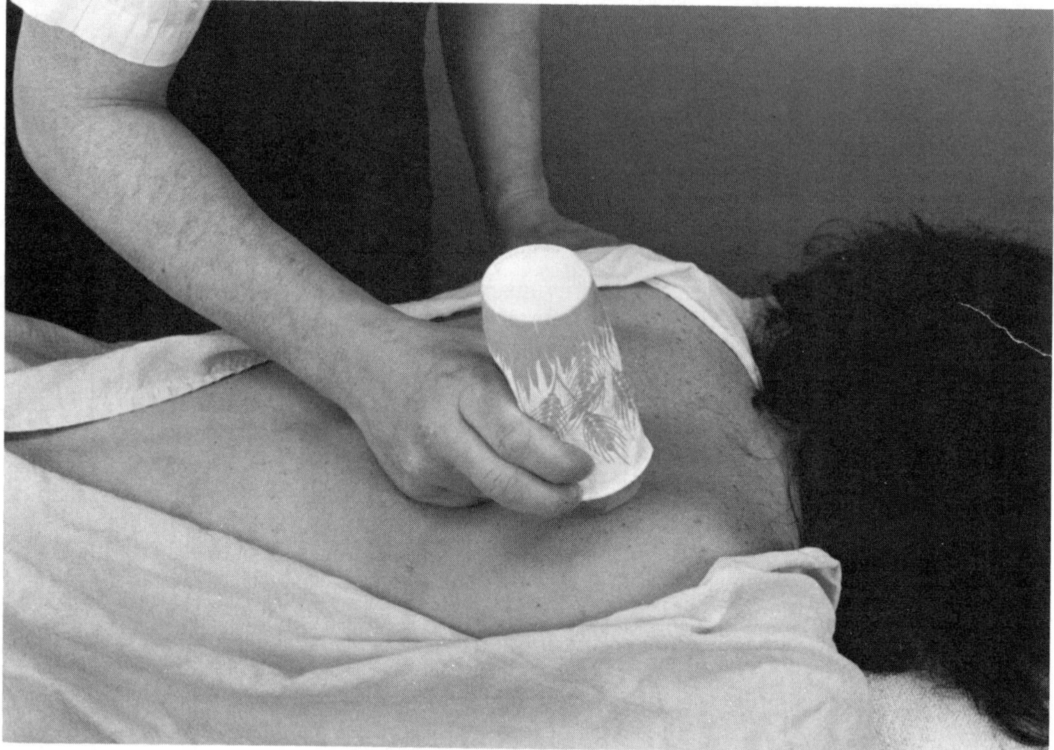

Figure 6.2. Ice massage to the right midthoracic area.

stage lasts about 3 minutes, whereafter Stage 3 occurs.

3. *Aching.* The aching sensation that follows Stage 2 is of short duration, but it signals the approach of the final and fourth stage.

4. *Numbness.* As the ice massage is continued, the area being treated becomes progressively numb (almost analgesic). When the reaction reaches this point or after 5 minutes (whichever occurs first), the ice massage should be terminated.

PRUDENT CONSIDERATIONS

The anticipated stages of response should be explained to the patient prior to application of the therapy.

Care should be exercised not to use ice for periods longer than 5 minutes and never on patients who have a hypersensitivity to cold (eg, cryesthesia) or on areas that have a history of frostbite. Caution should also be taken to avoid treating over poorly insulated parts (eg, bony areas). In addition, it is important to assure that the ice will never be held motionless at any one spot for longer than 2 minutes.

When the treatment is terminated, the area should be dried with a cloth (but not rubbed) and the status of the patient's skin recorded. If mobilization procedures are to be utilized, it is recommended that they be instigated immediately after the ice treatment is terminated.

Cold Packs

The most common way to apply cold therapy is to utilize commercially available cold pack equipment. The packs, which are similar in shape to hydrocollator hot packs, are stored in a refrigerated tank that has a preset temperature of 10 °F. Cold packs are available in a number of differently sized semiflexible units, which contain a special silicon material that helps to retain their degree of coolness. See Figures 6.3 and 6.4.

During application, the area of the patient's body must be exposed. The cooled pack may be (1) placed directly on the skin, (2) wrapped in or underlaid with a dry towel before placement (Fig. 6.5), or (3) wrapped in a warm moist towel before application. The latter method is often preferred when two goals are desired: gradual adaptation to the therapy followed by enhanced cooling. The initial warmth affords gradual physiologic accommodation, and the moisture within the towel has a tendency to intensify the later cooling effects of the pack.

Many chiropractic physicians find that the use of cold packs over the active and dispersive electrodes during high-volt electrotherapy enhances the benefits. See Figure 6.6.

Cold packs are usually applied for 20—30 minutes when maximum effect is to be achieved. After 30 minutes, the packs lose their necessary degree of therapeutic coolness and must be returned to the refrigerated tank. It then takes from 45 to 60 minutes for the pack to return to the therapeutic temperature. When new packs are purchased, however, they should be cooled at least 6 hours prior to their first use. See Figure 6.7.

The refrigeration units should be defrosted and cleaned monthly, and the packs being used should be defrosted, wiped clean, dried, and refrozen about every 6 months. A maintenance tag may be tied to the instrument to ensure that the procedure is completed at 6-month intervals.

Numerous types of cold packs are available for home use, which can be easily stored in the freezer compartment of a refrigerator. During application, they can be placed or strapped to the part to be treated. For acute problems, it is suggested that the patient use the pack for 10 minutes each hour when awake for the first 24—48 hours following injury. If such frequent applications are not practical for the patient, then a 15-minute treatment every 2—4 hours is recommended.

There are also "instant" chemical packs available that are activated by shaking or breaking an inner seal within the bag, which allows mixing of special chemicals. When improvisation is necessary in an emergency, crushed ice or a carton of frozen vegetables may be placed in a plastic bag and wrapped in a thin towel.

Vapocoolant Sprays

Several vapors have been available for many years that may be used to cool localized areas of the skin. The two that are in most common use are ethyl chloride and Fluori-methane.

Vapocoolant therapy can be defined as the intense localized cooling that is produced by the rapid evaporation of a hydrocarbon compound on the surface of the skin. Traditionally, these sprays have been used to increase active and passive ranges of motion in joints, sedate localized painful areas (especially trigger points), assist in the reduction of muscle spasm, act as a counterirritant, and serve as a local anesthetic (eg, small burns, insect bites).[15]

When a vapocoolant spray is used, it is important to assure that application is made in an open, well-ventilated area and that the patient's eyes are completely covered. The area to be treated must be exposed, and the surrounding area should be draped. The doctor should take care not to inhale the vapor during application.

A vapocoolant spray may also be used as a clinical aid in diagnosis in differentiating trigger-point disorders from other conditions. For example, if muscle spasm is secondary to

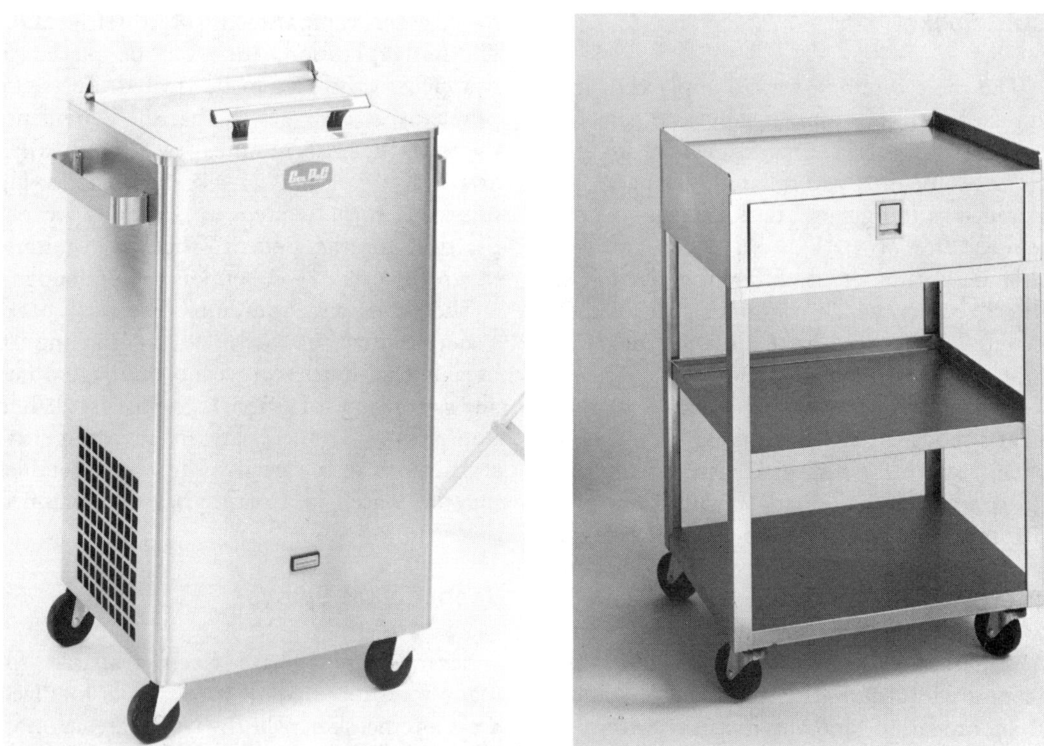

Figure 6.3. *Left,* a typical mobile cold pack modality; *right,* accessory stand.

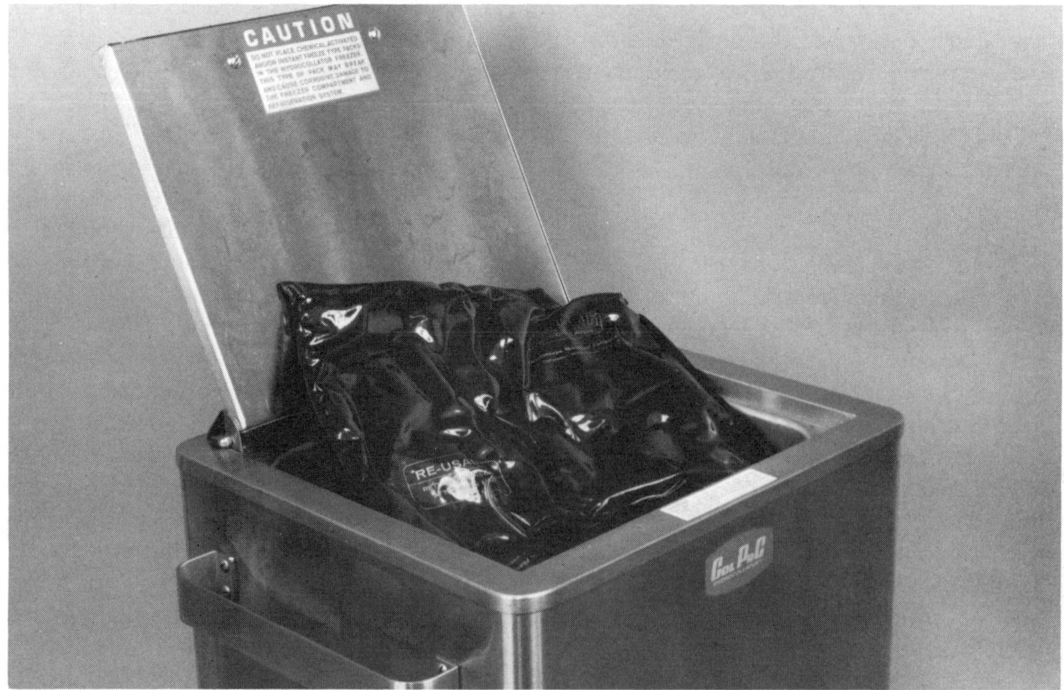

Figure 6.4. Lid open on a cold pack apparatus, exposing a cold pack.

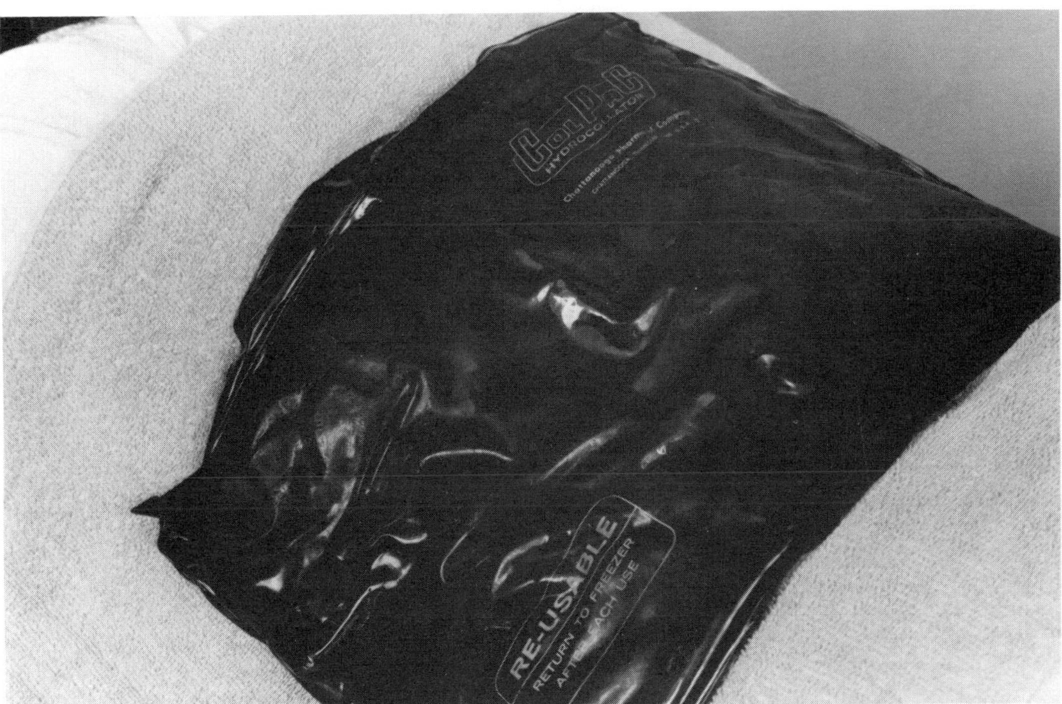

Figure 6.5. A cold pack application in which a towel has been placed between the pack and the patient's skin.

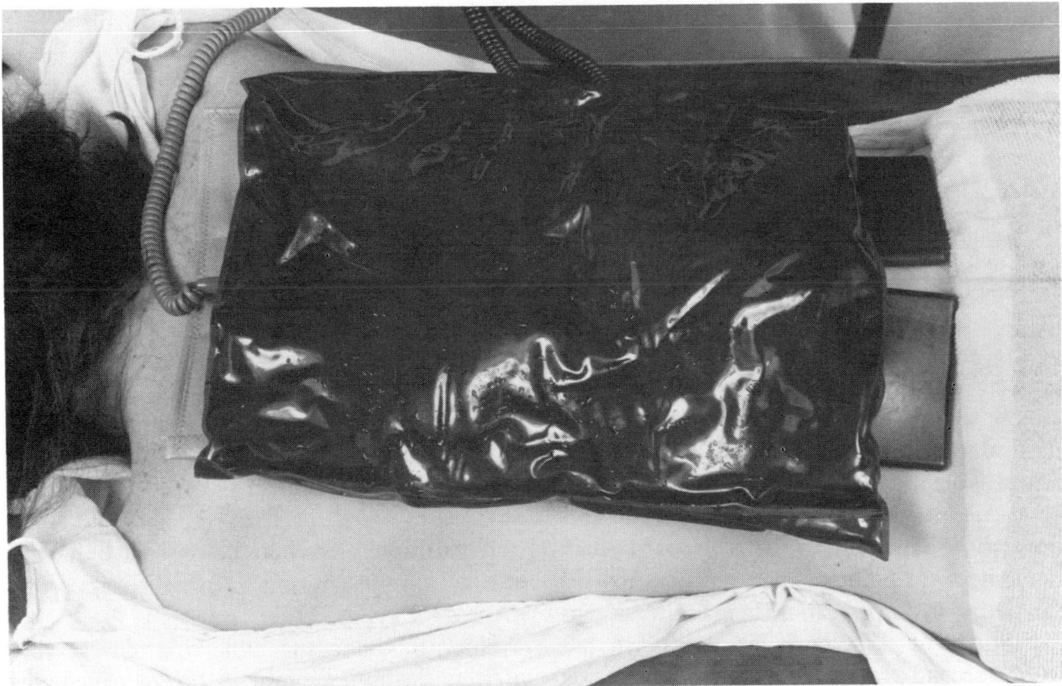

Figure 6.6. A large cold pack placed over both active and indifferent high-volt electrodes. The patient presented with an acute posttraumatic spinal strain.

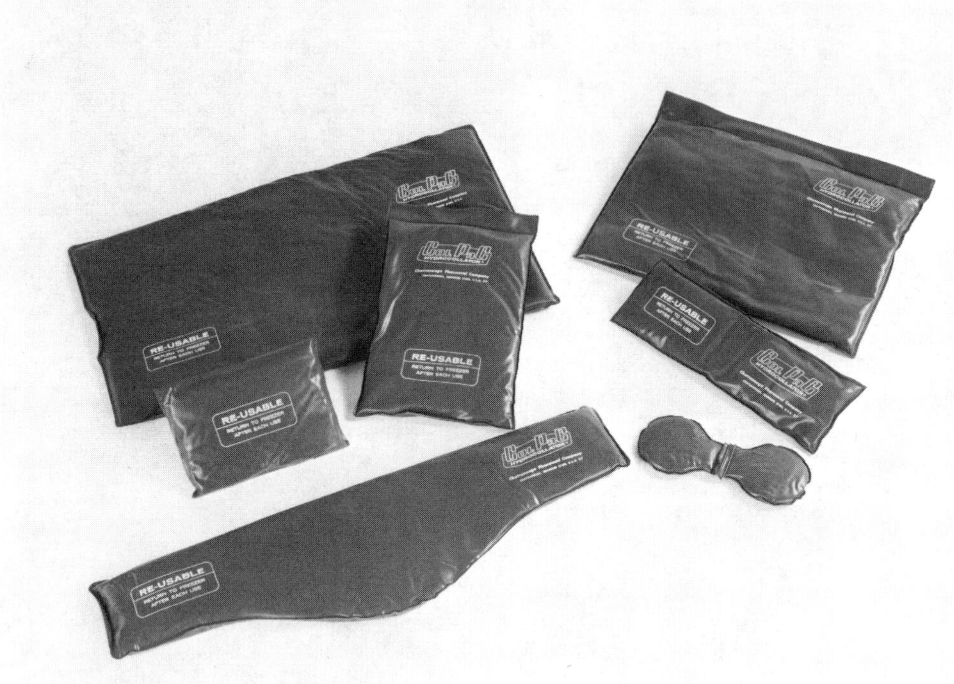

Figure 6.7. Reusable cryotherapy units are available in various shapes and sizes to fit almost any body part contour.

some other active cause of musculoskeletal pain or to a neurogenic cause, the relief of the spasm may make the patient's pain worse, pointing the way to a correct diagnosis.

GENERAL TECHNIQUE

During application, the pressurized bottle or can is held at a right angle to the part to be treated and at a distance of 2—3 feet from the patient's skin. It is best to spray from the focal point of pain outward toward the periphery. Application is made in sweeping bursts of 2 seconds each, interspaced with 3-second intervals. Such sweeps, made at approximately 4 inches per second, are continued until the pain dissipates or for 3 minutes, whichever occurs first. The stream should not be allowed to collect at any given site. If the skin becomes frosted or turns ivory white, application should be discontinued and the frost removed with a cloth.

One authority describes a method in which he applies a spray for 20 seconds and repeats the spraying at 10-second intervals.

Vapocoolant sprays work best for musculoskeletal complaints if massage or stretching procedures are utilized during their application. Multiple areas may be treated, but only one at a time, during each office appointment.

Fluori-methane and ethyl chloride may be used as a counterirritant in the management of myofascial pain, restricted motion, and muscle spasm with or without related trigger points. Fluori-methane is preferred to ethyl chloride in that it is less cold to the patient, noninflammable, not explosive, not a general anesthetic, and nontoxic when used correctly.[16]

SPRAY-AND-STRETCH TECHNIQUE

Travell, Nielsen, and others have conducted years of studies involving the use of volatile sprays and stretching in the treatment of musculoskeletal and referred pain syndromes.[17,18,19]

The vapocoolant is applied in one direction, never back and forth, at a distance of 18—24 inches and at the rate of 4 inches per second. A fine stream is used, not a mist. The rhythm should be a few seconds on and a few seconds off. When spraying near the face, precautions should be taken to cover the patient's eyes, nose, and mouth. The degree of cooling with from two to four unhurried, even, parallel, nonoverlapping sweeps with the spray, about ¼-inch apart, does not result in local anesthesia, but it is often enough to cause immediate and sometimes lasting disappearance of pain in acute joint sprain or muscle spasm precipitated by trauma.[20]

If an irritative trigger point is involved, the doctor should spray from the active trigger point to the referred pain zone. The therapy is continued until all trigger points found (several are common) have been sprayed.

To be most effective, passive movement must be used while spraying to gently stretch the muscle containing the trigger area. Spray and stretch is used until the muscle reaches its maximum or normal resting length. The stretch of the muscle should begin as spraying the affected area is started. It should be gentle but firmly applied by a sustaining passive stretch to the muscle while the patient remains relaxed.

Overchilling muscle tissue or overstretching will set up painful spasms that defeat the purpose of the therapy. During stretching, the doctor should feel a gradual increase in the range of motion of the affected muscle. Active motion in the direction of restriction should be tested after every one or two sweeps. This spraying and stretching may require from two to four applications to achieve the results desired.

Stop the treatment if there is no positive effect in 5 minutes. A few sweeps are usually sufficient to cover the skin overlying the affected muscle and extinguish the pain. Avoid skin frosting. The benefits may last several hours, days, or be permanent.

It takes about 5 minutes for skin and subcutaneous tissues to rewarm. During this time, moist hot packs can be applied to the area while the procedure is being conducted in another region. Following treatment, the patient should be given some simple exercises to be carried out several times each day. It is not uncommon to find on a follow-up visit that the original trigger points have vanished and the remaining discomfort can be traced to secondary trigger points not discovered on the first treatment.

The relief of pain facilitates early mobilization in restoration of muscle function. The benefits are apparently derived from the spray producing nociceptive impulses that propel faster from skin receptors along afferent nerves to higher centers than do noxious impulses from the muscle spindles, which travel along smaller afferents. The nociceptive impulses seem to set up a refractory state that blocks the slower muscle-pain impulses. Thus, the muscle is allowed to relax and be stretched to its normal resting length and pain-free state.

While vapocoolant sprays are quite beneficial in acute cases, chronic cases sometimes show better results with acupuncture. This is probably due to an acute case being a purely neurophysiologic disorder at the onset that in time develops organic changes that are benefited by the mechanical effects of the needling of the trigger areas but not by the cooling effect. Nevertheless, dramatic relief of painful motion of many years standing without structural deformity has been reported with only a few sprayings.

SPECIFIC SPRAY-AND-STRETCH TECHNIQUES

Grade I and II Strains and Sprains of the Elbow. The patient is placed in the sitting position with the elbow slightly flexed and abducted. Isolate trigger areas and site of major pain in the arm, elbow, and forearm, and spray sites. At the same time, ask the patient to extend his elbow and then slowly return it to the relaxed position. Repeat the spraying and active movement three or four times. Have the patient indicate with his finger the major source of pain. As the pain shifts position, spray the affected area. Once relief has been obtained in flexion-extension, add forearm pronation and supination in extension, spraying painful sites as necessary between movements. Have the patient attempt movements against resistance, and spray the painful area if necessary. Once relief is obtained, correct any subluxations isolated, apply an ace bandage or "tennis elbow" support, and instruct the patient in home exercises for 1—2 minutes each half hour during waking hours. Begin resistance and stretching exercises as soon as they are possible.[21]

Acute Low Back Muscle Spasms. The patient is placed in the lateral recumbent position with the involved side up and the knees slightly flexed. Isolate trigger areas and site of major pain, and spray sites. At the same time, ask the patient to pull his knees up toward his chest, and then slowly return them to the relaxed position. Repeat the spraying and active movement three or four times. Have the patient indicate with his finger the major source of pain. As the pain shifts position, spray the affected area. Once relief is obtained, have the patient turn to the other side if the condition is bilateral, and repeat the procedure. Once relief has been obtained in flexion-extension, add rotation and lateral flexion, spraying painful sites as necessary between movements. Have the patient attempt to walk, and spray the painful area if necessary. If possible, have the patient bend forward with his heels on the floor. Once relief is obtained, correct any subluxations isolated, support the area, and instruct the patient in home exercises for 1—2 minutes each half hour during the waking hours. Advise the patient to avoid remaining in any one position for too long. Begin resistance, stretching, and weight-bearing exercises as soon as acute symptoms subside.[22]

Grade I Knee Sprains. Place the patient supine with a pillow under the knee. Spray the painful and tender areas, and gently assist and resist the patient in knee flexion-extension, with emphasis on extension and quadriceps setting. As the pain shifts position, spray the affected area. Have the patient attempt to walk, semi-squat, and kneel, and spray the painful area if necessary. If possible, have the patient stand and bend forward, keeping the heels on the floor. Once relief is obtained, strap the joint, and instruct the patient in home exercises for 1—2 minutes each half hour during the waking hours. Full weight bearing should be restricted until the quadriceps indicate good strength. Begin resistance, stretching, and weight-bearing exercises as soon as they are possible.[23]

Grade I Ankle Sprains. The patient is placed supine with pillows under the knee and ankle. Spray the painful ankle area, and gently assist and resist the patient in ankle flexion-extension. As the pain shifts position, spray the affected area. Once relief has been obtained in flexion-extension, add inversion, eversion, and toe flexion-extension, spraying painful sites as necessary between movements. Have the patient attempt to walk, and spray painful areas if necessary. If possible, have the patient stand on his toes and bend forward with his heels on the floor. Once relief is obtained, correct any subluxations isolated, strap the ankle, and instruct the patient in home exercises for 1—2 minutes each half hour during the waking hours.

Begin resistance, stretching, and weight-bearing exercises as soon as they are possible. These should include toe standing, soleus muscle stretching, and eversion standing.[24]

Clay Compresses

In some areas, clay is used as a method of cold therapy because of its good insulation properties; ie, cooled clay retains its temperature for a relatively long period of time. The cold clay is spread on a towel that is applied directly to the skin.

The principles for use are much the same as those for using paraffin wax (eg, arthritis). Another common type of application is its use over a sprained ankle. After the cooled clay has been painted on the ankle, the ankle is bandaged and rested for about an hour.

Cryotherapy Units

One type of cold therapy apparatus that we have investigated is the Cryomatic unit. This refrigeration equipment permits application of a controlled temperature over a prolonged duration; thus offering a valuable aid in the treatment of conditions such as acute IVD syndromes where concentrated cryotherapy over a relatively long period of time is of value. See Figure 6.8.

The Cryomatic unit utilizes freon gas that is run through coils, similar to those of a common refrigerator or air conditioner. The thermostat may be set anywhere from 20 °F to 80 °F so that treatment of up to an hour or more at a time are possible without danger of adverse effects. See Figure 6.9. The danger of a cold "burn" is reduced because the intercoil spacing in the treatment pads is about 1 inch apart.

A Cryomatic modality is capable of maintaining a temperature constant that is lower than ice packs (eg, 20 °F) under like conditions and for a longer duration without the risk of frostbite. Studies have also shown that the therapy fires off a minimal amount of pain-evoking C fibers.[25]

All standard considerations, indications, and contraindications for the use of cold should be taken into account when a cold therapy apparatus is used. A cloth should always be placed between the treatment pads and the patient's skin. The patient should be checked periodically throughout the treatment to assure that the desired response is being achieved. Treatment duration may vary from 20 to 60 minutes or more.

Cold Immersion

Immersion in ice water or in an ice-water whirlpool has been reported by some as being highly effective in providing deep penetration into body tissues. Temperature reductions in deep muscle, where an average drop of 51.8 °F per hour have been detected, are similar to those following ice massage. The water is kept at about 50 °—60 °F, and the part being treated is immersed for 10—20 minutes. Exercises can easily be accomplished during the treatment.

For acute musculoskeletal conditions, especially extremity sprains or strains, active electrodes of a high-volt unit can be simultaneously incorporated into the water near the immersed part being treated.

Cryokinetics

The term *cryokinetics* was first coined by Hayden in 1964.[26] It refers to any situation where local cooling of a body part is followed by active exercise to mobilize the joint being treated. The spray-and-stretch technique is one example.

Alternating Heat and Cold

Some authorities suggest that the most successful applications and effects of therapeutic temperature control occur when heat and cold are alternated during the same treatment. The most common indication would be for patients presenting with acute

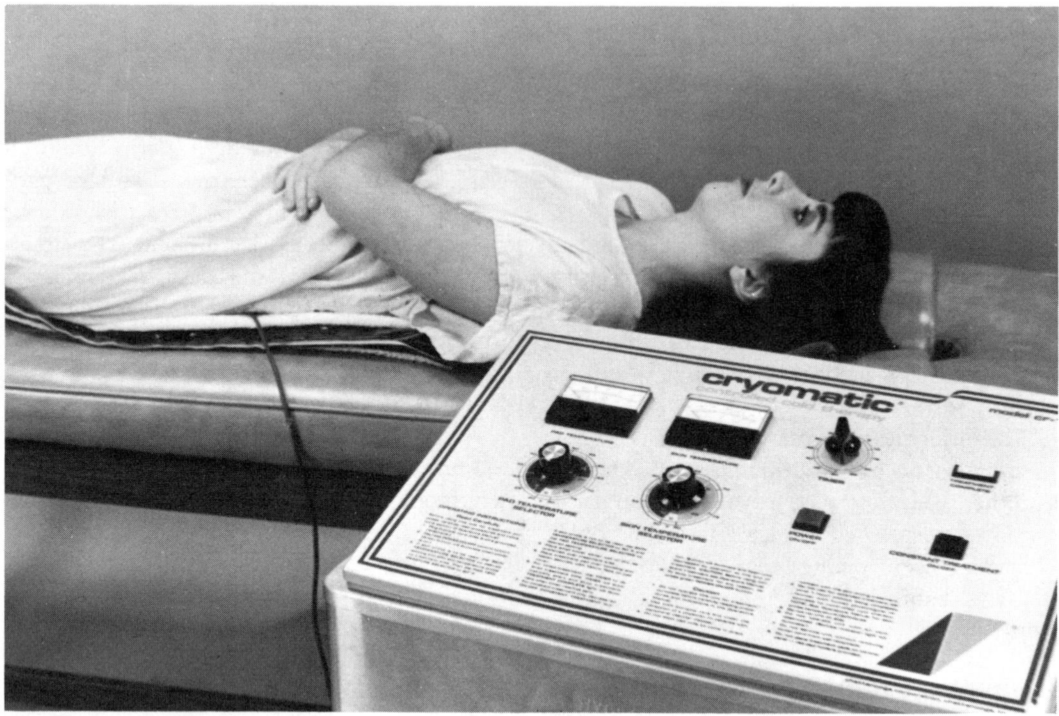

Figure 6.8. Controlled cryotherapy being applied to the lumbar area.

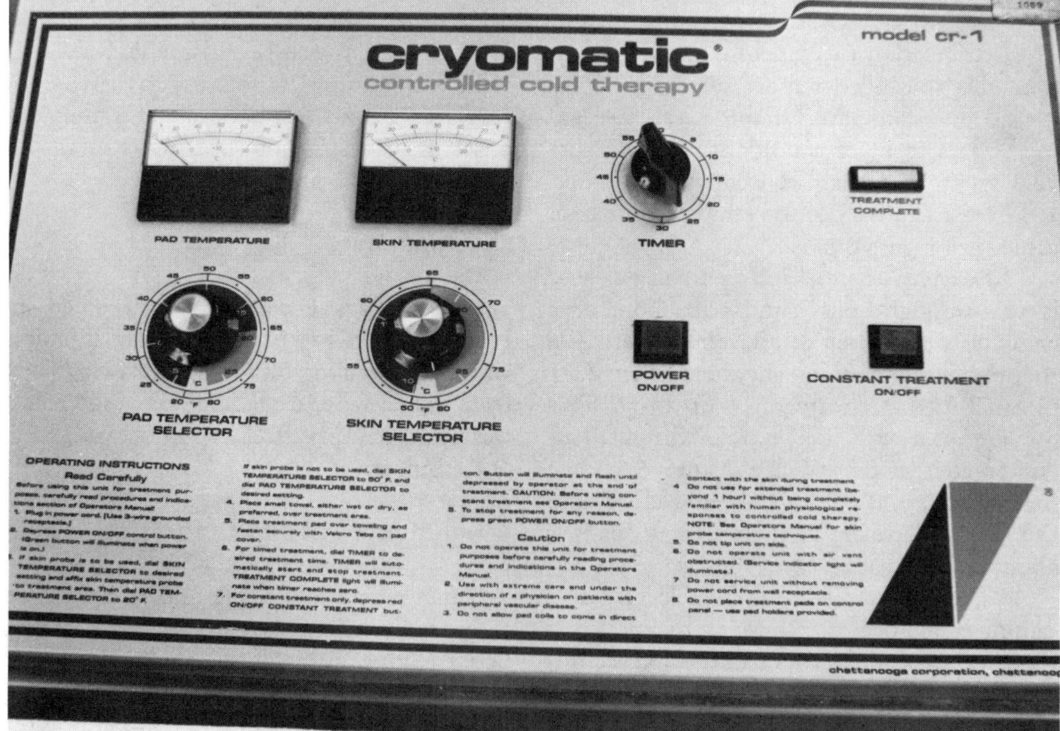

Figure 6.9. Control panel of a controlled Cryomatic cold therapy modality.

musculoskeletal complaints, especially posttraumatic swelling. The objective is to allow the patient to benefit from the effects of heat without the buildup of edema; hence, to elicit a "pumping" action to increase circulation and reduce stasis by alternating vasodilation and vasoconstriction.[27] The primary rule to remember is to always start and end the therapy with heat.

Applications of alternating heat and cold may be made by utilizing hot and cold packs, immersions into hot and cold water, or using two whirlpools of opposite therapeutic temperatures. In fact, almost any combination of acceptable modalities using these parameters may be considered. See Figure 6.10.

A modified form of alternating temperature therapy occurs when local cooling is combined with *remote* heating. This type of treatment is recommended as a possible way to reduce muscle spasm or states of spasticity. DonTigny and Sheldon believe that this method allows the core temperature of the patient to be maintained at a near normal level, thus minimizing undue effects to the CNS as might be reflected in shivering.[28]

Other Forms of Therapeutic Cold

Around the period of World War II, the use of liquid air and carbon dioxide snow was quite popular. However, these media to administer cold have given way to the other modalities described in this chapter because of their ease of application.

INDICATIONS

It has been stated that it is generally felt that cold is one of the best available therapies in the clinical management of patients with acute musculoskeletal complaints. After carefully examining the patient to rule out fractures or overt pathologies, cold therapy can be applied immediately along with compression and elevation (I-C-E).[29,30] This acronym refers to ice, compression, and elevation.

Cold is indicated whenever its physiologic effects are desired, thus readily appropriate in strains, sprains, bursitis, arthritis, tendinitis, fibrositis, myositis and splinting. Muscle "pulls" and cervical strains respond well to cold. Brief exposures of the skin to temperatures that are at or near freezing have been found to be most beneficial in relieving pain, removing edema, and relaxing muscle spasm. Cold also has been traditionally used to reduce the posttraumatic extravasation of blood and other tissue fluids.[31,32]

Many trainers report excellent results with cold therapy in the management of ligamentous irritations of the ankle, knee, hips, ribs, shoulder, elbow, and wrist. Because cold is effective in anesthetizing an area, reducing edema, and alleviating muscle spasm, it is an invaluable tool in the management of common athletic and recreational injuries.[33]

Cold compresses are extremely effective in the early stages of uncomplicated congestive disorders such as acute eye diseases, congestive headaches, laryngitis, pharyngitis, and tonsillitis. As a first-aid measure, an ice bag over the heart has been reported to check the violence of inflammation in acute pericarditis and relieve the pain of appendicitis.[34] The points shown in Table 6.4 summarize the basic indications for utilizing cryotherapy in most any form.

Bleeding and Swelling

Many musculoskeletal injuries require immediate attention for control of bleeding and/or the reduction of swelling. In any situation of bleeding or swelling, the I-C-E principle should be applied. In an emergency, the use of cold can serve as a substitute hemostat.

It is granted that research shows cold to produce a local vasodilation as an inevitable rebound phenomenon.[35] This is true, as in the case of ethyl chloride where the application is quick. Here, there is an immediate

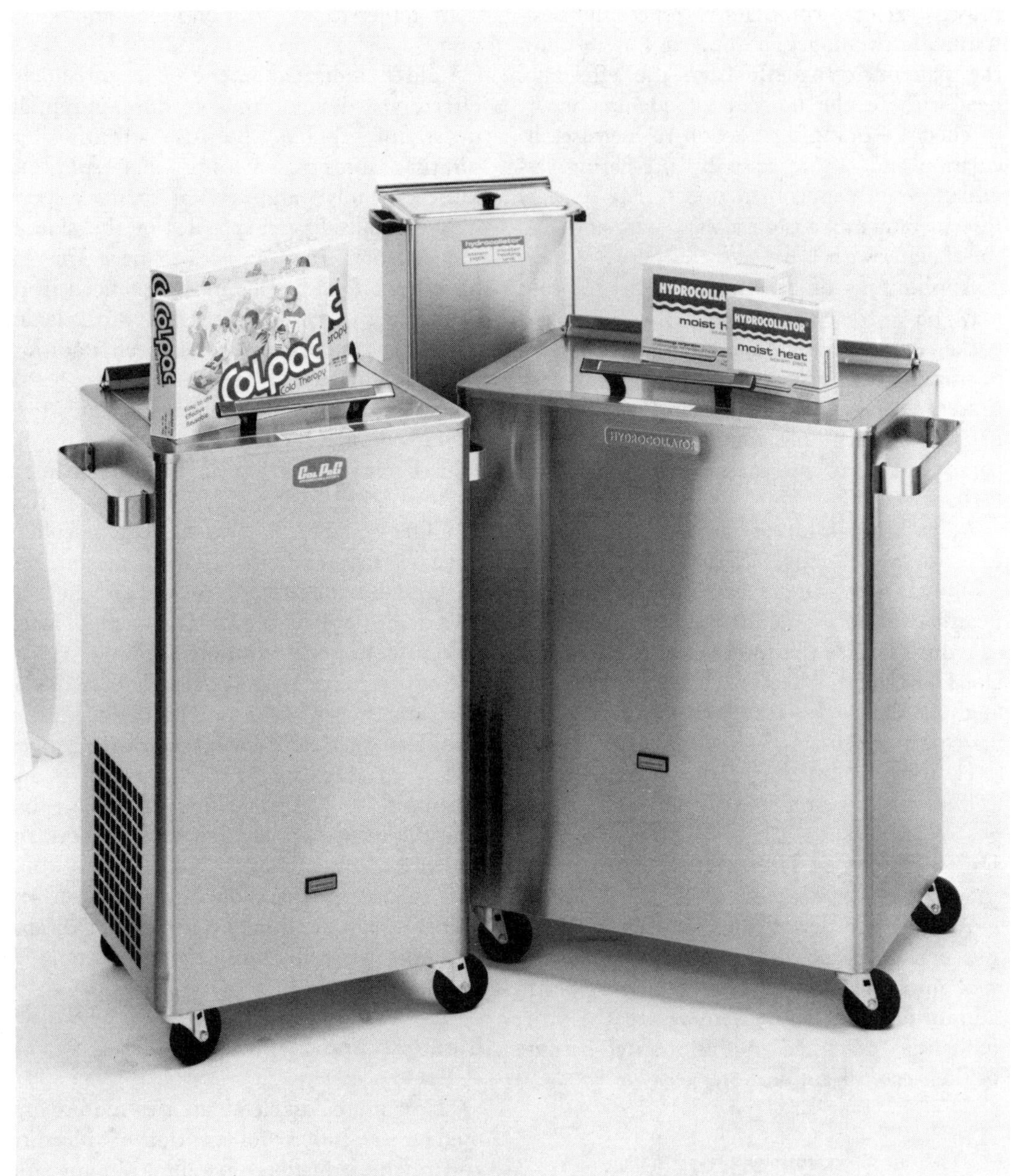

Figure 6.10. *Left,* Colpac apparatus, for the application of therapeutic cold; *right,* Hydrocollator equipment, for the application of therapeutic heat.

Table 6.4. General Indications and Contraindications to Cryotherapy

INDICATIONS

- Inhibit bleeding after acute trauma
- Relieve pain and reduce the accompanying reflex muscle spasm so often seen in acute musculoskeletal injuries
- Decrease blood flow to areas of acute inflammation
- Spasticity
- Burns
- Closed pressure sores
- Reduce adverse tissue changes and relieve pain in the first aid treatment of insect and snake bites
- Angiomas
- Boils and carbuncles
- Febrile states
- Herpes blisters
- Sprains and strains
- Varicose ulcers
- Warts

CONTRAINDICATIONS

- Raynaud's disease
- Chilblain (pernio)
- Coma
- Rheumatoid or gouty arthritis
- Cryesthesia
- Paroxysmal cold hemoglobinuria

vasoconstriction, followed by a visible rebound capillary flare. However, it takes more than a few seconds of superficial cold to stop bleeding.

The application of cold can often be applied for many hours in injuries prone to recurrent hemorrhage. The danger of frostbite is greatly minimized by placing a cloth or piece of clothing between the skin and the cold medium. It also helps to apply a skin lubricant.

Burns

First aid in burns obviously requires immediate removal from the source of heat. This should be immediately followed by cool washings, cold applications for at least 30 minutes to reduce blisters and pain, protection from infection, and management of the accompanying shock. Following therapy, topical vitamin E underlaid with diluted special waters (eg, DMSO) have been reported to be helpful in uncomplicated first- and second-degree burns.[36]

Fluori-methane or ethyl chloride may be used to alleviate the pain of first- and second-degree burns. The Spra-Pak nozzle should be used as it offers a mist-like spray to lessen the impact of the vapocoolant on the affected area. Spray lightly until the skin just beings to frost, but never frost the skin.

Inflammatory Edema

Cryotherapy is quite efficient in treating stubborn effusion such as that of chronic or recurring bursitis. See Figure 6.11.

When applied locally, cold produces arteriole vasoconstriction that reduces the associated secretions and exudation. Thus, as Andrews shows, it has a reverse effect on inflammation by decreasing capillary pressure and diminishing the amount of hemorrhage into tissue spaces, which facilitates lymphatic drainage to reduce swelling.[37]

In addition to vasoconstriction, prolonged cold also produces sedation, numbness, and increases muscle tone. A reflex vasoconstriction effect occurs in internal organs. If cold is

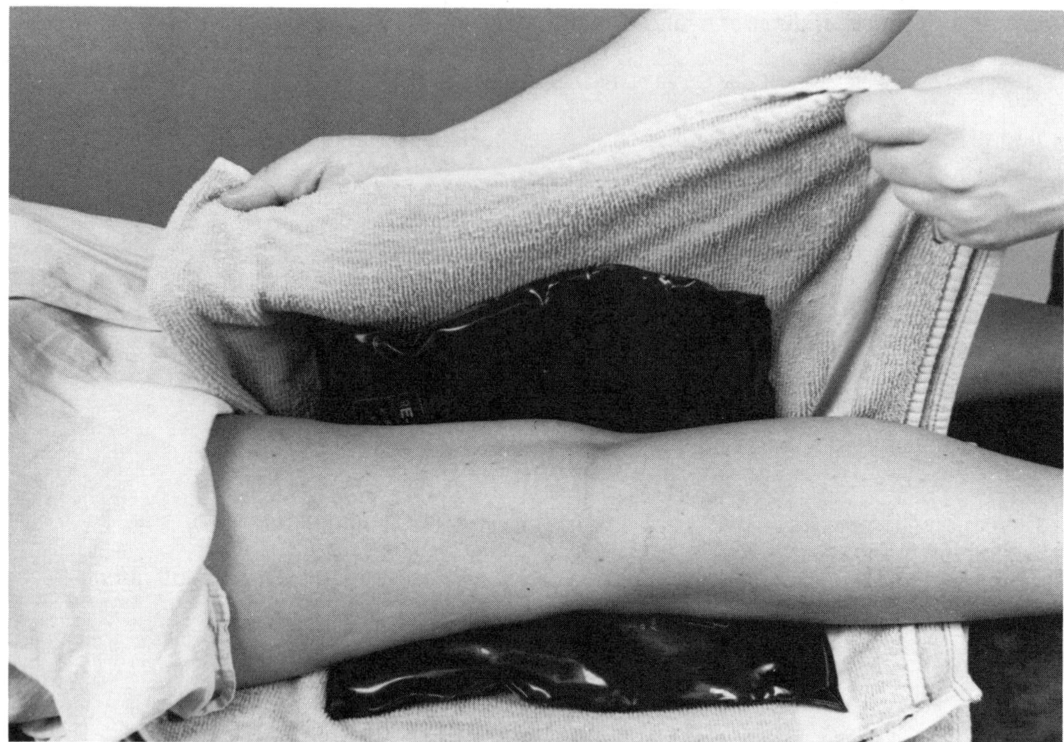

Figure 6.11. Application to the left knee of a cold pack wrapped in a warm moist towel (eg, for chronic effusion of prepatellar bursitis).

prolonged, the vasoconstrictive effects are fatigued and the opposite effects develop such as local vasodilation, reflex internal vasodilation, increased blood pressure, and decreased respiratory rate. The initial decreased capillary blood pressure is followed in 5—8 minutes by increased blood pressure and a slowed pulse.[38]

A study by Farry in 1980 of injured ligaments showed that the application of ice causes (1) increased subcutaneous swelling to injured and uninjured soft tissue and (2) a diminution of histologic evidence of inflammation in injured ligamentous tissue. This first point indicates that therapeutic cooling with ice to temperatures of 41°—59°F induces a degree of ischemia in soft tissues overlying injured ligaments that causes damaged vessels. This damage leads to some superficial posttherapy exudation and swelling. Regardless of this, it was noted that the inflammatory reaction in the deeper injured ligaments, including microscopic edema, was reduced. To gain the advantages of the anti-inflammatory reaction, the swelling of the overlying soft tissues can be minimized by using the standard practice of compression bandages.[39]

Pain and Reflex Muscle Spasm

As cold is a counterirritant and as the speed with which a nerve transmits an impulse is reduced in decreased temperatures, the pain threshold is increased. Complete elimination of conduction can be eliminated by depressing tissue temperatures 50°—59°F. This is one reason why cold applications allow a painful joint to be placed through greater angles of passive and active ranges of motion without undue discomfort.[40-44]

Spasticity

While cryotherapy has been used for centuries, its exact physiologic effects are not completely understood. Nevertheless, current research is beginning to solve the mystery of cryotherapy's actions and reactions.[45,46] It is evident, however, that involuntary muscle contractions require a large amount of nutrients, simultaneously create ischemic areas because of the compressed intramuscular capillaries, and produce pain.[47,48,49] Paradoxically, patients with rheumatic afflictions who have decreased joint mobility on cold damp days are benefited by ice massage.

Cryotherapy appears to be highly effective in the treatment of spasticity because cold tends to (1) bombard the CNS with impulses from cold receptors and initiate the Gate Theory of stimulus inhibition, (2) reduce the motor outflow in the site being treated, (3) initiate a reflex sympathetic influence on muscle spindles that decreases spasticity, and (4) depress the excitability of free nerve ending and the conductivity of peripheral nerves, which leads to analgesia.[50-53] The order of neurosusceptibility to cold is shown in Table 6.5.[54]

In cases of advanced multiple sclerosis, poliomyelitis, arthritis, and periarthritis, cold applications applied both proximal and distal to a joint tested have shown to offer a marked, but usually temporary, decrease in resistance to passive stretch, thus a marked increase in joint mobility, whether or not pain and tenderness are present. Such a decrease in resistance to passive stretch lasts from a few minutes up to 24 hours.[55,56]

Sprains and Strains

The initial effects of localized cooling (essentially from the vasoconstriction effect) are minimized swelling, reduced pain because of decreased nerve impulse conduction velocity, reduced tissue metabolism, increased neuromuscular function, reduced spasm because of reduced response of muscle afferents, and enhanced muscle contraction.[57,58,59] The greatest benefits of cold are achieved when sprains of Grade I and II levels have been of recent origin, especially if the level of temperature depression is controlled.[60,61]

Secondary swelling from vasodilation and increased profusion should be avoided. When tissue temperatures approach 60°F, vasodilation usually occurs as an innate survival response to avoid necrosis. Thus, prolonged cold must be carefully monitored.[62,63]

It is interesting to note, however, that a study of the effects of ice massage on delayed muscle soreness was conducted by Yackzan in 1981.[64] Soreness and range of motion evaluations were conducted at 0, 24, 48, and 72 hours following a single bout of eccentric exercises of the elbow flexors. The conclusion was that cryotherapy was *not* as effective in the treatment of delayed muscle soreness associated with strains as it has been reported in the pain associated with sprains.

Table 6.5. Comparative Motor Neurosensitivity Blockage to Cold

Motor Function of	*Conductivity Block Temperature, Fahrenheit*
Small medullated fibers. . .	71.6°
Large medullated fibers. . .	53.6°
Unmedullated fibers.	41.0°—50.0°
Primary spindle afferents .	82.4°
Monosynaptic reflex.	18.0°

Tumors

During the 1930s and 1940s, the use of focal freezing was quite popular in the treatment of readily accessible primary tumors. Use slowly faded when surgery and chemotherapy became more popular; however, recent experiments, especially by Osteopaths, are creating a renewed interest. For the sake of background information, it is well documented that regression of growth for several weeks or months may be expected in the size of the tumor mass, accompanied by degeneration of the tumor cells to the point of actual necrosis. Occasionally, the tumor may even disappear.[65]

A comprehensive study of experimental cryotherapy (carbon dioxide snow) in neoplastic cervical disease in 221 women and benign cervical disease in 317 women was reported by Sedlis in 1981. Temporary arrest in the neoplastic cases was achieved in 89.9% of the patients treated, according to 6-month follow-up Pap smears and/or biopsies. This figure, however, later dropped to 47.9% without subsequent treatment. In the benign group, only 2.5% of the cases progressed to cervical intraepithelial neoplasia.[66]

CONTRAINDICATIONS AND PRECAUTIONS

There are few contraindications to or precautions associated with the use of therapeutic cold as compared to other physiotherapies. In fact, it is one of the safest modalities that can be used. Refer to Table 6.4. Special caution, however, must be taken with volatile liquids. It should always be kept in mind that a volatile liquid (eg, ethyl chloride, ether, rhigolene, etc) is essentially a freezing agent and not a cooling agent as are some milder modalities (eg, a wrapped ice pack). Thus, any use of a volatile liquid should be used with caution and knowledge of its potential effects.

Ethyl chloride is highly volatile and flammable, thus no smoking can be allowed in the room. It must also be assured that no open flame or electric spark would be available that might cause an explosion.

A few cases of temporary nerve palsy have been reported when ice has been used for prolonged periods (eg, 30 minutes) and superficial nerves of the area were not protected.[67]

Some patients are unable to tolerate cold therapy. This cryesthesia may be due to a genetic factor, a neurologic disorder in which the receptors to cold are hypersensitive (eg, tooth decay and other forms of degenerative bone disease), or an underlying pathologic process (eg, impaired circulation states such as in autonomic vasospasm, diabetic neuropathy, arteriosclerosis, collagen disease, etc).

Patients with extreme sensitivity to cold may develop facial flushing, wheals or hives, and even syncope. It has been reported that some patients may faint after immersion of just one extremity in a cold bath of 5—6 minutes. In such hypersensitive individuals, it is best to select another modality than cold that would offer similar benefits.[68,69]

Special caution should also be exercised in utilizing therapeutic cold in the extremely young, weak, or elderly. In weak or debilitated individuals, the reaction to cold is either delayed or absent and, generally, there is a longer period of vital depression that is attended by subnormal nutrition and followed by a slow recovery.[70]

REFERENCES

1. Brown A: Physical medicine in rehabilitation. *Maryland State Medical Journal,* 19:61, 1970.
2. Haber WP: Therapeutic heat and cold. Lombard, IL, National College of Chiropractic, no date shown, pp 1-5.
3. Stillwell GK: Therapeutic heat and cold. In Krusen FH, et al (eds): *Handbook of Physical Medicine and Rehabilitation,* ed 2. Philadelphia, W.B. Saunders, 1971, pp 259-272.
4. Horton BT, et al: Hypersensitiveness to cold, with local and systemic manifestations of a histamine-

like character; its amenability to treatment. *Journal of the American Medical Association,* 107: 1263-1268, 1936.

5. Mohler HK: Cold and refrigeration. In Piersol GM, et al (eds): *The Cyclopedia of Medicine, Surgery and Specialties.* Philadelphia, F.A. Davis, 1949, vol 4, p 350.
6. Fox RH: Local cooling in man. *British Medical Bulletin,* 17:14-18, 1961.
7. Lowdon BJ, Moore RJ: Determinants and nature of intramuscular temperature changes during cold therapy. *American Journal of Physical Medicine,* 54:223-233, 1975.
8. Wolf SL, Basmajian JV: Intramuscular temperature changes deep to localized cutaneous cold stimulation. *Physical Therapy,* 53:1284-1288, 1973.
9. Bierman W, Friedlander M: The penetrative effect of cold. *Archives of Physical Medicine and Rehabilitation,* 21:585-592, 1940.
10. Schafer RC: *Chiropractic Management of Sports and Recreational Injuries.* Baltimore, Williams & Wilkins, 1982, pp 197-198.
11. Tepperman PS, Devlin M: Therapeutic heat and cold. *Postgraduate Medicine,* January 1983, pp 69-76.
12. Furnas D: Topical refrigeration and frost anesthesia. *Anesthesiology,* 26:344-347, 1965.
13. McMaster WC, et al: Laboratory evaluation of various cold therapy modalities. *American Journal of Sports Medicine,* 6:291-294, 1978.
14. Hill LL: *Parameters of Physiotherapy Modalities.* Lombard, IL, National Chiropractic College, class notes, date not shown, pp 21-23.
15. Halkovich LR, et al: Effect of fluori-methane spray on passive hip flexion. *Physical Therapy,* 61(2): 185-189, February 1981.
16. Hill LL: *Parameters of Physiotherapy Modalities.* Lombard, IL, National Chiropractic College, class notes, date not shown, p 26.
17. Nielsen AJ: Spray and stretch for myofascial pain. *Physical Therapy,* 58(5):567-569, May 1978.
18. Travell J: Basis for the multiple uses of local block of somatic trigger areas. *Mississippi Valley Medical Journal,* January 1949, pp 13-21.
19. Travell J: Myofascial trigger points: clinical view. In Bonica JJ, Albe-Fessard, D: *Advances in Pain Research and Therapy.* New York, Raven Press, vol 1, 1976.
20. Schafer RC: *Chiropractic Management of Sports and Recreational Injuries.* Baltimore, Williams & Wilkins, 1982, pp 254-255.
21. Ibid: pp 388-389.
22. Ibid: pp 440-441.
23. Ibid: pp 477-478.
24. Ibid: p 511.
25. Hill LL: *Parameters of Physiotherapy Modalities.* Lombard, IL, National Chiropractic College, class notes, date not shown, pp 24-25.
26. Hayden CA: Cryokinetics in an early treatment program. *Journal of the American Physical Therapy Association,* 44:990-993, 1964.
27. Knight KL, Londeree BR: Comparison of blood flow in the ankle of uninjured subjects during therapeutic applications of heat, cold, and exercise. *Medicine and Science in Sports and Exercise,* 12(1):76-80, 1980.
28. DonTigny RL, Sheldon KW: Simultaneous use of heat and cold in treatment of muscle spasm. *Archives of Physical Medicine,* 43:235-237, 1962.
29. McMaster WC: Literary review on ice therapy in injury. *American Journal of Sports Medicine,* 5: 124-126, 1977.
30. Olson JE, Stravino VD: A Review of cryotherapy. *Physical Therapy,* 52:840-843, 1972.
31. Betge G: *Physical Therapy in Chiropractic Practice.* Via Tesserete, Switzerland, published by author, 1975, pp 52.
32. Hocutt JE Jr, et al: Cryotherapy in ankle sprains. *American Journal of Sports Medicine.* 10:5, 1982.
33. Virtue RW: *Hypothermic Anesthesia.* Springfield, IL, Charles C. Thomas, 1955, pp 13-14.
34. Mohler HK: Cold and refrigeration. In Piersol GM, et al (eds): *The Cyclopedia of Medicine, Surgery and Specialties.* Philadelphia, F.A. Davis, 1949, vol 4, pp 353-354.
35. Schafer RC: *Chiropractic Management of Sports and Recreational Injuries.* Baltimore, Williams & Wilkins, 1982, pp 166-167.
36. Ibid: p 220.
37. Andrews FW: Discussion of ice therapy. *ACA Journal of Chiropractic,* April 1968.
38. Schafer RC: *Chiropractic Management of Sports and Recreational Injuries.* Baltimore, Williams & Wilkins, 1982, pp 197-198.
39. Farry PJ, et al: Ice treatment of injured ligaments: An experimental model. *New Zealand Medical Journal,* January 9, 1980, pp 12-14.
40. Schafer RC: *Chiropractic Management of Sports and Recreational Injuries.* Baltimore, Williams & Wilkins, 1982, pp 197-198.
41. Lee JM, et al: Effects of ice on nerve conduction velocity. *Physiotherapy,* 64:2-6, 1978.
42. Fox RH: Local cooling in man. *British Medical Bulletin,* 17:14-18, 1961.
43. Lehmann JF, et al: Effect of therapeutic temperatures on tendon extensibility. *Archives of Physical Medicine and Rehabilitation,* 51:481-487, 1970.
44. Bonica JJ, Albe-Fessard D: *Advances in Pain Research and Therapy.* New York, Raven Press, 1976.
45. Eldred E, et al: The effect of cooling on mammalian muscle spindle. *Experimental Neurology,* 2: 144-157, 1960.
46. Lightfoot E, et al: Neurophysiological effects of prolonged cooling of the calf in patients with complete spinal transsections. *Physical Therapy,* 55: 251-258, 1975.

47. Travell J: Ethyl chloride spray for painful muscle spasm. *Archives of Physical Medicine and Rehabilitation,* 33:291-298, 1952.
48. Nielsen AJ: Spray and stretch for myofascial pain. *Physical Therapy,* 58(5):567-569, May 1978.
49. Lehmann JF, et al: Therapeutic heat and cold. *Clinical Orthopaedics,* 99:207-245, 1974.
50. Wolf SL, et al: Effects of specific cutaneous cold stimulus on single motor unit activity of medial gastrocnemius muscle in man. *American Journal of Physical Medicine,* 55:177-183, 1976.
51. Miglietta O: Action of cold on spasticity. *American Journal of Physical Medicine,* 52:198-205, 1973.
52. Wolf SL, Letbetter WD: Effect of skin cooling on spontaneous EMG activity in triceps surae of the decerebrate cat. *Brain Research,* 91:151-155, 1975.
53. Haines J: A survey of recent developments in cold therapy. *Physiotherapy,* 53:222-229, 1967.
54. Henriksen JD: Conduction velocity of motor nerves in normal subjects and patients with neuromuscular disorders. Rochester, MN, Mayo Graduate School of Medicine (University of Minnesota), 1956. Thesis.
55. Schafer RC: *Chiropractic Management of Sports and Recreational Injuries.* Baltimore, Williams & Wilkins, 1982, p 198.
56. Kessler RM, Hertling D: *Management of Common Musculoskeletal Disorders: Physical Therapy Principles and Methods.* New York, Harper & Row, 1982, pp 122-127.
57. Ibid.
58. Clark R, et al: Vascular reaction of the human forearm to cold. *Clinical Science,* 17:165, 1958.
59. Hocutt JE Jr: Cryotherapy. *American Family Physician,* 23(3):141-144, March 1981.
60. Basur RL, et al: A cooling method in the treatment of ankle sprains. *Practitioner,* 215:708-711, 1976.
61. Starkey JA: Treatment of ankle sprains by simultaneous use of intermittent compression and ice packs. *American Journal of Sports Medicine,* 4: 142-144, 1976.
62. Matsen FA, et al: The effect of local cooling on post-fracture swelling. *Clinical Orthopaedics,* 109: 201-206, 1975.
63. Lewis T: Observations on some normal and injurious effects of cold on the skin and underlying tissues. *British Medical Journal,* 2:795-797, 1941.
64. Yackzan L, et al: The effects of ice massage on delayed muscle soreness. *The American Journal of Sports Medicine,* 12(2):159-165, 1984.
65. Mohler HK: Cold and refrigeration. In Piersol GM, et al (eds): *The Cyclopedia of Medicine, Surgery and Specialties.* Philadelphia, F.A. Davis, 1949, vol 4, pp 350-351.
66. Sedlis A, et al: Cryotherapy in cervical disease. *New York State Journal of Medicine,* November 1981, pp 1757-1760.
67. Drez D, et al: Cryotherapy and nerve palsy. *The American Journal of Sports Medicine,* 9(4):256-257, 1981.
68. Goldberg EA, Pittman DR: Cold sensitivity syndrome. *Annals of Internal Medicine,* 50:505, 1959.
69. Shelley WB, Caro WA: Cold erythema: a new hypersensitivity syndrome. *Journal of the American Medical Association,* 180:639-642, 1962.
70. Mohler HK: Cold and refrigeration. In Piersol GM, et al (eds): *The Cyclopedia of Medicine, Surgery and Specialties.* Philadelphia, F.A. Davis, 1949, vol 4, p 350.

Chapter 7

Low Frequency Currents

This chapter reviews basic electrotherapeutic principles and describes the more common wave forms available today for therapeutic and electrodiagnostic purposes; viz, galvanic current, sine wave, faradic current, electrical muscle stimulation, combination therapies, and transcutaneous electrical nerve stimulation (TENS). High-volt therapy will be covered separately in the following chapter.

INTRODUCTION

Low frequency currents are those electrical currents that can stimulate a patient at a frequency of under 1000 pulses per second (pps). Such currents are primarily used to exercise muscles after injury, develop muscular strength and tone, trigger chemical changes, alleviate pain, and break muscle spasm.

There are two chief types of low frequency units: those utilizing (1) direct (galvanic) current or (2) alternating current. The mechanism of action is determined in part on the wave form utilized and in part on the specific frequencies utilized.

ELECTROPHYSICS

To better appreciate the subject of the therapeutic application of low frequency currents, it is well to briefly review the following basic principles that relate to electric currents.

Structure of Matter

Matter is that which has weight and occupies space. All matter is made up of one or a combination of elements. An element may be generally defined as a basic substance that cannot be split into simpler substances under normal circumstances. Two or more elements unite to form a compound, and when this union takes place, a completely new substance is formed that may have quite different properties from its constituent (parent) elements.

A molecule is the smallest particle of any substance, compound, or element that can exist alone and still retain its basic properties. An atom is the smallest particle of an element that can take part in a chemical reaction, and it is made up of protons, neutrons, and electrons. A proton is a particle having an extremely small mass and bearing a positive (+) charge. A neutron has the same mass as a proton but no electrical charge. An electron has much less mass than a proton or neutron and bears a negative (−) charge.

The particles that form an atom are arranged like a minute solar system. The protons and neutrons are held together by a strong cohesive force to form the central nucleus of an atom, and the electrons revolve in orbits at high speeds around the nucleus. Electrons, negatively charged, are held in orbit by the force of attraction exerted on them by the positively charged nucleus. The number of electrons in an atom normally equal the number of protons; thus, the atom is electrically neutral.

In most instances, one or more electrons can readily be displaced from or added to an atom. When this occurs, the atom becomes *ionized.* The process of gaining electrons produces *negative* ions, while that of losing electrons produces *positive* ions.

The Electron Theory

Every object consists of an enormous number of protons and electrons. When opposite charges balance each other, the object is said to be electrically *neutral.* However, a generator of electricity, for instance, causes a disturbance of the electrons and the object either gains or loses electrons—thereby producing an electrical charge on the object. This form of electricity is said to be at rest (static electricity).

If a connection via a conducting medium is made between two objects with opposite charges, electrons will pass from the negative object to the positive object until there is an equal number of electrons in both. This flow of electrons constitutes an *electric current.*

FRICTION AND OTHER METHODS OF PRODUCING ELECTRICITY

The simplest way of producing static electricity is by friction between two dissimilar nonconductors (ie, insulators). Insulators are substances that do not readily allow electronic charges to pass through them. When electrons pass from one dry nonconductor to another, one becomes positively charged and the other becomes negatively charged.

Energy can be neither created nor destroyed, but it can be converted from one form of energy into another. Thus, electricity must always be produced from some other form of energy. When it is produced by friction, mechanical energy is converted into electrical energy.

Besides friction, electricity can also be produced by (1) chemical action (eg, in dry cells or batteries), (2) electromagnetic induction (eg, in a dynamo), (3) heat (eg, in a thermocouple), and (4) radiant energy (eg, in a photoelectric cell). These four processes are more commonly employed for the production of electric current than are static charges.

CHARACTERISTICS OF A CHARGED BODY

When considering an electrically charged body, two basic characteristics should be kept in mind:

1. *Distribution of the charge.* The electric charge is always held on the surface of the object, and it is from the surface that excess electrons can be lost or gained.
2. *Attractiveness.* Objects with like charges repel, while objects with unlike charges attract each other.

ELECTRIC FIELDS

An electric field is the area around a charged body in which the forces resulting from the charge are apparent. When one body is placed within the electric field of another: (1) the forces of attraction or repulsion are effective; (2) the closer the objects are together, the more marked are these forces. The forces resulting from the charge are distributed along definite lines called *electrical lines of force.* The term *electrostatic induction* refers to the production of electric or magnetic properties in one object by another *without direct contact.*

ELECTRICAL POTENTIAL AND CAPACITY

The properties exhibited by a charged body result from the stored up (potential) energy of its electric charges, and its electrical condition is called its electric *potential.* The unit of potential is the *volt,* which is also referred to as the electromotive force (EMF). A volt is defined as that EMF which produces a current of 1 ampere when applied to a conductor with a resistance of 1 ohm.

The electrical *capacity* of an object is its ability to hold an electric charge. It depends on (1) the material (eg, conductors have a relatively large storage capacity), (2) the surface area (ie, the greater the surface area, the greater the capacity), and (3) capacitance. The unit of capacitance is the *farad,* which is the capacity of an object that is charged to a potential of 1 volt by 1 coulomb of electricity. A *coulomb* is that quantity of electricity transferred by a current of 1 ampere in 1 second.

Current Electricity

An electric current is actually a flow of electrons. It is produced when a difference of potential exists between the ends of a conducting pathway. Thus, the essentials for producing an electric current are (1) a difference of potential and (2) a pathway along which electrons can flow.

ELECTROMOTIVE FORCE

When two objects are in a different state of electric charge, a difference of potential is said to exist between them. A difference of potential gives rise to an electromotive force that tends to produce a movement of electrons. If a pathway is provided, the EMF produces a flow of electrons; but, if there is no pathway, the potential EMF still exists. The greater the potential difference, the greater is the EMF; and both are measured in the same unit, the volt.

RESISTANCE

A pathway through which electrons can move is called a *circuit,* and the materials from which the conductor is made offers some inherent impedance to the movement of electrons. This impedance (resistance) factor is measured in *ohms.*

The amount of electrical resistance within a circuit depends on such factors as: (1) the material of the conductor (ie, some materials allow electrons to move through them more easily than others, thus they have a low resistance); (2) the length of the pathway (the longer the pathway, the more likely the greater number of impedance factors); (3) the cross-sectional area of the conductor (the greater the diameter of the pathway, the more room there is for the electrons to pass); (4) temperature (the higher the temperature of the conductor, the greater the resistance).

In addition to ''ohmic resistance,'' which is independent of current frequency, there is also ''capacitive resistance'' that must be considered. This latter factor is determined by the capacitance of the superficial tissues, and it is lowered by increasing the frequency of alternating current. See *Figure 7.1.*

CURRENT INTENSITY MEASUREMENT

The rate of flow of electrons through a conductor is known as the intensity of current, and it is measured in *amperes;* ie, an ampere is the unit for measuring the strength of an electric current. Because most modalities used in clinical practice are of extremely small amperage, the meters on the equipment are typically designed to measure in *milliamperes.* A milliampere (ma) is one 1000th of an ampere (0.001 ampere).

OHM'S LAW

According to Ohm's law, the intensity of an electric current varies directly with the EMF and inversely with the resistance of the pathway. When I is the intensity of current (measured in amperes), E is the EMF (measured in volts), and R is the resistance (measured in ohms), the formulae for Ohm's law may be written as $E = I \times R$, $R = E/I$, or $I = E/R$.

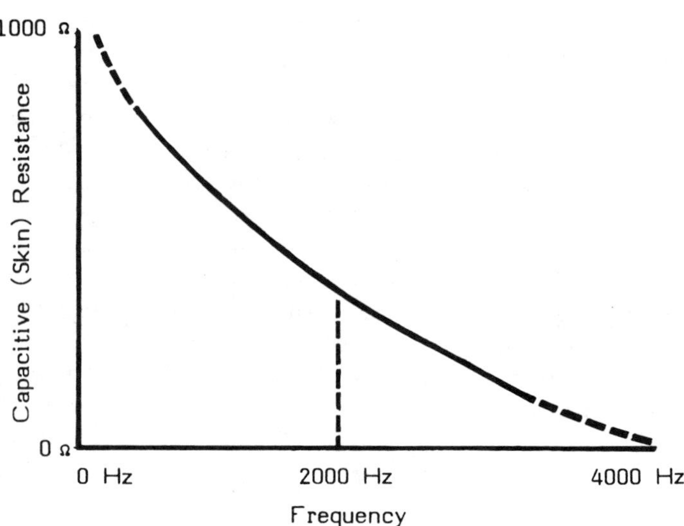

Figure 7.1. Graph showing the relationship between capacitive resistance and frequency. Note that skin resistance is inversely proportional to frequency.

DIRECT AND ALTERNATING CURRENTS

A generator of electricity may keep one end of the circuit negatively charged and the other end positively charged; then, the electrons always move in the same direction (ie, from the negative to the positive pole), and a direct current (dc) is produced. See Figure 7.2. Another type of generator (viz, a dynamo) causes a continual change in the polarity of the ends of a circuit; ie, at first one end is negative and the other positive, then the polarity is reversed. The electrons move first in one direction along the pathway and then in the other direction, producing an *alternating current* (ac). See Figure 7.3.

Each to and fro movement of electrons is one cycle, and the frequency of the current is the number of cycles per unit of time, which is usually measured in cycles per second (cps). The term *Hertz* (Hz) refers to a frequency of 1 cycle of *alternating* current per second. Typical house current is usually 60 Hz.

Magnetism

A magnet is a substance showing certain properties among which are (1) the power of attraction for certain materials and (2) the tendency (when free to rotate) to come to rest pointing in a North-South direction. Magnets may be composed of either natural or artifical substances:

1. *Natural magnets* are made of a type of iron ore with magnetic properties. The first known magnets, known as lodestones, consisted of this type of substance.
2. *Artificial magnets* are made of one or more types of material that can be magnetized such as iron and steel, and, to a lesser extent, nickel and cobalt. Soft iron readily acquires magnetic properties, but it also loses them quickly; thus, it is called a *temporary magnet.* Steel is much more difficult to magnetize, but it retains this property much longer than soft iron; thus, a steel magnet is called a *permanent magnet.* An electric current produces magnetic effects and a coil of wire carrying a current acts as an *electromagnet* while the current is flowing.

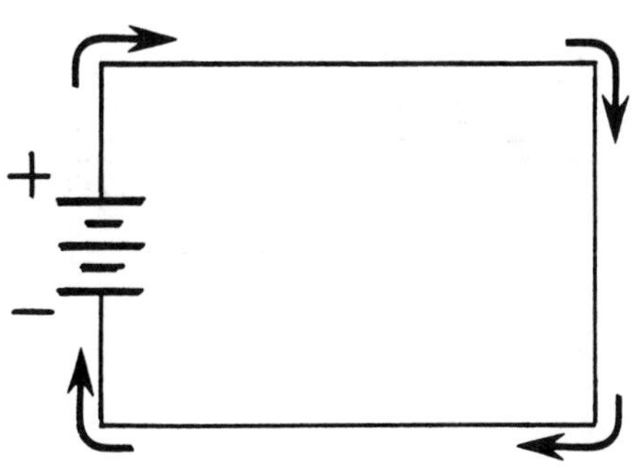

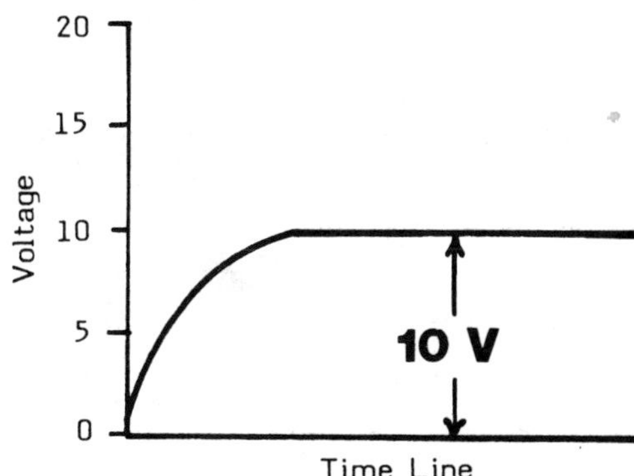

Figure 7.2. *Left,* diagram of a simple circuit within a generator. *Right,* graph of a 10-volt galvanic current.

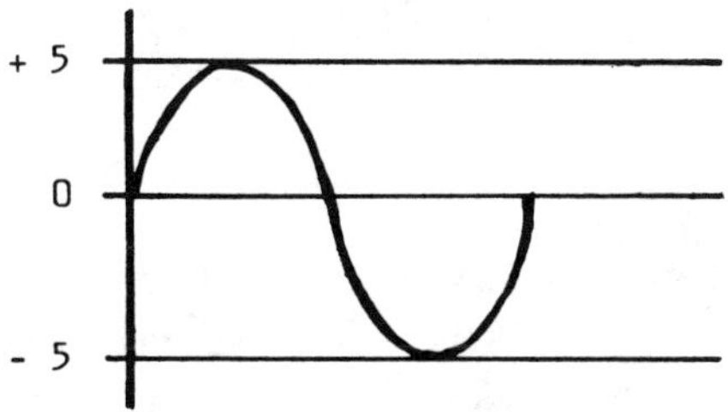

Figure 7.3. Schematic of a 5-volt alternating current wave.

MOLECULAR THEORY OF MAGNETISM

Like magnetic poles repel, and unlike poles attract. If a magnet is broken in half, each part forms a complete magnet no matter how often this process is repeated. It is therefore assumed that the individual molecules of magnetizable materials are tiny magnets. When the material is not magnetized, the molecules neutralize each other. But, when the material is magnetized, the effects augment each other.

TRANSMISSION OF PROPERTIES

Magnetization can occur by either contact or induction.

Magnetization by Contact. This process can be witnessed by stroking a piece of iron or steel with one pole of a bar magnet. The same pole is used throughout, and the strokes are always carried in the same direction. The end of the piece of material at which the stroke commences assumes the same polarity as the pole with which it was stroked. See Figure 7.4.

Magnetization by Induction. This refers to the production of magnetic properties in an object by a magnetic field; ie, direct physical contact is not made.

MAGNETIC FIELDS

The area around a magnet in which magnetic forces are apparent is known as the *magnetic field,* and these forces act along definite lines. See Figure 7.5. An electric current sets up a magnetic field around the conductor through which it is passing. When this occurs, three points should be remembered:

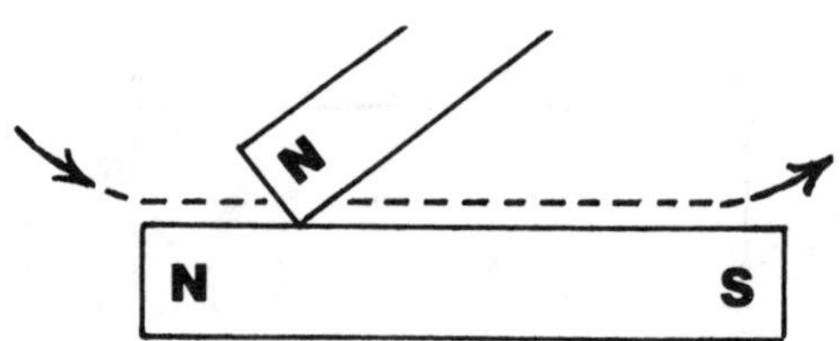

Figure 7.4. Magnetization by contact.

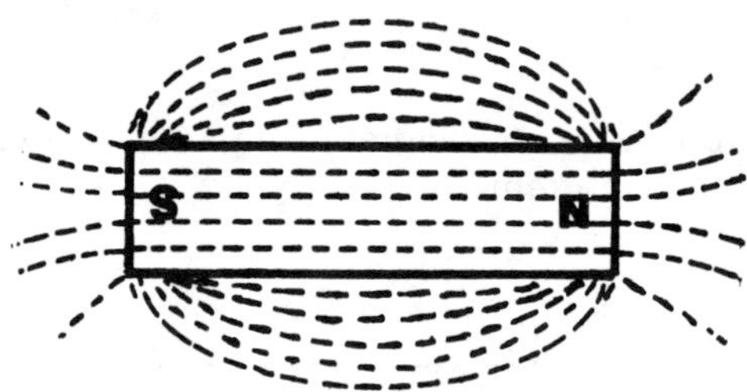

Figure 7.5. Schematic representation of a magnetic field.

1. When an electric current is passed through a coil of wire, magnetic lines of force are set up around each turn of wire and their combined effect forms a magnetic field around the whole coil.

2. Electromagnets consist of a coil of wire that is wound around a soft iron bar. When an electric current passes through the coil, a magnetic field is set up and the soft iron bar (core) becomes magnetized by induction.

3. An EMF can be induced in a closed circuit by bringing a magnet's lines of force in contact with a conductor that has been wound into the shape of a coil.

Principles of a Condenser (Capacitor)

A condenser is a device for storing an electric charge, and its operation is based on the principles of static electricity. For example, if a charged conductor is brought close to but not in contact with another conductor, its capacity is increased, especially if the other conductor has an opposite charge. When the objects approach each other, the charges concentrate on the adjacent surfaces and the electric field, which exists around any charged object, is concentrated between them. See Figure 7.6.

Placing a nonconductor (insulator) between the charged plates of a capacitor increases its capacitance. The simplest form of a capacitor consists of two metal plates that are separated by an insulator (dielectric).

General Characteristics of Currents

Most currents in use today are generally derived from commercial electric utility companies. With the exception of galvanic (direct) current, which is commonly obtained from dry cells or rectifiers, all other currents are obtained by various modifications of outlet current (ac) by means of transformers and other electromagnetic or thermionic devices.

If one keeps in mind that it is *current* that travels through a patient being treated by electrotherapy, such current is measured in amperage and receives its push via the voltage (electromotive force). As it travels through the circuit(s) of the unit or the patient's skin, its flow is impeded by resistance that is measured in ohms.

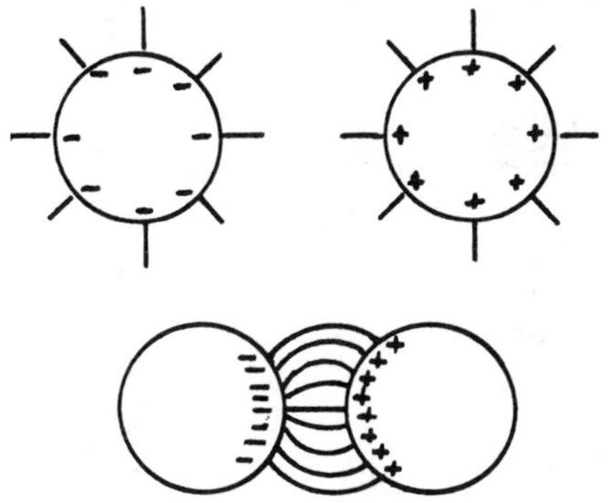

Figure 7.6. *Top,* diagram of two conductors, one charged negatively and the other positively. *Bottom,* the same conductors brought into approximation.

Many liken electric current to a simple water system. Table 7.1 lists some of the comparisons that can be made.

WAVE FORMS

In part, the physiologic effects triggered by low volt, low frequency currents are due to the wave form that is utilized. Figure 7.7 shows some of the basic wave forms in use today.

VOLTAGE

Voltage is the electromotive force that literally pushes current. It does not have a direct influence on the physiologic effects produced by electrotherapy—except that it must be sufficient to push the current into the patient (overcome inherent skin resistance). In a unit using high voltages, the intensity of stimulation (push) is regulated by turning a control knob that regulates the voltage. It should be noted that it is not voltage that burns patients; in fact, some early physical therapy modalities used an EMF exceeding 30,000 volts.

Low-volt or low-tension currents are those with a voltage of 100 or less; eg, galvanic, sine, faradic, and most TENS units. High-volt or high-tension currents have an EMF of over several hundred volts (eg, high-volt "galvanic" and high frequency currents).

CURRENT

Current is the electricity that flows through the patient, and it is measured in amperage. It is excessive current amperage that can burn a patient. Physiologically, current relates directly to the depth of penetration. The higher the peak current, the greater the depth of penetration. With high-volt units, the peak current typically reaches 2500 ma; whereas with low-volt galvanic units, the peak current ranges only from 1—30 ma.

Average current flow relates to the probability of a patient being burned. Average current per unit of time with high voltage is only about 1.5—2.0 ma; whereas with low-volt galvanic on the continuous setting, the average current equals the peak current and extreme care must be taken to avoid burning the patient. High-volt current and its physiologic effects are described further in Chapter 8.

PULSE RATE

Pulse rate refers to the number of times per second that a certain electrical flow or pulse is repeated. See Figure 7.8. It determines how frequently the patient is stimulated, and it has a direct effect on the physiologic effects that are triggered.

Table 7.1. Comparison of a Water System and Electric Current

Water System	***Electrical System***
Continuous water flow	Direct (galvanic) current
Gallons per second through pipe	Frequency (pulses per second) of current
Partial kink in the hose	Resistance (ohms)
Pipes	Wires or other conductors
Pressure	EMF or potential (voltage)
Pump	Dynamo or generator
Spurts of water	Pulsed current
Valves	Switches
Water	Current (amperage)

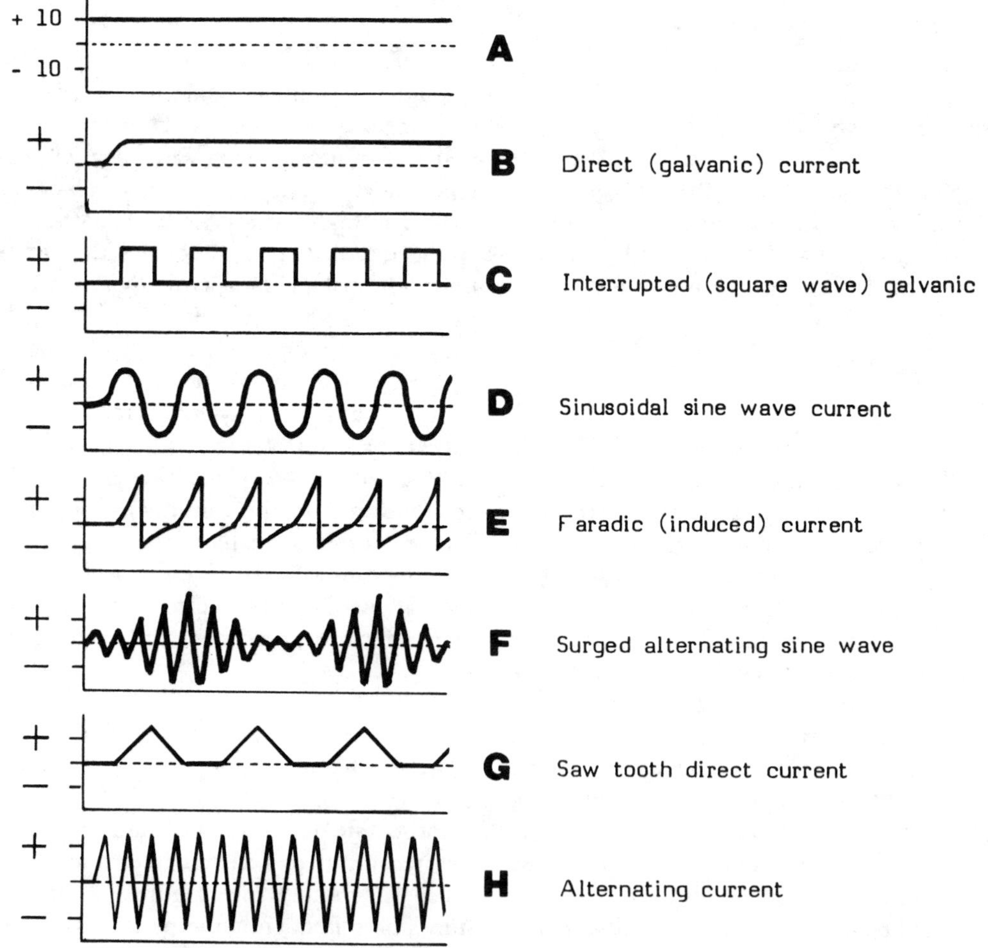

Figure 7.7. *A*, schematic of a 10-volt galvanic current. The voltage is represented by the distance above or below the zero line; *B through H*, various current wave forms.

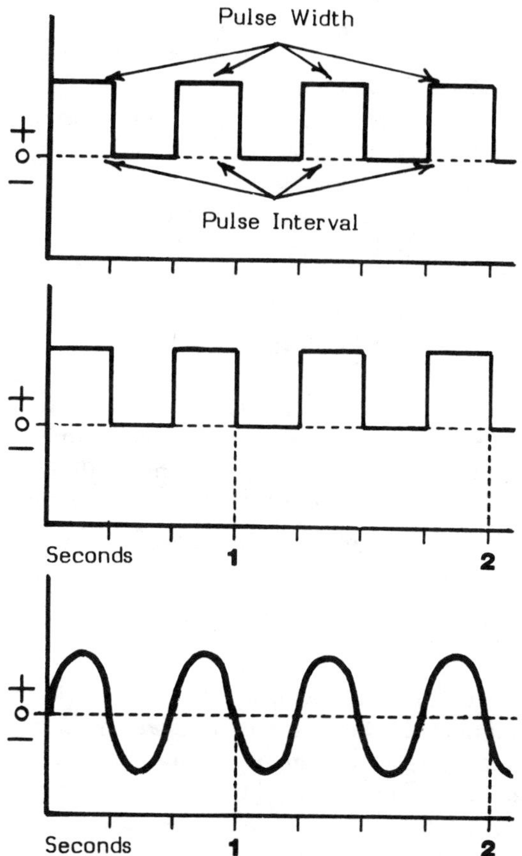

Figure 7.8. *Top diagram,* pulse width and interval. *Middle diagram,* schematic of a pulsed galvanic current where the pulse rate is 2 pps. *Bottom diagram,* in this example of sine wave, the pulse has two phases (alternations), and the pulse rate is 2 pps.

ELECTROPHYSIOLOGY OF ELECTRICAL MUSCLE STIMULATION

Low frequency currents can be direct or alternating. In this section, some basic physiology related to stimulation with alternating current or intermittent square wave galvanic current will be reviewed. Later in this chapter, the principles of stimulation related to the use of continuous galvanism will be reviewed.

Basic Considerations

RHEOBASE AND CHRONAXIE

Low frequency currents are used primarily to stimulate motor and sensory nerves. In order to trigger a muscle to contract, a current must have a minimal strength. When constant current is used to stimulate a muscle or nerve, the intensity that is just barely sufficient to trigger a threshold contraction is the *rheobase.* If the rheobase is doubled, then the *chronaxie* is the shortest time interval that is needed to produce a minimal contraction. In other words, the chronaxie is the minimal time required for excitation of a structure (eg, nerve cell) by a constant electric current of twice the threshold voltage. Thus, the rheobase is an intensity factor and the chronaxie is a factor of time. See Figure 7.9.

PHYSIOLOGIC EFFECTS OF ALTERNATING CURRENT

The basic effect on the body is muscle contraction if an alternating current of 1 Hz is applied to normal innervated muscle; ie, a single twitch-like contraction will occur. As the pulse rate (current on-off) is gradually increased, the rate of twitching correspondingly increases. As the frequency nears 20 Hz, the contractions merge until a tetanic contracture (persistent tonic spasm) results.

Therapeutic Physiology: Action Potential

DEPOLARIZATION

Every nerve cell fiber has its own voltage potential, which is about negative 80 millivolts (mv) and called the *resting voltage.* When stimulating a nerve fiber with a current (either ac or dc), the voltage potential of the nerve cell fiber increases as more voltage is added. The stimulation threshold is reached when the voltage potential reaches about negative 50 mv. When the voltage potential is increased to above negative 50 mv, the potential increases on its own to above zero, into the positive voltage area. In other words, the polarity of the nerve cell fiber changes from negative to positive (depolarization). The graph shown in Figure 7.10 depicts the change in voltage of a cell membrane when it is stimulated.

REFRACTORY PERIOD

After a nerve cell fiber undergoes depolarization, the polarity across the cell membrane drops from positive to slightly below its original resting voltage of 80 mv. The period of depolarization and return to the normal resting voltage of 80 mv is called the *relative refractory period.* Although stimulation can occur during the relative refractory period, it must be more intense than the "normal." Stimulation during the *absolute refractory period* has no effect whatsoever; ie, to create a second action potential, the nerve must be stimulated *after* the absolute and relative refractory periods of the first action potential have ended. Figure 7.11 shows various examples of current pulses.

WEDENSKY INHIBITION

When a nerve is stimulated for some time by a medium frequency current of constant amplitude (or maximum and minimum voltage value), the nerve cell responds with the maximum possible number of action potentials for that particular nerve fiber because the frequency of the stimulation is much higher than the frequency of the action potential. The maximum frequency of an action potential that lasts 10 ms is 100 times per second. When the frequency of the stimulation due to its shorter wavelength is faster than the frequency of the action potential and thus the ability of the nerve to recover, any stimulation that might occur during the absolute refractory period would have no effect. As the stimulation continues, the nerve fiber becomes partly insensitive to any stimulus. This decrease in sensitivity is called *Wedensky inhibition.*

Medium frequency currents of constant amplitude produce Wedensky inhibition and are of no therapeutic value. Such currents have little or no effect on nerves once Wedensky inhibition takes place.

Physiologic Basis of Electric Muscle Stimulation

To be effective, a muscle stimulus must have a certain intensity and duration. In addition, its final intensity must rise with adequate speed. Such a stimulus may be mechanical, electrical, thermal, or chemical in nature.

INTENSITY

Nothing will happen when a muscle is stimulated unless a certain *intensity* is obtained; eg, a certain point must be reached where a threshold level of current strength is delivered. A contraction will occur at or above this level; ie, complete contraction occurs above the threshold. This process reflects the "all-or-none law" of neuromuscular physiology. Each muscle fiber may have a different intensity threshold, however. If the true excitability level of muscle fibers is to be evaluated, the examiner must stay as close as possible to the threshold and work with the slightest contractions that are visible.

DURATION

The term *rheobase* refers to the intensity threshold for long-lasting stimuli. When the duration of muscle stimulation is decreased, a long-duration current at an intensity above the rheobase will result in a contraction. If the intensity of the current is the same, a time occurs when the stimulus abruptly loses its effectiveness. But increasing the intensity again will restore the effectiveness of the stimulus. The shorter the stimulus duration

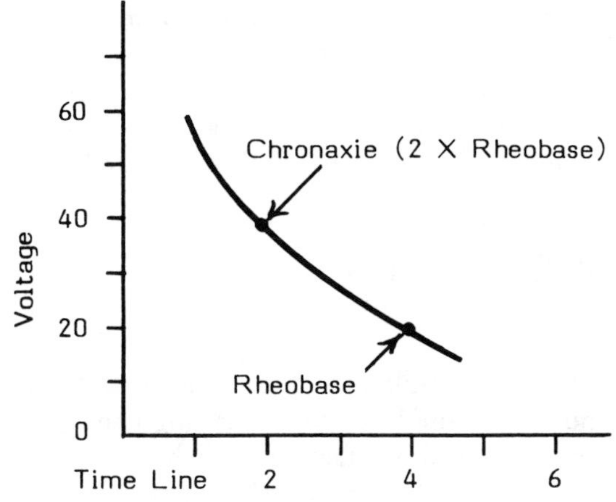

Figure 7.9. Diagram illustrating excitation time rheobase and chronaxie.

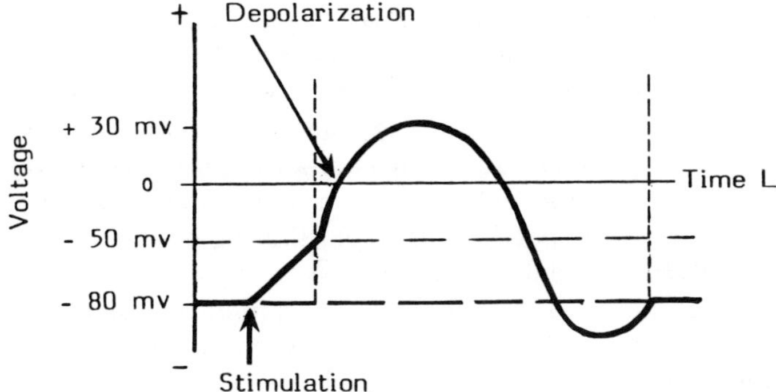

Figure 7.10. Diagram of the change in voltage when a call membrane is stimulated. This also portrays the voltage change during *any* nerve impulse.

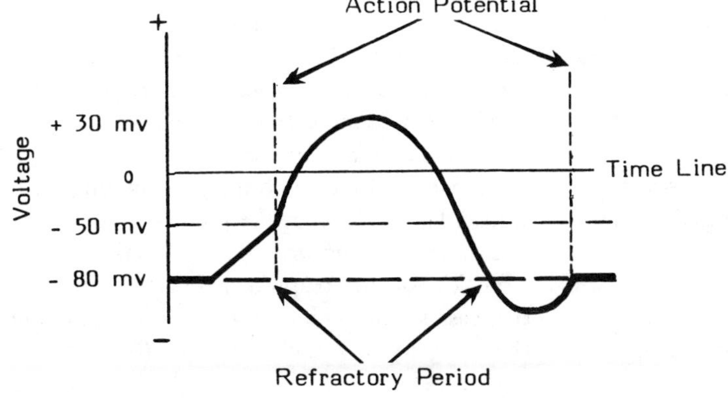

Figure 7.11. Schematic, similar to that of Figure 7.10. The arrows indicate the parameters of the *absolute refractory period* of the wave. The *relative refractory period* is that small period following, where the current falls below 80 mv.

below a certain value, the higher the stimulus intensity must be to be effective. The *utilization time* is the least time below which the decrease in efficiency of a stimulus occurs.

Utilization of Electric Muscle Stimulation

Any procedure used to stimulate muscle tissue by electricity falls under the general category of *electrical muscle stimulation.* Various types of modalities, frequencies, and wave forms can be utilized to stimulate muscle fibers electrically. Common objectives of electrical muscle stimulation include the reduction of spasticity, the exercise of weak muscles, and diagnostic evaluations to determine the state of a possible degree of degeneration. The therapy may be applied to normally innervated muscles or to muscles that are abnormally innervated or denervated.

INNERVATED MUSCLES

The reason for stimulating innervated muscles is to trigger forceful contractions, independent of the muscle(s) innervation, and these contractions should be of a tetanic nature. When innervated muscles are stimulated by way of their innervation, they will contract to stimuli of up to 2000 Hz. If the voltage is of sufficient intensity, the minimal effective duration of stimulus is about 0.02 ms. Impulses of faradic current of 1 ms readily trigger contractions in innervated muscle.

It has been found that even twitch contractions are of therapeutic value when one or more of the following goals are desired:

1. To relax "spastic" muscle tissue.
2. To reduce the spasticity of spastic paralysis; eg, following cranial or spinal cord injury.
3. To prevent disuse atrophy in muscle and to re-educate muscle.
4. To aid respiration by stimulating the abdominal wall and diaphragm.
5. To prevent phlebothrombosis by stimulating the calf muscles (eg, during the immediate postoperative period).

It should be noted that the above guidelines apply only to the application of low frequency currents on normally innervated muscle.

INDIVIDUAL MOTOR POINT STIMULATION TECHNIQUE

When stimulation of an individual motor point is desired, a stimulus strong enough to bring about a contraction must be applied to the motor point of the selected muscle or to a succession of involved motor points. A typical technique involves (1) placing a moist 2 × 4-inch dispersive pad on a site where there are no underlying muscle bellies, and (2) placing the active pad (1-inch or less in diameter) in the middle of the selected muscle belly where the muscle's motor point is located. Keep in mind that, once tissue resistance is overcome, an impulse that would not produce a contraction initially may then respond. Thus, rapid shifting of an electrode should be avoided.

The quantity of contractions to be induced per treatment depends on the type of response obtained and the degree of weakness present. For example, the number may vary from 3 to 10 in complete paralysis to possibly a dozen or more when simple weakness is present. Each of the first three contractions should be somewhat progressively stronger than the preceding one; after this, the contractions should be maintained at about the same strength. It is important to keep in mind that *once a contraction is achieved, sufficient relaxation must be obtained before the next impulse is initiated.*

Currents. Direct (galvanic), tetanizing, and sinusoidal currents are frequently used:

1. *Direct current.* The "make" and "break" of interrupted galvanic current is the easiest method to use for (a) evaluating the integrity of muscle tissue or (b) stimulating muscle tissue when single contractions are desired. See Figure 7.12. The negative

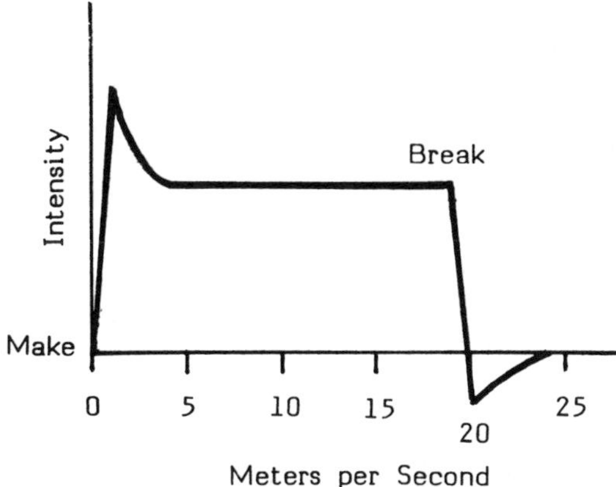

Figure 7.12. A typical "make" and "break" pattern when normal muscle tissue is stimulated by direct current. Note that the "make" response occurs between 0—3 ms and the less strong "break" occurs at 20—23 ms.

(−) pole is more stimulating under normal circumstances. Regardless of its diagnostic value, however, galvanic current is not the most effective method to use therapeutically as compared to other techniques.

2. *Tetanizing current.* A tetanizing current should be used when the objective is to give a normally innervated muscle passive exercise. Faradic current with an impulse frequency between 80 and 100 Hz is ideal for this purpose. Impulse duration is not of great significance.

3. *Sinusoidal current.* Refer to Figure 7.7. A frequency of 60 Hz is commonly used to produce tetany with a sine wave. Unfortunately, this technic is not tolerated well by most patients because of its strong sensory effects.

Bipolar Stimulation. Bipolar stimulation results from placing active electrodes (pads) of equal size at opposite sides of a selected muscle belly. This technique is commonly used when a muscle is so weak that, when monopolar stimulation is applied, the current strength necessary for a palpable response causes extremely strong contractions in neighboring muscles. This broad effect makes it impossible to evaluate the response of a specific muscle. Bipolar stimulation is typically indicated in radial nerve palsy or when stimulating the anterior muscles of the leg.

Muscle Group Stimulation. In normally innervated muscle, the stimulation of large groups of muscles is commonly used for the relief of muscle pain or spasm. The technique is also used occasionally for its psychologic effects.

DENERVATED MUSCLES

All normal reactions are slowed in a denervated muscle; however, an interrupted galvanic current can be used to obtain contractions. Even if just a flicker of tendon tension of a paralyzed muscle is achieved, it is clinically beneficial. It is common to find that the motor point has been displaced distally toward the tendon in denervated muscle.

Denervated muscles should be stimulated at a frequency of 0.5—40 Hz. The general guideline is: the longer the duration of denervation, the lower the frequency of stimulation. The aim is to trigger contractions that are as strong as possible so that optimal muscle tone will be maintained.

In comparison to an innervated muscle, a denervated muscle is slower to respond in all respects. See Figure 7.13. Thus, the operator should set a longer duration of stimulation, a higher current strength, and a lower frequency to trigger a contraction. Although the reaction threshold is sometimes lower than that of normal muscle in the early stages of nerve denervation, it will rise in the later stages.

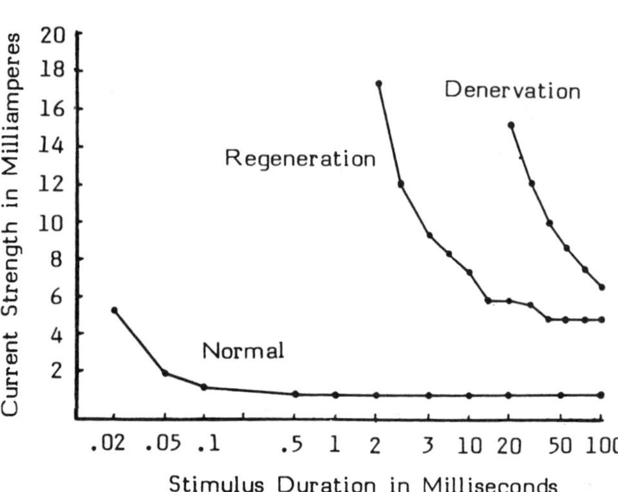

Figure 7.13. Graph showing the relationship between the strength and duration of a minimally effective stimulus for normal, regenerating (neurotized), and denervated muscle.

The major reasons for stimulating denervated muscle tissue are: (1) to enhance the circulation to and nutrition of affected muscle fibers; (2) to retard the development of fascicular agglutination and sclerosis of areolar tissue; and (3) to inhibit the progression of disuse atrophy. In addition, contractions greatly assist in correcting arteriovenous and lymphatic stasis within muscle tissue.

The recommended parameters for stimulating denervated muscle are shown in Table 7.2.

In summary, the best current for stimulating a denervated muscle is a tetanizing current that has a frequency of 5—10 pulses per second (pps), using a low-volt generator that produces a square wave. Denervated muscles respond best to a stimulus that lasts 1/1000 of a second, thereby reducing the sinusoidal frequency to 25 cycles per second (cps). Thus, this will be beneficial to paretic muscles.

Rationale of Electric Muscle Exercise

The primary reasons for applying electrical stimulation to muscle tissue are given below.

WEAKNESS OF INNERVATED MUSCLE

The stimulation of innervated muscle tissue is indicated when muscles are atonic or wasted from any cause and when voluntary exercise is not feasible. Such muscle contractions help to maintain an adequate circulation of blood and lymph of the part and lessen the formation of adhesions.[1]

MUSCLE SPASM

Muscle stimulation is an excellent therapy in situations of muscle spasticity if the spasm is *not* a protective (antalgic) spasm following trauma (eg, in fractures or acute arthritis). Such stimulation is also beneficial in fibrositis or myositis when a tetanizing current is used.

DYSFUNCTION OF DENERVATED MUSCLE

Muscle tissue supplied by an injured nerve does not contract voluntarily; thus, it tends to histologically regress into noncontractile

Table 7.2. Parameters for Stimulating Denervated Muscle

Type of Current	Direct current, rectangular waves, or sinusoidal current (if not too high in frequency). The duration of individual effective impulses for fully denervated muscle should be between 50 and 100 ms. The pulse in faradic current has a duration of only 1 ms and, for this reason, faradic current is not effective.
Strength of contraction	Try to trigger 25—50 strong contractions each patient visit because denervated muscles fatigue rapidly. It is best if a strong contraction is achieved against resistance.
Frequency of impulse	5—10 Hz for fully denervated muscle and 20 Hz during the beginning of regeneration. For normal muscle, a tetanic frequency is usually set at 50 Hz.
Schedule of treatment	3—4 treatments daily to retard atrophy is ideal. Home exercises are often the only other alternative. The application of therapeutic heat *may* also be beneficial.
Duration of treatment	Until the patient is able to produce reasonably good active contractions of the involved muscle(s).

connective tissue. For this reason, the physician must provide these muscles with nutrition and enable them to maintain their contractility through proper therapy.

Electrical Exercise. The rate of atrophy development may be slowed by electrical exercise. It will also improve tissue circulation, thus cellular nutrition will benefit. In order to be effective, the stimulating current must produce a sustained contraction of the denervated muscle, and it should be sufficient enough to produce a strong mechanical contraction—possibly against resistance. For optimal effect, 10 minutes of stimulation twice a day is required for each denervated muscle.

Signs of Overstimulation of Muscle Tissue

During muscle stimulation, careful monitoring of patient reactions is necessary to assure that adverse signs do not appear. The major signs of overstimulation include:

1. A slowed rate of contraction and relaxation.
2. A well-marked tremor during contraction.
3. Stiffness and pain instead of a prolonged feeling of comfort after the treatment is terminated.

BASIC CONSIDERATIONS WHEN UTILIZING LOW FREQUENCY STIMULATION

The general considerations, indications, and contraindications to acknowledge when using low frequency stimulation are described below.

Precautions Prior to Therapy

1. Initially, check skin sensation and for signs of possible diminished sensitivity. Constant monitoring, however, is not usually

necessary. Patients with debilitating diseases will require special monitoring and will not be able to tolerate a high intensity or a long duration of treatment.

2. Check to see that the unit is functioning properly.

3. Explain the therapy to the patient.

General Indications and Contraindications

See Tables 7.3 and 7.4.[2,3,4]

TECHNIQUES OF ELECTRICAL STIMULATION

The application of electrical stimulation is either monopolar or bipolar:

1. *Monopolar.* Two pads are used, with one of them being designated as the active pad. This technique is commonly used for iontophoresis, to trigger chemical changes in tissues by galvanism, and to exercise small muscle groups.

2. *Bipolar.* From two to four pads are used for stimulating large muscles or multiple groups of small muscles.

Rules of Application

1. Thoroughly moisten the sponge electrodes before use. Pain arising during application is usually due to uneven moisture at the electrode/skin interface.

2. Flexible electrodes mold more closely to the skin and are superior in performance to the older type of inflexible electrodes. Good electrode-patient contact is essential to ensure that the patient derives the maximum effect from the treatment.

3. Conducting solutions such as salt water improve the therapeutic results.

4. When stimulating innervated muscle, the active electrode should be placed over the motor point of the muscle.

5. Since denervated muscle does not have a functional motor point, the active electrode should be placed along the muscle belly or wherever the best response is achieved. Two electrodes of equal size may be placed at opposite ends of a muscle so that the current will stimulate along the muscle fibers and affect all parts of the muscle.

In the following sections, various types of low frequency currents will be described and some of the basic considerations of their effects will be reviewed.

Sinusoidal Current

Sinusoidal current is one type of alternating current. It elicits no polarity. By definition, it is a low voltage, low milliamperage, low frequency, alternating biphasic symmetrical current. Basically, it is utilized in four forms: (1) a continuous alternating current that varies from 1 to 2000 Hz; (2) a slow pulsating (variable) form; (3) a surged sinusoidal current; and (4) a tetanizing sinusoidal current. Refer to Figure 7.7.

With sinusoidal stimulation, the wave gradually increases from zero voltage on up to the maximum intensity set, then it recedes gradually through the zero point until it reaches a negative point that is equal to the previous maximum rise. It then returns to zero again, thus completing one cycle. Sinusoidal stimulation is a repetition of these cycles, and the alternations of the cycles are such that each cycle contains an equal amount of positive and negative charges. A sinusoidal current creates a muscular contraction with each impulse.[5,6,7]

The following points describe the usual variations made and settings used with sine wave therapy:

1. *Rapid sine.* Alternations of 40—80 Hz, with impulses that last about 1/100th of a second.

2. *Slow sine.* Alternations of 5—30 Hz, with single impulses lasting about 1/50th of a second.

3. *Surged sine.* The intensity of the current is gradually increased to a maximum value and then slowly decreased. This tech-

Table 7.3. Basic Indications and Contraindications of Low Frequency Therapy

GENERAL INDICATIONS		
Adhesions	Muscle spasm	Passive exercise
Circulatory stasis	Muscular atrophy	Restricted joint motion
Edema	Pain	Trigger points
GENERAL CONTRAINDICATIONS		
Areas of diminished sensation (extreme caution)	Over low back or abdomen during pregnancy	Pacemaker
Metallic implants	Over open wounds	Transcerebral applications
Metastatic carcinoma	Over or through heart	

Table 7.4. Unit Settings with and Clinical Indications of Low Frequency Therapy

Setting	*Indications/Comments*
Continuous (pulsed)*	Chemical changes; to decrease edema and/or congestion.
Tetanizing	To relieve pain (70—130 Hz) or to break muscle spasm.
Surge	To exercise muscles; build strength and tone in muscles, tendons, and ligaments.
Reciprocal	To exercise joints by alternately stimulating agonist and antagonist muscles.
Automatic	Usually provides 1 minute each of tetanizing, surge, and pulsed cycles, and then repeats.

*The continuous setting on high-volt units relates to the electrodes, not the type of wave form produced. Please refer to the chapter on high-volt therapy.

nique is primarily used to develop strength and tone in muscles, tendons, and ligaments.

4. *Tetanizing sine.* This setting is primarily effective in breaking muscle spasm and relieving the associated pain.

When sinusoidal stimulation is applied to normally innervated muscles, the muscles contract and relax with each cycle. Each completed cycle of sinusoidal current passes through four phases: (1) anode opening, (2) cathode closing, (3) cathode opening, and (4) anode closing.

Faradic or Induced Current

True faradic current, which is a second type of alternating current, is not often used today. Basically, a faradic current is a biphasic asymmetrical pulse; ie, a low frequency alternating current with pulses in two directions, with one immediately following the other. One pulse is of high intensity and short duration and the other (following) pulse is of low intensity and long duration. Refer to Figure 7.7. Since the total amount of electricity is the same in either direction, there are no polarity effects.

When a faradic stimulus is used either to the motor point of a muscle or anywhere along its nerve, the intervals between current flow are too short to allow for relaxation of the muscle tissue. Thus, a continuous contraction is produced. Contractions with faradic current occur at the breaks that are set, ranging up to 100 per second. What happens, essentially, is that muscles with normal innervation have no time to relax and a smooth tetany is produced.

When faradic current is used, a flow of current for just 1/1000th of a second is sufficient to trigger a contraction in innervated muscles but not in paralyzed muscles. This is because a paralyzed muscle still possesses the ability to respond to sufficiently long stimuli. As a result of its lack of innervation, paralyzed muscle will not respond to the stimuli of current. This fact forms the basis for electrodiagnostic applications. Thus, faradic current has two primary functions: (1) to stimulate contractions in muscles that have normal innervation but poor tonicity and (2) to test muscles for reaction of degeneration.

Galvanic Current

When galvanic current was referred to years ago, it was described as a current that was characterized by a continuous, waveless flow of unidirectional electricity of low voltage. Refer to Figure 7.7.

The emphasis on high-volt stimulators, which are in common use today, has confused some as to the use and relationship between low-volt and high-volt units. However, we believe that there is only one type of therapeutic galvanism; ie, direct, unidirectional, waveless, low-volt galvanic current. Since high-volt stimulators do not strictly match this classical definition and, more importantly, because the action of high-volt units on the body is so much different, we will describe their use in a separate chapter (Chapter 8) and classify them as a separate type of modality.

HISTORICAL PERSPECTIVE

Classically, direct (galvanic) current was the first known form of current flow. Its use dates back to 1789 when Professor Galvani, at the University of Bologna, noticed that whenever a spark jumped between the electrodes of a friction machine, a frog's leg placed on a metal plate near the spark would suddenly twitch. Galvani hypothesized that this reaction was due to the fact that the frog's body was a source of electricity and that the metal plate, in some way, served to discharge the flow of electricity. Twenty years later, Volta, another Italian scientist, proved that Galvani's experiment represented a flow of electricity that did not arise from the animal but arose from a current produced at the contact of two dissimilar metals. In other words, it was due to the sudden "make" of a flow of electricity. Volta then constructed the first electric cell, using these observed principles. The cell was comprised of alternate discs of copper and zinc, separated from one another by porous discs made of paper that were soaked in vinegar.

Galvanism as a therapeutic procedure came into popular use in the late 1800s, when it was chiefly utilized to observe and evaluate the functions of nerves and muscles. It was at this time that the basic laws of electrophysiology were firmly established by such famous names as Faraday, d'Arsonval, Duchenne, DuBois-Reymond, Erb, Kellogg, and Telsa.

Galvanism has since been used throughout the health care fields. During the first half of this century, the work of the pioneers was refined and expanded by Clark, deKraft, Nagelschnidt, Schereschewsky, Schliephake, Tisdale, Whitney, Zeynek, etc, into the areas of high frequency currents, microwaves, shortwave diathermy, and surgical galvanism.

PHYSICS OF LOW VOLT GALVANISM

It has been previously explained that low-volt galvanism is defined as a direct flow of electrons that is unidirectional and uninterrupted. The terms direct current and galvanic current are synonymous. Direct currents are low frequency currents; ie, they have a rate of oscillation that is less than 1000 per second. This direct flow of electrons can be generated from several different sources such as batteries, cells, generators, induction coils, metallic rectifiers, motors, and vacuum or valve tube rectifiers.

Cells and Batteries: Chemical. Two common, yet relatively expensive, methods for generating electricity are by means of cells and batteries:

1. *Wet cells.* The chemical production of electric current is effected by the freeing of electrons when metals are allowed to go into solution. For example, if plates of zinc and copper, which are neutral in their normal solid state, are immersed into a dilute solution of sulfuric acid and joined by wires that are outside of the solution, a milliammeter that is connected in-line will register electron flow from the zinc plate to the copper plate through the sulfuric acid medium. In such a solution, positive ions are freed from the zinc plate (making that plate negative). These positive zinc ions repel the positive ions of hydrogen toward the copper plate, because like charges repel. These hydrogen ions are thereafter found on the copper plate as free hydrogen molecules. In this manner, the copper plate becomes positively charged while the zinc plate becomes negatively charged.[8] In other words, a "wet" galvanic cell may be defined as two metals such as copper and zinc that have been immersed into an electrolytic solution, where current emits from the positive terminal (the anode) and the negative terminal (the cathode) is the binding pole to which the current returns.

It should be emphasized that the current always flows from the positively charged copper anode to the negatively charged zinc cathode. Conversely, the electrons themselves always flow from the cathode to the anode. Thus, in summary, current flows from the anode to the cathode, while electrons flow from the cathode (−) to the anode (+).

See Figure 7.14. Because of their relatively large size and weight and the effected polarization, wet cells are no longer in popular use clinically. They have commonly been replaced by smaller, lighter dry cells.

2. *Dry cells.* Dry cells essentially consist of a zinc container lined with thin blotting paper, which serves as the negative electrode, and a centrally located carbon rod, which serves as the positive electrode. A paste made up of manganese dioxide, zinc chloride, ammonium chloride, water, and granulated carbon fills the space between the electrodes: the zinc shell and the carbon rod. Such an arrangement prevents polarization and forms an electric cell that is relatively light in weight and small in size.

The small, round dry cell batteries commonly used today have a power of 1.5 volts. Because the average resistance offered by the

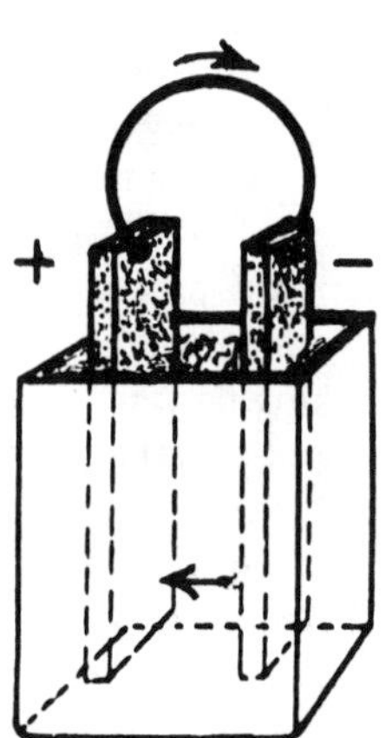

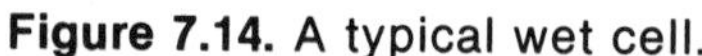

Figure 7.14. A typical wet cell.

human body is 1000 ohms, one dry cell will create in the vicinity of 0.0015 amperes (1.5 ma) of current in a patient. See Figure 7.15.

Generators. The early studies of Faraday made several ways possible to economically convert mechanical energy into electrical energy by means of a generator. An electric generator (dynamo) may be defined as an apparatus that converts mechanical energy into electric power. See Figure 7.16. It is usually made of the following components: a magnetic field created by electromagnets, an armature consisting of insulated wires coiled around a soft iron core, metallic brushes that serve as a collecting mechanism, copper slip rings (in ac generators) that rotate with the armature or a split-ring commutator (in dc generators), and an activating power source to keep the magnets or armature moving.

Motors. An electric motor is the exact reverse of a generator, for a motor converts electrical energy into mechanical energy. Like a generator, however, it essentially consists of an armature rotating within a magnetic field. It is the rotating armature that creates the mechanical energy that is transferred, usually via gears or a pulley (belt). Motors can be built to operate on either direct or alternating current.

Motor Generators. Motor generators consist of a motor and a dynamo. The motor (either ac or dc) drives the dynamo, which, in turn, furnishes a galvanic current and a number of low frequency currents.

Metallic Rectifiers. Rectifiers are devices (rotary converters) that change alternating current into unidirectional current by allowing an appreciable flow of current in one direction only. Metallic rectifiers, also called *semiconductor diodes,* conduct electricity if there is a charge present.

Vacuum or Valve Tube Rectifiers. Vacuum tube or valve tube rectifiers consist of thermionic tubes that function by changing an alternating current into a smooth direct current. See Figure 7.17. There are virtually hundreds of types of vacuum tubes in use today, having from two to seven electrodes. The tubes in common use employ an indirectly heated cathode as the source of the thermal ("boiled off") electrons.

Induction Coils. Induction coils produce a large induced or faradic current flow from a direct current source. Because early faradic coils delivered an alternating current of only a brief duration, they were frequently used as tools in the differential diagnosis of lower motor neuron diseases.

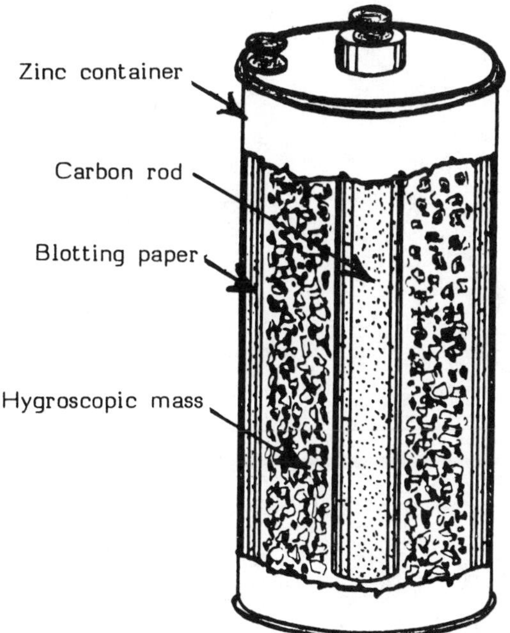

Figure 7.15. A typical dry cell.

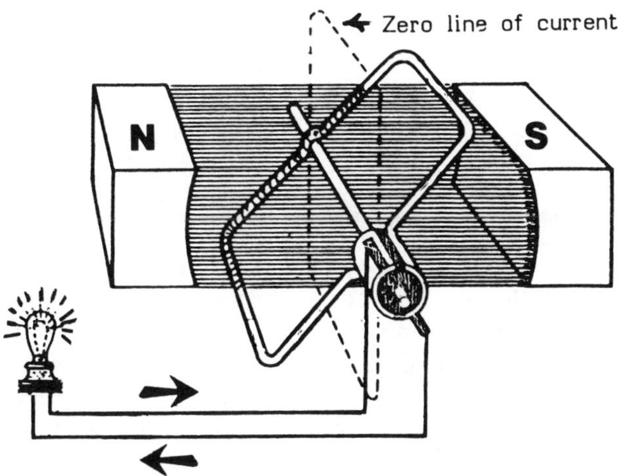

Figure 7.16. Schematic of a simple dynamo, where a wire loop rotates within a magnetic field to light an incandescent bulb.

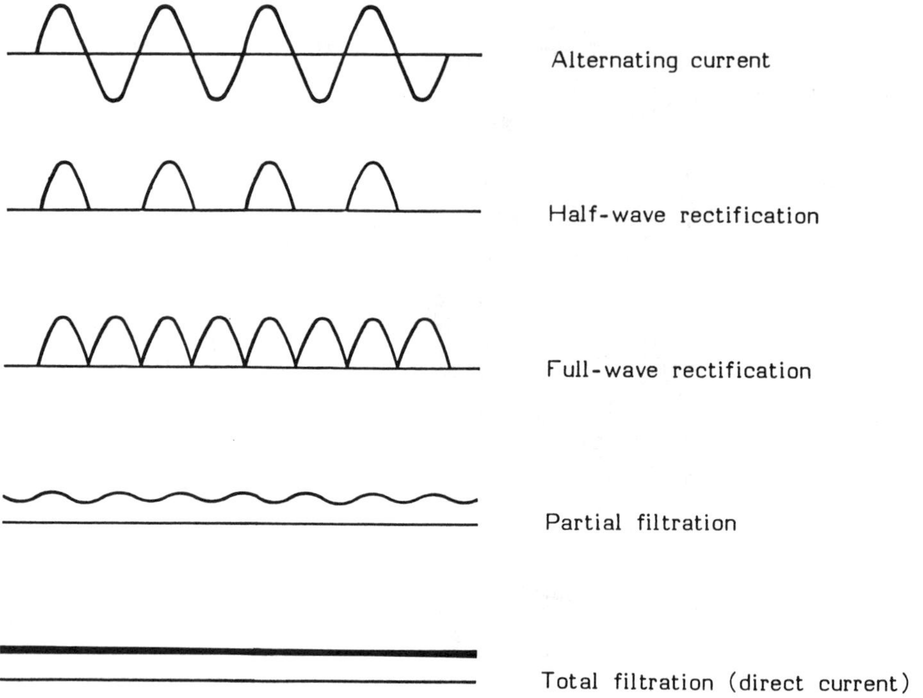

Figure 7.17. Diagrams showing how alternating current is transformed through various steps, from top to bottom, into direct current by a rectifier.

THE PHYSIOLOGIC EFFECTS OF LOW VOLT GALVANISM

The primary physical actions of low-volt galvanic stimulation are: (1) electrochemical effects and (2) electrokinetic effects. These actions produce or trigger certain physiologic changes, based on their influences on body tissues. These changes, which are described below, consist of changes in polarity, thermal changes, pain control effects, and miscellaneous effects.

Polarity. The primary action of galvanic current on body tissues is chemical, and these chemical actions trigger certain physiologic alterations. From an electrobiologic viewpoint, the human body can be crudely likened to a container of dilute salt water. When NaCl molecules dissolve in water, they dissociate into sodium ions that bear a positive charge and chloride ions that carry a negative charge. When a direct current is passed through body tissues (or any salt solution), the positive sodium ions move toward the negative pole (cathode) and the negative chlorine ions move toward the positive pole (anode). This process is known as ion transfer or, more appropriately, *iontophoresis.*

In a classic experiment, the student takes a beaker filled with salt water and passes a low-volt galvanic current through it. The hydrogen and sodium ions migrate to the cathode and the oxygen and chlorine ions migrate to the anode. Due to electrical ionization, hydrogen chloride collects at the positive pole and sodium chloride forms at the negative pole. Thus, it can be said that the primary effect of ion transfer by galvanic current is an acid reaction at the positive pole and an alkaline reaction at the negative pole.

These actions at the respective poles are referred to as *polar effects* because they occur only at the electrodes (poles).

Polarity can be checked by using one or more of three different testing procedures:

1. *The water bubble test.* A pinch of salt is added to a beaker of water, and electrodes from a galvanic unit are placed within the beaker on opposite sides. After the flow of current begins, the student should observe any bubble formation on the electrodes. Twice as many bubbles will appear at the negative pole (the cathode) due to the formation of hydrogen gas (free hydrogen molecules). Oxygen produces about half as many bubbles at the positive pole (the anode).

2. *The litmus paper test.* The initially blue paper will turn red when placed near the positive pole and the initially pink paper will turn blue when held near the negative pole.

3. *The phenolphthalein test.* A strip of blotting paper is moistened with a dilute solution of phenolphthalein, and the two electrodes of a galvanic unit are touched at opposite ends of the strip. After the current is turned on, a red dot will appear where the negative pole touches the damp blotter.

Two other associated electrobiologic reactions are worthy of consideration; ie, cataphoresis and electro-osmosis.

1. *Cataphoresis.* In addition to the polar effects of galvanic current caused by ion transfer, other nondissociated colloid molecules move under the influence of the direct current toward the cathode. This process is known as *cataphoresis,* which involves the movement of fat globules, blood cells, bacteria, albumin, starch particles, and any other single cells that carry an electrical charge due to their absorption of ions.

2. *Electro-osmosis.* Another reaction that occurs as a result of direct current is a shifting of the water content of tissues through membrane structures. This process is called *electro-osmosis.*

The major physiochemical and physiologic effects of direct current are shown in Table 7.5. Although the primary effects of galvanic current are from polar changes, other physiologic effects (eg, thermal, analgesic) may occur independent of polarity. Both the anode and the cathode can trigger some vasomotor stimulation.

Thermal Changes. Both the anode and the cathode may trigger a modest amount of increase in skin temperature. It should be pointed out, however, that such effects are minimal and would not in themselves warrant the use of galvanic current to therapeutically produce superficial heat.

Pain Control. The positive pole is used to treat acute pain because the acid reaction acts as a sedative on the alkaline tissues often seen in acute pain. However, the negative pole is used as the active electrode in situations of chronic pain. The negative electrode tends to soften, relax, and liquefy indurated, taut, and mineralized soft tissues—signs so often associated with tissues emitting chronic pain.

In addition to the polar effects that relate to pain, it has been well established that galvanic current stimulates some enkephalin production for pain control, whether a positive or negative polarity is used. Clinical studies indicate, however, that spiked currents such as those utilized in high-volt and TENS units are far more efficient in this regard than are waveless unidirectional currents.

Miscellaneous Effects. Galvanic currents may be delivered to the patient in a continuous flow, a pulsed current, or a tetanizing setting. Accordingly, galvanic stimulation can be used to move fluids, exercise muscles, or relax spasticity. A typical unit for applying galvanic current is shown in Figure 7.18.

STIMULATION VIA DIRECT CURRENT

When galvanic current is suddenly started or interrupted (referred to as "make" or "break" points) in muscle or nerve tissues, a muscular contraction or some phenomenon

Table 7.5. Major Physiochemical and Physiologic Effects of Direct Current

Type of Effect	*Positive Pole (Anode*	*Negative Pole (Cathode)*
Physiochemical	Attracts acids	Attracts alkaloids (bases)
	Repels alkaloids	Repels acids
	Attracts oxygen	Attracts hydrogen
	Corrodes metals by oxidation	Does not corrode metals
Physiologic	Hardens scar tissue	Softens tissues
	Decreases nerve irritability	Increases nerve irritability
	Dehydrates tissue	Congests tissues
	Produces vasoconstriction	Produces vasodilatation
	Retards bleeding	Enhances bleeding
	Produces ischemia	Produces hyperemia
	Tends to be analgesic	Tends to increase pain at low intensities
	Germicidal effect	

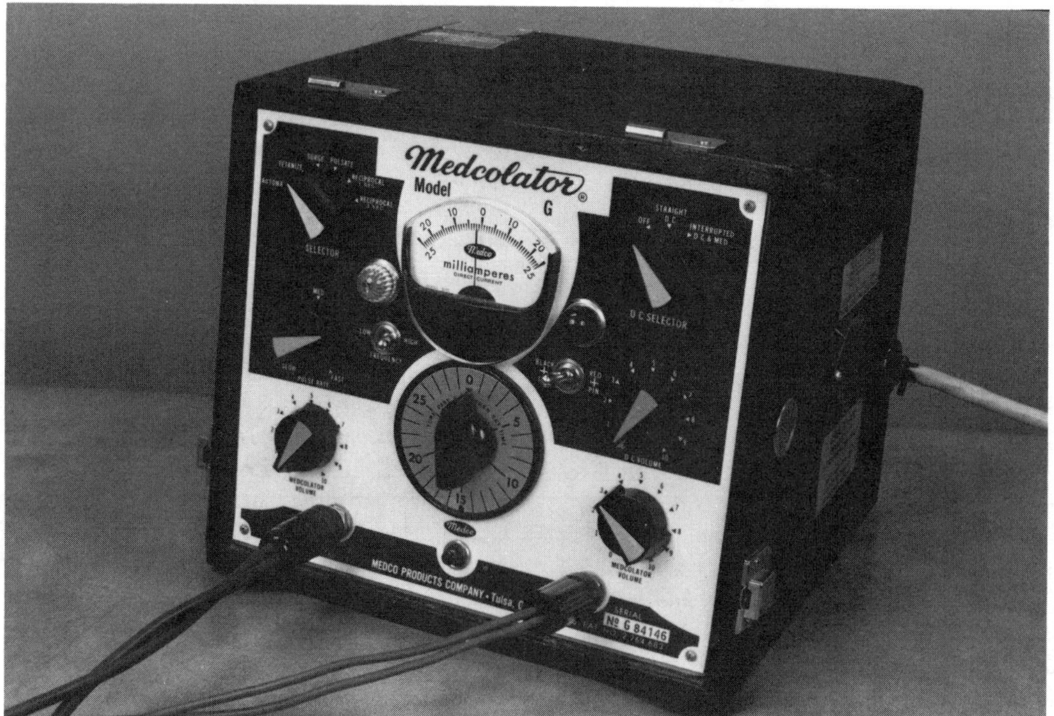

Figure 7.18. A Medcolator galvanic therapy unit.

of a sensory character (eg, a slight shock or tingling sensation) will be produced. Refer to Figure 7.12. This reaction first occurs under the negative electrode and then, as current strength is increased, it also manifests under the positive electrode.

To fully appreciate what occurs when stimulation is made by direct current, the electrobiologic postulates of DuBois-Reymond, Nernst, and Pfluger are summarized below.[9]

DuBois-Reymond's Law. The intensity of the stimulus and the following muscular contraction are directly proportional to the magnitude and change in current strength, or, in the presence of the same current strength, the intensity is proportional to the rate of fluctuation.

Nernst's Postulate. Muscle or nerve stimulation is triggered by changes in ionic concentration at the cell membrane. Ions migrate at different velocities through the two media of the body (interstitial fluid and cellular protoplasm) in which they are soluble, according to the strength and duration of the current applied.

Pfluger's Law. The closing (''make'') of a galvanic current on a nerve triggers an increase in irritability at the negative pole, called *catelectrotonus,* and a decrease in nerve irritability at the positive pole, called *analectrotonus.*

It is presently thought that the initial reaction at the cathode (eg, contraction) is primarily due to the excessive concentration of hydrogen because hydrogen ions have a much higher velocity as compared to other ions, according to Nernst's postulate. Thus, contractions at the cathode are greater than at the anode. That is, cathode closing current (CCC) is greater than anode closing current (ACC); but on opening the circuit, the contraction at the anode (AOC) is greater than at the cathode (COC).

COMMON CLINICAL APPLICATIONS

Great care should be taken in the application of low-volt galvanic to avoid burning the patient. The practitioner should be certain that a delegated therapist completely understands the parameters for patient care when the therapy is applied.

Preparation. Two electrodes are usually used in galvanic treatments, and the therapy is delivered via moistened sponges that cover bare metal electrodes. See Figure 7.19. These sponges (usually 3 or 4 square inches in size) must be thoroughly moistened or uneven stimulation will occur that might cause a burn. In fact, the most common cause for a patient feeling a painful or burning sensation is failure to completely soak the sponges prior to application—soaked to the point where they will not float. Conductivity during treatment can be improved when the sponges are soaked in a warm saline solution. After soaking the electrodes, they should be firmly squeezed so that they will not drip water. If the sponges were previously used for ion transfer, special care must be taken to remove all chemical residue by several thorough rinsings.

Technique. The following general rules apply to any treatment with galvanic current:

1. The maximum current intensity is 1 ma for every square inch of active electrode or to patient tolerance, whichever comes first. Thus, if the active electrode size is 3 × 3 inches, the *maximum* intensity is 9 ma. If a 4 × 4-inch pad is used, the maximum intensity is 16 ma. Even if a patient does not feel the current at 9 ma when a 3 × 3-inch pad is used, the amperage should not be increased. To do so may result in a severe burn to the patient. It should also be noted that lengthening the treatment time increases the net buildup of charge and thus the net effects of the therapy.

2. Once the intensity has been set for the treatment, it should not be increased later during the therapy. After a few minutes of stimulation, the patient's thermoreceptors and nociceptors under the electrodes quickly accommodate to the stimulation. Accompanying this adaptive accommodation is a slight degree of analgesia that decreases the pa-

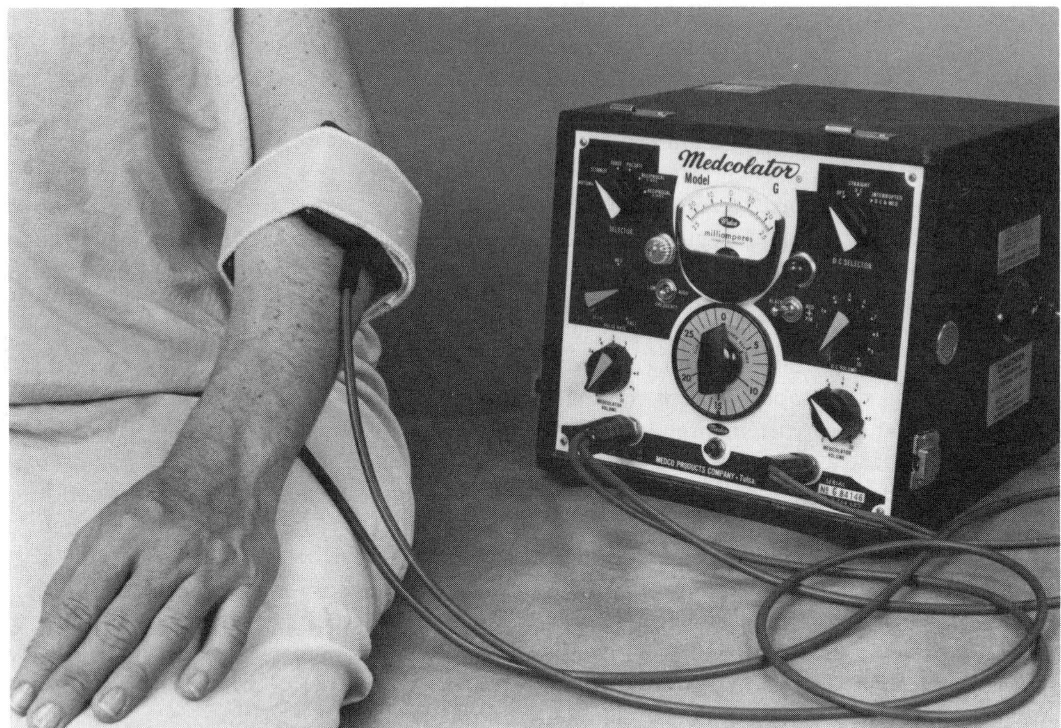

Figure 7.19. Galvanic therapy being applied to a patient's proximal forearm.

tient's usual acuity of cutaneous sensations. Thus, increasing current intensity after the first several minutes of therapy can easily result in a burn.

3. The electrode that is placed over the site requiring treatment is called the *active* electrode. The other electrode is referred to as the *indifferent* or *dispersive* electrode. The only function of the latter is to complete the unidirectional circuit. See Figure 7.20.

4. If the active and dispersive electrode are of equal size, the polarity effects (the primary reason for selecting galvanic current) are diminished tremendously. With such a pad selection, electrical stimulation occurs under both poles but it is minimal. The indifferent electrode should be as large as is conveniently possible to provide for maximal dispersive effects. Most authorities believe that the dispersive pad should be at least four times larger that the active electrode. Thus, if a 4 × 4-inch (16 sq inches) active electrode is used, a dispersive electrode of 64 square inches or more is recommended.

5. Both the active and dispersive electrode should make full contact with the skin of the patient. Areas where uneven contact occurs may readily become sites of a burn because current will concentrate around these points.

6. When the polarity switch of the unit is set at the positive setting, the active electrode will be the positive pole and the indifferent electrode will be the negative pole. When the polarity switch is set at the negative setting, the active electrode will be the negative pole and the indifferent electrode will be the positive pole.

Cutaneous Reaction. As the galvanic current begins to flow, the patient should perceive a gentle tingling or prickling sensation under the electrodes. As the skin resistance is gradually overcome, a slight sensation of warmth will be felt. At the conclusion of the treatment, a flushing of the skin will be ap-

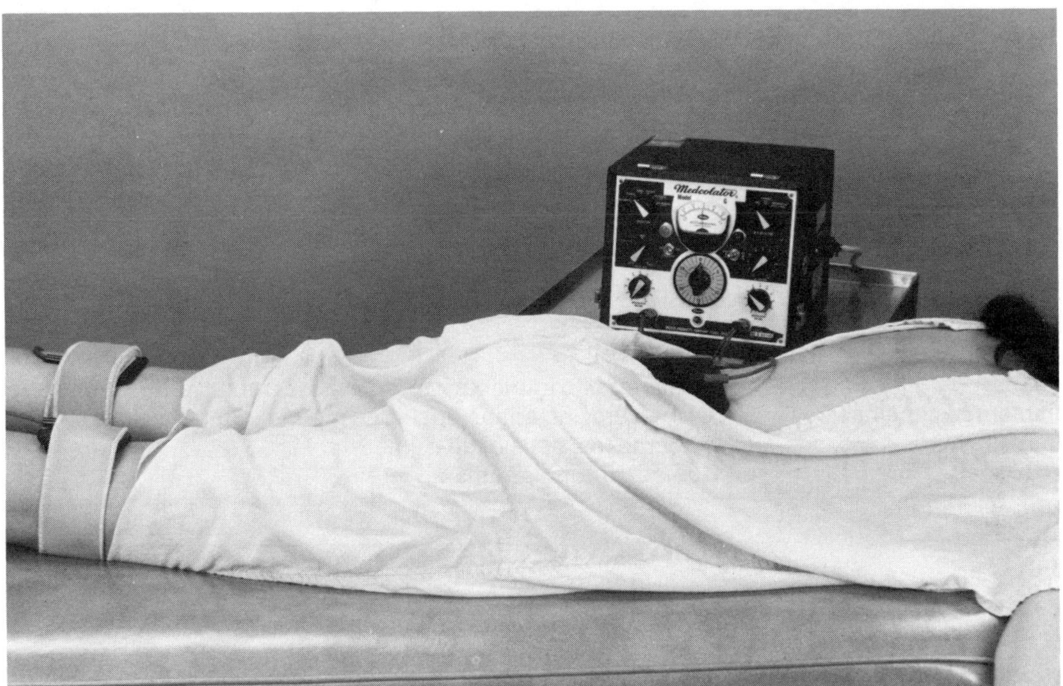

Figure 7.20. In the above photograph, galvanic therapy is being applied for a low back pain complaint. Note that the active electrode is placed on the lumbosacral area while indifferent electrodes are placed distally in the popliteal spaces so that the current is distributed through the sciatic nerve trucks.

parent where the electrodes were placed. This flush, referred to as *galvanic hyperemia,* is due to the chemical stimulation of cutaneous capillaries. This vasomotor effect gradually fades after the treatment has been concluded; however, it may reappear some hours later if moist heat is applied to the same area. An identical reaction may be seen in the extreme when an excessive intensity has been used or when the treatment duration has been prolonged far beyond typical limits; ie, a chemical burn of the skin will likely result.

INDICATIONS AND USE

Direct current stimulates chemical and vasomotor changes in the underlying skin, and some increased local circulation occurs below the electrodes. It is important to note that the current does not flow directly from electrode to electrode, as often pictured in textbook descriptions, but follows the path of least resistance along the nerve fibers of the body and/or through the connecting integument. The actual depth of penetration as the current travels along the skin is quite minimal, rarely deeper than the corium.

Historically, galvanic current has been used therapeutically for many musculoskeletal conditions. See Table 7.6. Most galvanic units in use today have several settings that permit muscle exercise or tetanic contraction. In recent years, however, the use of galvanism has become more and more limited to ion transfer via iontophoresis as high-volt and interferential modalities have become popular.

Special Considerations During Application. The following points should be consid-

Table 7.6. Basic Indications and Contraindications of Galvanic Stimulation

GENERAL INDICATIONS		
Acute trauma	Joint pain	Sciatica
Adhesions	Neuralgia	Sprains
Arthritic complaints	Neuritis	Strains
IVD syndromes	Myalgia	
GENERAL CONTRAINDICATIONS		
Impaired cutaneous sensation	Near the heart	Metastatic carcinoma
Implanted pacemaker	Over metallic implants	Transcerebral applications
Metallic joints, pins, or IUDs	Over scars and adhesions	Treatment on a metallic table
	Over the low back or abdomen during pregnancy	

ered whenever direct current is used as a therapy:

1. Turn the intensity on and off gradually. If the electrodes are removed before the intensity is reduced to zero or if any other rapid change in intensity occurs, the patient is likely to suffer a shock or burn.

2. Never place a patient over a direct current electrode. Electrodes should be fixed in place by weights (eg, sand bags) or straps.

3. Never alter the polarity switch during treatment. A change in polarity made after the intensity control is turned on can result in a severe burn.

4. Be sure that the connecting wires are well insulated; ie, that there are no frayed or naked wires.

5. Treatment should never be given on metallic tables, and electrodes should never be allowed to touch metal objects (eg, adjacent equipment) during current flow.

6. If the patient complains of any unpleasant sensation, discontinue the treatment until the cause can be determined and evaluated. *All* metallic jewelry and objects (eg, rings, watches, underwear clips) must be removed from the treatment area prior to therapy.

Therapy Duration. Treatment times with galvanism are generally for 10—20 minutes. A duration of less than 10 minutes will not be adequate to trigger desirable chemical changes.

Contraindications. See Table 7.6.

SPECIAL APPLICATIONS: IONTOPHORESIS

The term *iontophoresis* refers to the introduction of chemical ions into superficial tissues of the body for therapeutic purposes by means of a direct low-volt galvanic current.

The most important physiochemical effect of galvanic current is the migration of ions that occurs when direct current passes through chemical solutions (eg, tissues). Positive charges are attracted to the negative pole, and negative charges are attracted to the positive pole. This physiochemical principle is the basis of the ion transfer that takes place in iontophoresis.[10]

Two classic experiments have been used to demonstrate ion transfer via iontophoresis:

1. *The potato experiment.* In this experiment, a hole is cut into the top of a raw potato and a potassium iodide solution is put

into the hole. The positive and negative electrodes of a galvanic unit are then inserted directly into the potato on opposite sides of the hole containing the electrolytic solution. As the galvanic current flows, it attracts the iodine anions toward the positive pole. The free iodine that forms there in the starch creates a blue stain. This can readily be appreciated when the current is shut off and the potato is cut open.

2. *LeDuc's rabbit experiment.* LeDuc placed two rabbits in series so that a direct current would flow through both of them. The setup was such that the current from the positive electrode entered the first rabbit after the electrode had been saturated in a solution of strychnine sulfate. It then left the first rabbit via a water-soaked negative electrode and entered the second rabbit by a water-soaked anode. The current finally left the second rabbit via a cathode that had been saturated with a solution of potassium cyanide. When a current of 40—50 ma was turned on, the first rabbit was seized by tetanic contractions, courtesy of the strychnine ions, and the second rabbit quickly expired of cyanide poisoning. However, if the two rabbits are replaced and the experiment is repeated with the flow of ions reversed, there are no ionic changes and neither rabbit is harmed.

Table 7.7 lists some general guidelines for the therapeutic indications of iontophoresis.

Clinical Technique. The sponge of the active electrode is covered with gauze which has been soaked in a solution (1% minimum, 2% usual maximum) to be introduced into the underlying skin. If positive ions are to be introduced, then the positive pole is selected as the active electrode because ions of like charge repel. If negative ions are to be introduced, they will be driven into the skin when then the negative electrode is used as the active pole.

It is good practice to use a quantity of absorbent gauze that is about a half an inch thick; however, cotton felt or asbestos paper of the same thickness may be substituted. Soaking the sponge in the electrolytic solution will often damage a sponge; thus, when substances like vasodilators are to be introduced, gauze or blotting paper are used to hold the solution prior to introduction.

Special Concerns. The major concern when one utilizes iontophoresis is the possibility of chemical burns of the skin or destruction of mucous membranes that may occur if the current intensity has been set too high. There is also the possibility that the patient may have an allergic reaction to the ion or even an untoward systemic reaction as might occur with certain chemicals.

Iontophoresis can only be achieved with low-volt continuous galvanic current. High-volt and interferential modalities do not have a sufficiently long pulse duration to allow ions to be driven into the skin. Even with galvanic current, the depth of penetration is minimal, and it is highly unlikely that ions will be driven to such a great depth as into a bursa of a deep joint or to break up periarticular calcium deposits as has been claimed by some authors.

Applications. Table 7.8, whose data have

Table 7.7. General Indications for Iontophoresis

Type of Ion(s)	*Indications*
Chlorine	Superficial scars and adhesions
Heavy metals (eg, zinc or copper)	Some skin infections, sinus problems
Vasodilators (eg, histamine)	Arthritis (chronic)

Table 7.8. A Summary of Ions Commonly Utilized in Therapeutic Iontophoresis

Ion(s)	*Polarity*	*Source*	*Action(s)*	*Indications*
Acetate	Negative	Acetic acid, 5%—10% white vinegar	Acid radical production in alkaline areas	Bursitis (chronic) Calcium deposits Frozen shoulder
Calcium	Positive	Calcium chloride, 2%, or calcium lactate, 2%	Stabilizes irritability threshold	Adhesive capsulitis Spasticity
Chlorine	Negative	Sodium chloride, 2%	Sclerolytic	Adhesions Capsulitis Scar tissue
Copper	Positive	Copper sulphate, 2%	Caustic antiseptic Astringent	Allergic rhinitis Fungus infections Gynecologic conditions Hemorrhoids Skin disorders
Hesperidin	Negative	Hesperidin, Bioflavinoid complex, 5%	Increases capillary strength	Ecchymosis Minute varicosities Myofascial capillary fragility Subepidermal bleeding
Hyaluronidase	Positive	Wyadase, 1%—2%	Aids absorption	Edema Posttraumatic swelling
Hydrocortisone	Positive	Acusone, 0.5% cream	Anti-inflammatory	Acute sprains Bell's palsy (early) Bursitis Chronic back pain Degenerative joint disease Epicondylitis Frozen shoulder IVD syndromes Myositis Peripheral neuropathy Rheumatoid arthritis Skin disorders Sprains (subacute) Tenosynovitis

Table 7.8, continued

Ion(s)	*Polarity*	*Source*	*Action(s)*	*Indications*
Iodine	Negative	Iodex with methyl salicylate, 2%; potassium iodide, 2%; lugal solution, 2-5%	Sclerolytic Antiseptic Analgesic	Adhesions Bell's palsy (late) Fibrositis Frozen shoulder Myofibrositis Peripheral neuropathy Scar tissue Skin disorders
Magnesium	Positive	Magnesium sulphate, 2%; or magnesium aspartate, 2%	Antispasmodic Analgesic	Acute pain Degenerative joint disease IVD syndromes Myositis Neuritis Osteoarthritis Periarthritis Peripheral neuropathy Rheumatoid arthritis Spasms Sprains (chronic)
Niacin	Negative	Niacin, 5%	Vasodilation Analgesic	Arthritis Peripheral vascular disease Spasm
PABA	Negative	Para-amino benzoic acid, 5%	Sclerolytic	Myofascial sclerotic conditions Peyronie's disease Scleroderma
Proteolytic enzymes	Negative	Amylase Bromelain Chymotrypsin Pancreatic lipase Pancreatin Papayotin Rutin Trypsin (all 5%)	Sclerolytic Anti-inflammatory Proteolytic	Acute myofascial pain Adhesions Arthritis Bursitis Chronic pain Inflammation Tendinitis

Table 7.8, continued

Ion(s)	*Polarity*	*Source*	*Action(s)*	*Indications*
Salicylate	Negative	Sodium salicylate, 2%; dissolved aspirin	Analgesic Decongestive	Back pain (acute or chronic) Callosities Degenerative joint disease Epicondylitis IVD syndromes Myalgia Peripheral neuropathy Rheumatoid arthritis Sprains (subacute) Tenosynovitis
SOD	Negative	Super-oxide dismutase, type G, 5%	Sclerolytic Proteolytic Anti-inflammatory	Adhesions Arthritis Bursitis Inflammation Skin disorders Sprains/strains Swelling Tendinitis
Xylocaine	Positive	Xylocaine, 5% ointment	Analgesic Anesthetic	Bursitis (acute) Epicondylitis IVD syndromes Myositis Neuritis Painful joint restriction Spinal pain (acute) Sprains (acute) Tenosynovitis Vascular conditions
Zinc	Positive	Zinc oxide, 1%—2%	Caustic antiseptic	ENT disorders Gynecologic conditions Skin disorders Ulcers

been taken from several sources, shows a tabulation of ions frequently used for specific entities.[11-14]

Treatment Duration. The usual treatment time during iontophoresis is 10—15 minutes, but it may be up to 20 minutes when such chemicals as mecholyl are driven into the skin and as much as 30 minutes when xylocaine is used to ease severe pain.

ELECTRODIAGNOSIS

Electrodiagnosis is the use of electrical modalities to test the integrity of muscles and nerves. It has become a valuable tool in evaluating whether or not partial degeneration of a nerve or muscle fibers is suspected. Low voltage currents are used in the process, and the degree of reaction gives the practitioner an idea of the extent of disability present.

Innervated muscles normally react to electrical stimulation; however, several situations exist where normal responses are not seen. These will be described in this section.

Reaction of Degeneration

If the conduction of impulses through a peripheral nerve has become impaired because of disease, trauma to the nerve trunks or anterior roots, or a lesion in the spinal cord, changes occur in the electrical reaction of the muscles innervated. Such reactive changes usually occur within 10 days after the initial insult, and they are known as the reaction of degeneration (RD).

With a RD, two responses may be seen: (1) no response to brief impulses of faradic tetanizing current; or (2) a sluggish response to galvanism. See Figure 7.21.

PARTIAL DEGENERATION

This situation exists when a muscle is partially denervated or when some of the nerve fibers are normal and others are denervated. Greater amounts of current are required to elicit a response in such instances. In *partial reaction of degeneration:* (1) the nerve shows a decrease of both tetanic and galvanic responses; and (2) the involved muscles show (a) decreased tetanic excitability, (b) increased galvanic excitability, (c) a slow response, but not as pronounced as in full RD, (d) polar response changes, and possibly, (e) a displacement of the motor point.

COMPLETE DENERVATION

In this situation, there is complete denervation of the muscle. If reinnervation does not occur, fibrosis of the fibers will eventually take place. In *full reaction of degeneration:* (1) the nerve does not respond to either faradic (tetanic) or galvanic stimulation; (2) after about 10 days, the involved muscle tissue does not respond to faradic (tetanic) stimulation; (3) the muscle will respond to galvanic stimuli with a slow, sluggish response but only when greater current intensity is applied; (4) the motor point is displaced toward the periphery where the fibers of the muscle attach to the tendon, and (5) the formula for polar response may change.

In *complete reaction of degeneration,* there is absolutely no response to any current in either the nerve or the muscle. See Table 7.9. Thus, these signs exhibit the final stage of full RD.

There are three distinct stages in the course of reaction of degeneration:

1. *First stage:* 10 days to 2 weeks. Following the first week, the nerve loses all response to tetanic stimulation. If the muscle responds at all to tetanic current, it is quite feeble. Galvanic testing elicits only a slow, weak contraction in the muscle(s) involved, rather than the normal brisk contractions. The cathodal closing contraction is greater than the anodal closing contraction—the reverse of the normal response.

2. *Second stage:* the stage of full RD, which lasts from a few weeks to 1 year or more.

3. *Final stage:* In this stage, there is either

Table 7.9. Electrical Reactions of Muscles and Nerves

Status	*Tissue*	*Galvanic Stimulation*	*Tetanizing Faradic*
Normal reaction	Muscle	Brisk single contraction	Tetanic contraction
	Nerve	Brisk single contraction	Tetanic contraction
Partial reaction of degeneration	Muscle	Sluggish contraction	Diminished response
	Nerve	Diminished response	Diminished response
Full reaction of degeneration	Muscle	Sluggish response	No response
	Nerve	No response	No response
Complete reaction of degeneration	Muscle	No response	No response
	Nerve	No response	No response

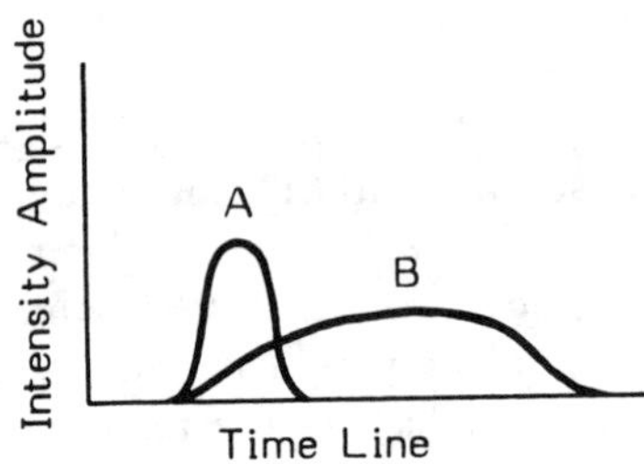

Figure 7.21. Simple graph contrasting the brisk response in normal muscle to a direct current, *A,* and the slow sluggish response to a direct current during degeneration, *B.*

a gradual return of voluntary function with an electrical response or an absolute irreversible RD develops.

Miscellaneous Electrical Muscle Testing Procedures

With the use of electromyography in neuromuscular diagnosis, a more positive prognosis is offered. In cases of peripheral nerve injuries, electrotherapy is indicated in order to maintain muscle tone and to prevent muscle atrophy. In such cases, muscle testing should become an integral part of therapy to evaluate progress. Accordingly, muscle stimulators should provide features to conduct the following tests along with their therapeutic modes.

Accommodativeness Test. According to the established principles of electrophysiology, neuromuscular units have the ability to accommodate to a gradually increasing current (ie, an *exponentially progressive current*). Totally denervated muscles lose this ability, and this fact permits a simple but reliable test for establishing the degree of denervation.

Faradic Excitability Test. Innervated neuromuscular units should respond by contraction when currents of short duration (eg, 1 ms) are applied. For this test, a simple sine wave would do, but sophisticated variable frequency generators allow for more precise evaluation.

Galvanic Excitability (Rheobase) Test. In this test where direct current pulses of long duration are used (eg, 500—1000 ms or interrupted dc), the actual amount of current strength (measured in milliamperage) necessary to contract a muscle is measured. Variable frequency generators permit the application of true square wave current and a more precise measurement, but simpler units can also be used for this test.

Chronaxie Test. This test requires a variable frequency generator that incorporates precise timing and current intensity measurements. The chronaxie determines the impulse time necessary for a muscle to contract with double the current strength of the rheobase. Most healthy neuromuscular units have a chronaxie of 1 ms or less.

Strength Duration Curves. This test can be performed with a variable frequency generator, measuring the current intensity in milliamperage, at different impulse settings; eg, 1000 ms (rheobase), 500 ms, 250 ms, 100 ms, 50 ms, 25 ms, 5 ms, 1 ms, 0.1 ms, and 0.05 ms. These measurements can be plotted graphically and provide detailed objective data about the excitability of any selected neuromuscular unit. The chronaxie is obtained from this test graphically. With experience, a physician or therapist can perform the test in less than 5 minutes, particularly when it is used in conjunction with subsequent treatments.[15] See Figure 7.22.

TENS

According to most authorities, the acronym TENS refers to *transcutaneous electrical nerve stimulation,* a procedure where an electrical current is passed across the skin.[16-19] In its broadest sense, TENS refers to many types of therapeutic devices, including high-volt modalities. However, the term is generally reserved for those small portable electrical units that the patient wears to control pain.

TENS devices became popular following Melzack and Wall's classic article, published in 1965, where they outlined their now famous "gate control" theory of pain.[20,21] In 1967, Mortimer and Shealy developed a dorsal column stimulator that they surgically implanted. Later, it was found that it wasn't necessary to surgically implant the device; rather, it could simply be worn by the patient.

Application

A great deal has been written about TENS, and there are many fine charts available as a guide for the placement of electrodes. See Figure 7.23. Many excellent types of stimulators are available for home and professional use.

The following features are common to most pain control TENS devices:

1. They are designed to provide sensory and not motor stimulation. This fact is important because motor stimulation will initiate or produce muscle contractions in many cases of severe pain that may aggravate the patient's complaint.

2. Because afferent nerve fibers differ greatly from efferent nerve fibers in (a) length of refractory period, (b) accommodation to stimuli, (c) threshold of firing, and (d) response to different wave forms, TENS wave form widths are 40—500 ms or less (usually under 130 ms), while pulse widths for triggering motor responses are 500 ms or better, and frequencies can usually be set in the 70—150 pps range for effective pain control.[22]

3. Wave forms are usually spiked; ie, they are not smooth symmetrical waves. Most units have a wave that alternates and is a variation on the faradic or square wave.

4. Electrode placement should be on the same dermatome(s) as is the patient's perception of pain, preferably over or proximal to the site of pain.[23] In radiating pain, electrodes may additionally be placed over the major nerve pathways (eg, in sciatica). In cases of nerve damage, electrodes should be placed proximal (never distal) to the site of pain.[24] If the site of pain is so sensitive that the slightest stimulation is excruciating, the

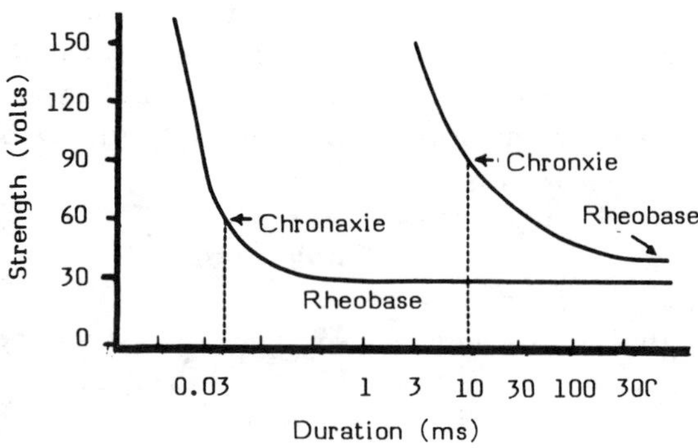

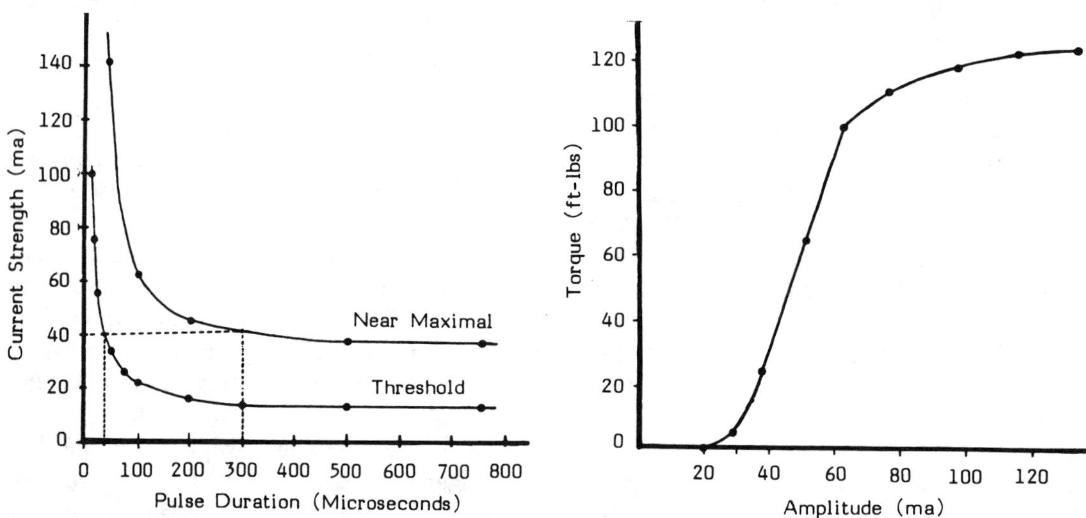

Figure 7.22. *Top diagram,* strength duration curve showing the relationship between pulse duration and amplitude necessary to excite (minimally) muscle tissue. *Bottom left diagram,* a modified strength duration curve of wrist extensors with an intact neuromuscular unit, showing amplitude and duration characteristics of a threshold contraction and near maximum contraction. *Bottom right diagram,* strength amplitude curve of a quadriceps femoris, showing that the force of contraction is dependent on electrical stimulus current amplitude. Note that no torque is produced until a threshold value is reached.

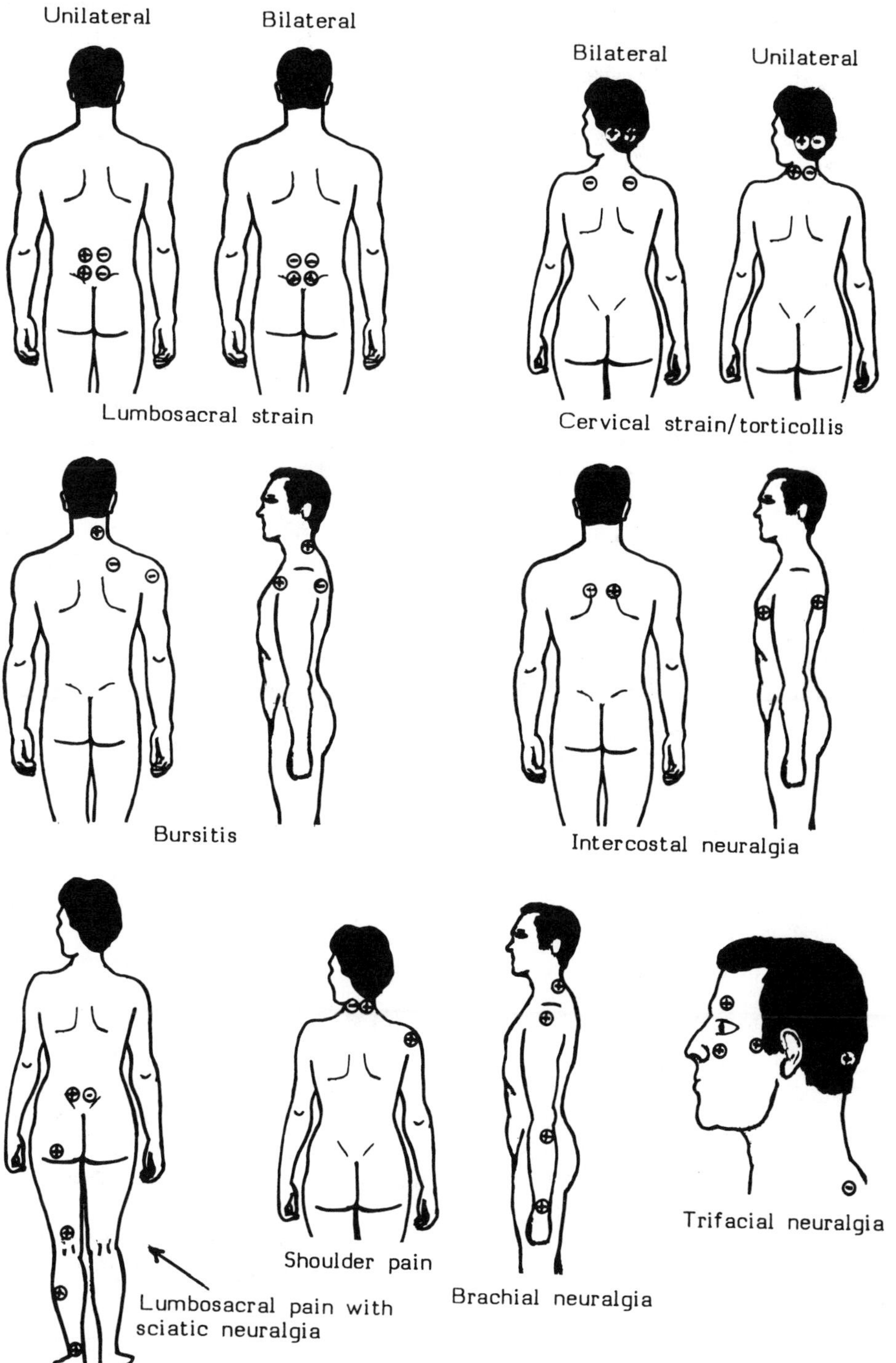

Figure 7.23. Some examples of TENS electrode pad placement (courtesy of Associated Chiropractic Academic Press). Refer to manufacturer's guidelines for detailed instructions.

stimulation of the contralateral area will initially provide partial relief that tends to become more effective after a few days. Acupuncture points far distant from the site of pain have also proved to be successful sites of stimulation.[25-29] In fact, Fox and Melzack have suggested that Tens and acupuncture have a similar mode of action.[30]

5. In treating postsurgical pain, the electrode should be placed as close to the incision as possible.

6. Pain modulation usually lasts only while the current is turned on; ie, it has no residual posttherapy effects.

TENS is intended for the symptomatic relief of a large number of painful syndromes until the cause can be found, the relief of chronic intractable pain syndromes, or cases where analgesic drugs would be contraindicated.[31,32,33] Obviously, electrical stimulation of any type should be used with caution in undiagnosed pain syndromes where the etiology has not been firmly established. Table 7.10 shows a general listing of pain syndromes that have been reported to be relieved by TENS analgesia.[34-37]

Precautions

The only contraindication known, when used with a physician's prescription, is in patient's using a demand-type pacemaker.[38] However, stimulation over the carotid sinus, the heart in patients with known arrhythmias or myocardial disease, the pregnant uterus, open wounds, or the pharyngeal/laryngeal muscles would undoubtedly be hazardous.[39]

COMBINATION THERAPIES

Several modalities have been developed as combination therapies. It is believed by many that two modalities in combination may significantly augment the patient's recovery. Although some question exists as to their true value, we will briefly review the two most commonly used of these combined therapies: (1) ultrasound with sine wave currents and (2) ultrasound with high-volt currents.

Ultrasound with Sine Waves

For years, one of the more popular modalities in use has been the Medco-Sonalator, which permits the simultaneous treatment of a patient with ultrasound and sine wave. The original rationale for the development of this unit centered on the fact that patients receiving ultrasound therapy could not feel the current, and thus often failed to appreciate the therapy. To overcome this psychologic obstacle, the manufacturer came up with the concept of combining sound with sine waves that could be felt by the patient. However, the true clinical value of the combination lies in the fact that ultrasound, a high frequency current that quickly overcomes skin resistance, allows for a more rapid and efficient penetration and stimulation of sine waves. Thus, the ultrasonic waves augment the production of muscle exercise or tetany that occur with sine wave, but the sine wave in no way improves the therapeutic efficacy of the ultrasound waves.

Ultrasound combined with sine waves has also been found to be of considerable clinical value in locating and dissipating trigger points. An intense, almost painful, sensation is felt by the patient as the combined sound/sine head is moved over a trigger point. The area can then be treated, using the tetanizing setting, directly over the hypersensitive area for 3—5 minutes. Several examples of common trigger-point sites and their areas of referred pain are shown in Figures 7.24 and 7.25.[40,41]

It should be noted that when combined sound/sine therapy is used, the ultrasound is delivered as a high frequency pulsed stimulation. Such stimuli have as their primary effect the removal of edema, but those effects commonly associated with continuous ultrasound stimulation do not occur.

The pulse rates used with combined sound/

sine techniques do not exceed 60 pps, which does not fall into those ranges or parameters that are commonly related to pain control. The sine wave can be tetanized, pulsed, surged, or be placed on a reciprocal setting.

Ultrasound with High-Volt Current

The combination of ultrasound with high-volt current is something of extremely questionable value. In our literature search, we have been unable to find any study that documents deeper penetration, more effective results, or any added value in combining ultrasound with high-volt currents simultaneously—especially when the ultrasound is administered in the pulsed mode.

Physiologically, pulsed ultrasound triggers actions that are very similar to pulsed high-volt currents. Again, as with ultrasound/sine combinations, the supposed purpose of the ultrasound is to quickly overcome skin resistance to permit deeper penetration and more effective stimulation.

We have found some added value in treating trigger points. However, in our opinion, this value is not sufficient to warrant purchase of a combined sound/high-volt unit.

Multiple Therapy Stimulation

Although some would like us to tout the use of multiple therapies to a patient at the same session, the reader is carefully cautioned to review exactly how each modality affects the body before prescribing multiple therapies during any given office visit. One doctor of whom we are aware has an ultraviolet light in the waiting room, an infrared lamp in the dressing room, plus uses four modalities per patient visit. This is multiple therapy in its extreme. Another practitioner uses condensor field diathermy simultaneously with low-volt galvanic on the same area, which is contraindicated and quite dangerous.

A conscientious practitioner should ask the following questions before prescribing multiple therapies:

1. *Is the primary physical effect the same?* Hot moist packs, induction field diathermy, and microwave all build up superficial heat. To follow one with the next during the same visit represents a redundant duplication of therapy and is not indicated. One may find it advantageous, however, to use a pain control device (eg, TENS) over an area of musculoskeletal pain and then treat with a modality that is effective for tetanizing spastic muscles. Likewise, mobilization procedures (eg, intersegmental traction) can be of considerable value following therapy with a physical therapy modality that effects soft-tissue relaxation.

2. *Do the modalities complement each other?* When treating over the buttocks region of obese patients, for example, there is little penetration through the fatty tissues when high-volt current is used alone. Hot moist packs placed over the electrodes, however, will help to permit more effective penetration by promoting perspiration and a mild hyperemia in the area.

3. *Has the correct modality been chosen?* Ultrasound in the pulsed setting is extremely effective for removing edema and sine wave is excellent for breaking spasticity in muscles. However, high-volt by itself accomplishes both of these functions effectively.

4. *Will multiple therapies shorten the treatment time or improve the effects of the treatment?* The answer to this will often be found within professional literature and/or accredited seminars. If not, a decision based solely on personal observations that do not parallel the rules of logic is difficult to justify.

FREQUENCY OF TREATMENTS

The specific modality used; the patient's age, sex, and physical condition; and the severity and duration of each complaint—all play a part in determining the number and frequency of treatments that will be required.

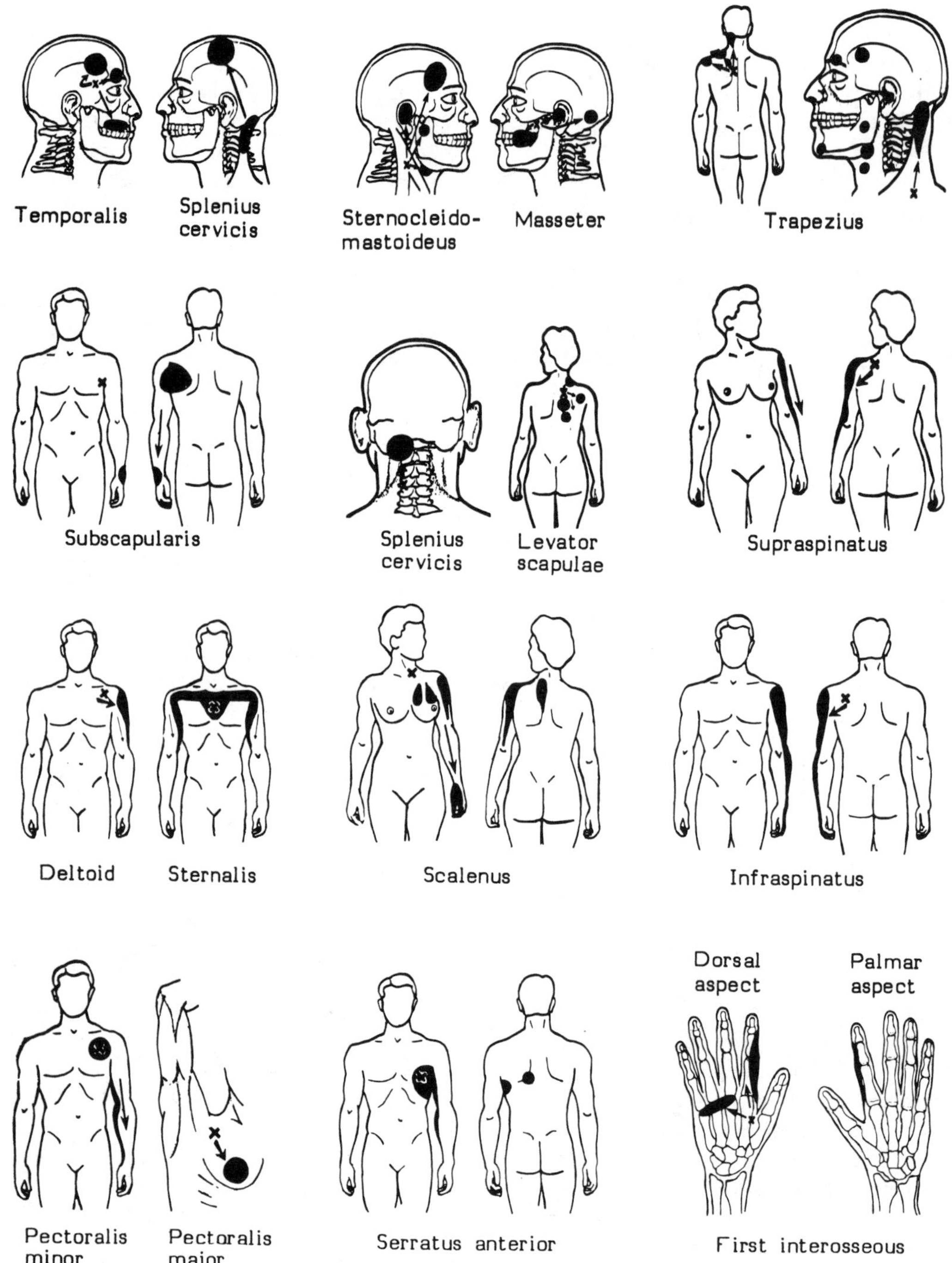

Figure 7.24. Some examples of common trigger points; where X, indicates the common site of the trigger point, and the blackened areas indicate typical areas of referred pain (courtesy of Associated Chiropractic Academic Press). Refer to a specific text on this subject if more information desired.

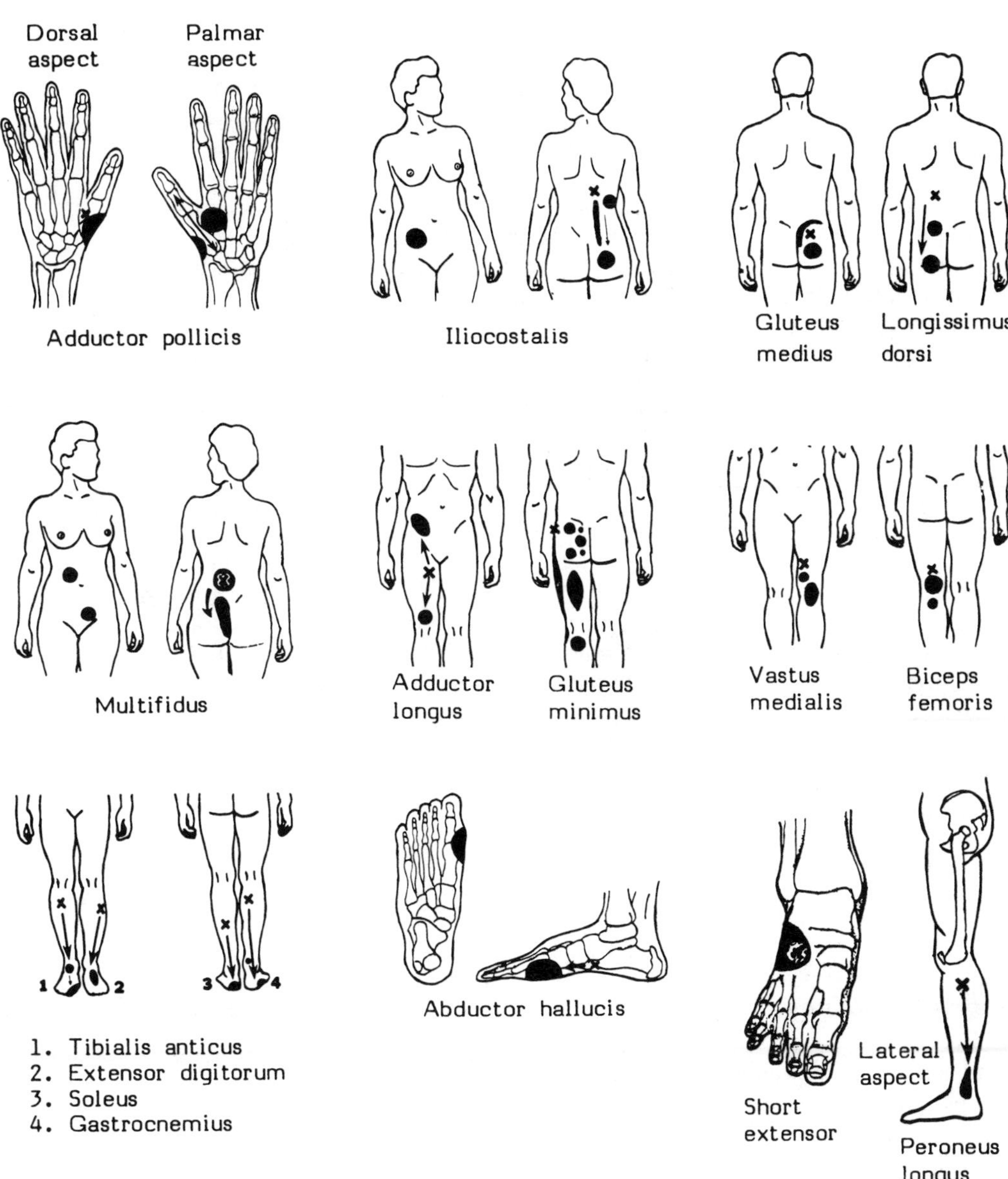

Figure 7.25. Other common trigger points (courtesy of Associated Chiropractic Academic Press).

Table 7.10. Typical Pain Syndromes That Are Usually Relieved by TENS Analgesia

Systemic Pain	*Head and Neck*	*Abdomen*
Bursitis	Cluster headaches	Bladder pain
Cancer	Dental disorders	Bowel stasis
Causalgia	Migraine	Diverticulosis
Multiple sclerosis	Spondylosis	Dysmenorrhea
Neuralgia	Sprains/strains	Labor
Osteoarthritis	Suboccipital headaches	Postoperative pain
Phantom limb syndrome	TMJ syndrome	
Raynaud's syndrome	Tic douloureux	
Rheumatoid arthritis	Torticollis	
Synovitis	Trigeminal neuralgia	
	Whiplash	
Back Pain	***Lower Extremities***	***Upper Extremities***
Coccydynia	Ankle pain	Epicondylitis
Facet syndrome	Foot pain	Frozen shoulder
Intercostal neuralgia	Fractures	Hand pain
IVD syndrome	Ischialgia	Peripheral nerve injury
Lumbago	Joint mobilization	Sprains/strains
Lumbosacral pain	Knee pain	Subdeltoid bursitis
Radiculitis	Passive stretch pain	Wrist pain
Sprains/strains	Sciatica	
Thoracodynia	Sprains/strains	
Whole back pain	Tendinitis	
	Thrombophlebitis	

General Guidelines

The following extremely general guidelines for musculoskeletal complaints may be used in developing a treatment program for a patient. However, each individual practitioner must remain responsible for basing every therapeutic program on an individual patient's current physical condition.

PHASES OF THERAPY

1. *Acute stage.* Following an acute musculoskeletal injury, especially during the first 24—48 hours, it may be necessary to treat the patient once or several times each day until the pain subsides. In some patients with severe IVD injuries, multiple treatments or concentrated care combined with bed rest is often the regimen of choice.

Note: If a patient truly requires daily treatment for 5 consecutive days and is first seen on a Thursday, for example, treatment should be given Thursday, Friday, Saturday, Sunday, and Monday. A treatment schedule of Thursday, Friday, Monday, Tuesday, and Wednesday would be difficult to clinically justify. A patient's pain does not stop just because a holiday weekend intervenes. Health insurance companies and professional review committees are well aware of this.

2. *Postacute healing stage.* Treatments for musculoskeletal complaints after the acute pain has subsided need not be spaced as

close together as during the acute stage. Treatment is usually administered on a daily basis, then every other day, and eventually to about once per week. If pain persists after 10—15 visits, it is probably advisable to completely re-examine the patient and re-evaluate the initial diagnosis, seek consultation, or refer the patient for further specialized evaluation before therapy is continued.

3. *Strengthening stage.* As healing becomes more complete, the therapy should be directed to developing strength and tone in the injured muscle, tendons, and ligaments. Therapy during this stage is frequently scheduled once (possibly twice) a week and is usually combined with a specific exercise program that is given to the patient (by demonstration/explanation and writing) to apply at home.

RESPONSE TO THERAPY

Results should not be expected with just one or two applications of a modality. Changing therapies after each one or two visits when a patient is not responding is not practical and serves no useful purpose. If 8—10 treatments with one specific modality have been given with no apparent results, re-examination, an alternative therapy, or referral should be seriously considered. Modalities such as ultrasound or shortwave diathermy usually have a cumulative effect, and results are usually minimal until after 2—4 visits.

Prognosis

If denervation occurs in patients with motor disturbances, therapy should be instituted as soon as possible. The process of atrophy begins immediately and will be apparent within 7—14 days without care. With peripheral nerve injuries, low-volt galvanic is the *only* effective wave form because of its long pulse duration. Treatment time in the acute stage should be about 3—5 minutes. Frequent therapy (5—6 times a day) or a supplemented vigorous exercise regimen to prevent atrophy is often necessary.

If regeneration occurs within the first year, the prognosis is good. The prognosis after 2—3 years without results is dismal. The objective is always to retard the process of atrophy somehow so that the degree of recovery can be increased as far as possible.

CLOSING COMMENTS

In summary, low frequency stimulation is primarily used for the following reasons:

1. *Pain control.* TENS units are most beneficial because of their short pulse durations and specific analgesic effects on sensory fibers.
2. *Relief of spasticity.* To relieve spasm, tetanizing currents are used.
3. *Edema.* Pulsed currents are effective in moving fluids and reducing areas of congestion.
4. *Electrodiagnosis.* The reaction of degeneration may be ascertained using electrodiagnostic evaluations.

REFERENCES

1. McQuire WA: Electrotherapy and exercises for stress incontinence and urinary frequency. *Physiotherapy,* 61(10):305-307.
2. Melzack R: Pain mechanisms, Parts I—III. Paper presented to the Second Annual Seminar on Chronic Pain, New Orleans, LA, May 4-6, 1979.
3. Zimmerman M: Neurophysiology of nociception. *Pain Abstracts,* Second World Congress on Pain, International Association for the Study of Pain, September 1978, vol 1, pp 173-174.
4. Kahn J: *Low Volt Technique,* ed 4. Syosset, NY, published by author, 1983.
5. Haber WP: Sinusoidal current. Monograph published by the National College of Chiropractic, Lombard, IL, date not shown.
6. Scott BO: *The Principles and Practice of Electrotherapy and Actinotherapy.* Springfield, IL, Charles C. Thomas, 1959.
7. Fields HL, Basbaum AI: Anatomy and physiology of a descending pain control system. In Bonica JJ, et al (eds): *Advances in Pain Research and Therapy.* New York, Raven Press, 1979, vol 3, pp 427-440.

8. Watkins AL: *A Manual of Electrotherapy,* ed 3. Philadelphia, Lea & Febiger, 1968, p 83-84.
9. Ibid: p 135-136.
10. Stillwell GK: Electrical stimulation and iontophoresis. In Krusen FH, et al (eds): *Handbook of Physical Medicine and Rehabilitation,* ed 2. Philadelphia, W.B. Saunders, 1971, pp 374-380.
11. ACA Council on Physiological Therapeutics: Physiotherapy guidelines for the chiropractic profession. *ACA Journal of Chiropractic,* IX:S-74, June 1975.
12. Kahn A, Kahn J: in *Journal of the New York State Society of Physiotherapists, Inc,* annual issue, June 1959.
13. Hill LL: *Parameters of Physiotherapy Modalities.* Lombard, IL, National chiropractic College, class notes, date not shown, p 88.G.
14. Lerner FN: Adjunctive procedure: iontophoresis. *The American Chiropractor,* November 1984.
15. Wolf SL (ed): *Clinics in Physical Therapy: Electrotherapy.* New York, Churchhill Livingstone, 1981.
16. Lister MJ (ed): Transcutaneous electrical nerve stimulation. *Physical Therapy,* 58:1441-1492, 1978.
17. Long DM, et al: Transcutaneous electrical stimulation in pain research and therapy. In Bonica JJ, et al (eds): *Advances in Pain Research and Therapy.* New York, Raven Press, 1979, vol 3, pp 569-585.
18. Sternback RA: TENS: A pain management alternative. Monograph published by LaJolla Technology, Inc, San Diego, CA, 1984, pp 3-18.
19. Transcutaneous electrical nerve stimulation. Monograph published as a special issue of *Physical Therapy,* 58:1441-1492, 1978.
20. Melzack R, Wall PD: Pain mechanisms: a new theory. *Science,* 150:971-979, 1965.
21. Mowry EA: Transcutaneous neural stimulation: for the relief of acute pain. Reprint from *The North Carolina Chiropractic Journal,* date and issue not shown.
22. Zimmermann M: Peripheral and central nervous mechanisms of nociception, pain, and pain therapy. In Bonica JJ, et al (eds): *Advances in Pain Research and Therapy.* New York, Raven Press, 1979, vol 3, pp 3-32.
23. Eriksson MBE: *Transcutaneous Nerve Stimulation and Chronic Pain.* Lund, Liber Forlag, 1983.
24. Sternbach RA: TENS: A pain management alternative. Monograph published by LaJolla Technology, Inc, San Diego, CA, 1984, p 12.
25. Merskey H, et al: Pain terms: a list with definitions and notes on usage, recommended by the IASP subcommittee on taxonomy. *Pain,* 6:249-252, 1979.
26. Wagman IH, Price DD: Responses of dorsal horn cells of M. mulatta to cutaneous and sural nerve A and C fiber stimuli. *Journal of Neurophysiology,* 32:803-817, 1969.
27. Hillman P, Wall PD: Inhibitory and excitatory factors influencing the receptive fields of lamina V spinal cord cells. *Experimental Brain Research,* 9: 284-306, 1969.
28. Cheng R, et al: A controlled study shows that electro-acupuncture elevates cortisone levels in blood plasma. *International Journal of Neuroscience,* 10, 1979.
29. Foreman RD, et al: Effects of dorsal column on stimulation on primate spinothalamic tract neurons. *Journal of Neurophysiology,* 39:543-546, 1976.
30. Fox EJ, Melzack R: Transcutaneous stimulation and acupuncture; comparison of treatment for low back pain. *Pain,* 2:141-148, 1979.
31. Thurman BF, Christian EL: Case report: response of a serious circulatory lesion to electrical stimulation. *Physical Therapy,* 51(10):1107-1110, October 1971.
32. Mayer DJ, Liebeskind JC: Pain reduction by focal electrical stimulation of the brain: An anatomical and behavioral analysis. *Brain Research,* 68:73-93, 1974.
33. Terman GW, et al: Intrinsic mechanisms of pain inhibition: activation by stress. *Science,* 226: 1270-1277, December 14, 1984.
34. Sternbach RA: TENS: A pain management alternative. Monograph published by LaJolla Technology, Inc, San Diego, CA, 1984, p 11.
35. Peterson B: TENS at St. Cloud Hospital. No other publication data shown, pp 5-24.
36. Eriksson M, et al: Long term results of peripheral conditioning stimulation as an analgesic measure in chronic pain. *Pain,* 6:335-347, 1979.
37. McKelvy PL: Clinical report of the use of specific TENS units. *Physical Therapy,* 58(12):1474-1477, December 1978.
38. Eriksson M, et al: Hazard from transcutaneous nerve stimulation in patients with pacemakers. *Lancet,* 1:1319, 1978.
39. Peterson B: TENS at St. Cloud Hospital. No other publication data shown, p 1.
40. Schafer RC: *Chiropractic Management of Sports and Recreational Injuries,* Baltimore, Williams & Wilkins, 1982, part four.
41. Travel J, Rinzler SH: The myofascial genesis of pain. *Postgraduate Medicine,* No. 11, 1952.

Chapter 8

High Voltage Therapy

This chapter reviews the basic guidelines and principles that relate to the high voltage stimulators. There are at least six good units on the market today, and those concepts that pertain in general to most of them will be emphasized. The advantages and disadvantages of high voltage units will be compared to those of low voltage units. How the units specifically affect pain, muscle spasm, and edema will be explained in light of present knowledge. Also described will be clinical applications, contraindications to be considered, and other practical concerns.

INTRODUCTION

One of the more popular modalities on the market today is a device that was originally termed *high voltage galvanism* and is now popularly called *high voltage monophasic pulsed stimulation.* These devices have revolutionized the field during the past 30 years in their effective management of musculoskeletal complaints. An example of a unit is shown in Figure 8.1.

Utilization of high voltage therapies has spread across most disciplines. Their effectiveness in pain control has led to their use by several professional athletic teams and in the offices of many private practitioners who see a high percentage of musculoskeletal cases.[1,2] Dentists have found them to be effective for treating pain associated with the TMJ syndrome, veterinarians are using them for pain modulation, and their use can be seen in many burn centers throughout the United States.

Because high voltage units were originally referred to as galvanic units, much confusion was created in clinical practice. There has been considerable debate as to what ionic chemical changes, if any, actually take place. Some people taught that there was no polarity effects, while others preached about distinct iontophoretic reactions. Some talked about stimulating denervated muscles, while others said the therapy was useless for this purpose. Even today, there are many unanswered questions as to just exactly how these units affect the body. Thus, while definitive answers will not be claimed here, personal observations and empirical results will be shared with the reader, as will the conclusions drawn from the few clinical studies reported. Credit for most of the principles that are being widely accepted goes principally to Dr. Gad Alon of the University of Maryland.[3]

HIGH VOLTAGE STIMULATION: COMPARATIVE FEATURES

Strictly speaking, high-volt units are not galvanic in action, nor are they similar in some other ways to low voltage units.

The low-volt galvanic units in use today produce a unidirectional low voltage monophasic direct current that may or may not be pulsed. If pulsed, the pulse is on for a relatively long period of time. The time and the exact number of pulses per second is permanently preset, and they cannot be varied by the operator. These units have a relatively high amperage current, usually ranging from 0—20 milliamperes (ma).

High-volt units, on the other hand, generate an electromotive force of up to 500 volts. They utilize unidirectional, monophasic, interrupted (noncontinuous) currents. The current flow consists of twin spikes (pulses). See Figure 8.2. The total pulses per second (pps) can be manually varied by the operator by rotating a dial. In comparison to pulsed low-volt units, the pulses of high-volt units are on for a very short time and this interval may be controlled to some extent in some units. High-volt units have a relatively low current amperage, averaging between 1.0 and 1.5 ma.

Basic Characteristics

In order to understand the question of polarity and how high-volt units function, we must examine the various characteristics of the current and the pulse. A number of studies have explored these properties.[4,5,6]

When a continuous galvanic current is utilized in a low-volt galvanic unit, the current must be carefully set at a particular level so as not to burn the patient. It is usually recommended that the maximum current with low voltage units be set at 1 milliampere for every square inch of active electrode or to patient tolerance, whichever is less. If the active pad (electrode) has dimensions of 3-inches × 3-inches, for example,

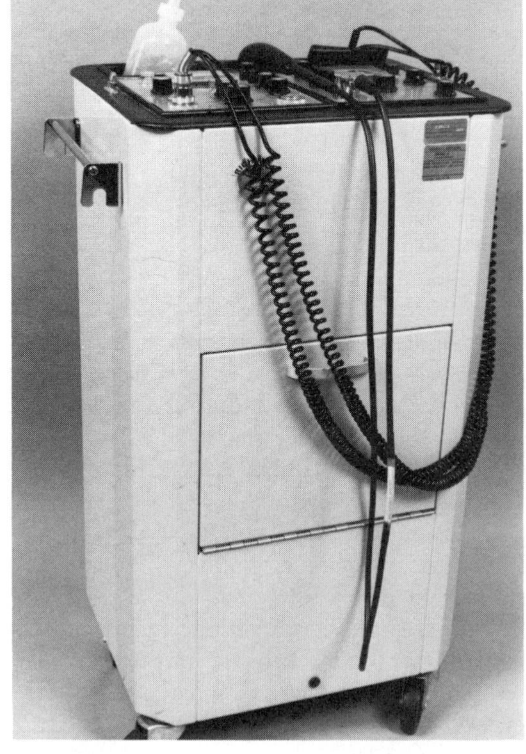

Figure 8.1. A. Richmar high-volt unit and cabinet.

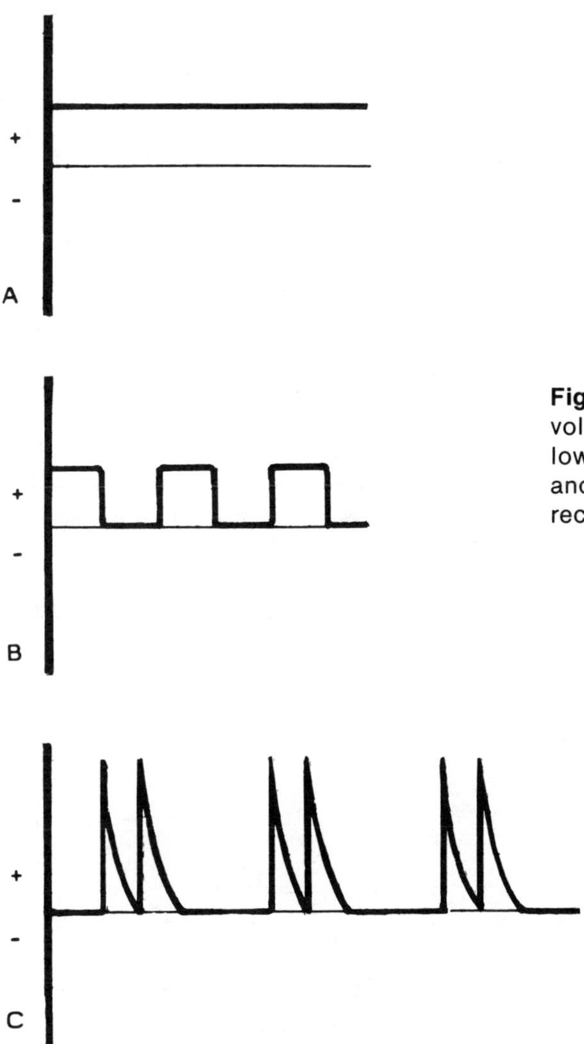

Figure 8.2. Comparison of (A) positive low-volt direct galvanic current, (B) positive low-volt "square wave" galvanic current, and (C) high-volt monophasic pulsating direct current.

then the maximum current would be set at 9 ma. As it is *amperage* and not *voltage* that causes a burn during electrotherapy, a setting above this 9-ma level (optimal peak) would be dangerous if a burn is to be avoided. Another point should also be considered here. As the setting in this example using low-volt galvanism is in the continuous mode, the peak current will be exactly the same as the average current; ie, current averaged within a timeframe. Thus, peak current and average current are always the same when continuous low-volt galvanism is used.

During pulsed electrotherapy, the depth of tissue penetration is proportional to the magnitude (pulse amplitude) of the current that is generated by the unit. As long as the conductivity of the body tissue does not change, increasing the amplitude of wave peaks will result in the current reaching deeper structures.

High-volt stimulators have a distinct advantage over low-volt units in that the former have the ability to reach much higher wave peaks. The ability to achieve this without burning the patient is possible in high-volt units because the *pulse duration* is extremely short; ie, a low average current is produced. In other words, high-volt units generate a relatively high-peak wave with a low-average current amperage.

The various controls on a typical high-volt unit are shown in Figure 8.3.

Studies conducted with one particular commercial unit have indicated that the unit reaches a peak current of about 2,500 ma, but it generates an average current that reaches a maximum of only 1.5—2.0 ma. This permits a relatively deep depth of penetration without danger of burning the patient. In fact, there was no danger of burning the patient even when the high-volt unit was set on maximum because the average current never built to an intensity level that would cause a burn. See Figure 8.4.

PENETRATION

Several factors determine the depth of high-volt energy penetration, and this causes various tissues to be influenced in different ways.[7,8,9]

1. *Peak Current.* As previously described, the peak current is directly proportional to the depth of penetration. High-volt units may reach peaks of 2,500 ma.

2. *Tissue Conductivity.* The depth of tissue penetration is also influenced by the conductivity properties of different tissues.

A. *Bone and Cartilage.* Bone and dense connective tissue are practically nonconductors because of their low fluid levels. When a high-volt electrode is placed over osseous tissue (eg, patella), the current will not transverse the bone, but it will travel around it.

PULSE
INDICATOR
PADS
BLACK
RED
POWER ON
5
10
15
20
30
40
60
80
PULSES/SEC.
0
100
200
300
400
500
VOLTS
10
20
5
25
OFF
MINUTES
CAUTION
HAZARDOUS ELECTRICAL OUTPUT
THIS EQUIPMENT FOR USE ONLY BY QUALIFIED MEDICAL PERSONNEL
DO NOT USE ON INDIVIDUALS THAT ARE PREGNANT OR HAVE A PACEMAKER
PROBE
PADS
CONT.
MIN
RESET
MAX

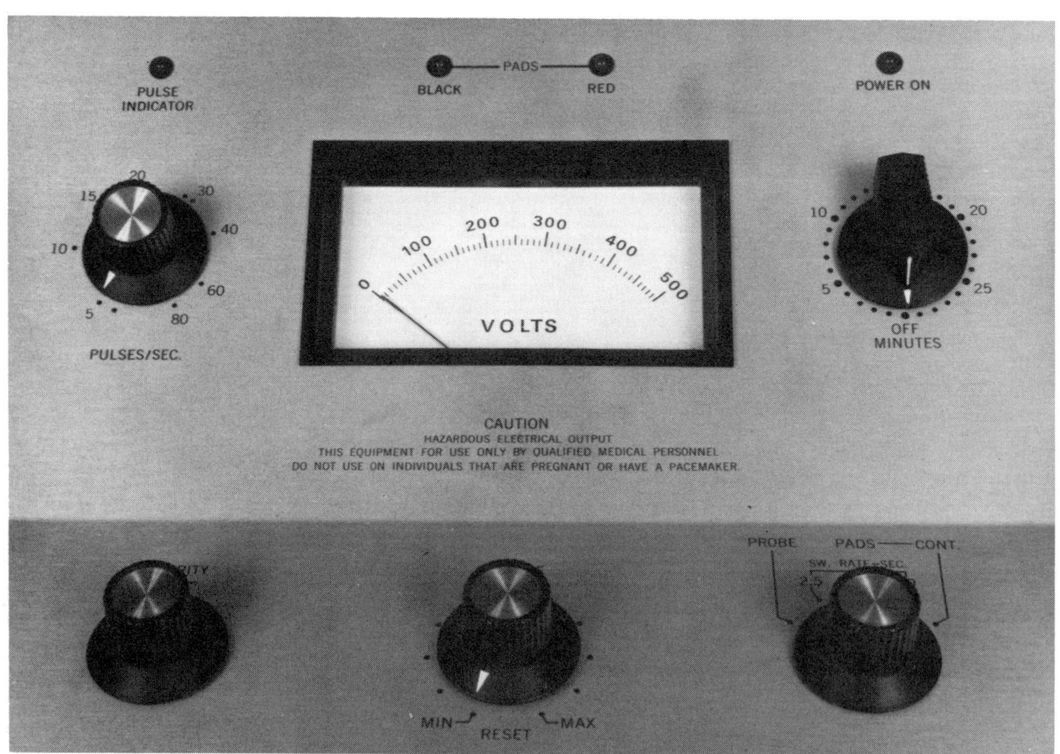

Figure 8.3. Dials on a typical high-volt unit.

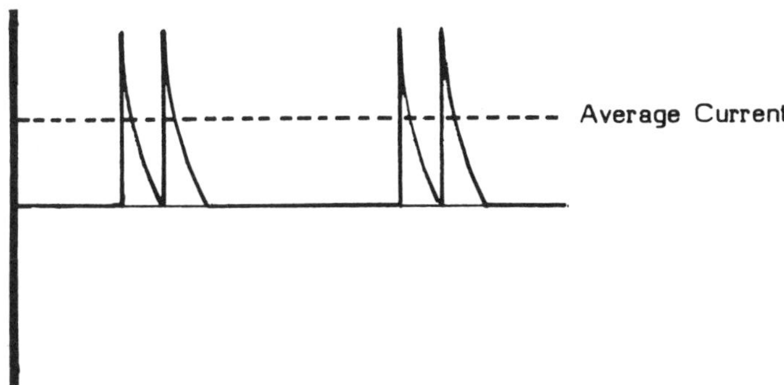

Figure 8.4. Diagram of a high-volt pulsed direct current. Note that with high voltage the average current is considerably lower than the peak current.

Even when peak currents reach maximum levels, there is poor penetration into bone.

B. *Fat.* Thick adipose tissue is also a relatively poor conductor of high-volt current. For this reason, it is sometimes difficult to achieve good therapeutic results with obese patients, especially when treating the gluteal area. In such cases, it might be useful to use hot packs over the electrodes to help promote sweating that would slightly improve conductivity.

C. *Muscle.* Muscle tissue is a relatively good conductor. As higher current peaks are reached, transmission enters into deeper layers of muscle. This permits activation (contraction) of deep muscle fibers.

3. *Neuroselectivity.* Low peak currents (eg, those of low-volt galvanic units) trigger the excitation of all types of peripheral nerve fibers simultaneously. This factor underscores a distinct advantage of high-volt therapy. That is, as the intensity (peak current) is gradually increased, (a) there is excitation of nonpain sensory fibers, (b) next there is stimulation of the motor fibers, and (c) only at the extremely high levels is there activation of nociceptors.

When first using a high-volt unit, the operator should test this effect on himself or herself. As the intensity control is slowly increased, the first sensation will be of mild stimulation. This is the effect of stimulation to light touch, pressure, and possibly temperature receptors. As the intensity is increased further, motor fibers will be activated. If the pulse rate has been set at 80 pps, then this stimulation will trigger enkephalin production for pain control. When motor fibers are strongly activated, tetany will be produced. If the intensity is increased still further, pain will be produced.

4. *Visceral Reactions.* The ability of high-volt units to penetrate body tissue is not limited to the excitation of skeletal muscle fibers or peripheral somatic nerves. The deeper penetration made possible by the higher peak current may also affect the smooth muscles and glands of internal organs directly or via autonomic nerve fibers.

PULSE RATE

Pulse rate is another factor that has a direct influence on the therapeutic results of electrotherapy. Pulse rate can be defined on a clinical basis as the number of times each second the body tissues are being stimulated during treatment.

Before we describe the pulse rate of a high-volt unit, it would be well to review the characteristics of a low-volt unit. With a low-volt galvanic generator, the pulse rate is preset and options fall into one of three selections:

1. *Continuous Current.* With this setting, there is a continuous flow of electrons from one pole (electrode) to the other. Continuous low-volt galvanism is utilized primarily to promote the chemical changes that occur, drive specific ions into the skin (iontophoresis), and enhance subcutaneous circulation.

2. *Pulsed Current.* The predetermined monophasic pulse rate of a low-volt galvanic unit is preset at a level to excite, and thereby exercise, peripheral muscle fibers. This is especially effective when reaction of degeneration is present.

3. *Tetanizing Current.* This predetermined setting is set at a rate to tetanize, therefore fatigue, muscle fibers when the clinical objective is to relieve spasticity.

Varying the Pulse Rate on a High Voltage Unit

In contrast, the pulse rate of a high-volt unit can be manually set any place from 1—120 pps, depending upon the particular unit used. It is important to realize that a high-volt unit is *always* pulsed because its nature is to be a pulsed current and not a continuous current. If it were not pulsed, a severe burn would occur almost instantly.

The way that the pulse of a high-volt unit is delivered to the patient can be varied, depending on what clinical effect is desired. Variables are determined by the specific control setting used. See Figure 8.5.

Most units allow three general types of settings: (1) a "Continuous" mode, where the active electrodes emit a continuous current,

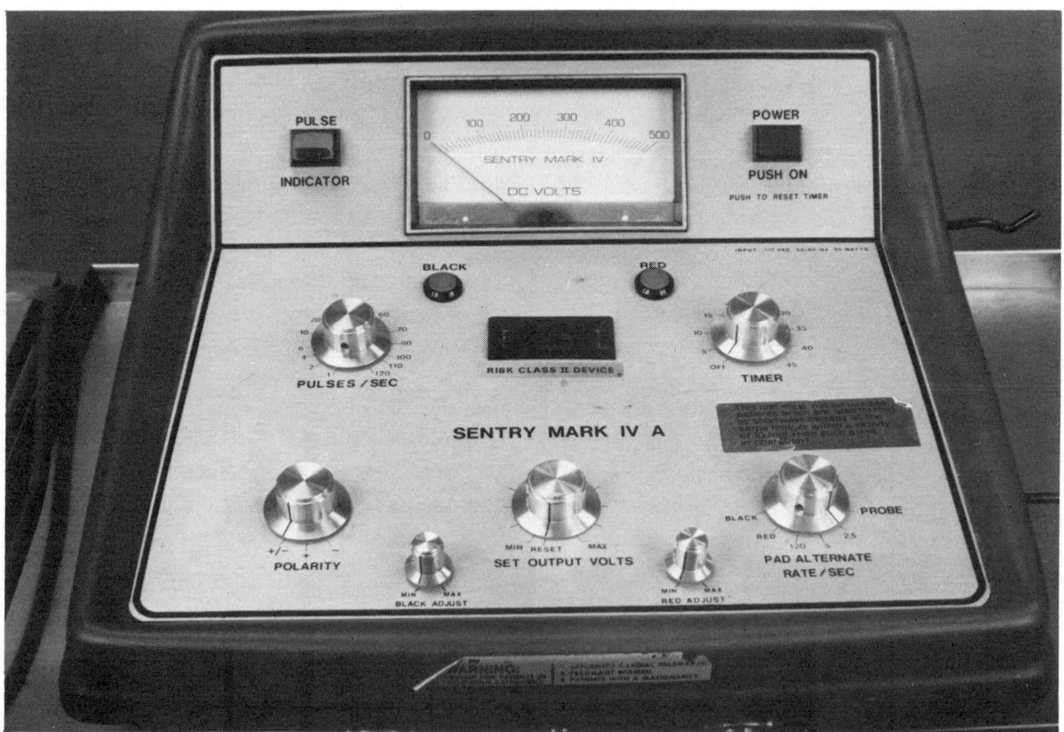

Figure 8.5. Control panel of a Sentry high-volt unit.

(2) a "Switch Rate" mode, where the separate active electrodes operate alternately, and (3) an "Interrupted" mode, where the current of both active electrodes is simultaneously turned on and off.

CONTINUOUS RATE MODE

The "Continuous" setting on some high-volt units is confusing to many operators. The pps rate may be delivered at a constant pace on the dial labeled "Continuous." This means that the patient is continuously being stimulated. It does not infer that the wave form (shape) is continuous (ie, the wave is always pulsed); rather, it means that a continuous stimulus will be delivered at the particular frequency (pulse rate) set by the operator. For example, if the mode control is set on "Continuous" and the pulse rate is set at 30, the patient will be stimulated continuously at a rate of 30 times every second during application. This is in direct contrast to the next type of setting, which is called the "Switch Rate" mode. The "Continuous" setting is recommended whenever the objective of the treatment is the reduction of edema, pain modulation, or stimulation of nervous tissue. It is generally not used if the goal is to fatigue spastic muscles.

SWITCH RATE MODE

This control permits the operator to alternately switch the current on or off under one or more specific electrodes. An application example might be in the paraspinal treatment of the lumbar spine where the active electrodes are placed over the left and right loins. A "Switch Rate" setting permits the contraction (exercise) of first one side and then the other on an alternating basis. That is, one side is allowed to relax while the other side is active.

This setting has two important advantages: (1) It permits alternating tetany bilaterally; ie, first one side and then the other. This is a more effective method of breaking muscle spasm than the "Continuous Rate" mode. (2) It limits accommodation of the tissues to the stimulation. See Figure 8.6.

Parameters for Setting the Switch Rate. Keeping in mind that there are no specific clinical studies at this writing that prove

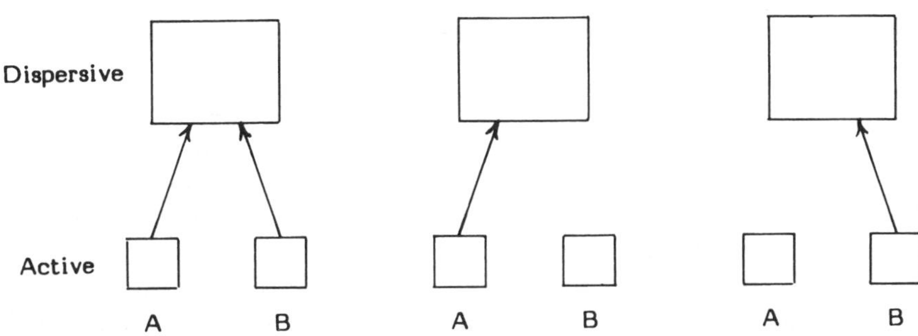

Figure 8.6. *Left diagram,* on the "Continuous" setting of a high-volt unit, the current flows without interruption from the active electrodes to the indifferent electrode. *Middle and right diagrams,* with the cyclic "Switch Rate" mode, the current from Electrode A flows to the indifferent electrode for 5 seconds while Electrode B is inactive; then the current from Electrode B flows to the indifferent electrode for 5 seconds while Electrode A is inactive.

without question that one particular switch rate has an advantage over another, the following guidelines that are based on the authors' empirical findings can be used in setting particular control dials on a high-volt unit:

1. *The 2.5-second switch rate.* A particular clinical entity that responds well to this setting has not as yet been found. To date, it has received minimal attention except by some in extremely acute cases; but even then, it has not been found to be as effective as the "Continuous" mode for treating acute disorders.

2. *The 5.0-second switch rate.* Patients with moderate—acute pain seem to tolerate this setting well. Therefore, this is the preferred setting for the great majority of cases when high-volt therapy is selected.

3. *The 10.0-second (or more) switch rate.* This setting is used for patients with stubbornly chronic musculoskeletal complaints; however, it is generally far too harsh for patients in acute pain.

INTERRUPTED MODE

This technique is sometimes called a "Surge On" and "Surge Off" setting. That is, the pulses delivered to the patient are interrupted from all active electrodes on a regular basis. With this particular setting, for example, the unit can be set at 50 pps for 5-second active and 10-second inactive intervals. This means that 50 pulses per second will be delivered to the patient for 5 seconds, the current is then turned off for 10 seconds, and the cycle is repeated. On most units, the "On" and "Off" phases can be set anywhere from 1 to 40 seconds.

The effect of an interrupted mode is alternating bilateral activation and relaxation. This technique has been shown to be valuable when muscle reeducation or strengthening is the objective.

PARAMETERS FOR SETTING THE PULSE RATE

1. *1—10 pps.* This setting, especially around 5 pps, is used frequently for muscle stimulation or pain modulation when a small diameter electrode is used. If the correct site is located and stimulation is at an intensity above the sensory level, good results will be achieved in producing muscle contraction under the electrode. This procedure also appears to be the most efficient for triggering the production of endogenous endorphins by high voltage modalities. Although high-volt units do not seem to be as effective as low-volt alternating currents in triggering endorphin release, they are still highly effective for this purpose.

2. *10—15 pps.* At this pulse rate, a twitching form of muscle contraction may be achieved; thus, a setting in this range is used whenever muscle exercise is the objective. High-volt therapy is not effective, however, for exercising muscle tissue if there has been a complete reaction of degeneration in peripheral nerves. When the development of strength and tone in muscles, tendons, and ligaments is desired, whatever passive exercise is accomplished with a modality should be with a surged setting (if it is available with the unit).

Note: Electrical stimulation for muscle exercise should never be a replacement for a well developed exercise program done by the patient periodically throughout the day.

3. *15 pps and Greater.* Muscles tend to tetanize when the pulse rate progressively exceeds 15 pps. The degree of tetany achieved depends on the number of muscle fibers or motor units that are stimulated. Once most all motor units of a part have been excited, full tetany will be achieved and a further increase in pulse rate will have no additional effect on tetany. If muscle tetany is desired without the effect of muscle fatigue, then a pulse rate of 20—80 pps is generally recommended. See Figure 8.7.

4. *70—110 pps.* A number of studies have

indicated that a pulse rate in the 70—110 pps range is the most advantageous for triggering *enkephalin* production for the purpose of pain control. This does not contradict the fact, previously described above (1.), that the 1—10 pps rate is recommended for triggering *endorphin* production.

Pulse Duration

Pulse duration, more appropriately termed *pulse width,* represents that period of time when spikes are created in the current wave. It is measured at 50% of the peak pulse amplitude. In contrast with high-volt units, the pulse in low-volt units exists for a relatively long period (eg, 1—300 milliseconds or longer).

PULSE DURATION IN HIGH-VOLT UNITS

In high-volt stimulators, the duration of the pulses is much shorter than the intervals between the pulses. One of the effects of this is that the average current is increased as the pulse rate is increased. See Figure 8.8. For this reason, it is important to remember that as the pulse rate is increased, the current intensity should be lowered proportionately or patient discomfort will reach an intolerable level. The average current in high-volt units does not exceed 2 ma. Any amount over this would burn the patient. As the voltage (electromotive force) is increased, the pressure (push) driving the minimal current that the unit has into the patient is increased. If the

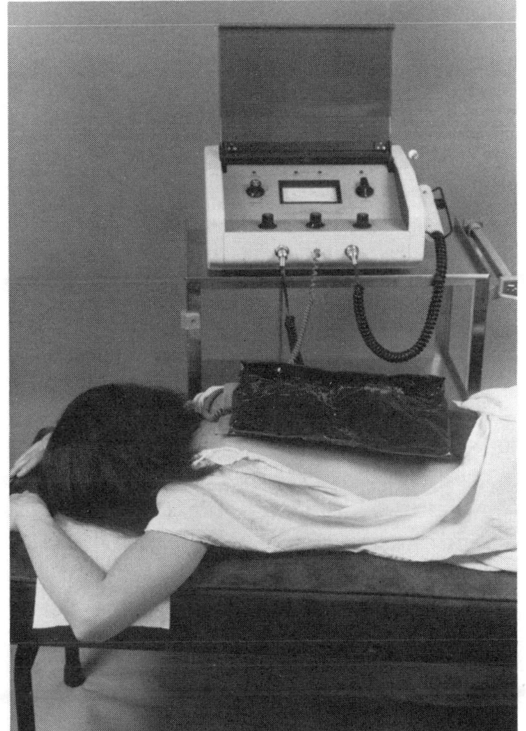

Figure 8.7. The application of high-volt therapy for a problem in the upper lumbar area.

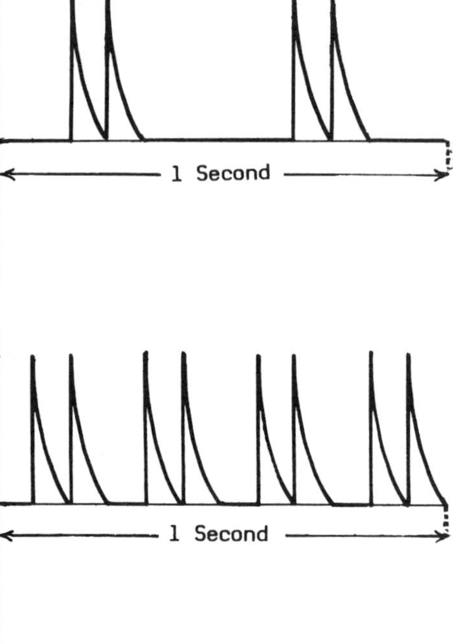

Figure 8.8. Effects of an increased pulse rate on average current in high-volt units. *Top diagram,* the pulse rate is set at 2 pps. *Bottom diagram,* when the pps is doubled to 4 pps, the average current the patient receives becomes doubled.

current force is increased too rapidly, tissue resistance to this becomes highly painful to the patient.

COMPARATIVE PULSE DURATION IN LOW-VOLT UNITS

The relatively long duration that is characteristic of the pulses in low-volt units is associated with several salient features:

1. The longer the pulse duration, the more buildup of chemical charges below the electrodes. In addition, pulses that are polarity symmetrical (as in a sine wave) have no buildup of chemical charges. This effect is referred to as Zero Net Charge (ZNC). See Figure 8.9. Pulses that are not equal symmetrically may develop a net charge equivalent to their parameters(+/−).

With low-volt continuous galvanic current, the monophasic wave precipitates the buildup of considerable electric charges that are associated with well-defined chemical and thermal changes. In comparison, the current in high-volt units is monophasic and is always a pulsed wave. There has been considerable debate as to whether or not this wave produced by high-volt units is associated with an accumulation of chemical changes. A study conducted at the University of Virginia that measured skin pH following high-volt stimulation demonstrated that no statistically significant changes occurred.[10] The pulse durations that are delivered with high-volt units are extremely short, measured in microseconds. It has been postulated that a pulse wave must be "on" for at least 1 millisecond in order to achieve any significant chemical changes.

In addition to the pulse duration being extremely short in high-volt units, the duration between the pulses is relatively long. This further decreases the possibility of the buildup of chemical charges. The body's normal

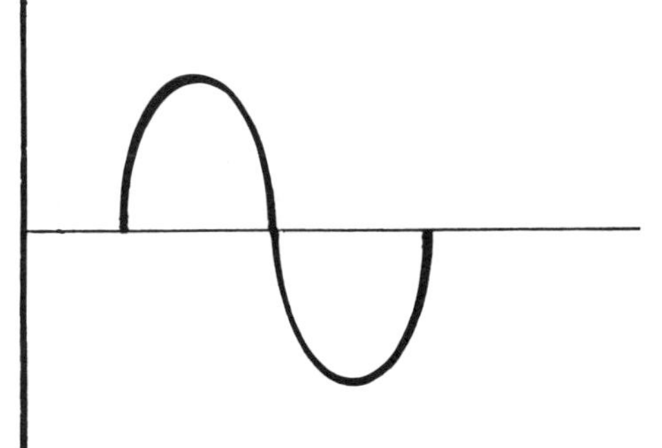

Figure 8.9. Diagram of a sine wave. A sine wave is an example of a symmetrical pulse. The current under the positive and negative electrodes is equal, and there is no net buildup of chemical charges within the involved tissues.

homeostatic mechanisms readily neutralize the slight charges that might occur, thus decreasing the chance of accumulation. See Figure 8.10.

Although there are apparently no "net" charges with high-volt therapy (hence, no or insignificant iontophoresis), there is definitely a different perception (sensation) when the polarity of the current entering the patient is altered. It has been contended that the temporary buildup of charge below the electrodes is a "trigger factor" that stimulates some of the changes with which high-volt stimulation is credited; viz, enhanced tissue regeneration and healing.

2. Short pulse durations are less irritating to body tissue than long pulse durations. Thus, high-volt therapy stimulation is more comfortable to the patient. This feature is more than likely a result of the fact that there is no significant net chemical buildup or pH changes, and, hence, minimal adverse irritation.

3. As has been noted earlier, the short pulse duration during high-volt stimulation permits the excitation of nervous tissue in a specific progression: first light sensory fibers, then motor fibers, and finally the pain-provoking fibers. This effect, which offers the patient the ability to discriminate, is one of the most valuable features of high-volt units in that it permits the operator to activate or stimulate just sensory fibers when only pain control (via stimulation of the dorsal columns of the spinal cord) is desired.

4. Another factor closely associated to pulse duration is the *interpulse duration.* These intervals in high-volt units are relatively long, and this also has the effect of decreasing the chemical changes and their byproduct accumulations in the tissues beneath the electrodes.

Microinterval Spacing

Some high-volt units have a setting that controls the interval between the twin pulses. These intervals are adjusted within a range of from 5 to 125 microseconds, depending on the particular unit. Most units preset the interval duration at a setting of 65—75 microseconds. However, this setting is currently being debated as to its value. Few operators have noted significant, if any, physiologic changes or better results in units utilizing this setting. In fact, some investigators have noted that there is no clinical value to the second spike and, thus, no clinical significance to a microsecond interval setting.

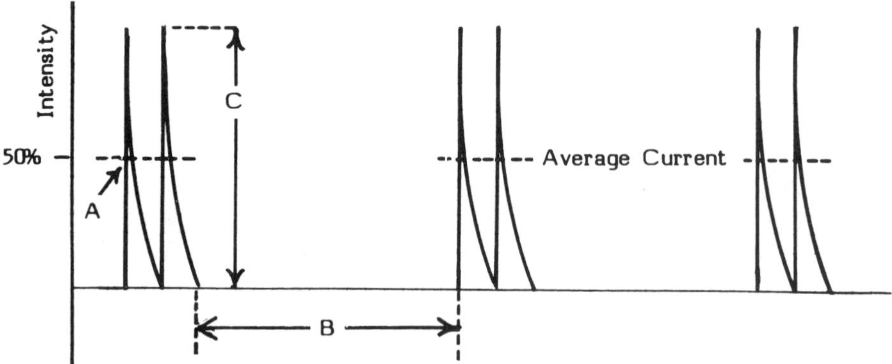

Figure 8.10. Diagram of the pulse duration, interpulse interval, and amplitude peak of the current generated by a high-volt unit. *A,* pulse duration, measured at 50% of peak amplitude; *B,* interpulse interval; *C,* peak current, representing the highest magnitude of the pulse amplitude.

Since patient comfort is definitely influenced by this setting, those parameters that might be considered if the unit has this setting are listed below:

1. Lower the microsecond interval setting to bring the twin pulse peaks closer together, thereby increasing the current concentration and bringing about increased excitation.
2. The microsecond interval setting can be increased for patients who are hypersensitive or in acute pain. Increasing the setting widens the twin peaks, and the stimulation feels more comfortable to the patient. This will permit the operator to increase the peak intensity without producing undue irritation.
3. The usual range of spacing (eg, from 50—75 microseconds) permits stimulation mainly of sensory and motor fibers, with minimal stimulation to those fibers that conduct pain-producing impulses.

Charge of the Pulses

Pulse charge is represented by the total amount of actual electricity that is absorbed by the tissues of the body with each individual pulse. The pulse charge is a factor that is inherent to each specific piece of equipment, and it cannot be controlled by the operator. It should be noted, however, that this charge should not exceed 20—100 microcoulombs per pulse/cm^2 of electrode size. This rarely exceeds 25 microcoulombs in high-volt units. The amount of charge determines, in part, the type of nerve fibers that are excited (ie, nonpainful sensory, motor, nociceptive).

PHYSIOLOGIC EFFECTS AND APPLICATIONS

In general, it can be said that high-volt therapy affects body tissues in certain specific ways to modulate pain, muscle spasm, inflammation, tissue healing and repair, based on the way that the control settings on the unit are adjusted. The major effects may be summarized as follows:

1. Pain reduction
2. Muscle spasm reduction
3. Muscular exercise and reeducation
4. Circulation enhancement

5. Edema reduction
6. Insignificant chemical changes without appreciable iontophoresis.

Pain

High-volt stimulation is one of the major therapies that may be used for pain control.[11-15] At 70—110 pps, when the active electrodes are placed over the site involved (ie, the same dermatomal level), analgesia may take place via the postulates of the Gate Control Theory.

Since pain reactions occur in an alkaline area, positive polarity is recommended when using the 3-inch × 3-inch or 4-inch × 4-inch electrodes over the site of pain (eg, sprain, strain, stasis). The area under the positive pole tends to become acidic. Trigger points, on the other hand, are localized areas that are acidic. This is due to the abundance of hyaluronic acid, P factor, bradykinin, histamine, mucopolysaccharides, and water (70%) within a trigger point. Thus, the acidic trigger point is best resolved by using a small diameter electrode that emits a negative polarity and produces an alkaline reaction.

Some doctors prefer to dissipate trigger areas by using ultrasound in combination with a high-volt current whenever a combination unit is available.

Pain modulation may only be achieved during the time of therapy. Thus, its effect is greatest preparatory to any adjustive procedure. If the pain is acute, the intensity is increased only to the point where the patient barely perceives a sensation of stimulation. After the acute stage has passed and the patient is out of immediate distress, which is usually by the second or third visit, the intensity can be increased to patient tolerance in an attempt to fatigue spastic musculature.

At the conclusion of treatment, pain can also be controlled by using the small diameter probe over the most tender trigger point (called the *ah shi* point by Orientals) and one of three acupuncture sites (LI-4, HC-6, or BL-51), depending on where the tender site is located. Stimulation should be applied at each of these two sites for about 20—30 seconds, using a small electrode with a negative polarity at an intensity up to patient tolerance.

Muscle Spasm and Muscle Weakness

According to the situation at hand, motor stimulation may be used to tetanize muscles or to exercise muscles. When the patient has passed the acute stage, muscles can be tetanized at a 70—110 pulse rate. Although most muscles are in tetany at 15—20 pps, the higher setting is preferred (along with a 2.5, 5.0, or 10.0 Switch Rate) in an attempt to also trigger the production of enkephalins for pain control.

Care must be taken not to tetanize muscle fibers that are in acute spasm. A tetanizing current applied early in the treatment regimen may severely aggravate the patient's condition and prolong healing.

Once the problem of muscle spasm has been resolved, especially following a musculoskeletal injury, attention may be directed toward building up strength in the involved muscles, tendons, and ligaments.[16] As a general rule in muscle reeducation, a negative polarity is used and the pulse rate is set at 100 pps with a "Surge Off" time that is from three to four times longer than the "Surge On" time. Thus, if the intensity surges "On" for 3 seconds, the rest period ("Off" time) should be set at 10 or 11 seconds. Allowing a rest period that is several times longer than the "On" time reduces the chance of excessively fatiguing the muscles being treated. See Figure 8.11.

Note: When muscle reeducation is attempted in cases where the CNS is involved a much slower pulse rate is preferred (eg about 15 pps).

Specific muscles or muscle groups may also be exercised by using a high-volt current to stimulate motor nerve points (eg, in facial paralysis). In such cases, a pulse rate of 4—5 pps applied for 10 seconds to each point i

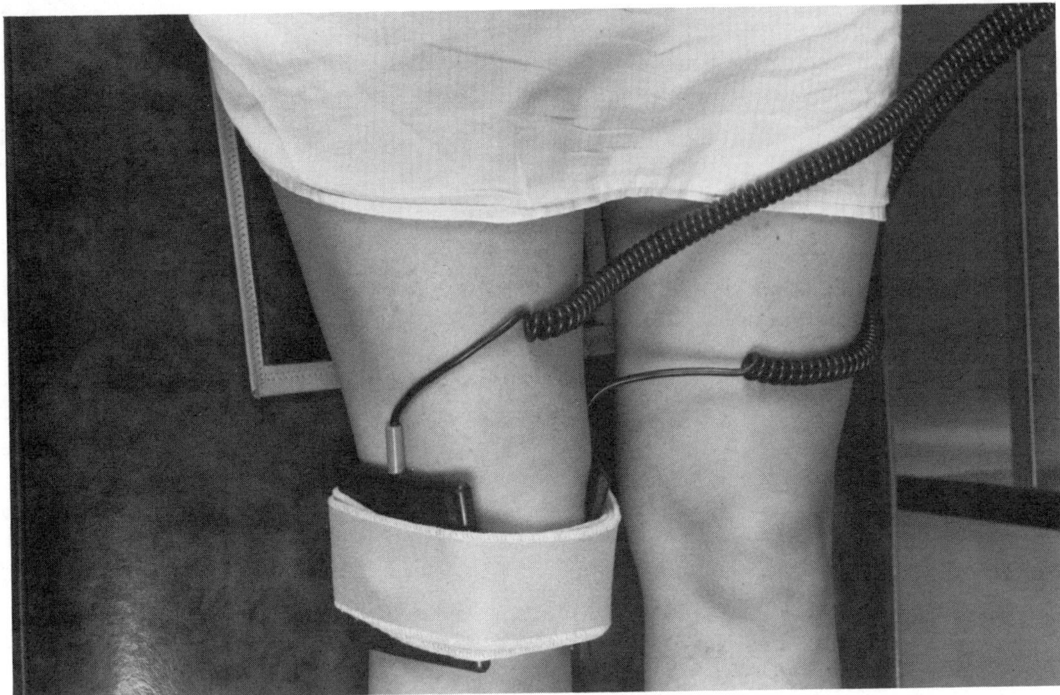

Figure 8.11. Pad placement for applying high-volt therapy to a knee disorder.

recommended. The usual procedure is to treat the contralateral (unaffected) side first, then the involved side.

Most functional palsies show no motor deficit. It should be noted, however, that high-volt therapy has not proved to be of clinical value in patients who have suffered a peripheral nerve injury and show signs of highly deficient innervation to specific muscles.

Increasing Circulation

It has been our experience that high voltage currents appear to stimulate a slight increase in the microcirculation by means of a reflex effect following excitation of autonomic nerves. However, this slight effect seems to have no appreciable clinical significance and present claims to the contrary are unwarranted according to the data available. Considerably more investigation is needed in this area.

Reduction of Edema

High-volt currents as a modality used to remove edema have proved to be highly efficient. As a pulsed stimulator, in contrast to a continuous current applicator, the "pumping" effect of a high-volt unit is excellent when acute posttraumatic edema is present.[17]

When edema reduction is the sole objective of adjunctive therapy, a low pulse rate (eg, below 10 pps) is recommended. It is helpful to add pressure to the active electrodes (placed over the edematous area) with cold packs to enhance the therapeutic effect. See Figure 8.12.

In treating a sprained ankle or wrist, for example, the part can be placed in a plastic tub filled with cold water and the active electrodes can be submerged into the water at the sides of the injured joint. Care should be taken not to increase the intensity above the light sensory level, as this will have a tenden-

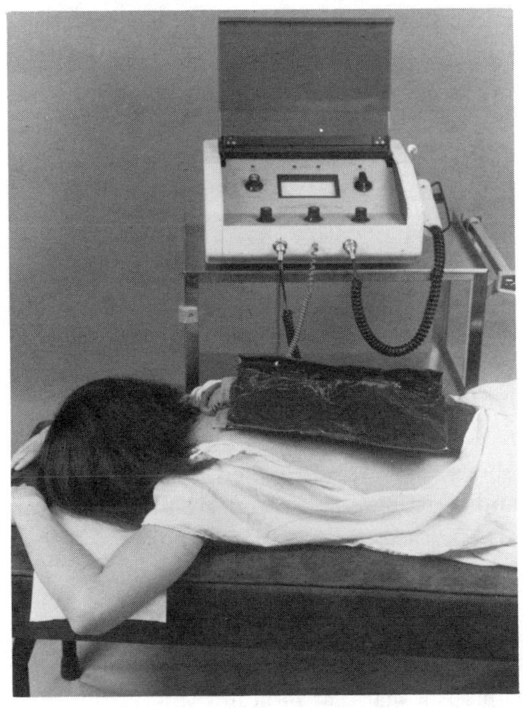

Figure 8.12. Active high-volt pads being secured by cold packs.

cy to aggravate the patient's condition. Polarity does not seem to have a major effect in such cases; however, it has been generally found empirically that results are better when therapy is started with a negative polarity and finished with a positive polarity. See Figure 8.13.

Tissue Healing

There have been some reports as to the possible healing effects of high voltage currents. Some hospitals have been using positive polarity sensory stimulation on the continuous mode with good results in the treatment of severe burns. Although some minimal documentation of these beneficial effects have been published, it is unlikely that healing could occur unless there was a temporary buildup of chemical changes associated with a high peak current to permit deep penetration. It is widely believed that studies in the near future will document the effects of high-volt currents in the healing of damaged soft-tissue, fractured bone, and injured nerves.

CONTRAINDICATIONS

A high-volt unit is one of the safest modalities in use today. It seems that the worst effects possible are caused by increasing the intensity too rapidly, thereby pushing the current at such a rapid rate that tissue accommodation cannot occur. When this happens, considerable discomfort is administered to the patient even though a burn does not occur.

The three standard contraindications to high-volt therapy are:

1. Applications over the low back or abdomen during pregnancy.
2. Over neoplastic areas.
3. Using on patients wearing a pacemaker.

It should also be mentioned that extreme

caution must be used if application is made near the heart or carotid sinus, and any possible clinical value of applying high-volt transcerebrally is highly questionable.

UTILIZING A HIGH-VOLT UNIT

High-volt units are available in both cabinet and portable units. Some portable units are shown in Figure 8.14.

Although the use of different adjustments on high-volt modalities has been described previously, the effects of adjusting the control dials found on most units are worthy of summarization here to underscore the results that can be expected.

Timer/Treatment Time

The timer on the unit sets the treatment duration and automatically shuts the current off when the time parameter is reached. The treatment times generally used with pads vary from 15 to 25 minutes. Treatments of less than 15 minutes are of limited clinical value when 3 × 3 or 4 × 4 electrode pads are used. When a probe is used to exercise small muscle groups (eg, hand, face, foot), 3—5 minutes is usually sufficient. Acupuncture points can be effectively stimulated in 20—30 seconds. In some stubborn cases (eg, unremitting chronic sciatica), treatment durations of 30—45 minutes with pads have proved to be highly significant.

Polarity Switch

All high-volt units have positive and negative polarity switches. When the switch is set on positive (+), the active pads are positive and the indifferent dispersal pad serves as the negative pole. The opposite is true if the switch is set on negative (−).

The intensity level should always be greatly decreased prior to changing polarity. In addition, as a safety factor, most units will automatically shut off if the polarity switch is changed during a treatment. If this occurs, the operator should turn the intensity dial back to zero and reset it after the polarity switch has been set.

POSITIVE POLARITY

A positive polarity is used with 3 × 3 or 4 × 4 pads (active electrodes). It has an analgesic effect over areas of pain, tends to constrict blood vessels, and has a mild germicidal effect.

NEGATIVE POLARITY

A negative polarity is used to treat trigger points, dilate blood vessels, soften adhesions, and to exercise and reeducate muscles. It can also be used to locate trigger points.

Intensity

The intensity control in most high-volt units is a dial that indicates volt output from 0 to 500. One unit also has a milliamperage reading from 0 to 2500.

The following guidelines are generally applicable:

1. Increase the intensity level just to where the patient barely senses the sensory stimulation effect if pain control, edema reduction, or tissue healing of burns or wounds is the objective.
2. Slowly increase the intensity level to patient tolerance when muscle exercise or a tetanizing current is desired.
3. The intensity level should be set at the high motor or the pain threshold when acupuncture points are treated with the small diameter electrode.

Most of the newer units have an intensity balance switch that permits the operator to increase the intensity level at either active pad to achieve the balance desired. The level of intensity may be increased any time after the treatment has been initiated without danger of burning the patient. As previously described, this is because the maximum average current with a high-volt modality never exceeds 1.5—2.0 milliamperes.

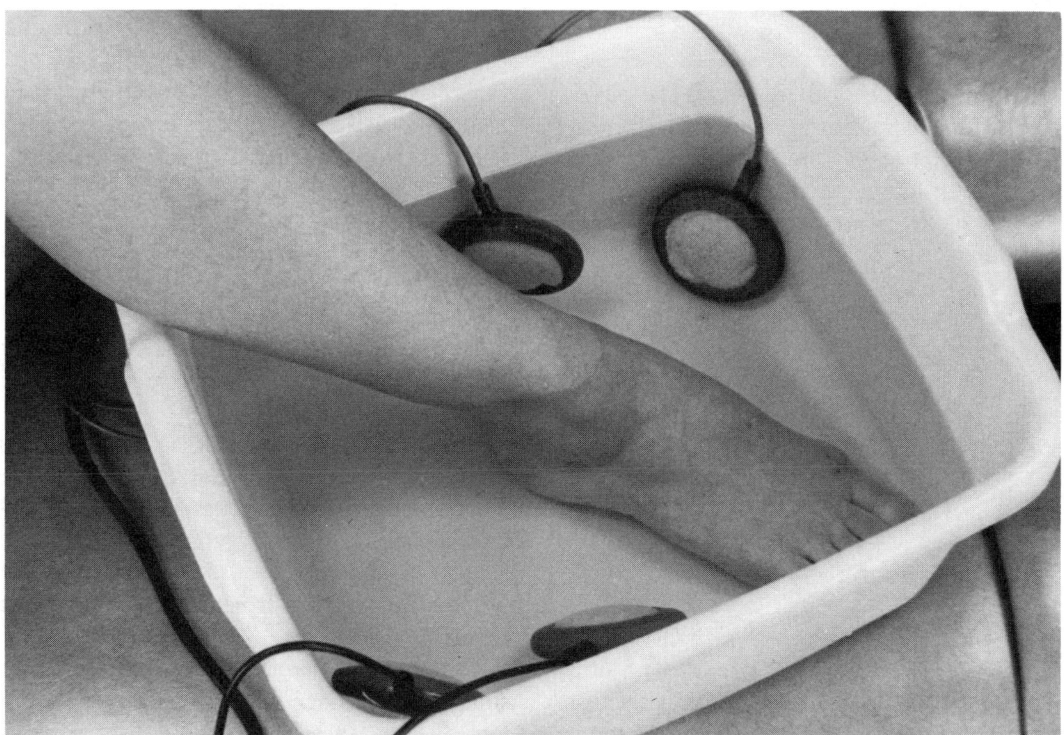

Figure 8.13. Use of high-volt electrodes under water. Although the photograph depicts sponge inserts within the electrodes, some operators feel that better conductivity is achieved if they are removed.

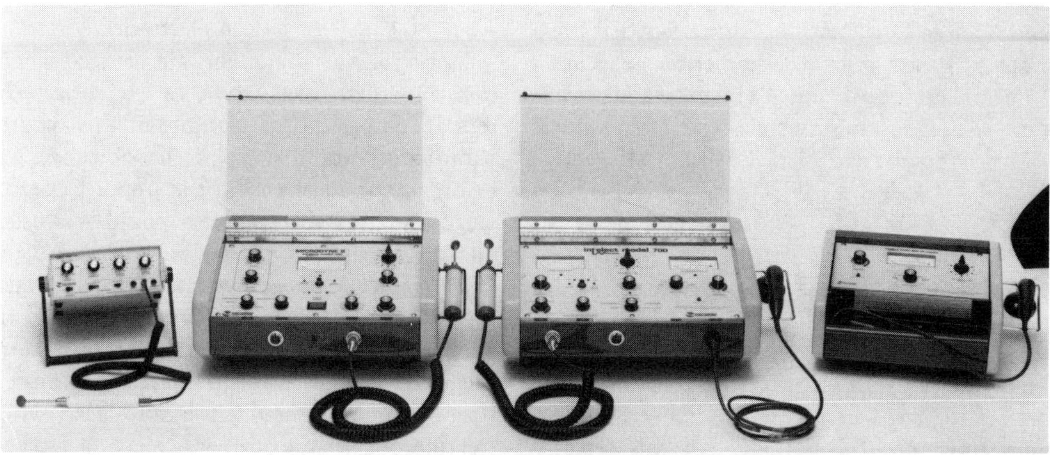

Figure 8.14. Shown from left to right are a portable HV unit, a Microdyne II HV unit, an Intelect HV unit with ultrasound, and a portable ultrasound unit.

Pad Switch Rate

The current being delivered to the patient can be altered so that it either flows continuously or alternately through the active pads. The "Continuous" mode is generally used for edema reduction, light sensory stimulation, and the promotion of healing. The "Switch Rate" mode is usually used alternately to exercise or tetanize one muscle group and then another.

For more information, please refer to an earlier section in this chapter titled "Varying the Pulse Rate on a High Voltage Unit."

Pulses per Second

The current frequency of a high-volt unit is measured in pulses per second. The original low frequency high-volt units ranged only from 1 to 28 pps. Those who first manufactured these units stated that 20 pps had been found to be the ideal setting for tetanizing muscle groups. However, later research and clinical indications led to today's standards that require units with ranges of up to 120 pps.

Parameters for setting the pulse rate, the microsecond interval spacing of the twin spikes of the pulse, and the "Surge On" and "Surge Off" settings were described previously. Please refer to the section headings, "Pulse Duration" and "Microinterval Spacing." Surge rates were described under "Muscle Spasm and Muscle Weakness."

Electrodes and Pad Placement

Several recent studies indicate that rigid electrodes are less effective than flexible electrodes in terms of efficiently delivering current flow into the patient. For this reason, most companies that were supplying rigid electrodes with sponge inserts are now supplying more flexible electrodes that readily conform to anatomical contours.

As a general rule, it can be stated that the closer the active electrodes are to the dispersive electrode, the less depth of penetration. For example in treating a superficial lumbar strain or sprain, the dispersive electrode is placed as near as possible to the active electrodes. If a disc syndrome is being treated, however, the dispersive electrode is placed quite far from the active pads (eg, anterior thigh or abdomen). General suggestions are shown in Table 8.1.[18]

One, two, three, or four active electrodes (of various sizes) can be used, depending on whether the operator desires to stimulate specific points or treat a large area diffusely. Appliance cabinets are usually constructed to hold a number of accessories, as shown in Figure 8.15.

Following are some general guidelines that should be considered when placing monopolar, bipolar, specific small diameter, or dispersive electrodes.

MONOPOLAR PAD PLACEMENT

With this technique, a large dispersive pad is used in conjunction with one, two, three, or four active pads of smaller though not necessarily of equal size. Small diameter (ECG-like) electrodes can also be used in place of 3 × 3 or 4 × 4 electrodes.

Monopolar arrangements are utilized whenever a "splash over" type of excitatory pattern is indicated. An example of this type of stimulation would occur if the objective was to break muscle spasm in the upper trapezius area. Two active electrodes could be used: one on either side of the trapezius, with the dispersive pad placed over the upper thoracic spine. This arrangement brings about fairly deep penetration of current and is recommended whenever deep nerve or muscle stimulation is desired. It is also used when treating edematous areas, relaxing spastic areas, muscle reeducation, and treating disuse atrophy of specific muscle groups.

Table 8.1. General Guidelines in Applying High-Volt Stimulation*

Condition	*Mode*	*Where to Apply*	*Rate (sec)*	*Polarity*	*Pulse*	*Time (min)*
Soft tissue	Pads or water	Over affected area	10	-	60—80	15—20
Acute spasm	Pads or hands applicator	Bilateral agonist and antagonist; use 4 pulses for 3 min to reeducate	10	- +	60—80 4—5	8—10 8—10
Neuritis, radiculitis, nonmuscular pain	Pads, water, hand applicator	Source of innervation; trace along nerve to affected area	10	+	80	15—20
Trigger point therapy	Hand applicator	Locate trigger point at moderate intensity; repeat to tolerance if necessary. Reduce intensity before going to another point		- +	80	⅓—1
Bursitis	Pads, hand applicator	Place pads over affected area; use hand applicator over related trigger points and areas of residual pain after pad treatment	10	- +	60—80	15—20
Sciatica, nonradiating	Pads, hand applicator	Two pads over lumbar spine; hand applicator to desensitize areas of residual pain	10	- +	80	15—20
Sciatica, radiating	Pads, hand applicator	One pad over lumbar spine and one pad over extremity pain, iliac crest, or buttock	10	- +	60—80	15—20
Arthritic joint (hands or feet)	Water, hand applicator	Place part in water if possible; palpate for painful areas. Use hand applicator in positive	10	- +	80	8—10
Edema with pain	Pads, water	Place over affected area. Intensity to tolerance at 15 min, 80 pulses or 5 min at lower pulse setting	5	-	80	20

Table 8.1, continued

Condition	*Mode*	*Where to Apply*	*Rate (sec)*	*Polarity*	*Pulse*	*Time (min)*
Edema without pain	Pads, water	Same as above except with a lower pulse rate	5—10	-	4—5	20
Scars, adhesions	Pads	Place over affected area	10	-	60—80	15—20
Wry neck or shoulders	Pads, hand applicator	Pads over both trapezius muscles; hand applicator over cervicals and thoracic spine, scapulae. Passive joint ROM exercise	10	- +	80	15—20
Bells palsy	Hand applicator, small electrode	Treat unaffected side first; 10 sec at each motor point		-	4—5	
Trifacial neuralgia	Hand applicator	Trace trigeminal nerve. Intensity to patient tolerance		+	80	
Open wounds, burns, skin ulcers	Pads, water	Remove sponges, use a sterile gauze pad to cover the wound. If water is used: 2% saline or Zephrian solution	10			20

*Based on Sentry Mark IV HV Unit.

BIPOLAR PAD PLACEMENT

In this arrangement, the active and dispersive electrodes used are of equal size. This method of stimulation is used when contractions of a specific muscle rather than of muscle groups are desired. The electrodes are placed at each end of the muscle selected to stimulate the motor nerve point, reeducate a specific muscle group, prevent atrophy, or promote posttraumatic healing in specific muscle(s).

SPECIFIC POINT TECHNIQUES

A variety of small diameter hand-held electrodes have been developed for use with the larger indifferent pad. See Figure 8.16. These small electrodes can be used for stimulating acupuncture points, auricular points, trigger points, motor nerve points, and mucous membranes. They are also helpful in treating small muscle groups on the face, hands, and feet.[19] A device is also available that can be rolled across the skin. The inten-

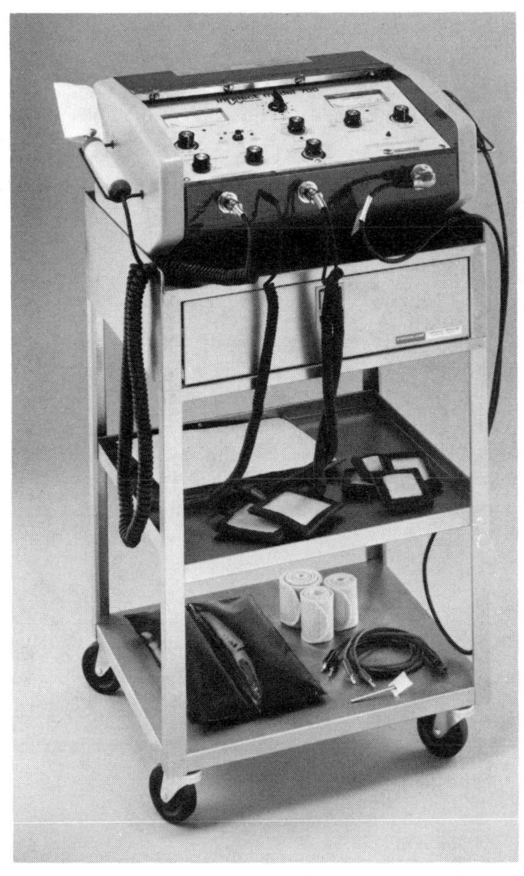

Figure 8.15. A Chattanooga high-volt unit with accessory stand.

sity and activating controls for a hand-held electrode are usually built into the handle of the instrument so that the operator has digital control of the intensity level desired and the ability to turn the applicator on or off.

THE DISPERSIVE PAD

The dispersive pad is typically an 8-inch × 10-inch flexible electrode. The contact area in the older types was a sponge that required saturation to assure good contact and conductivity. The newer pads are made of a flexible rubber-like material that only require an initial wiping with a damp cloth or sponge. During therapy, patient perspiration beneath the electrode maintains an efficient fluid interface for good conductivity.

The dispersive pad may be placed over most any broad body surface except the head, and it does not have to make total contact with the skin as long as the contact surface is larger than that of the sum of the active electrodes used. See Figure 8.17. For example, when trigger points are being treated with a small hand-held electrode, the patient need only place a palm on the dispersive pad.

Some patients feel uncomfortable when the dispersive pad is placed upon the abdomen. Thus, most operators avoid this arrangement when possible.

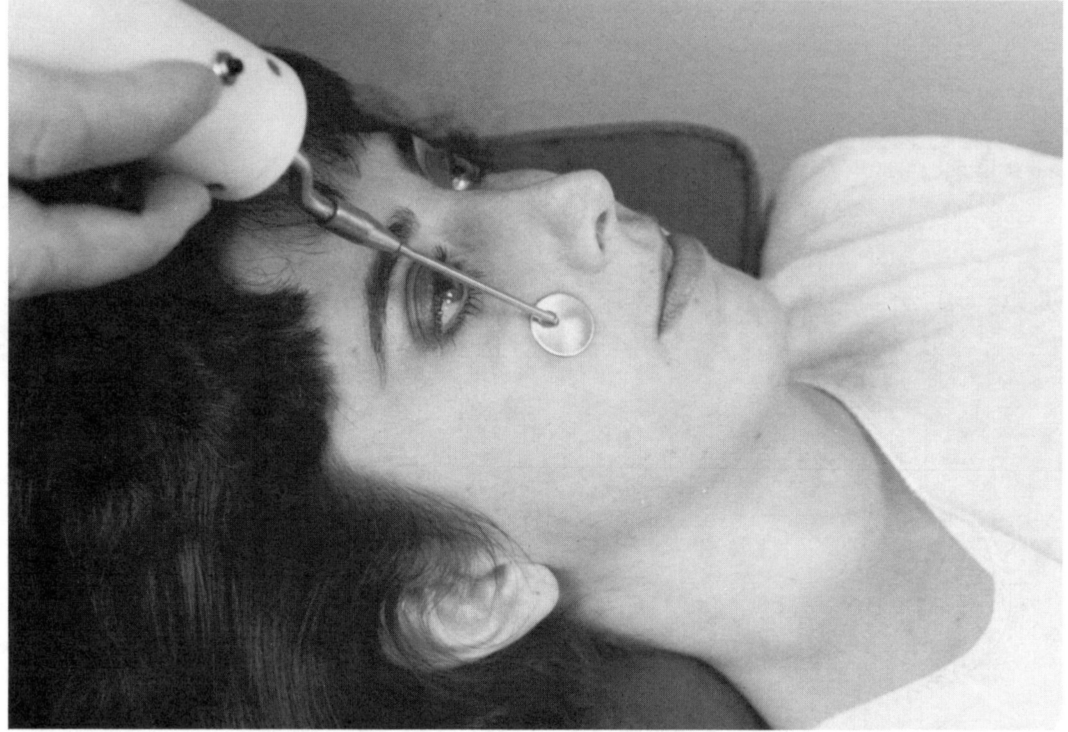

Figure 8.16. A small high-volt probe being used over the right maxillary sinus.

REFERENCES

1. Griffin JE, Karselis TC: *Physical Agents for Physical Therapists*. Springfield, IL, Charles C. Thomas, 1979.
2. Massey BH, et al: Effects of high frequency electrical stimulation on the size and strength of skeletal muscle. *Journal of Sports Medicine and Physical Fitness*, 5:136-144, 1965.
3. Alon G: High voltage stimulation (high voltage pulsating direct current). Monograph published by the Chattanooga Corporation, 1984.
4. Ghaznavi C: An investigation of pulse characteristics in the electrical stimulation of acupuncture loci. Paper presented to the Twelfth Annual Meeting of the Association for the Advancement of Medical Instrumentation, Arlington, VA, 1977.
5. Munsat TL, et al: Effects of nerve stimulation on human muscle. *Archives of Neurology*, 33:608-617, 1976.
6. Wolf SL (ed): *Electrotherapy*. New York, Churchill Livingston, 1982, pp 7-16.
7. Cooper IS, et al: Safety and efficacy of chronic stimulation. *Neurosurgery*, 1:203-205, 1977.
8. Howson DC: Peripheral neural excitability. *Physical Therapy*, 58:1467-1473, 1978.
9. Roth MG, Wolf SL: Monitoring stimulation parameters from clinical transcutaneous nerve stimulators. *Physical Therapy*, 58:586-587, 1978.
10. Newton RA, Karselis TC: Skin pH following high voltage pulsed galvanic stimulation. *Physical Therapy*, 63:1593-1596, 1983.
11. Gracanin F, Trnkoczy A: Optimal stimulus parameters for minimum pain in the chronic stimulation of innervated muscle. *Archives of Physical Medicine and Rehabilitation*, 53:243-249, 1975.
12. Vodovnik L, et al: Pain response to different tetanizing currents. *Archives of Physical Medicine and Rehabilitation*, 46:187-192, 1965.
13. Lampe GM: Introduction to the use of transcutaneous electrical stimulation devices. *Physical Ther-*

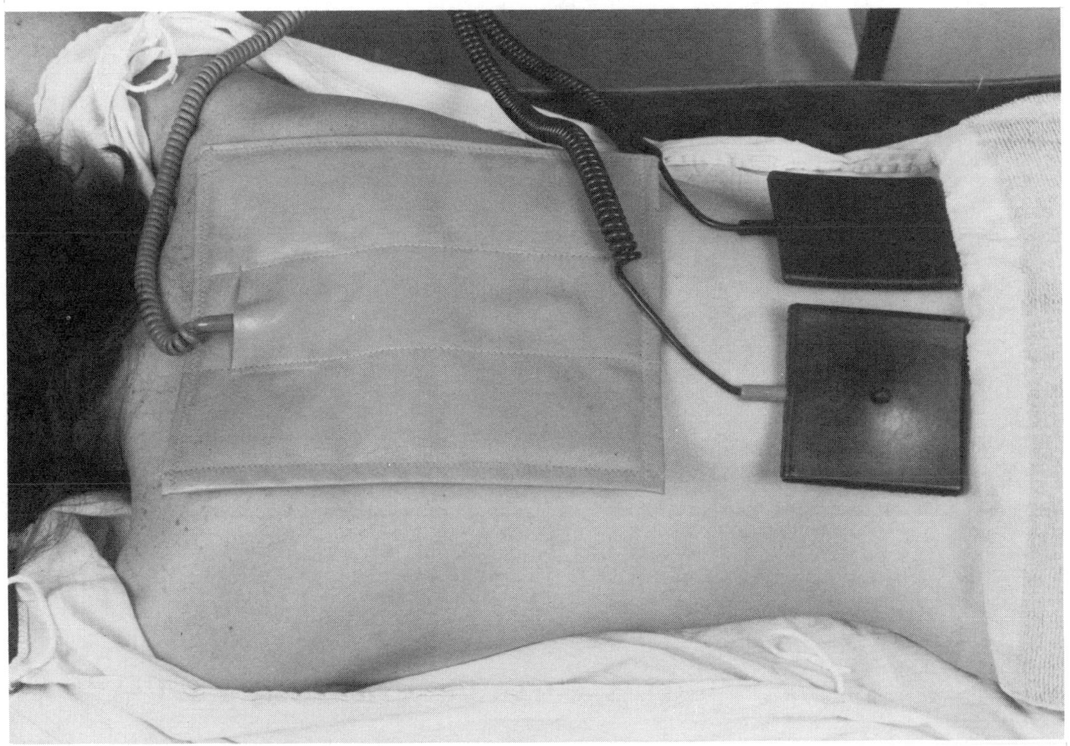

Figure 8.17. The indifferent (dispersive) pad is placed close to the active electrodes in cases of superficial muscle strain.

apy, 58:1450-1454, 1978.
14. Bishop B: Pain: its physiology and rationale for management. *Physical Therapy,* 60:13-37, 1980.
15. Wolf SL: Perspectives on central nervous system responsiveness to transcutaneous electrical nerve stimulation. *Physical Therapy,* 58:1443-1449, 1978.
16. Currier DP, et al: Electrical stimulation in exercise of the quadriceps femoris muscle. *Physical Therapy,* 59:1508-1512, 1979.
17. Genendlis R, et al: High voltage pulsed direct current effect on peripheral blood flow. Paper presented to the annual meeting of the Maryland Physical Therapy Association, Friedriksburg, MD, 1980.
18. Hill LL: *Parameters of Physiotherapy Modalities.* Lombard, IL, National Chiropractic College, class notes, date not shown, pp 115-116.
19. Milner M, et al: Force, pain, and electrode size in the electrical stimulation of leg muscles. *Nature,* 223:645, 1974.

Chapter 9

Interferential-Interference Current Therapy

One of the newest modalities being utilized today is interferential (interference) current therapy. Although this modality has been available in Europe since the 1950s, its use has gained widespread popularity in the United States only during the past decade or so.

This chapter describes the background, physiological basis, effects, application techniques, indications, and contraindications in the therapeutic use of interferential current.

INTRODUCTION

In previous chapters, high frequency and low frequency currents have been described, as well as such useful adjuncts as hot and cold packs, infrared and ultraviolet, etc. These previously described modalities have one basic principle in common: they all have their principal effects on the skin and, based on how efficiently or effectively the modality broke down skin resistance, they bring about certain specific effects on deeper tissues. In other words, each of these modalities produce their effects from the *outside to the inside;* thus, we can call these modalities *exogenous* physiotherapeutic approaches.

Mode Rationale

As each of the previous specific modalities were described, the effects that each had on breaking down skin resistance were explained and each modality could be classified according to the particular type of tissue in which the major effects occurred—skin, subcutaneous fat, muscle, bone, viscera, and the various tissue interfaces. Interferential current, on the other hand, is totally different from the other modalities that have been described. It consists of two medium frequency currents that cross deep within a body part, and, in so doing, trigger the formation of a *third* current that radiates from the *inside to the outside,* thus creating an *endogenous* physiotherapeutic approach.[1]

Historical Perspective

The modern therapeutic use of interferential current was first introduced in the early 1950s in Vienna by Nemec. Gildemeister had earlier introduced the term *medium frequency* in 1944, and his studies generally concentrated on medium frequencies from 2,000 to 3,000 cycles per second (Hz). Drawing from the studies made by Gildemeister,

Nemec utilized two crossed medium frequency currents.[2] Unfortunately, Gildemeister's and Nemec's work received little attention initially. It was not until the late 1970s and early 1980s that general interest among American clinicians developed to a significant extent.

THE PHYSIOLOGICAL BASIS

To fully appreciate this type of therapy, the reader should recall that one of the major effects of high frequency stimulation is that the frequency or rapidity with which the stimulus bombards the skin (eg, 100,000 Hz or more; with shortwave, 27 MHz) is so rapid that skin resistance is immediately overcome, allowing for deep penetration of the therapy. See Figure 9.1. Low frequency currents, in contrast, have frequencies of under 1,000 Hz and do not produce such deep penetration, but they do have a profound effect on electroexcitable tissues (eg, muscles, nerves).[3-7]

Background

For clinical purposes, the skin and its underlying tissues can be likened to electrical capacitors. As the frequency of a modality increases, the impedance of the "biological capacitor" decreases. Thus, with high frequency therapies, the impedance is quite low and a large percentage of the energy sup-

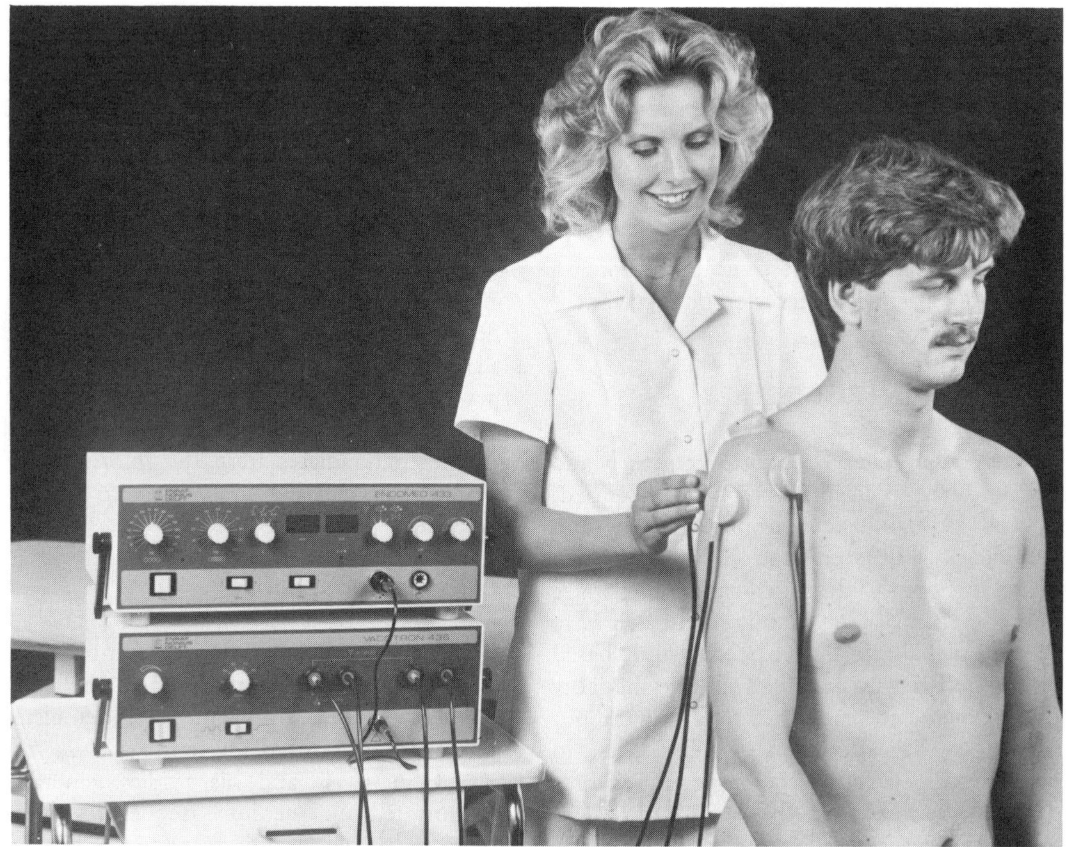

Figure 9.1. Application of interferential therapy to a patient's right shoulder.

plied by the generator is dissipated in the body tissues being treated.

It should also be noted that because of the nature of high frequency shortwave modalities, the electrodes do not make direct contact with the skin. Thus, it may be stated that the energy is capacitively coupled with the body via an electrode-skin interface. This is in sharp contrast with low frequency modalities wherein excitable tissues permit a passage of ions (flow of electric current) as the permeability of their membranes changes. The flow of current creates an electric field that reflects, to some degree, the activity of excitable tissues. Certain tissues (eg, nerve) readily conduct this current, while other tissues (eg, adipose, osseous) tend to resist the flow of current.

It has been established through numerous studies that different types of body tissues propagate impulses at different frequencies.[8] See Table 9.1.

Currents Commonly Used in Therapy

Different types of electric current are often used in therapy to treat various situations. For comparison of their wave characteristics, some of the most common types are shown in Figure 9.2.

INTERFERENTIAL CURRENT UTILIZATION

The currents used in interferential therapy are medium frequency alternating sine waves. Therapeutically, these currents are between 1,000 and 100,000 Hz.[9] The definition of the medium frequency range of therapy is based on electrophysiologic criteria; ie, the effects of these currents on the excitable tissues of the body.

Skin Impedance

It has been well established that skin impedance (resistance) is quite high in the low frequency ranges, with the resistance decreasing dramatically as the frequency increases. In addition, skin resistance decreases further when alternating currents are used, and Nippel shows that this process can be expressed mathematically.[10] In this context, skin resistance can be divided into two categories:

1. *Ohmic resistance.* This factor is independent of the frequency of the current.
2. *Capacitive resistance.* This factor is the patient's resistance to the current flow, and it is determined by the capacitance of superficial tissues. Capacitive resistance lowers as current frequency is increased.

Table 9.1. Comparison of Optimal Frequency to Achieve Maximum Tissue Response

Tissue Type	*Frequency*
Sympathetic nerves	0—5 Hz
Smooth muscle	0—10 Hz
Motor nerves	10—50 Hz
Parasympathetic nerves	10—150 Hz
Sensory nerves	90—110 Hz
Nociceptive system	130 Hz

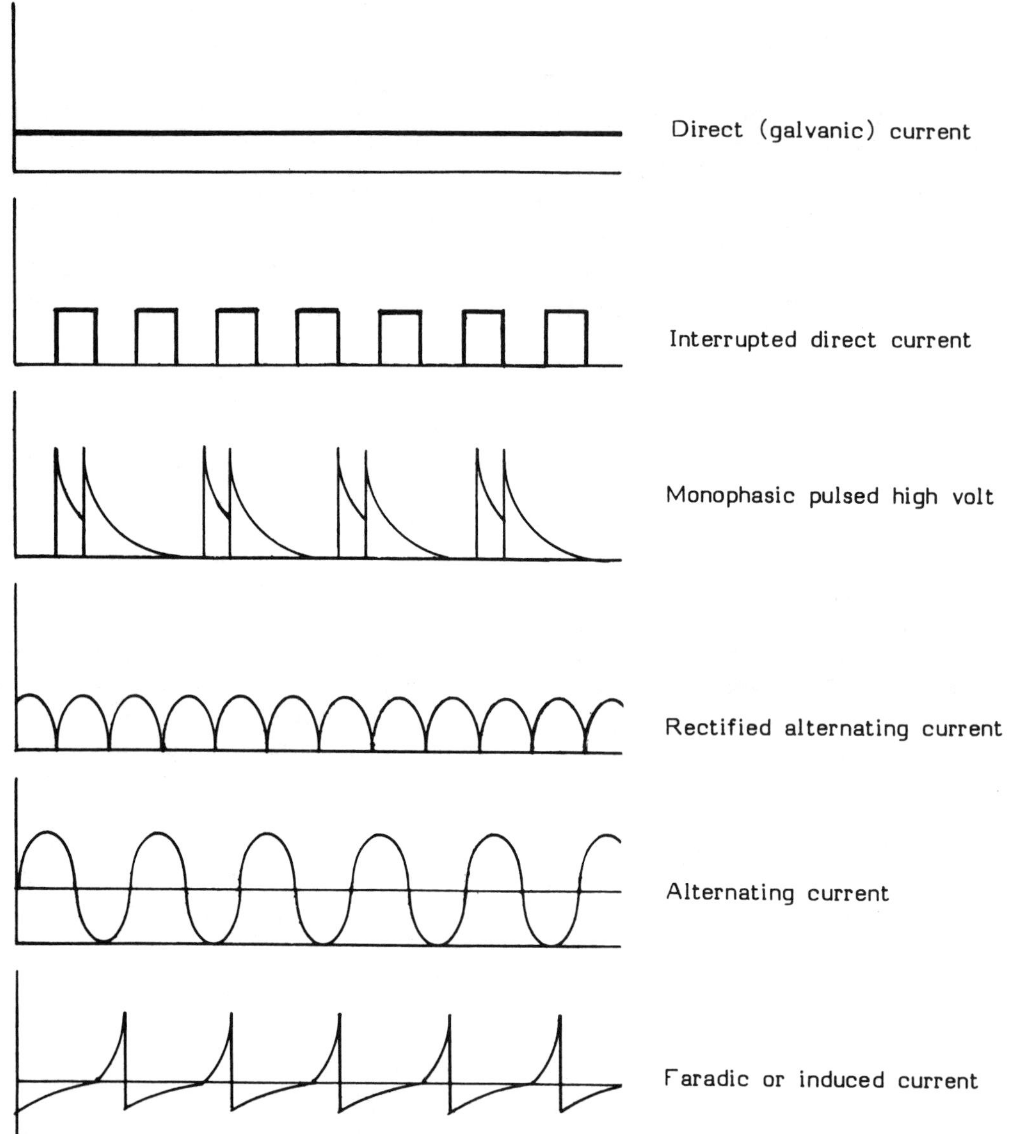

Figure 9.2. Schematics of common types of therapeutic currents.

Depolarization Factors

Thus, as opposed to low frequency currents, stimulation of body tissues with medium frequency currents brings about different effects. Based on which frequency of stimulation is used, depolarization can occur in one of two fashions:

1. *Cycle synchronous depolarization.* With a direct or alternating current, each pulse triggers a depolarization of involved nerve fibers (ie, providing the duration and strength of the pulse are adequate). This process is referred to as "cycle synchronous depolarization." Each nerve fiber, however, will have a maximal depolarization frequency that is determined by the refractory period. This will be in the vicinity of 800—1000 Hz for heavily myelinated nerve fibers.

2. *Asynchronous depolarization.* As the frequency of stimulation increases, some of the pulses will occur during the refractory period. Thus, the involved nerve will not react to every pulse, but it will react to the stimulation current at its own frequency. Asynchronous depolarization therefore occurs. The depolarization frequency of the nerve does not coincide with the frequency of the current, nor does it coincide with the depolarization frequency of the other nerve fibers in the nerve bundle.

With medium frequency alternating currents, not every cycle will result in a depolarization of the nerve fiber. In order to depolarize the fibers, the summation of several cycles is required. The depolarization of nerve fibers, according to the summation principle, is known as the *Gildemeister effect.*

As nerves are stimulated with medium frequency alternating currents, the fibers will mutually discharge with their maximum frequency. In fact, if the intensity of the current is high enough, depolarization may even occur during the relative refractory period. However, as stimulation continues, the motor end-plates become fatigued and transmission of the stimulus may not take place. Eventually, the involved muscle will cease to contract.

The phenomenon where continuous stimulation with a medium frequency current leads to inhibition of the reaction or a complete blockage throughout the duration of the stimulation is called *Wedensky inhibition.* To prevent Wedensky inhibition and fatigue of the motor end-plates, it is essential after each depolarization to interrupt the current. A rhythmic interruption will cause the fibers in the nerve bundle to depolarize at the frequency of the interruption.

Intersection

Interferential therapy actually occurs when two alternating medium frequency currents are superimposed. By definition, *interferential current* is the phenomenon that occurs when two or more oscillations are applied simultaneously to the same point (or series of points) in a medium (eg, a body part).

The medium frequencies that are applied with interferential current are generally 4,000 cps sine wave currents which are crossed simultaneously (triggered by two generators). However, they cross at slightly different frequencies. One of the sine waves has a fixed frequency (generally, 4000 Hz), and the frequency of the other current can be set at a variable amount that is usually between 4000 and 4250 Hz.

The linear superimposition of the second wave on the first wave is called *interference.* See Figure 9.3.[11] In Figure 4, it can be seen that the placement of four electrodes on the skin, as shown, will establish the specific location where current intersection takes place. By placing the two currents close to one another, the depth of penetration is kept superficial, while placing the electrodes farther apart will increase the depth of penetration. The density of the body tissues involved will also alter the depth of penetration and the locale of intersection.

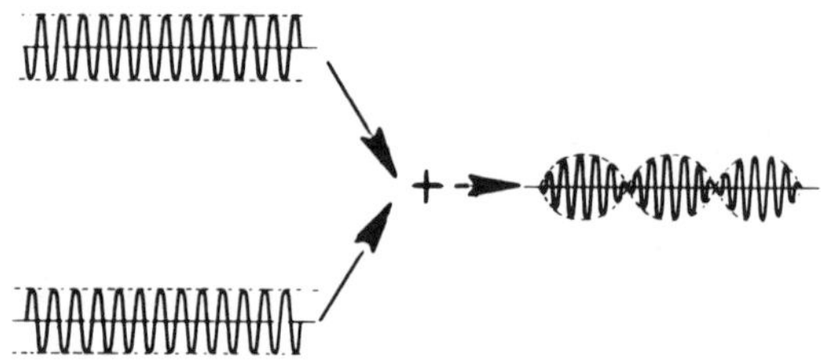

Figure 9.3. Schematic of linear superimposition.

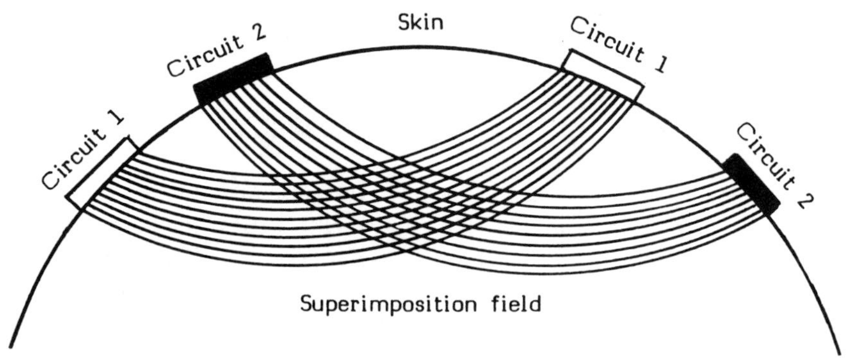

Figure 9.4. Schematic of superimposition field.

At the area of intersection, a low frequency endogenous current will be generated. This endogenous current, for all practical purposes, has a frequency that is the difference of the two frequencies which were originally applied. Thus, if one current has a frequency of 4000 Hz and another has a frequency of 4100 Hz, an endogenous low frequency current having a frequency of 100 pulses per second will be generated. This means that the amplitude of stimulation (eg, 4000 cycles) varies after intersection occurs, from zero on up to the maximum amplitude value of 100 cycles.

It should be noted that most interferential units do not indicate the 4000 Hz frequency setting on the dials of the control panel. If the setting on the interferential has a scale of 0—100, this actually means 4000—4100 Hz.

Because interference current therapy is a by-product of a superimposition of two alternating sine wave currents, there will be no direct current effects within the involved tissues. Chemical alterations and polar changes do not occur as they do with direct current; thus, an operator need not be especially concerned about burning the patient with interferential therapy.[12] As just explained, the placement of electrodes predetermines the exact site and degree of interference.

In Figure 9.5, it can be seen that when two currents are placed at right angles to one another, 100% interference occurs. As a result of mathematical computations, a schematic of the stimulation may be drawn that occurs in the form of a four-leaf clover pattern. See Figure 9.6. The length of the arrow heads shown in Figure 9.7 represent the

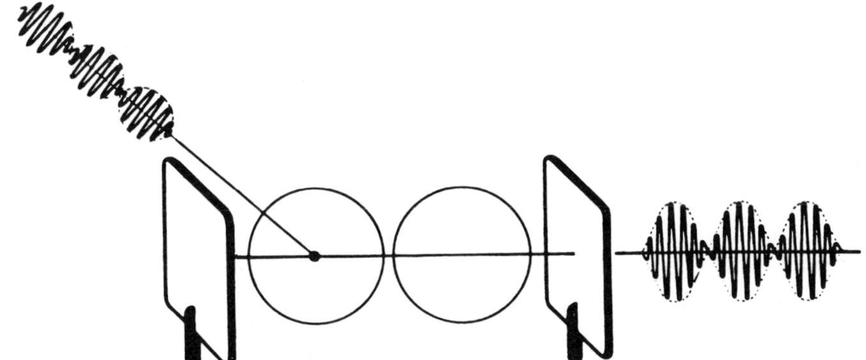

Figure 9.5. Distribution of current intensity with linear current superimposition.

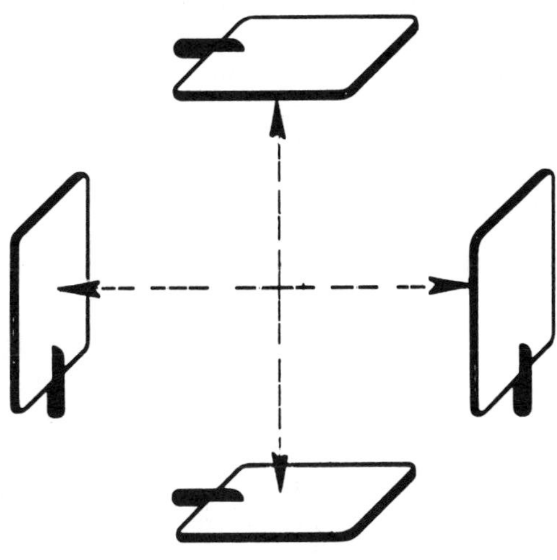

Figure 9.6. Perpendicular superimposition using a 4-pole technique. Interference occurs where these currents intersect, and the depth of modulation depends on the direction of the currents. Current amplitude can vary from 0 to 100%.

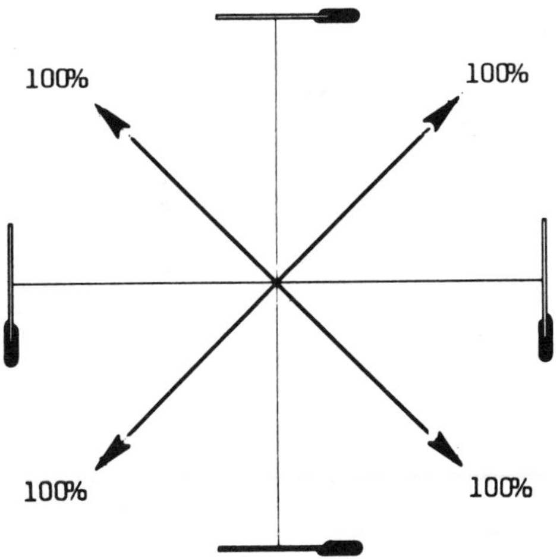

Figure 9.7. The modulation depth is 100% on the 45° diagonals in perpendicular superimposition when a 4-pole technique is used.

stimulation intensity that occurs, and the extent of modulation depth ocurring in various directions is shown in Figure 9.8.

Treatment frequency is determined by those physiologic effects that occur at various frequencies; thus, it is based on the effects desired. The parameters shown in Table 9.2 are generally recommended when interferential therapy is used.

Modulation

If a patient is stimulated over a lengthy period, body tissues have a natural tendency to adapt by accommodating to the stimulus; eg, the patient might say after a prolonged application, "I no longer feel the stimulation." For this reason, interferential current units are designed to allow for a modulation of frequency.

The rhythmic increase and decrease of intensity in interferential therapy is referred to as *amplitude modulation,* and the treatment frequency is called the *amplitude modulation frequency* (AMF).

EFFECTS OF MODULATION

Frequency modulation to prevent accommodation was first used by Bernard who used modulation currents CP (courtes periodes) and LP (longues periodes) in which the modulation alternated on a regular basis between 50 and 100 Hz.[13]

A modulated frequency produces two major effects:

1. Interferential therapy provides a modulation of therapy. To allow for optimal repolarization, (a) the current has to be interrupted after every depolarization or (b) the intensity of the current has to be decreased significantly. The frequency of the amplitude modulation (ie, the treatment frequency) determines the frequency of depolarization.[14]

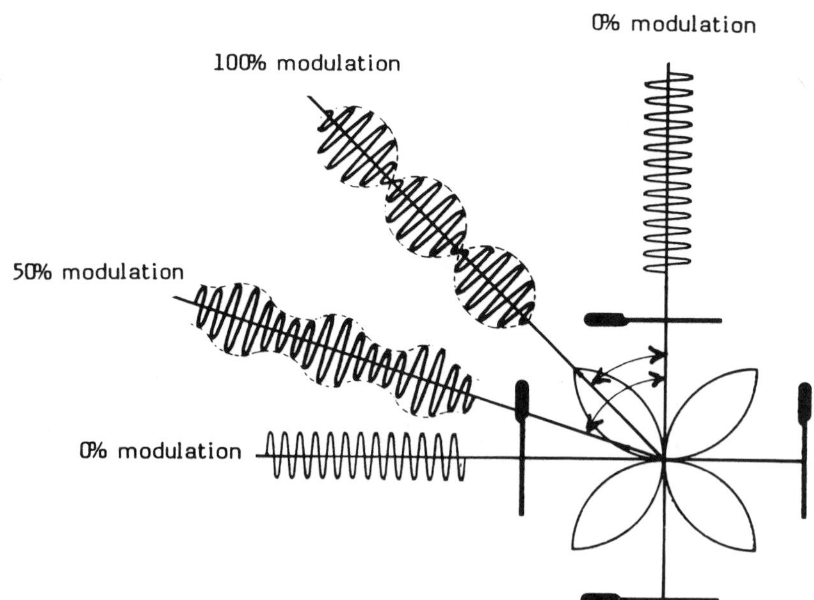

Figure 9.8. The maximum resultant force is halfway (ie, 45° diagonally from each circuit) between the two forces when two equal circuits intersect at 90°.

Table 9.2. Typical Interferential Therapy Parameters

Range	*Comments*
0—100 Hz	General muscle toning with increased deep blood and lymph flow. It may also be helpful in reducing edema. Used for stimulation of the contents of the pelvic cavity.
1—5 Hz	A constant frequency of 1—5 pps may elicit a twitch in denervated muscle.
1—10 Hz	When set on constant stimulation, single contractions at the specific pulse rate setting take place. This frequency range is used in the stimulation of exercise in innervated striated muscles (eg, bronchial walls, sphincters) and to initiate stretching of joint contractures. This frequency range has also been recommended in the treatment of some visceral complaints, patients with atonic bowel, patients with stress incontinence. This frequency range also has a direct effect on smooth muscle; eg, producing a contraction and relaxation of blood vessel walls. Frequencies in this range may trigger endorphin production. At least one of the various interferential units available has a small diameter electrode for use with a two electrode technique to trigger endorphin production. On a constant setting, this frequency range produces contraction of individual muscles innervated by motor nerves.
5—60 Hz	May stimulate partially denervated muscle tissue.
10—100 Hz	This frequency range is thought to have a profound effect on the vegetative portions of the nervous system.
40—90 Hz	Increases circulation rate.
50 Hz	Stimulates striated muscle tissue.
90—100 Hz	Many consider this frequency range to be the most effective in triggering enkephalin production for pain control; however, some recent studies have extended the range for this purpose to 130 pps. This range may provoke reversible muscle contractions.
100 Hz	A constant frequency of 100 Hz depresses the sympathetic portion of the autonomic nervous system. It is also effective for analgesia, lessening tonus, and may slightly increase circulation. A rhythmical frequency of 100 Hz is thought to be effective for building up muscle tissue in cases of myopathy, and it enables individual isometric exercise to be performed until fatigue sets in.

2. Modulation of the frequency prevents accommodation from occurring.

It should be kept in mind that the frequency of the "black" circuit is fixed at 4000 Hz. It is the frequency through the "red" circuit that is variable (able to be voluntarily modulated).

SPECTRUM CONTROL

In interferential therapy, the word *spectrum* indicates the range of frequencies through which the alternating current can be made to swing rhythmically above a preset base frequency. With the Dutch Enraf-Nonius equipment (Endomed unit), for example, the frequency is modulated by means of two spectrum variant switches that can be adjusted, based on the results the operator wishes to achieve. See Figure 9.9. When the first spectrum dial is preset at 150 Hz and the second is set at 100 Hz in the Endomed unit, the frequency will modulate from 150 Hz on up to 250 Hz; ie, the total range of modulation is the sum of the two dial settings. If the first dial is set at 0 Hz and the second dial at 100 Hz, the frequency will modulate from 0 up to 100 Hz.

The Endomed unit has three spectrum variants that can utilized:

1. In the first position setting (aggressive), the frequency modulates from the setting on the first dial, which is held for 1 second, on up to the higher frequency of the setting of the second dial, which is also held for 1 second. See Figure 9.10.

2. In the second position setting (moderate), the base frequency is retained for a 5-second period. Then, over a period of 1 second, all frequencies in the set spectrum are increased up to the highest frequency, which is then maintained for 5 seconds. Subsequently, the frequency gradually returns to the lower frequency during a 1-second period. See Figure 9.11.

3. In the third spectrum setting (mild), the frequencies are never at a constant setting. They continually change from the higher to the lower setting at 6-second intervals. See Figure 9.12.

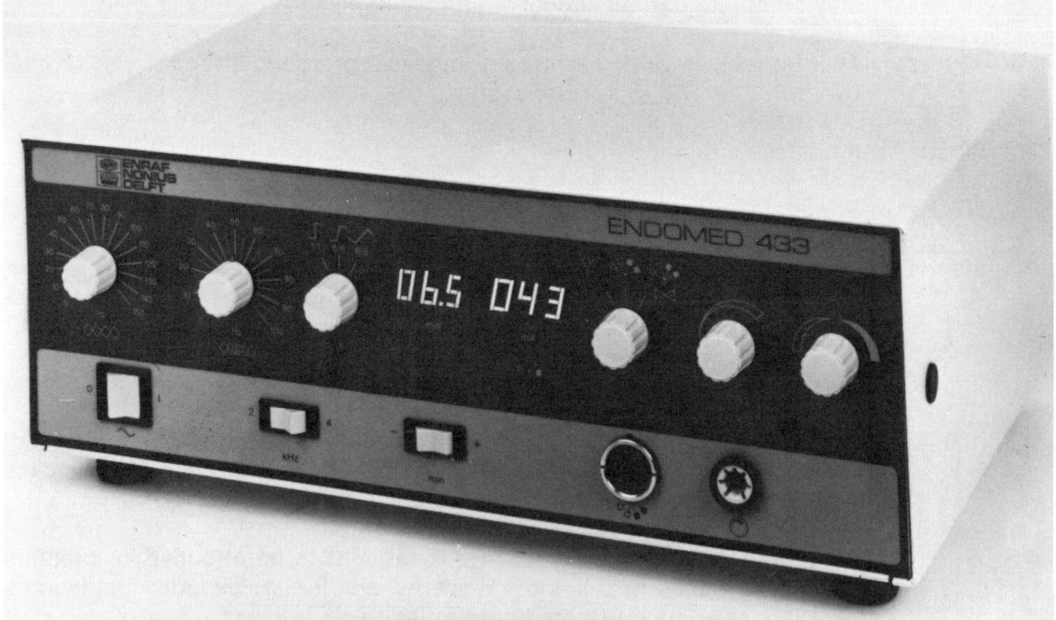

Figure 9.9. Control panel of an Endomed 433 unit.

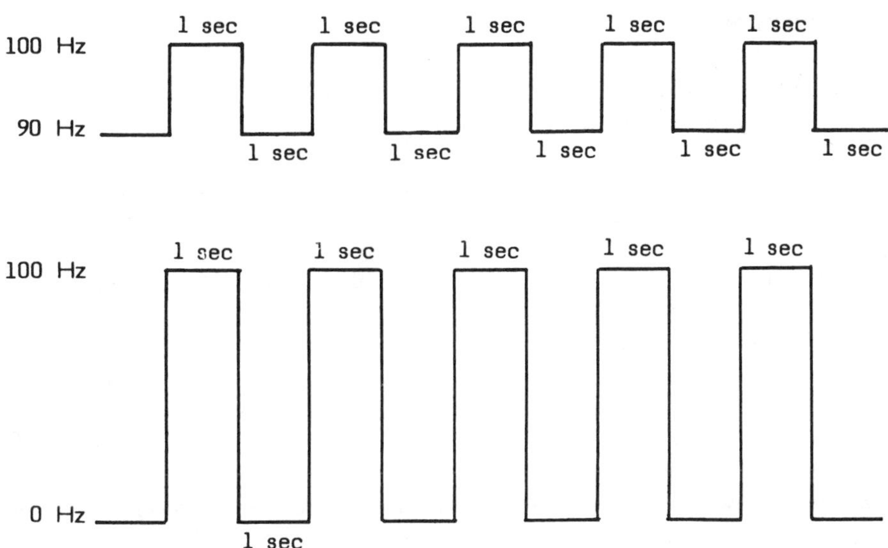

Figure 9.10. *Top,* diagram of a current pattern when the first dial is set at 90 Hz and the second dial is set at 10 Hz, with 1-second intervals. *Bottom,* current pattern when the first dial is set at 0 Hz and the second dial is set at 100 Hz, with 1-second intervals. This setting is quite irritating to the patient and should only be used in situations of a stubbornly chronic nature.

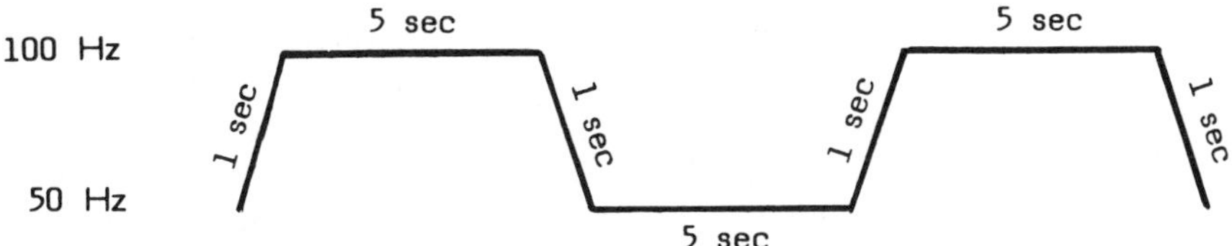

Figure 9.11. Diagram of a current pattern when both the first and second dials are set at 50 Hz. This setting is used for most clinical situations because it is generally tolerable to most patients and allows for specific stimulation to occur, based on the frequency setting.

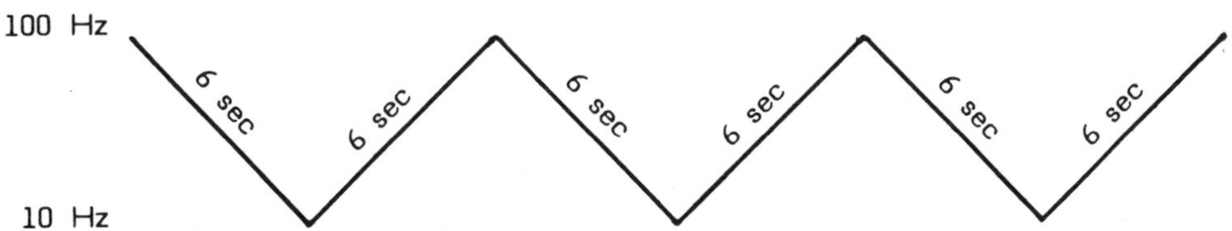

Figure 9.12. Diagram of a current pattern when the first dial is set at 10 Hz and the second dial is set at 90 Hz. This setting is usually extremely comfortable to the patient; however, the constant sweep does not permit optimal therapeutic effects to occur as a direct offshoot of the frequency. This setting is recommended in highly acute conditions, utilizing an extremely narrow sweep (eg, 90—100 Hz) for analgesia.

Electrode Placement

Interferential electrodes come in a large variety of sizes and types (eg, pads, gloves, discs, pens). Either two or four electrodes may be used in the treatment of a patient, and the techniques are of equal importance.

BASIC TECHNIQUES

1. *Two-pole technique.* Using two electrodes emitting alternating current, superimposition occurs within the machine itself. The modulation current leaving the machine has the same value in all directions, and the modulation depth is always 100%. However, the amplitude varies between zero and 100%, being greatest in the direction of a straight line joining the two electrodes and zero in the direction perpendicular to that line. Refer to Figure 9.5.

It should be noted that some authorities have questioned whether or not interference occurs with the two-pole technique. Additional studies will need to be undertaken before a conclusive statement can be made.

2. *Four-pole technique.* Two unmodulated currents are generated, with current crossing occurring within the part being treated. At the point of superimposition, a modulated current arises whose modulation depth varies between zero and 100%, depending on where the electrodes have been placed. The modulation depth is only 100% on the 45° diagonals. Refer to Figures 9.6, 9.7, and 9.8.

Searching for a specific location is easier with the two-pole technique. The four-pole technique has the advantage of lower strain on the skin, if this factor is important.

Various examples of electrode position for specific disorders are shown in Figures 9.13 and 9.14, and some examples of various treatment protocols are listed in Table 9.3.

ARRANGEMENT GUIDELINES

Electrode arrangement determines where the therapeutic effects will be concentrated. The following general rules will aid an operator in making decisions as to specific placement; however, most manufacturers supply a more detailed electrode placement guide with each unit.

1. Red and black electrodes must be crisscrossed when a four-pole technique is used. See Figure 9.15.
2. When electrodes are placed close together, treatment current is more superficial and greater stimulation occurs in the affected muscles, tendons, and ligaments.
3. Electrodes that are placed at a considerable distance apart allow deeper penetration. This arrangement is more beneficial for treatment of deep joints, viscera, or the spine.
4. Two-pole techniques stimulate in a straight line and are highly helpful when treating across a joint such as an elbow or knee.

Vectoring

The ideal situation exists when the patient is able to pinpoint the site of pain or dysfunction. When this is the situation, the electrodes are placed at the site, and the patient can then indicate whether or not the therapy feels the strongest at the subjectively perceived location of the problem. Regretfully, this is not always possible, and adjustments need to be made to vector or move the location of current crossing (superimposition) from one site to another to permit therapy to multiple areas.

An automatic vector scan is usually incorporated in an interferential unit to increase the region of effective stimulation or to treat an extremely large area. The site of optimal stimulation rotates within the area of current intersection. Thus, if specific localization is desired, it would be preferable to use a four-pole technique without a vector scan.

Specifically, vectoring, which is activated by a switch on the control panel, enables a rotation of the "four-leaf clover" (refer to

Fig. 9.8) within the body rather than having constant superimposition at one site. During a vector scan, the patient should perceive the varying sensation of the current.

Dosage

As a general rule, the intensity should be adjusted to the patient's tolerance.

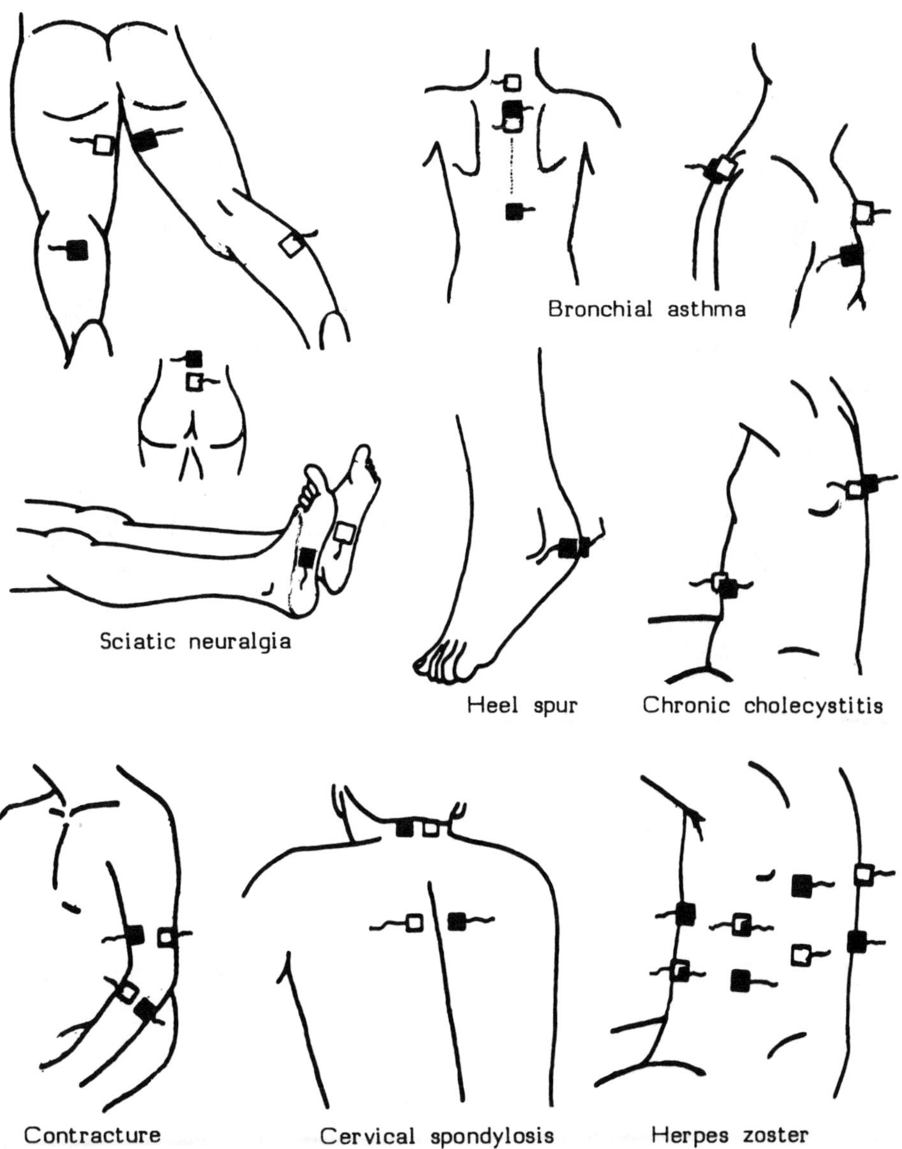

Figure 9.13. Some examples of electrode placement.

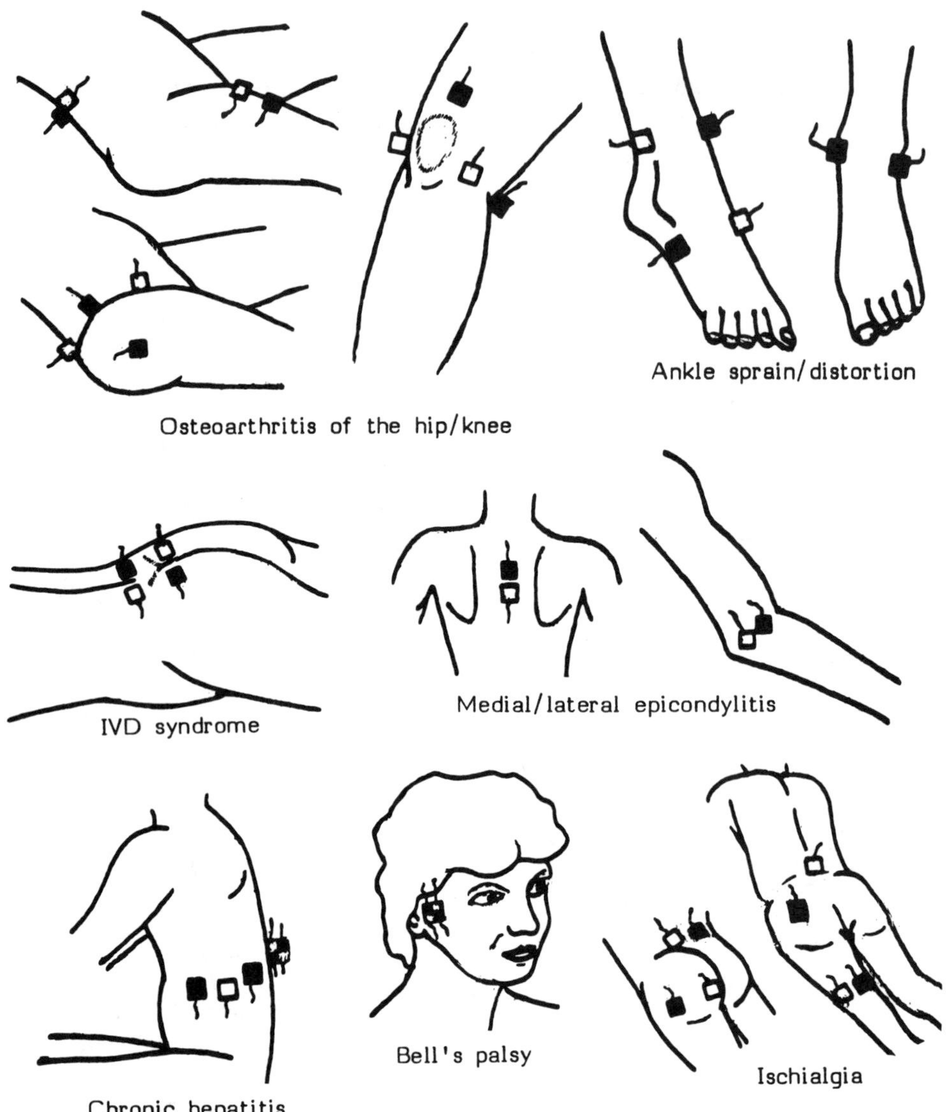

Figure 9.14. Additional examples of electrode placement.

THERAPEUTIC LEVELS

Based on the effects desired, one of the following dosage levels should be considered:

1. *Submitis dose (gentle).* A very weak intensity that is set under the patient's sensory threshold.
2. *Dosis mitis (mild).* A weak intensity in which the intensity of stimulation is just barely perceived. This dosage level is usually used in situations of acute pain where the primary objective of the therapy is to trigger enkephalin production for pain control.
3. *Dosis normalis (average).* Intensity brought up to the patient's easy tolerance.
4. *Dosis fortis (aggressive).* This is the

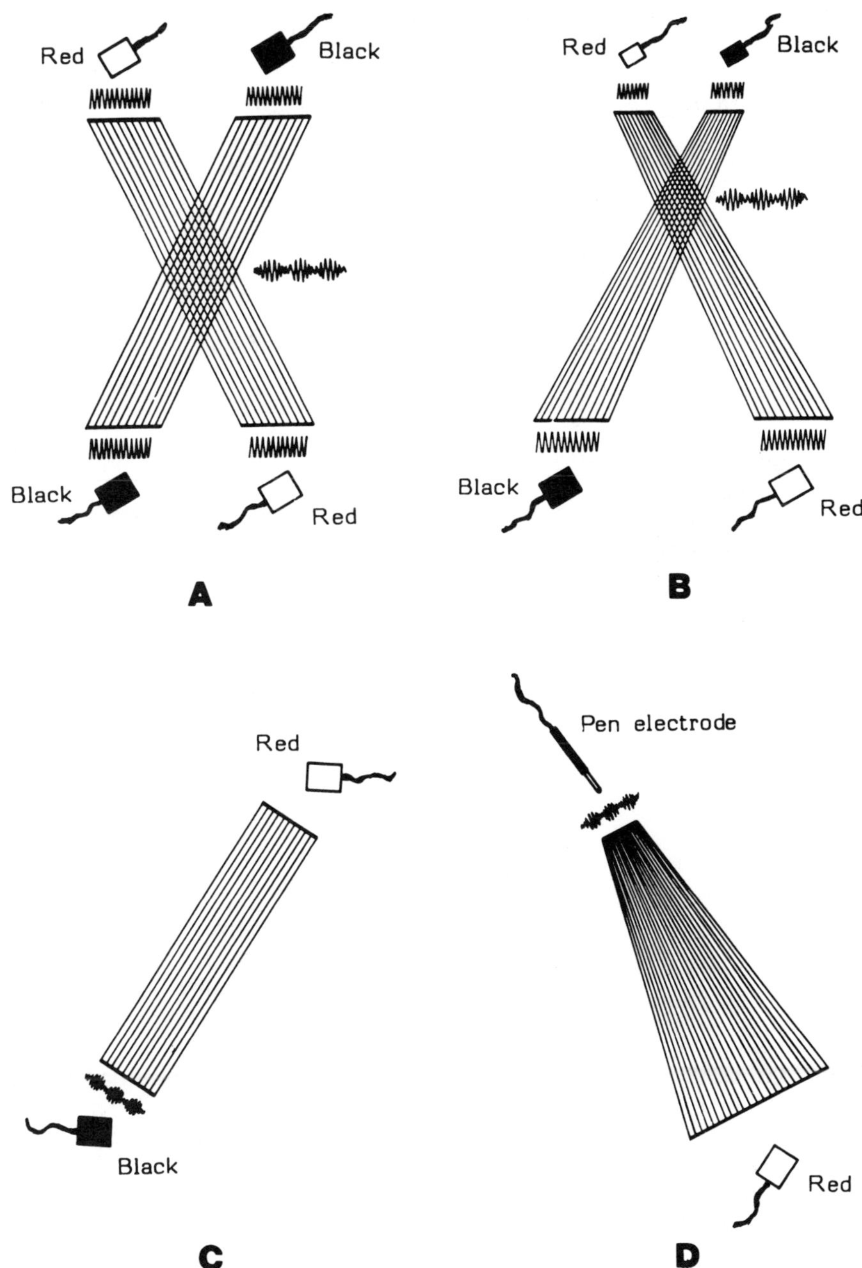

Figure 9.15. Some examples of electrode placement and its effect on current density: A, four-pole technique with electrodes of equal size; B, four-pole technique with electrodes of unequal size; C, two-pole technique with electrodes of equal size; D, two-pole technique with electrodes of unequal size.

Table 9.3. Examples of Interferential Treatment Regimens

Disorder	***Electrodes***	***Frequency (Hz)***	***Duration (minutes)***	***Dosage***	***Carrying Frequency***
Ankle/foot distortion or dislocation	Local: 4	Acute: 100 or 90—150 spectrum Chronic: 0—100 spectrum	12—15	Mitis—normalis	4000 Hz
Bell's palsy, TMJ dysfunction	Local: 4	20—100, depending on severity	8—11	Mitis	4000 Hz
Bronchial asthma	Segmental: 4 Level: C8, T2, T3, T10, with pairs staggered bilaterally in dermatomes	90—150	12—15	Mitis	4000 Hz
Cervical spondyloarthrosis	Local: 4	Acute: 90—150 spectrum Subacute or chronic: 100 or 0—100 spectrum	5—15	Mitis	4000 Hz
Contracture	Local: 2 or 4	0—10 or 0—100 (#1) 100 (#2) 0—100 (#3)	5—15	Mitis if pain, fortis if no pain	2000 to 4000 Hz
Epicondylitis, lateral or medial	Local: 2 Segmental: T4, T7, using smaller pole on involved side	90—150 or 0—100 spectrum	1—15	Mitis if pain, fortis if no pain	4000 Hz
Heel spur	Local: 2	90—100 spectrum, increase to 0—100 when tenderness decreases	5—10	Mitis to fortis	4000 Hz

Table 9.3, continued

Disorder	*Electrodes*	*Frequency (Hz)*	*Duration (minutes)*	*Dosage*	*Carrying Frequency*
Herpes zoster	4 covering dermatome	90—150 spectrum or 50—100 spectrum	10—15	Mitis	4000 Hz
Ischialgia	Local: 2 or 4 on nerve path*	100 or 90—150 spectrum	12—15	Mitis to normalis, using vector scan	4000 Hz
IVD protrusion	Local: 2 or 4	Acute: 100 or 90—150 spectrum Chronic: 0—120 spectrum	12—15	Mitis, normalis later	4000 Hz
Osteoarthrosis deformans, hip or knee	Local: 2 or 4 Segmental: 4 Level: L2—L3	Acute: 100 or 90—150 spectrum Chronic: 0—100 spectrum	12—15	Mitis to fortis	4000 Hz

*After analgesia is produced, treat spinal level.

strongest intensity that the patient can tolerate. It is used for treating chronic, resistant cases.

MENSURATION

The intensity of interferential current is measured in milliamperes. Most treatments will be in the range of 5—30 ma; however, many patients will react differently to the stimulation because of various social, familial, emotional, experience, and other conditioning or pathophysiologic factors. Should the patient accommodate during the treatment, the intensity can be safely increased without danger of burning the patient.

Although little can be gleaned from the intensity level that the patient is able to tolerate, it should be recorded in the patient's progress records during each visit. Data of the previous reaction can be used as a general guideline as to whether or not the patient is responding; ie, acute conditions are intolerant of relatively high intensities.

CONTROL

Some units have a switch that allows the patient to increase or decrease the intensity voluntarily. This practice is strongly discouraged in this country because of the danger of malpractice. The physician should be in control of the therapy at all times: the patient is not trained in proper application. The physician prescribes the treatment, not the patient. Several court actions have resulted after a doctor had delegated control of the unit to the patient, even though *no harm* had been done to the patient.

Duration

Treatment times of 10—15 minutes are typically recommended. However, Nikolova-Troeva suggests that treatments of up to 30 minutes can be highly desirable.[15] As a general rule, the more chronic the case, the longer the therapy should be applied.

Suction

Interferential therapy is frequently administered to the patient through suction cups that are, in turn, connected to a vacuum pump. Although the vacuum is not essential for the interferential current to be effective, it has generally been found to be beneficial. Our clinical studies have shown it to be a tremendous advantage during applications of the therapy. See Figure 9.16.

The suction mode, which is entirely independent from the interferential circuit, allows the electrodes to tightly adhere to the patient's skin. The major advantage of this is that it permits active or passive exercise of the part being treated *during* therapy. When desirable, another primary effect of using suction applicators is that extravasated fluids (edema) are drawn peripherally to the surface of the skin during the therapy. This effect is quite beneficial in patients when deep swelling is present in acute musculoskeletal injuries.

A caution exists with some of the older units in that setting the suction at too high a level may lead to unsightly skin bruises. Care should be taken to avoid such a reaction.

FREQUENCY OF PULSES

The suction unit can usually be set to provide continuous suction or it may be regulated from 10—80 pulses per minute, if this would be clinically beneficial. The control dial should be set at a sufficient intensity that the suction cups do not "pop off" yet take patient tolerance into consideration.

APPLICATION

Interferential therapy has many applications and is one of the better modalities available for treating musculoskeletal complaints or for affecting the internal organs, especially those of a deep-seated nature. Although some authorities suggest that interferential currents can replace the use of high-volt stimulation, this has not been true in our experience. This false belief of interferential replacing high-volt therapy possibly stems from a lack of understanding the full nature of the two modalities.

Interferential vs High-Volt Therapy

Interferential current has its effect by an intersection (superimposition) that occurs within the tissues, the depth of which is determined by where the electrodes are applied. Although intersection may occur in muscles, tendons, and ligaments, its effect is not dramatic. High-volt therapy is preferred when a dramatic effect would be desirable. On the other hand, high-volt currents do not penetrate as deeply. Thus, interferential is preferred in the treatment of deep joints such as the shoulder, hip, knee, or spine. See Figure 9.17.

The general rules to apply are: (1) if it's a deep or large joint problem, interferential is the modality of choice; (2) if it's a soft-tissue injury of muscles, tendons, ligaments, and/or other pariarticular tissues, then high-volt therapy is the preferred modality.

PAIN CONTROL

Another significant difference between interferential and high-volt therapy is in the area of pain control. Reference to the chapter on high-volt therapy will elucidate the pro-

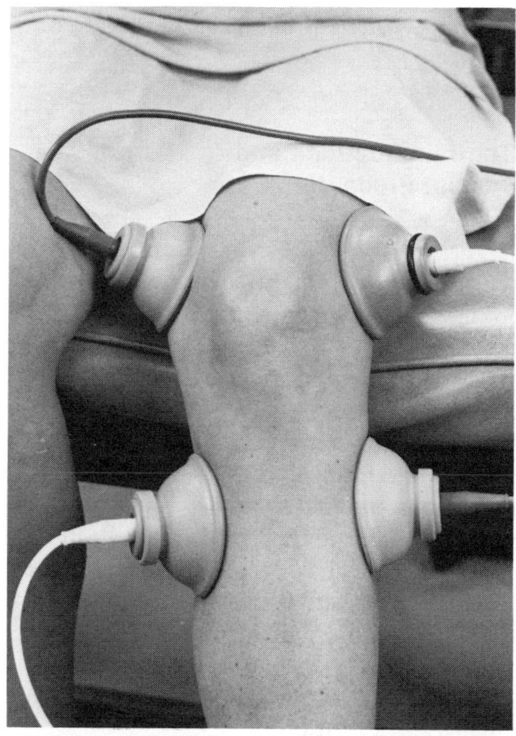

Figure 9.16. An example of suction cup applicators used in four-pole interferential therapy to a knee.

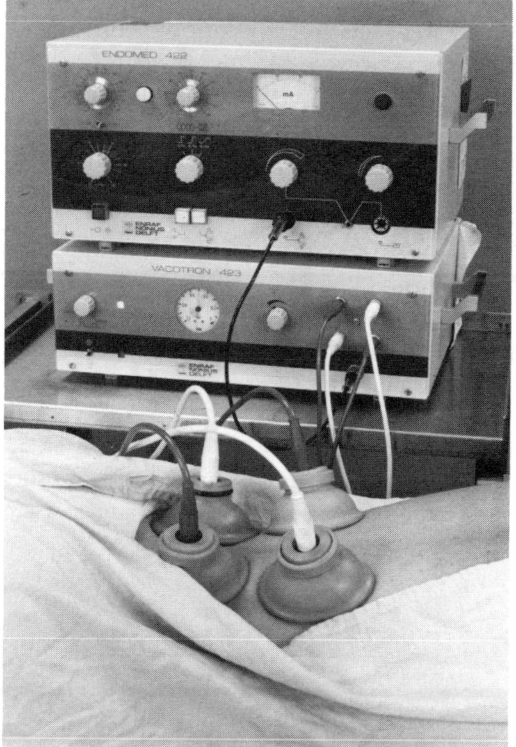

Figure 9.17. Application of interferential therapy to the lower back.

found advantage that high-volt current has if the patient can discriminate between sensory and motor stimulation. Although this may also occur with interferential therapy, subjective discrimination is not as keen.

High-volt therapy is quite effective in triggering endorphin production with the small-diameter electrode, and more so, according to our experience, than is interferential therapy. However, we have found interferential therapy to be more beneficial in blocking deep-seated pain or pain arising from visceral dysfunction. Again, the general rules stated previously should be considered.

OTHER APPLICATIONS

Interferential therapy is quite useful for building strength in muscles, tendons, and ligaments, especially during postinjury rehabilitation. It is not, however, the modality of choice to use for passive exercise when denervation is present. Interferential therapy may also prove to be of value in many other clinical entities. Future research may establish more specific parameters.

General Indications

The following points are considered to be some of the primary advantages of interferential therapy:[16-19]

1. Endogenous stimulation.[20]
2. Slight or no danger of burns from therapy.
3. Can be used over areas with nonelectronic metallic implants.[21-23]
4. Great depth of penetration.
5. Resistance of the skin is minimal between 3000 and 4000 Hz, thus higher intensities can be provided without patient discomfort.
6. Hypesthesia is not a contraindication.

Contraindications and Special Precautions

The following special concerns and contraindications should always be taken into account prior to treatment with interferential current:[24-26]

1. Metastatic carcinoma
2. Implanted pacemaker
3. Pregnant uterus
4. Over carotid sinus
5. Transcerebrally
6. Through the chest or over the heart.

Special care and consideration should likewise be given before interferential therapy is administered in the following cases:

1. Localized inflammatory processes
2. Thrombosis, decreased vascularity, poor circulation, varicosities
3. Tendency to hemorrhage
4. Tuberculosis
5. Over pelvic organs during menstruation
6. Hyperpyrexia.

Suction applicators are contraindicated in situations of possible superficial hemorrhage (eg, purpura, hemophilia) or superficial hyperesthesia (eg, raw contusions, adiposis dolorosa).

A more comprehensive list of indications and contraindications is shown in Table 9.4, representing a composite of various authoritative opinions.[27-35]

Care should be taken to see that an interferential unit is not within 20 feet of an activated shortwave diathermy machine. If an activated diathermy unit is turned off, the sudden surge of energy may easily damage a circuit and injure a patient or operator.[36]

Table 9.4. General Indications and Contraindications of Interferential Therapy

GENERAL INDICATIONS		
Anterior tibial syndrome	Incontinence	Psoas syndrome
Bell's palsy	Intermittent claudication	Rheumatic disorders
Bronchial asthma	Ischialgia	Sciatica
Bursitis	IVD syndromes	Shoulder-arm syndrome
Capsulitis	Joint deformity	Spasm
Causal myopathies	Lumbago	Spondylitis
Causalgia	Lymphedema	Spondylosis
Cholecystitis (chronic)	Migraine	Sprains/strains
Contractures	Myalgia	Spurs
Decubitus ulcers	Myositis	Stiffness
Effusions	Neuralgia	Stump pain
Epicondylitis	Neuritis (chronic)	Subluxation syndromes
Facet syndrome	Neuroma	Sudeck's atrophy
Facial palsy	Osteoarthritis	Synovitis
Fibrositis	Pain (idiopathic)	Tendinitis
Frozen shoulder	Periarthritis	Thoracodynia
Heel/ankle spur	Posttraumatic edema	TMJ dysfunction
Hematoma calcification	Prostatitis	Trigger points
Hemiplegia	Psoas syndrome	Vasospasm
Herpes zoster	Prostatitis	
GENERAL CONTRAINDICATIONS		
Abscess	Hyperpyrexia	Pregnant uterus
Carotid sinus area	Implanted pacemaker	Thrombophlebitis
Circulation block	Menstruating uterus	Transcerebral current
Heart area	Metastatic carcinoma	Tuberculosis
Hemorrhagic dyscrasias	Patient hyperanxiety	Varicosities

REFERENCES

1. Mayer DJ: Endogenous analgesia systems: neural and behavioral mechanisms. In Bonica JJ, et al (eds): *Advances in Pain Research and Therapy*. New York, Raven Press, 1979, vol 3, pp 385-410.
2. Ganne JM: Interferential therapy. *The Australian Journal of Physiotherapy*, 22(3):101-110, September 1976.
3. Ganne JM: Some aspects of treatment of pain by counter irritation. *Australian Journal of Physiotherapy*, 10(3):90-95, 1961.
4. Andersson SA: Pain control by sensory stimulation. In Bonica JJ, et al (eds): *Advances in Pain Research and Therapy*. New York, Raven Press, 1979, vol 3, pp 569-585.
5. Cauthen JC, Renner EJ: Transcutaneous and peripheral nerve stimulation for chronic pain states. *Surgical Neurology*, 4:102-104, 1975.
6. Handwerker HO, et al: Segmental and supraspinal actions on dorsal horn neurons responding to noxious and nonnoxious skin stimuli. *Pain*, 1:147-165, 1975.
7. Melzack R: *The Puzzle of Pain: Revolution in Theory and Treatment*. Harmondsworth (Middle-

sex), England, Penguin Education Books, 1973.
8. Savage B: *Interferential Therapy*. Boston, Faber & Faber, 1984, p 17.
9. Nippel FJ: Interferential current therapy: an advanced method in the management of pain. Paper presented to the Annual Conference of the American Physical Therapy Association, Veterans Administration Special Interest Group, Atlanta, June 9, 1979.
10. Ibid.
11. Hogenkamp M, et al: *Interferential Therapy*. Delft, Holland, B.V. Enraf-Nonius, October 1983, p 9.
12. Hansjurgens A, May, H-U: Differences between dynamic interference current (DIC) analgesia and TENS-analgesia. Paper presented to the Dynamic Interference Current Therapy Workshop, Milwaukee, Wisconsin; sponsored by the Program in Physical Therapy (Marquette University) and The Physical Therapy Education Institute; April 12-13, 1980.
13. Bernard PD: La therapie diadynamique, editions "PHYSIO." Paris, France, 1962.
14. Bolomey de Zwart EM, et al: *Instruction Manual: Interferential Therapy*. Delft, Holland, B.V. Enraf-Nonius, date not shown, p 4.
15. Nikolova-Troeva L: Comparative studies on therapeutic results obtained by means of interference therapy and other methods in arthrosis deformans. *Physical Medicine and Rehabilitation,* 8(3), March 1967.
16. Eigler E: Success achieved by treatment with interferential current on patients with epicondylitis humeri. Paper presented to the 84th Congress of the German Society for Physical Medicine and Rehabilitation, Hannover, Germany, October 12—14, 1979.
17. Indeck W: Skin application of electrical impulses for relief of pain in chronic orthopaedic conditions. Paper presented to the Scientific Session of the American Academy of Orthopaedic Surgeons, January 1974.
18. Schoeler H: Physical block of the sympathetic chain. *Technik in Der Medizin,* 1:16-18, 1972.
19. Willie CD: Interferential therapy. *Physiotherapy,* 55(12):503-505, 1969.
20. Mayer DJ: Endogenous analgesia systems: Neural and behavioral mechanisms. In Bonica JJ, et al (eds): *Advances in Pain Research and Therapy*. New York, Raven Press, 1979, vol 3, pp 385-410.
21. Nikolova-Troeva L: Interference-current therapy in distortions, contusions and luxations of the joints. *Munchener Medizinische Wochenschrift,* 11:579-582, 1967.
22. Leeb H: Experience with the application of interfering alternating currents in inflammatory diseases of the female genital organs. *Wiener Medizinische Wochenschrift,* 105(47):972-975, 1955.
23. Kinsman AJ: Clinical effects and uses of interferential current therapy. Paper presented to the Australian Physiotherapy Association Congress, Sidney, Australia, August 1975.
24. Kloth L: Interferential current therapy. Paper presented to the 49th Annual Scientific Session of the American Physical Therapy Association, Phoenix, Arizona, June 16-19, 1980.
25. Hill LL: *Parameters of Physiotherapy Modalities.* Lombard, IL, National Chiropractic College, class notes, date not shown, pp 91-102.
26. Shealy CN, et al: Electrical inhibition of pain: experimental evaluation. *Anesthesia and Analgesia, Current Researches,* 46(4):299-304, 1967.
27. Hogenkamp M, et al: *Interferential Therapy*. Delft, Holland, B.V. Enraf-Nonius, October 1983, p 30.
28. Bolomey de Zwart EM, et al: *Instruction Manual: Interferential Therapy*. Delft, Holland, B.V. Enraf-Nonius, date not shown, pp 8-9.
29. Savage B: *Interferential Therapy*. Boston, Faber & Faber, 1984, pp 55-110.
30. Kinsman AJ: Clinical effects and uses of interferential current therapy. Paper presented to the Australian Physiotherapy Association Congress, Sidney, Australia, August 1975.
31. Hill LL: *Parameters of Physiotherapy Modalities.* Lombard, IL, National Chiropractic College, class notes, date not shown, pp 91-92.
32. Sjolund BH, Eriksson ME: Endorphins and analgesia produced by peripheral conditioning stimulation. In Bonica JJ, et al (eds): *Advances in Pain Research and Therapy*. New York, Raven Press, 1979, vol 3, pp 587-592.
33. Shealy CN, et al: Dorsal column electro-analgesia. *Journal of Neurosurgery,* 32:500-564, 1970.
34. Guenthner R, et al: Comparative studies of physical therapy in cervical and lumbar vertebral column syndromes. *Physikalische Medizin,* 5(6):239-241, 1976.
35. Ganne JM: Report on the results of treatment of pain with sustained sinusoidal current on 100 patients during 1961 and 1965. *Australian Journal of Physiotherapy,* 14(2):47-53, 1968.
36. Savage B: *Interferential Therapy*. Boston, Faber & Faber, 1984, p 56.

Chapter 10

Hydrotherapy

The chapter describes the physiologic basis for using water as a therapy and the clinical contraindications associated. The more common specific applications such as whirlpools, Hubbard tanks, and therapeutic baths are explained.

INTRODUCTION

The term *hydrotherapy* (or hydrotherapeutics) is derived from the two Greek words that mean *water* and *heal;* thus, by definition, it refers to the use of water in the treatment of disease or trauma.

Scope of Hydrotherapy

In a broad sense, hydrotherapy, whether it is used internally or externally, includes water treatment utilizing any of the three natural forms of water; ie, solid (ice), liquid (water), or vapor (steam). Years ago, physicians generally limited the term only to the therapeutic effects of cold water. This concept originated with Priessnitz, who is considered by many as the "Apostle of Cold Water." In recent decades, however, the therapeutic use of water (hydrotherapy) and its study have been expanded to include both cold and heated water.

Various related terms are often associated with hydrotherapy. For example, the term *hydropathy,* which is actually a misnomer, is generally reserved to indicate the therapeutic effects that are obtained when large amounts of cold water are used, internally or externally. *Hydrosudotherapy* refers to the treatment of disease by sweating and hydrotherapy; and when water in the form of vapor or moisture is applied therapeutically, the technique is sometimes referred to as *hygrotherapy.*

General Therapeutic Rationale

Water is an excellent medium for therapy because of its high specific heat. This property allows for (1) slow absorption of heat by the body through the process of conduction and (2) slow cooling of the body or any of its exposed parts. Water is quite versatile to use because it permits full or partial immersion of a part or it can be specifically directed by spraying an isolated area of the skin.

The most common technique for hydrotherapy involves the use of the small whirlpool tank, which permits immersion within agitated water of one or more extremities or the patient may sit in the tub. See Figure 10.1. Larger therapy units (eg, a Hubbard tank), incorporating larger whirlpools, can accommodate both a patient and a therapist. See Figure 10.2. This latter type of therapy is beneficial when passive exercise is indicated during the treatment.

TYPES OF HYDROTHERAPY

A number of commonly utilized forms of hydrotherapy are briefly described below:

Whirlpool. This form of therapy is characterized by partial immersion of the patient into water that is rapidly agitated and mixed with air to superficially stimulate the immersed part. Other effects include cleansing

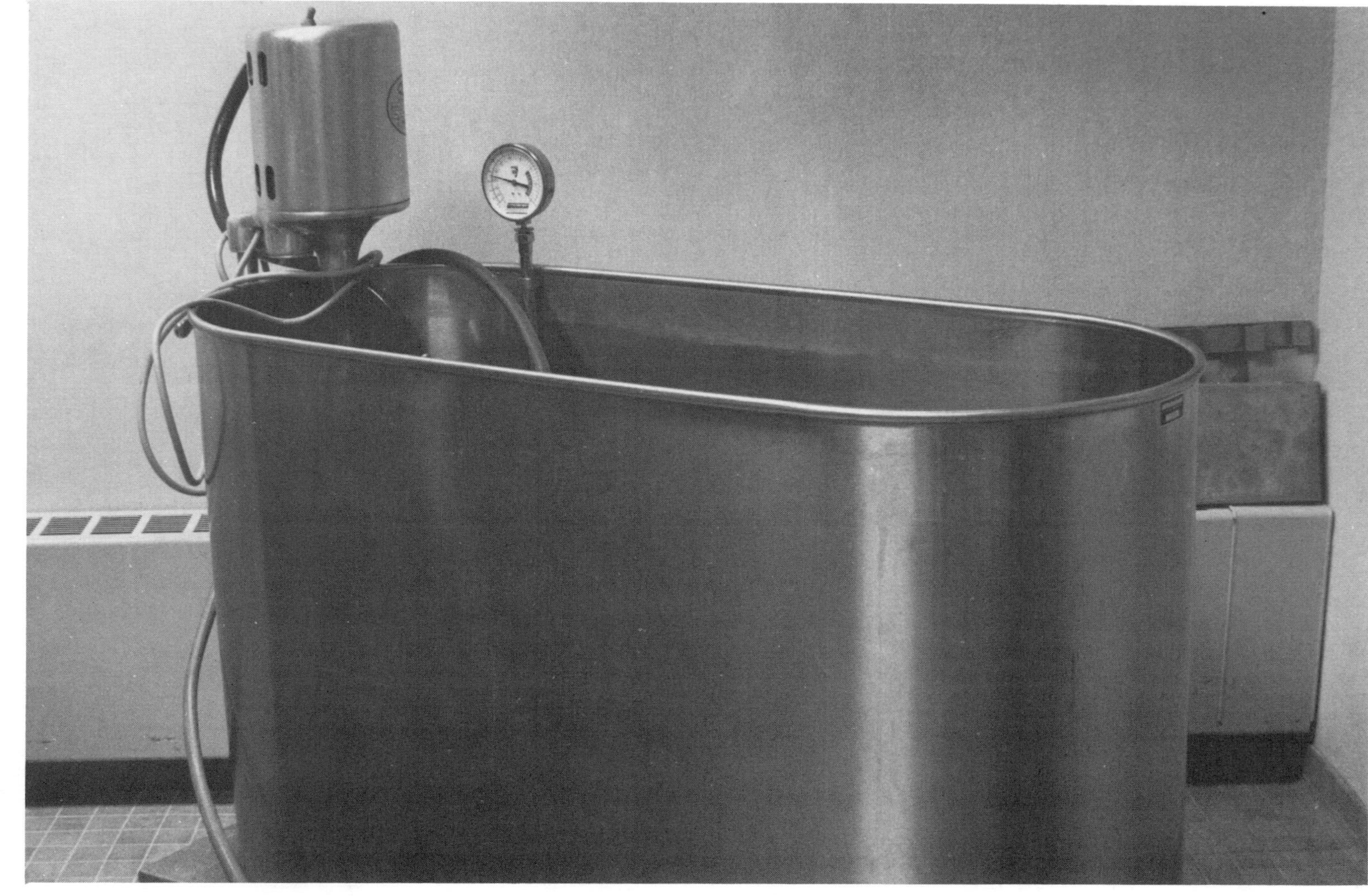

Figure 10.1. A small whirlpool tank.

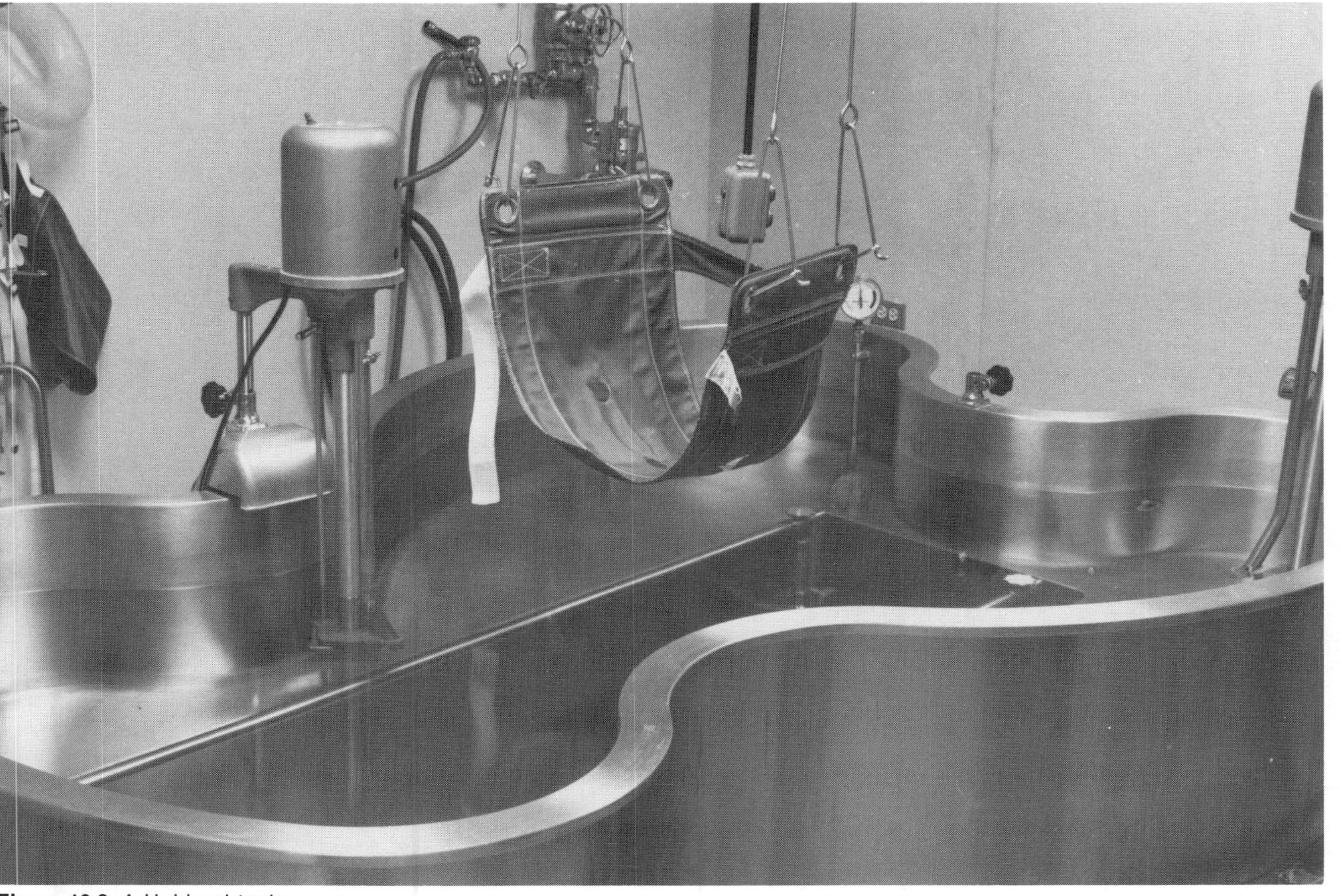

Figure 10.2. A Hubbard tank.

(eg, wounds), sedation, and passive exercise.

Sitz Bath. A sitz bath is utilized in the treatment of the pelvic region, especially the rectal, perineal, and genital regions.

Hot and Cold Sprays and Douches. This therapy involves the application of water from multiple "needle-spray" nozzles that strike the body or body part from various (usually horizontal) directions to produce stimulating and cleansing effects.

Steam. The inhalation of warm vapors (medicated or nonmedicated) are often used in some cases of nasal congestion, sinusitis, and other upper respiratory disorders.

Miscellaneous Therapies. Some authorities include several other modalities of care under the general classification of hydrotherapy, including applications of ice; hot or cold moist packs, compresses, and dressings. These applications are described in other chapters of this manual (see Index). The common procedure of prescribing a certain quantity of drinking water each day (eg, dehydration states, kidney and bladder disorders, constipation, toxicosis, fever) can also be broadly listed as hydrotherapy.

THE PHYSIOLOGIC BASIS FOR USING WATER AS A THERAPY

Water as a therapeutic agent allows for several remarkable possibilities. There are many reasons why water can be utilized successfully as a method of therapy for a patient in distress. The ten major properties that serve as the basis for intelligent application are briefly described below.

Buoyancy

Water is extremely buoyant. In fact, as *Archimedes principle* indicates; ie, a body that is fully or partially immersed in a liquid experiences an upward thrust which is equal in force to the weight of the liquid that it displaces. Thus, when a body or a part of a body is placed in water, there will be only a minimal strain on the weight-bearing joints of the part(s) immersed.[1] This fact is extremely valuable in the treatment of patients when full weight-bearing is contraindicated such as in various types of paralysis or painful joint irritations. Another factor to be considered regarding the buoyancy property of water is the ease with which the patient can actively exercise or be passively exercised when the involved part is underwater.

When a Hubbard tank is used, the patient can exercise the extremities underwater against the resistance that is offered by the water (quantity and velocity) being used. As in other neuromuscular therapies and techniques for grading patients with motor deficits, additional criteria would include the number and speed of the exercise bouts and the range of joint motion achieved.

Cohesion and Viscosity

When a patient is placed in water, the liquid has a tendency to adhere to the skin. This cohesive effect, together with the viscosity and friction of the water at the water-skin interface, tends to resist movement of the immersed part.

The properties of cohesion and viscosity must be considered in many forms of hydrotherapy. For example whenever *hydrogymnastics* (underwater exercises) are prescribed for the patient, it is best to have the patient begin the movements slowly and gradually increase the speed to the optimal level.

Hydrostatic Pressure

Closely related to the cohesiveness and viscosity of water is the effect that water pressure has on the immersed part(s). Some authors believe that the hydrostatic pressure of water increases the venous and lymphatic flow from the periphery, which, in turn, ultimately increases the patient's urinary output.[2,3]

Mechanical Stimulation

Jets or sprays of pressurized water can be incorporated in a whirlpool, Hubbard tank, or directed toward the patient in the form of a shower, bath, douche, or spray. One of the effects of the resulting stimulation is increased molecular motion in the skin that may aid the healing process. This technique may also be used to cleanse or debride an open wound and combat secondary infection, treat pressure sores, or influence viscera reflexly.

Conductivity

Water is an efficient conductor of heat, and this fact is related to its relatively high specific gravity when compared to that of other substances. It takes 1 calorie of heat to raise 1 gram of water 1 °C; thus, water is used as the standard. See Table 10.1.[4]

Versatility

Water is readily transformed from its solid, liquid, and gaseous states, and each state has its peculiar mechanisms of use. As a solid (ice), it serves as a cooling agent. As a liquid, it can be used in packs, baths, sprays, and douches. As a vapor, it can be used in steam baths and inhalation therapy.

It should be noted that when water vapor or steam reverts to a liquid, a large quantity of calories (540) are liberated. This fact, unfortunately, is dramatically illustrated by the severe burns that may occur when steam comes in contact with the skin and condenses on it.

Temperature

Water influences the body's homeostatic environment in several different ways. One significant manner is by variance of temperature. As a general rule, those physiologic responses to treatment are in direct proportion to the extent of the homeostatic changes produced; ie, the greater the temperature change, the greater the physiologic response, both locally and systemically.

WATERBEDS

A patient who sleeps on a waterbed at or near (within a degree) of body temperature will usually sleep well and awaken refreshed. If the temperature of the bed is increased to over 101 °F, however, most people will awake with complaints of stiffness and soreness. This is partly because the change in environmental temperature dramatically affects the body but primarily because of the prolonged absorption of heat, coupled with inactivity, during sleep. In addition, some people with gross physical misalignments may find that their symptoms will become aggravated because of the lack of firm support of a waterbed.

WATERBATHS

A patient placed in a waterbath of 98 °F has minimal, if any, physiologic responses

Table 10.1. Relationship of Specific Heat to Specific Heat Conductivity

Substance	*Specific Heat*	*Specific Heat Conductivity*
Water	1.0	1.000
Paraffin wax	0.69	0.450
Alcohol	0.59	0.330
Glycerin	0.57	0.500
Air	0.23	0.043

because of the temperature of the waterbath. If the temperature of the water is increased to 110 °F, however, marked physiologic changes take place.[5]

Effects of Prolonged Exposure to Heated Water. The following major changes occur when a patient who is immersed in water is exposed to increases of temperature:[6]

1. Increased pulse rate
2. Slight increase in body temperature
3. Increased temperature of those parts that are immersed, as evidenced by flushing of the skin
4. Increased metabolism
5. Increased leukocytosis
6. Slight tissue, blood, and urine hyperalkalization.

As stated previously, the degree of temperature change from pretherapy body temperature is directly related to the therapeutic effects on the patient. Water temperatures between 92 °F and 97 °F, as a general rule, are considered neutral because the patient usually perceives them as being neither warm or cool, as surface temperature perception is usually related to body temperature. Table 10.2 shows various temperature levels and their typical subjective descriptions.[7]

Chemical Effects

Chemical changes may occur when water is taken by mouth or when chemicals are introduced internally during lavage.

Reflex Effects

The application of heat or cold in any form to one area of the body has an effect on circulation in other areas.

Several factors determine the extent of the effects of water as a therapeutic agent that should be taken into consideration prior to the use of water as a modality:

1. The degree of temperature change desired
2. The water temperature itself
3. The suddenness with which the water therapy is applied
4. The duration and pressure of application
5. The extent of body surface treated
6. The frequency of application
7. The age, weight, and general condition of the patient.

INDICATIONS

The major physiologic effects of hydrotherapy and the corresponding indications for care may be summarized as follows:

1. Thermal or hypothermal effects
2. Increase or decrease in circulation
3. Increase in mobility, especially when exercise is performed underwater
4. Relaxation
5. Analgesia or sedation, especially during cold water therapy

Table 10.2. Temperature Levels and Their Subjective Interpretations

Typical Perception	*Degrees Fahrenheit*	*Degrees Celsius*
Very hot	104—115	40—46
Hot	98—104	36.5—40
Warm	96—98	35.5—36.5
Neutral	92—96	33.5—35.5
Tepid	80—92	27—33.5
Cool	65—80	18—27
Cold	55—65	13—18
Very cold	34—55	1—13

6. Debridement (eg, open wounds)
7. Promotion of tissue healing and repair
8. Relief of muscle spasm.

The general indications for hydrotherapy are shown in Table 10.3. Water also has variable cleansing, diaphoretic, diuretic, emetic, hypnotic, and purgative effects.

CONTRAINDICATIONS

Special considerations and contraindications for hydrotherapy are listed in Table 10.4.

THERAPEUTIC BATHS: APPLICATIONS

Various types of baths have been used for many years—with full or partial immersion, with or without added minerals or chemicals, and with heated or chilled water. The medicinal value of *balneotherapy,* the use of baths in the treatment of disease, has been extolled for centuries. Paracelsus called the bath "the Archaeus (the inner physician)." From the times of the famous Roman baths, many spas and mineral springs of the world have become meccas for the afflicted who seek a "miracle" cure. Certainly, no one can deny the value of regular bathing and cleansing; however, many of the claims made over the years for such "treatments" are highly questionable.

In this section, we shall describe the more common types of baths in use today and a few less commonly utilized techniques. The avid student of this subject should also refer to the many detailed texts on this subject that are available.

Whirlpools and Hubbard Tanks

One of the most common applications of hydrotherapy is with the whirlpool or the larger Hubbard tank. A whirlpool or Hubbard can be an extremely beneficial modality. Its primary and unique therapeutic value is in the opportunity to provide active or passive exercise of an injured part within water. Although the requirement to constantly change or disinfect a large amount of water is relatively expensive, this expense is justified by the extraordinary benefits that can be obtained.

WHIRLPOOLS

A whirlpool unit is a partial immersion bath in which the water may be agitated and mixed with air. The agitated water can be specifically directed toward an affected part. A whirlpool bath has the advantage of (1) patient immersion, in part or as a whole, (2) temperature effects, and (3) mechanical effects as a result of the agitated water.[8] The degree of water agitation is controlled by an aerator on the unit, and the temperature of the water can be maintained at a constant setting by a thermostat control.

Indications. In general, whirlpools are indicated in the following situations:

1. When exercise to a part under water is desirable. For example:
   a. Low back injuries
   b. After the first 3 days in strains and sprains
   c. Postoperative orthopedic conditions
   d. The treatment of arthritis and fibrositis
   e. Peripheral nerve injuries.
2. Burns.[9-12]
3. Peripheral vascular injuries (Note: temperature should not exceed 105 °F in venous disorders, including indolent ulcers; 93 °F in arterial disorders).[13]
4. Miscellaneous applications; eg, gentle massage, cleans wounds and stimulates healing, relieves pain and relaxes muscles, and softens soft tissues prior to stretching, exercise, or manipulation.

Therapeutic Temperature. Temperature parameters are shown in Table 10.5.

Treatment Duration. Treatment time with a whirlpool should be from 15 to 20 minutes.

Table 10.3. General Indications of Common Hydrotherapy Techniques

Technique	***Effects***
Hot baths or applications	Relaxes capillaries and other soft tissues; draws blood from deep tissues to surface; relieves pain and muscle spasm; increases core temperature; increases joint mobility, especially when exercise is performed underwater; increases circulatory and metabolic rates; increases blood volume and oxygen consumption; produces slight alkalinity; relieves pain of myositis and neuritis.
Warm baths or applications	Soothes irritated cutaneous nerves; soothes nerves of visceral organs that are related reflexly with the area of skin that is warmed; promotion of tissue healing and repair; increases pulse rate; increases kidney function; lessens general nervous sensibility; relaxes muscles; increases perspiration; lowers blood pressure; dilates blood vessels.
Brief hot tub or shower baths	Produces general relaxation; relieves fatigue.
Gradually elevated hot tub or vapor baths	Relaxes muscles generally; calms emotions.
Warm sprays	Debridement of open wounds.
Hot and cold applications	When applied in sequence 4—6 times, the cardiovascular system is stimulated both generally and locally. The final immersion should always be in the hot water.
Neutral baths	Sedation, muscle relaxation, general vasodilation; quiets emotional excitability.
Cold baths or applications	Cools the body part; contracts small blood vessels when applied locally; stimulates the part, especially when followed by friction and percussion massage; analgesia and sedation; decreases core temperature; raises blood pressure; increases muscle tone; decreases heart rate and lengthens period of diastole; produces hyperpnea; increases basal metabolism in proportion to duration of the therapy.

Table 10.4. Precautions in the Use of Hydrotherapy

External Hydrotherapy (eg, baths, whirlpool, Hubbard tanks, sprays).

1. Care should be taken whenever treating the very young or elderly.
2. Be certain with all patients to explain what the treatment consists of and what should be expected during therapy.
3. Patients with heart conditions, hypertension, or diabetes should be treated with great caution.
4. Care should be taken in treating any patient who has sustained a cardiovascular accident.
5. Patients with rashes or dermatologic diseases should not be treated in a Hubbard tank or whirlpool unless the unit is sterilized and the water is changed after use.
6. If a patient becomes dizzy, nauseous, or weak, therapy should be discontinued immediately.

Table 10.5. Temperature Parameters for Whirlpool Baths

Area/Disorder	*Water Temperature*
Upper extremity	104°—108°F
Lower extremity	102°—104°F
Full body immersion	99°—104°F
Arthritic complaints*	100°—104°F
Acute musculoskeletal complaints	55°—70°F
Postacute musculoskeletal complaints**	99°—110°F
Burns	Below 96°F

*Not acute rheumatoid or inflammatory arthritis.
**After 48—72 hours.

Sterilization. A whirlpool should be drained and cleaned after each treatment. Either betadine or zephiran chloride can be used to disinfect the tank. However, if an open wound has been treated, more elaborate sterilization procedures should be administered.

HUBBARD TANKS

A Hubbard tank is another form of full immersion therapy, although the tank is much larger than a typical whirlpool. The water can be agitated by one or more aerators located on the side(s) of the unit. A therapist can enter the tank with the patient to provide close supervision or passive exercise. The tank is large enough to allow walking exercises in the water. A crane is usually provided above the unit so that a weak or paralyzed patient may be passively transferred by a hoist to a canvas plinth in the tank.[14,15] See Figure 10.3.

Indications. In general, Hubbard tanks are indicated in the following situations:

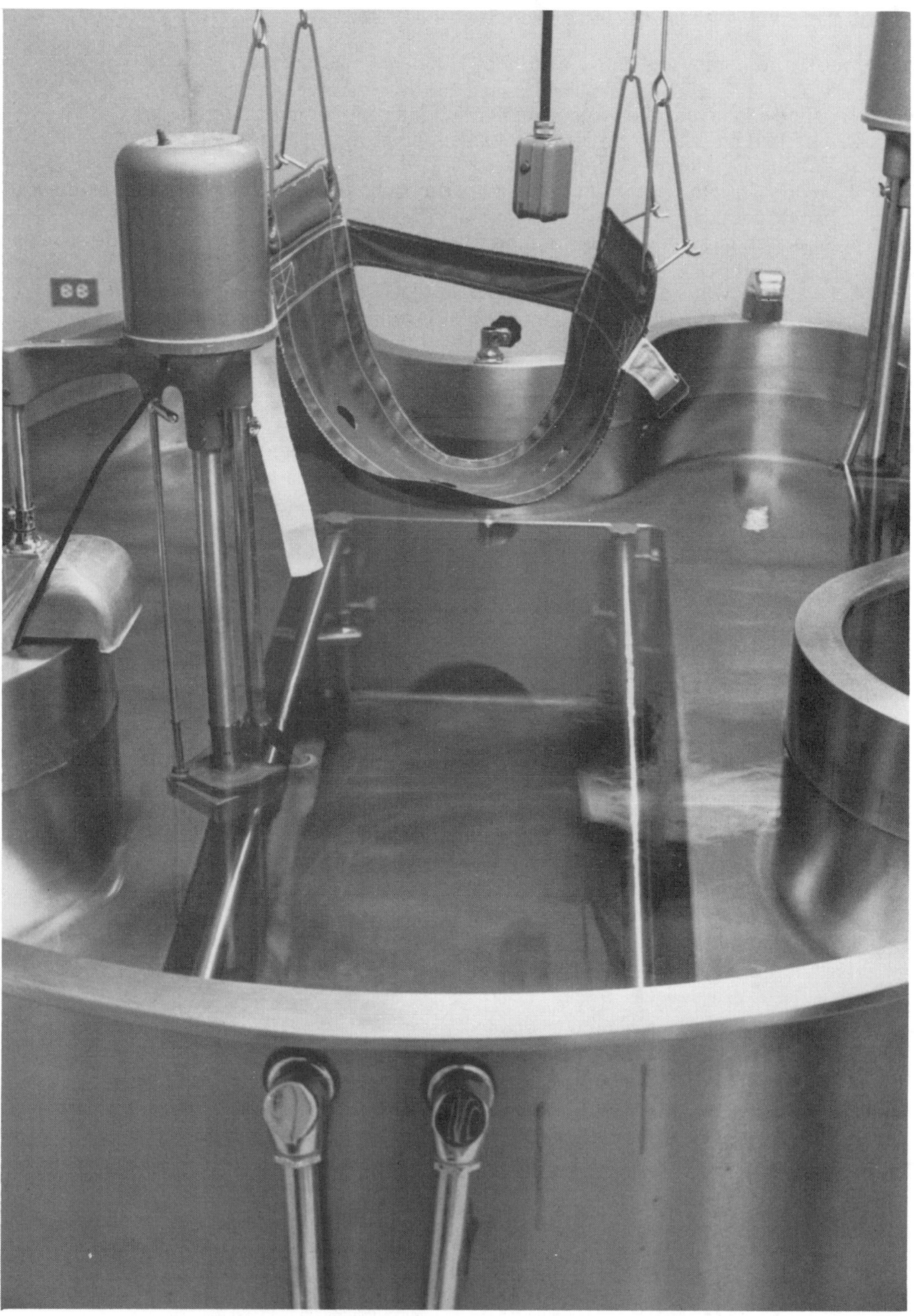

Figure 10.3. A different view of a Hubbard tank.

1. All indications previously listed for whirlpool baths
2. When underwater exercise is desirable
3. When underwater passive range of motion exercises can only be performed if the therapist is in the water
4. When debridement and cleaning of large areas of burned tissue is desirable
5. Various applications in postoperative rehabilitation.

Special Considerations. Three points deserve special mention: (1) Care should be taken with patients exhibiting contagious skin diseases (eg, athlete's foot) so that cross-contamination to other patients is avoided. (2) Patients undergoing hydrotherapy for the treatment of burns should be carefully monitored to prevent an excessive depletion of sodium salts.[16,17] (3) When saline solutions are used with water agitation, extremely effective therapeutic results can be achieved in treating patients with skin grafts.

Contrast Baths

Alterations of hot and cold have been used for many years, especially in the care of patients with acute musculoskeletal injuries. The effected alternating contraction and dilatation of blood vessels has been found to be quite beneficial in hastening healing. Blood flow is markedly increased both locally and reflexly and metabolism is increased locally.[18,19]

Also see Chapter 6, Cryotherapies, where contrast baths are further described.

Sitz Baths

Sitz is the German word for *sit.* A sitz bath is defined as a partial immersion that is designed to affect primarily the circulation of the pelvic region; ie, the patient sits in water whose level covers the hips. Sometimes, a specially constructed "sitz" tub is provided that is shaped to allow the legs to be out of the water.

Indications. A warm sitz bath is generally indicated in the treatment of painful hemorrhoids; however, it has also been found useful in treating patients with prostatic complaints, sciatica, cystitis, urinary retention, dysmenorrhea, postpartum distress, and following certain types of pelvic surgery. A cold sitz tends to tone pelvic muscles (eg, atonic constipation, subinvoluted uterus) and viscera and lessens pelvic bleeding (eg, uterine, rectal).[20]

Therapeutic Temperature and Treatment Duration. The temperature of the water is varied depending on the effect desired. Typical parameters are shown in Table 10.6.

Other Types of Baths

A partial listing of some of the many types of baths used throughout the years is shown in Table 10.7.[21]

Douches and Sprays

One or multiple streams can be directed against a specific part of the body or against the body as a whole. The technique is quite popular in Europe. The purpose is to combine (1) water, with a static or variable temperature, and (2) pressure or friction against the skin. Due to the necessary nozzle-skin distance and the "splash" effect, a large treating area (eg, large shower stall) is required.

A therapeutic spray is essentially an application of water (85°—115°F) from multiple needle nozzles that is usually directed horizontally to the body (except the head) from multiple directions. Such applications are both cleansing and stimulating, inducing a general tonic effect. The effect of the spray can be varied by altering the temperature, pressure, and duration.

A *scotch douche* is a spray directed against a localized area, usually by a percussion jet or fanned spray. A common *water pik* can be used to cleanse the nose, tonsils, and gums.

Table 10.8 summarizes the parameters, indications, and treatment times of some of the more popular douches and sprays.[22,23,24]

Table 10.6. Suggested Sitz Bath Temperature and Duration Parameters

	Temperature	*Treatment Duration*
Cold sitz	55°—75°F	2—10 minutes
Hot sitz	105°—115°F	2—10 minutes
Contrast sitz:		
Hot phase	105°—115°F	3 minutes (3 times)
Cold phase*	55°—85°F	30 seconds (3 times)

*Always finish with cold.

Table 10.7. Miscellaneous Types of Therapeutic Baths

Name of Bath	*Temperature*	*Traditional Indication**
Cold	55°—70°F	Following acute injury
Neutral	92°—97°F	Sedation, relaxation, general vasodilation
Hot	100°—115°F	Stiffness (eg, arthritis)
Alkaline	94°—98°F	Dermatologic disorders, insect bites
Alpha Keri	94°—98°F	Itching
Ascorbic acid powder	94°—98°F	Allergy, infection, hemorrhoids
Aveeno (oatmeal)	96°—98°F	Skin irritations (less drying than starch), hives, chafing, itching, windburn, sunburn
Balpine (pine oil)	96°—98°F	Fatigue, relaxation, sedation, slight hyperemia, skin cleansing
Borax	94°—98°F	Antiseptic, skin irritations, drying
Bran	94°—98°F	Itching, softens skin, relaxation
Bromine-valerian	92°—98°F	Nervous disorders
Chamomile	94°—98°F	Antiseptic, insomnia, digestive problems
Epsom salts	92°—100°F	Fatigue, induces perspiration, relaxes muscles, detoxifier, relieves catarrh
Hayflower/oatstraw	94°—98°F	Promotes perspiration, releases impurities, detoxifier
Mineral steel	92°—98°F	Convalescence
Oil of Cade (juniper oil, Almay tar)	94°—100°F	Itching
Oxygen	96°—98°F	Visceral disorders
Potassium permanganate	94°—98°F	Astringent, antiseptic, deodorant
Saline	94°—98°F	Tonic, first aid for burns
Sodium bicarbonate	94°—98°F	Itching, opens pores, cleanses skin
Sulphur	90°—102°F	Arthritis, acne, scabies, promotes healing
Tea	70°—92°F	First degree burns
Vinegar	96°—98°F	Fatigue, restores skin's acid mantle, poison ivy
Vinegar-borax	96°—98°F	Ringworm

*Several traditional uses listed above have not been verified scientifically.

Table 10.8. Traditional Parameters for Douches and Sprays

Name	*Temperature Guidelines*	*Special Indications*	*Therapy Duration*
Neutral spray.......	Begin at 100°F and slowly lower to 94°F	General relaxation, sedation	3—5 minutes
Hot spray:			
Phase 1...........	Begin at 100°F and slowly raise to tolerance	Cleansing	1—2 minutes
Phase 2...........	Cool rapidly to 85°F	Tonic	1—2 minutes
Alternating hot and cold:			
Phase 1...........	Begin at 100°—110°F for 1 minute, then lower quickly to 90°F for .5—1 minute	Vigorous tonic	
Phase 2...........	Increase to 112°F for 1 minute, then decrease to 85°F for .5—1 minute	Vigorous tonic	4—6 minutes
Phase 3...........	Increase to 115°F for 1 minute, then end with 94°F for 2—3 minutes	Vigorous tonic	
Scotch douche	Hot: 105°—118°F	Stimulation, reflex dilatation	3—6 minutes
	Neutral: 94°—97°F	Sedation	3—6 minutes
	Cold: 90°—85°F	Stimulant, tonic	.5—1 minute

Gargles

A gargle is a wash for the throat, especially the tonsillar area. It is conducted by tipping the head back so that the liquid will accumulate toward the back of the pharynx and then agitating the fluid by the exhalation of air.

A saline or salt-vinegar gargle is the most common type used (eg, for pharyngitis, tonsillitis, postnasal drip, laryngitis). Some vitamin-mineral distributing companies offer a mineral solution that has strong astringent qualities.

REFERENCES

1. Zislis JM: Hydrotherapy. In Krusen FH, et al (eds): *Handbook of Physical Medicine and Rehabilitation,* ed 2. Philadelphia, W.B. Saunders, 1971, p 346.
2. Moor FB, et al: *Manual of Hydrotherapy and Massage.* Mountain View, CA, Pacific Press, 1964, p 4.
3. Fischer E, Solomon S: Physiological responses to heat and cold. In Licht S (ed): *Therapeutic Heat.* New Haven, Elizabeth Licht, 1958.
4. Moor FB, et al: *Manual of Hydrotherapy and Massage.* Mountain View, CA, Pacific Press, 1964, pp 2-3.
5. Ibid: pp 1-2.
6. Ibid: pp 15-16.
7. Buchman DD: *The Complete Book of Water Therapy.* New York, E.P. Dutton, 1979, p 103.
8. Kaplan CM: A whirlpool chair. *Physical Therapy,* vol 49, August, 1969.
9. Smith EI, De Weese HMS: The topical therapy of burns in children. *Archives of Surgery,* vol 98, April 1969.
10. Whiting WB, et al: Hydrotherapy at burn center. *Western Medicine,* March 1966.
11. Rose HW: Initial cold water treatment of burns. *Northwest Medicine,* 35:267, June 1936.
12. Ofeigsson OJ: First aid treatment of scalds and burns by water cooling. *Postgraduate Medicine,* 30:330, October 1961.
13. Finnerty GB, Corbitt T: *Hydrotherapy.* New York, Frederick Ungar, 1960, pp 61-71.
14. Zislis JM: Hydrotherapy. In Krusen FH, et al (eds): *Handbook of Physical Medicine and Rehabilitation,* ed 2. Philadelphia, W.B. Saunders, 1971, p 352.
15. Downer AH: *Physical Therapy Procedures: Selected Techniques,* ed 2. Springfield, IL, Charles C. Thomas, 1974, pp 182-184.
16. Gotshall RA: Sodium depletion related to hydrotherapy for burn injury. *Journal of the American Medical Association,* 203:101-105, 1968.
17. Shulman AG: Ice water in the primary treatment of burns. *Journal of the American Medical Association,* 173:1916, August 27, 1960.
18. Abbott GK, et al: *Physical Therapy in Nursing Care.* Washington, DC, Review & Herald Publishing Association, 1941, pp 114-116.
19. Bierman W: *Physical Medicine in General Practice.* New York, Paul B. Hoeber, 1947, pp 36-38.
20. Moor FB, et al: *Manual of Hydrotherapy and Massage.* Mountain View, CA, Pacific Press, 1964, pp 41-42, 45.
21. Buchman DD: *The Complete Book of Water Therapy.* New York, E.P. Dutton, 1979, pp 73-85.
22. Fuerst EV, Wolff LV: *Fundamentals of Nursing.* Philadelphia, J.B. Lippincott, 1959, p 233.
23. Moor FB, et al: *Manual of Hydrotherapy and Massage.* Mountain View, CA, Pacific Press, 1964, pp 69-74.
24. Harmer B, Henderson V: *Textbook of the Principles and Practice of Nursing,* ed 5. New York, Macmillan, p 331.

Chapter 11

Traction, Stretching, Vibration, And Bracing

We have previously described ways that modalities could be utilized to control pain, effect muscle spasm, reduce edema, relieve neurologic symptomatologies, and produce other therapeutic effects. In addition, the principles of heat, cold, and electrotherapy have been described. This final chapter reviews traction, stretching, and vibration procedures commonly in use today, emphasizing those procedures used to elongate compressed or shortened body tissues and to stimulate physiologic reactions through the use of vibration. The chapter concludes with a brief explanation of the more common procedures utilizing orthotics.

TRACTION

Traction is the act of drawing or pulling a body part or parts by any means. Typical forms include:

1. *Axial traction,* where traction is made in line with the long axis of a course through which a body or body part is drawn.
2. *Weight traction,* where traction is exerted by means of weights.
3. *Elastic traction,* where traction is exerted by elastic devices such as rubber bands, elastic bandages, or elastic stockings.
4. *Head or lumbopelvic traction,* where traction is applied to the cranium or lower back such as in the treatment of cervical or lumbosacral injuries or disorders.
5. *Extremity traction,* where traction is applied to a fracture/dislocation following reduction.

Skin traction, as opposed to that where connection is made to surgically implanted pins or hooks, is both a definitive conservative treatment method as well as a first-aid measure. Traction forces applied to the skin are transmitted to bone via underlying ligaments, strong fascia, and muscle-tendon units. The next two sections review the basic principles associated with stretching and traction, the types commonly used, and the general parameters for their use.

Historical Perspective

Treatment procedures utilizing stretching or traction forces have been used since before the time of Hippocrates. They have been used to relieve pain, to set fractures and dislocations, and to cause pain and torture. As with many of the innovations that have been ascribed to Hippocrates, he is honored by historians as having been the first to use isometric traction in treating fractures of the femur. More than likely, however, forms of therapeutic structural pulling and stretching have been used since the beginning of civilization.[1]

It is a normal inclination to stretch when a part of the body feels stiff or cramped. We commonly see people stretch tired necks, massage sore arms, or crack their knuckles. Ancient artwork depicts that it was probably early in recorded time that people tried to "set" a fracture by using some form of stretching or leverage force. See Figures 1.1, 1.2, and 1.3.[2]

Isometric traction procedures were still being used during the last century when Hamilton published a text on "fracture tables." However, fracture therapy utilizing isometric forces alone was unsatisfactory, and doctors sought more efficient procedures. It was not until many years later that isotonic traction was used on femur fractures in an attempt to try to overcome the spasm of heavy thigh muscles. Similar isotonic traction techniques are still in use today.

During the mid-1800s, Crosby was the first person to really promote a form of isotonic skin traction on the leg and the technique came to be known as Buck's extension. Later, traction devices included the use of tongs, hooks, pins, and other devices for treating fractures. Skeletal traction has also been used for centuries in treating scoliosis, kyphosis, and other spinal deformities.

In recent years, traction procedures have been developed for managing lumbar disc lesions (Cyriax), lumbar strain (Christie), cervical pain (Goldie and Lindquist), sciatica (Weber, Mathhews, and Hickling), and in the management of dislocations. In spite of such wide use over the years, there are many who are not convinced that traction has any physiologic benefit. As recently as 1976, Weinberger wrote that traction is "irrational, counterproductive, nonphysiologic, and traumatic." He feels that "traction perpetuates new and aggravates already present skeletal abnormalities.

Some clinicians would limit the use of traction forces to patients with fractures. Others feel that nerve root signs should be evident before traction is considered in spinal disorders. At the other extreme of viewpoint, we find those who would use the forces of traction for virtually any musculoskeletal complaint. Regardless of personal belief, there is a paucity of firm scientific evidence to substantiate *or* repudiate the effects of traction on the body.

Physiologic Basis

The term *traction* is a derivative of the Latin word *tractico,* which refers to the act of drawing or pulling.[3] It is commonly thought of as any procedure in which a longitudinal tensile force is applied to a part of the body in an effort to stretch soft tissues or separate articular surfaces. Thus, traction is the opposite of joint approximation (compressed joint surfaces). Traction involves exactly the opposite process of compressive approximation; ie, traction forces promote mobility, and approximation of joints promotes stability. It should be well noted that, in either case, joint receptors are responsive to alterations in joint position.[4]

There is no question that traction forces have a profound effect on joint receptors, which respond to changes in joint position and tensile stress. It is believed that the effect of joint receptor discharge upon motor neurons responses depends on the position of the joint and the type of joint movement associated.

In order to achieve a traction effect, the forces used must be of sufficient strength and duration. Traction forces may be delivered manually, by weights and a pulley system, or by several types of mechanical devices. See Figure 11.1.

In general, the application of traction is utilized primarily to trigger the following physiologic responses:

1. To separate or stretch spinal segments and/or extraspinal joint surfaces.

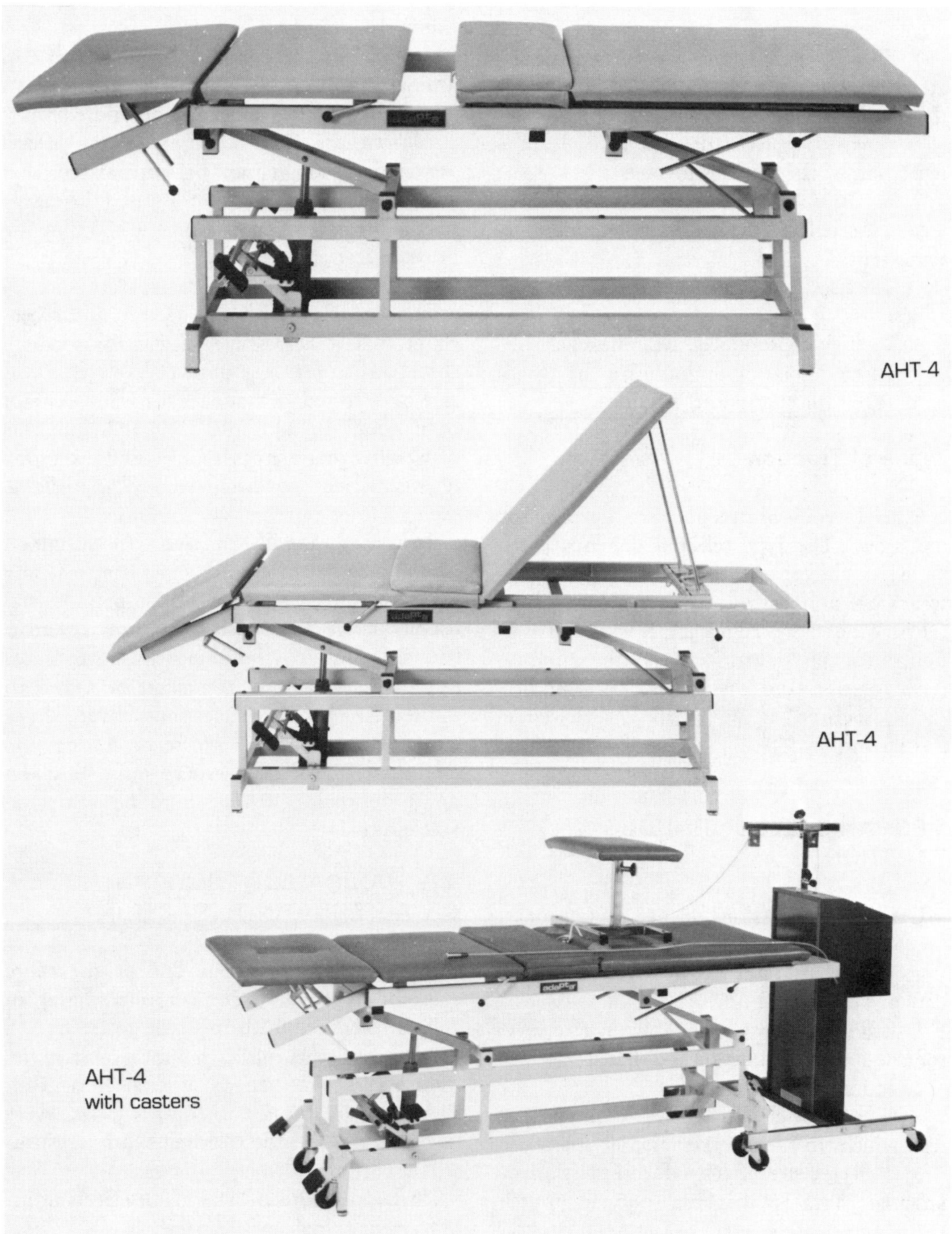

Figure 11.1. The AHT-4 Adapta traction table, with and without casters (courtesy of the Chattanooga Corporation).

2. To promote distraction and gliding of joint facets.

3. To relieve muscle spasm. When moderate continuous stretch is applied to a part, the muscles assume a position of physiologic rest. This rest period may, in turn, lead to relaxation of the muscles involved.

4. To dissipate edema or congestion in an area, especially if the traction is applied intermittently.

5. To stretch fibrotic tissues and break adhesions.

6. To trigger proprioceptive reflexes.

7. To temporarily immobilize or splint parts (eg, with continuous traction).

Types of Traction

Several types of traction are in common use today. The type selected depends partly on what objective(s) the practitioner wishes to achieve and partly on the patient's physical condition. See Figure 11.2. Types of traction, their physiologic effects, their indications for use, and the specific contraindications associated, if any, will be reviewed in this section.

MECHANICAL CONTINUOUS TRACTION

Continuous traction to the spine makes use of a constant pull that may be applied from several minutes up to several hours or days at a time.

Physiologic Effects. The major effects of continuous spinal traction are that it:

1. Immobilizes tissues.

2. Places muscles in a state of physiologic rest, which, in turn, relaxes muscle spasm.

3. Relieves the effects of compression on articular surfaces that are due to muscle spasm or other compressive factors.

4. Stimulates proprioceptive reflexes.

5. Stretches fibrotic tissues and adhesions.

6. Reduces the circumference of the intervertebral disc (IVD) and thus aids in restoring its position to one that allows for normal biomechanics.

7. Relieves the compression effects of foraminal distortion (eg, encroachment).

8. Helps to relieve congestion and edema.

Indications. Once the physiologic effects are recognized, it can be appreciated that continuous spinal traction is used primarily in the treatment of patients to (1) provide immobilization in severe sprains, strains, or fractures; (2) relieve muscle spasm; and (3) reduce edema. Although some authorities claim that it is possible to actually separate spinal structures, it is most unlikely that this can be effected without creating more harm than good. In addition, the small amounts of weights that are commonly used are grossly insufficient to bring about appreciable separation of vertebral motion units.

Sustained Spinal Traction. In sustained (static) traction of ambulatory cases, a steady pull is applied to the spine for periods that usually range from a few minutes up to a half an hour. It is important that a constant pull is applied, and care must be taken to assure that slippage does not occur. Once taut soft tissues start to relax during the treatment, the slack produced must be taken up if optimal benefits are to be achieved. See Figure 11.3.

MECHANICAL INTERMITTENT OR ALTERNATING TRACTION

Intermittent traction is one of the more common types of traction applied today in general practice. With this type of traction, a mechanical unit applies a series of stretches interspaced with periods of relaxation. Tensile forces are applied to the body part every few seconds, and the treatment duration usually lasts from 15 to 30 minutes.

Physiologic Effects. The major effects of intermittent spinal traction are:

1. The pumping action created by the alternating traction increases vascular flow and lymphatic drainage, thus reducing edema and congestion.

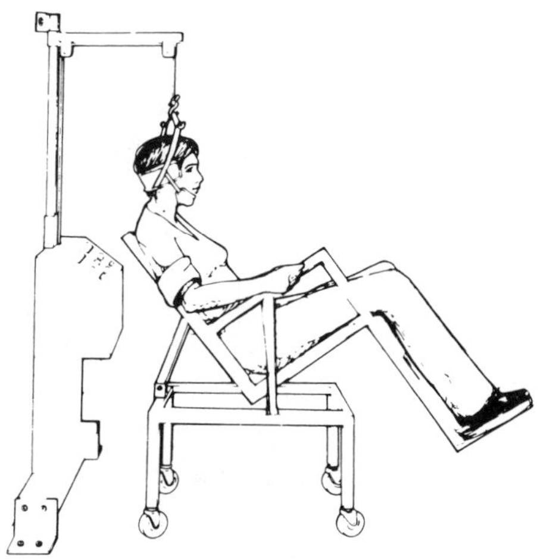

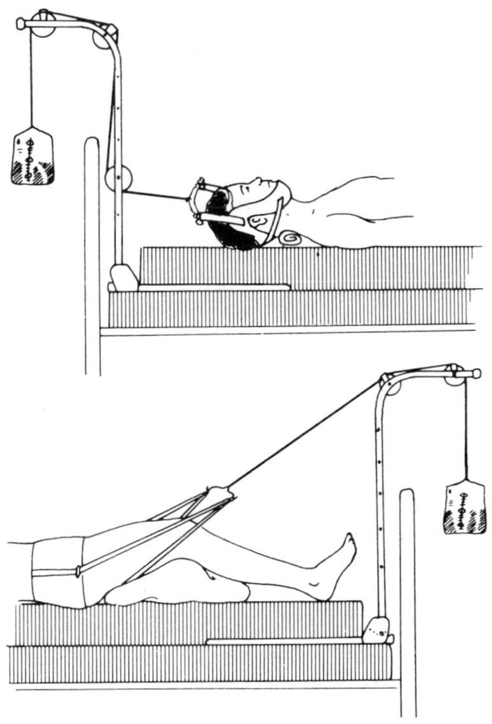

Figure 11.2. *Top diagram,* some mobile traction units offer four modes of treatment: intermittent, progressive intermittent, static, or progressive static. *Middle diagram,* a portable traction unit applying continuous cervical traction. *Bottom diagram,* continuous lumbopelvic traction (courtesy of STC, Inc).

2. There is a stimulating effect that helps to tone muscles, thereby reducing fatigue and tending to restore normal elasticity and resiliency.

3. Stretching of adhesions and fibrotic tissues occurs.

4. The alternate pull and relaxation periods promote IVD hydration.

5. Proprioceptive reflexes are stimulated.

Indications. Intermittent spinal traction is used primarily to (1) reduce congestion in chronic musculoskeletal disorders and (2) provide increased mobility in patients with arthritic complaints.

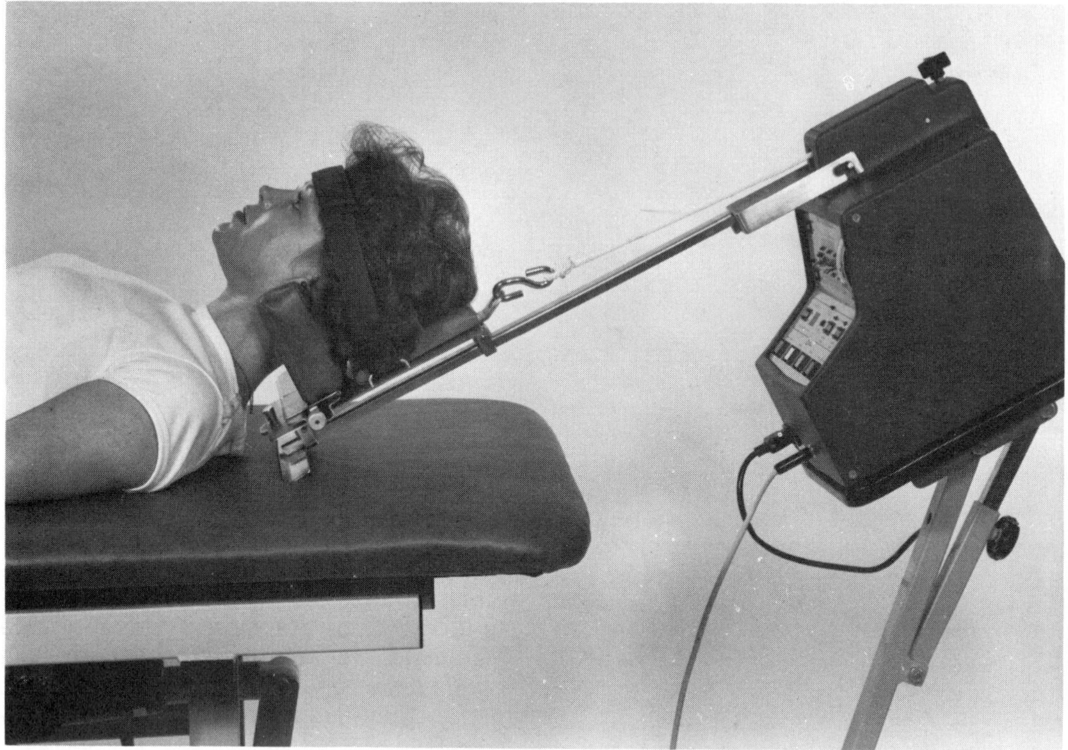

Figure 11.3. One form of cervical traction, with the patient in the horizontal position (courtesy of the Chattanooga Corporation).

MANUAL TRACTION

Traction can also be applied without the use of a mechanical device — usually by a therapist. It may be desirable to apply a continuous steady pull, intermittent pulls, or just a few quick pulls. Care must be taken not to exacerbate chronic complaints and to avoid sudden twists or turns of the patient, especially when applying manual traction to the cervical spine. See Figure 11.4.

MISCELLANEOUS TYPES OF TRACTION

Many other types of traction are in use today, including devices that the patient wears. See Figure 11.5. Other types include special traction benches, gravity lumbar traction, traction on split tables or inclined surfaces, positional traction, and, more recently, gravity inversion traction.

Intersegmental Traction

POSITIONAL TRACTION

Positional traction utilizes pillows, sandbags, rolls, or blocks, which are placed in such a way that a tensile force is placed on the involved perivertebral structures. The technique is usually performed to affect only one side of the spinal region being treated.

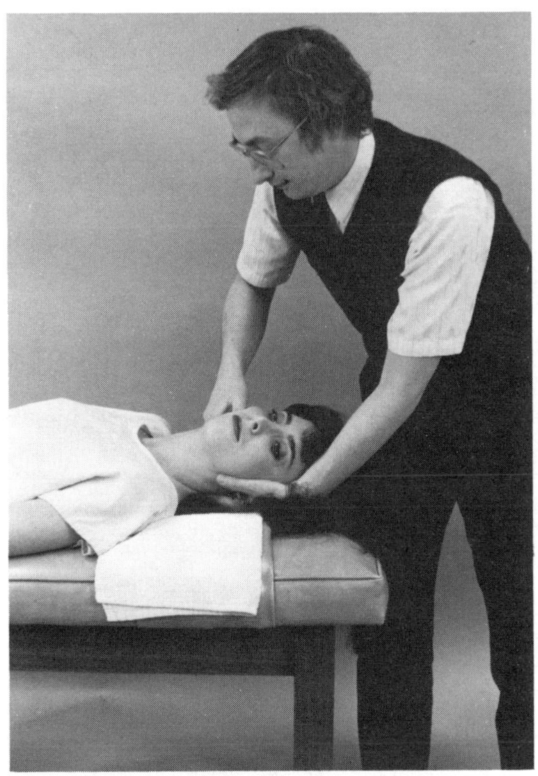

Figure 11.4. Manual traction being applied simultaneously with a cervical rotary adjustment.

GRAVITY INVERSION

Gravity inversion boots are specially made devices that are tightened around the ankles to allow a patient to hang from a stationary horizontal bar in a totally upside down (head caudad) position. Therapeutic inversion boots were first designed by an orthopedic surgeon, R. M. Martin, to relieve interspinal disc pressure. Since their introduction in the 1960s, they have been utilized for specific weight lifting exercises and are popularly used in the treatment of certain musculoskeletal disorders.[5]

Principles of Applying Traction

To effect even a minimal separation of spinal segments by traction, the applied forces must have sufficient magnitude and be applied over an adequate duration.[6,7,8,9] The resistance offered by the patient to the traction forces depends on the weight of the patient plus other factors such as the size, contour, and texture of the two congruent surfaces (ie, the patient's skin and the table surface). Surface resistance is usually equal to about half the weight of the patient's body or body segment. Thus, when traction is to be applied, a force equal to about half the patient's body weight is necessary to overcome the effects of friction.[10]

WEIGHT POUNDAGE

As a general rule, the following guidelines apply to the application of spinal traction:

- *Cervical (sustained) traction:* start at 10 lbs and increase poundage gradually (eg, 5-lb units) to patient tolerance. Do not exceed 30 lbs.
- *Lumbar traction:* apply 25%—50% of

the patient's total body weight. Do not exceed 120 lbs.

• *Intermittent traction:* use approximately 5%—10% of the patient's total body weight. The usual range is from 15 to 30 lbs.

Experience has shown that (1) traction weight is relative to treatment duration; ie, less weight should be used for longer treatment times, and (2) heavier poundage can be used for shorter periods of intermittent traction.[11]

DIRECTIONS OF PULL

The most common way to apply the forces of traction is to have the patient in a horizontal or modified horizontal position. With the patient in this position, longitudinal tensile forces can readily be effected to the cervical or lumbar regions. An adjustable table designed for this purpose is shown in Figure 11.6.

Vertical traction forces can also be applied to the cervical region by using a harness, straps, weights, and a pulley system. In recent years, as previously described, there has been growing interest in reverse or antigravity traction where the patient is inverted—keeping in mind the contraindications involved.

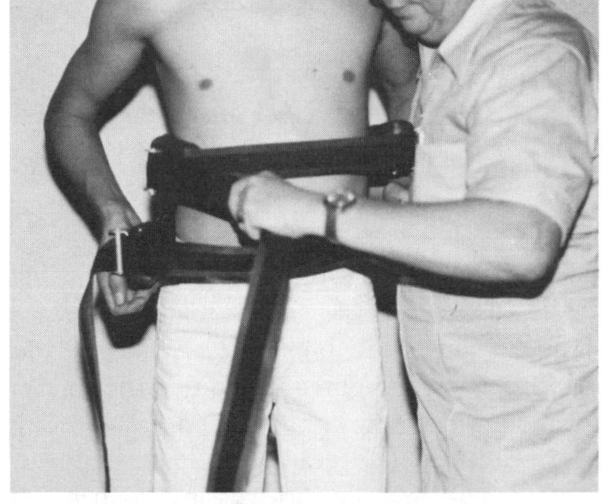

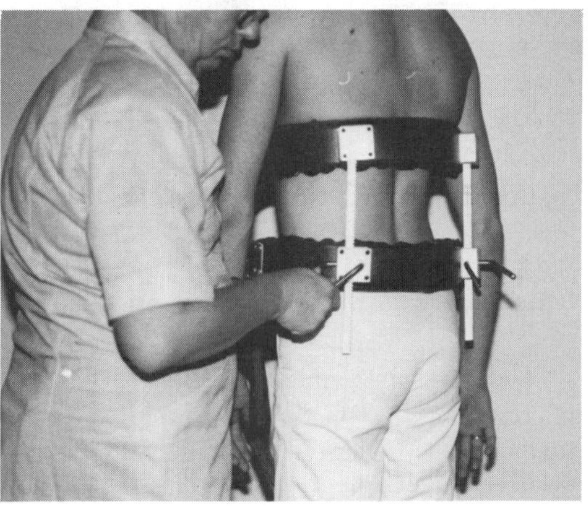

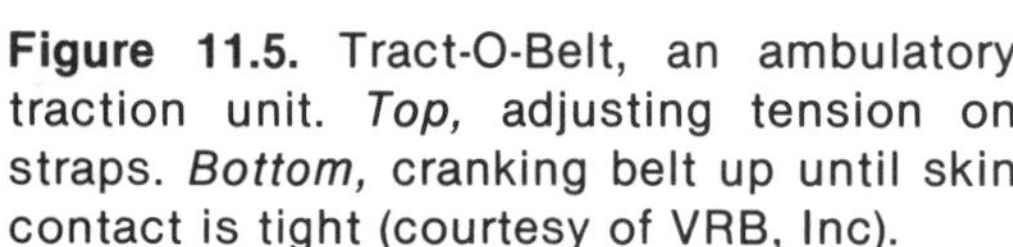

Figure 11.5. Tract-O-Belt, an ambulatory traction unit. *Top,* adjusting tension on straps. *Bottom,* cranking belt up until skin contact is tight (courtesy of VRB, Inc).

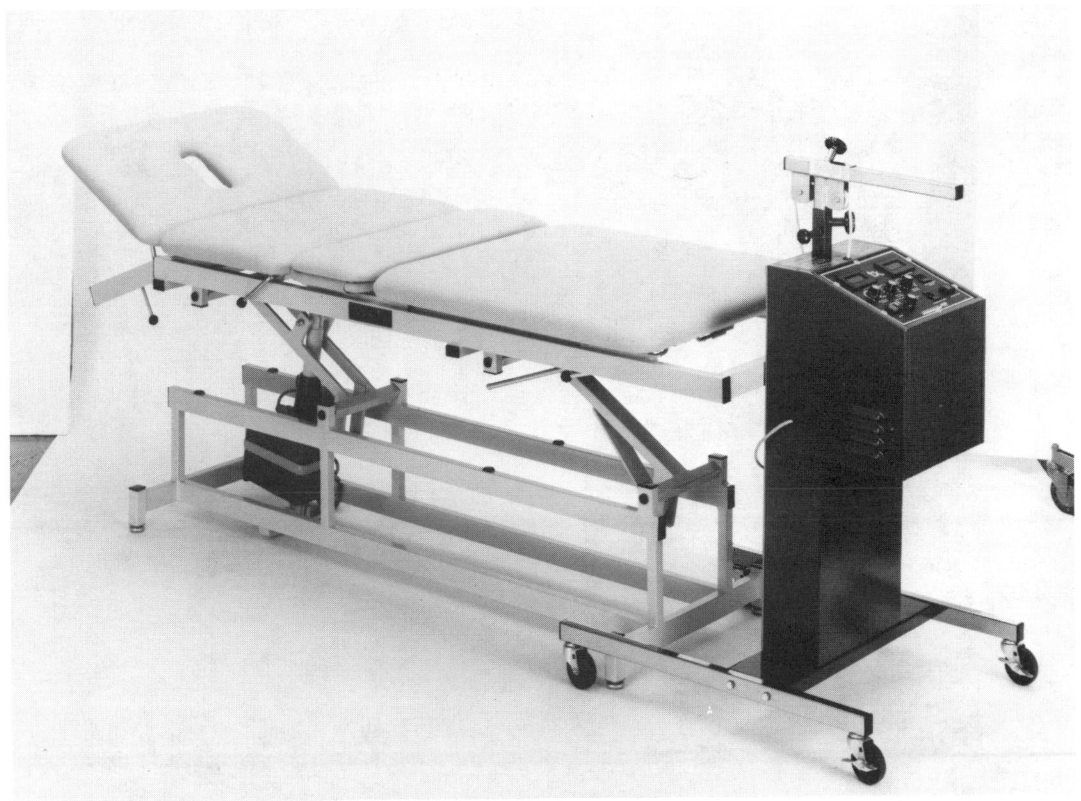

Figure 11.6. Several types of professionally designed horizontal tables are available that include split midsections and various angles of body tilt. This photograph shows the AHT-4 Adapta traction table (courtesy of the Chattanooga Corporation).

ANGLES OF PULL

- *Cervical region.* When applying the forces of traction to the cervical region, the head should be placed in 25°—30° of flexion when the forces are applied to affect C3—C7 or in 0° of flexion when the forces are applied to affect the occiput, atlas, or axis.
- *Lumbar region prone.* The amount of flexion is determined by the size of the pillow under the patient's abdomen.
- *Lumbar region supine.* The patient's hips and knees are flexed and a support is placed under the patient's legs. See Figure 11.7.

The above examples refer to traction forces applied bilaterally. However, in some instances, unilateral traction is indicated such as in unilateral joint hypomobility, spasticity, or spinal curvatures. When a protective (antalgic) scoliosis is present, traction is applied to the contralateral side of pain. In a lumbar scoliosis that is caused by unilateral muscle spasm, traction is applied on the concave side of the lordosis.[12,13]

DURATION

The time length of therapy depends on the specific condition being treated, the physical status of the patient, and patient tolerance. Intermittent traction is rarely applied for more than 30 minutes, while sustained traction of up to several hours may be appropriate.

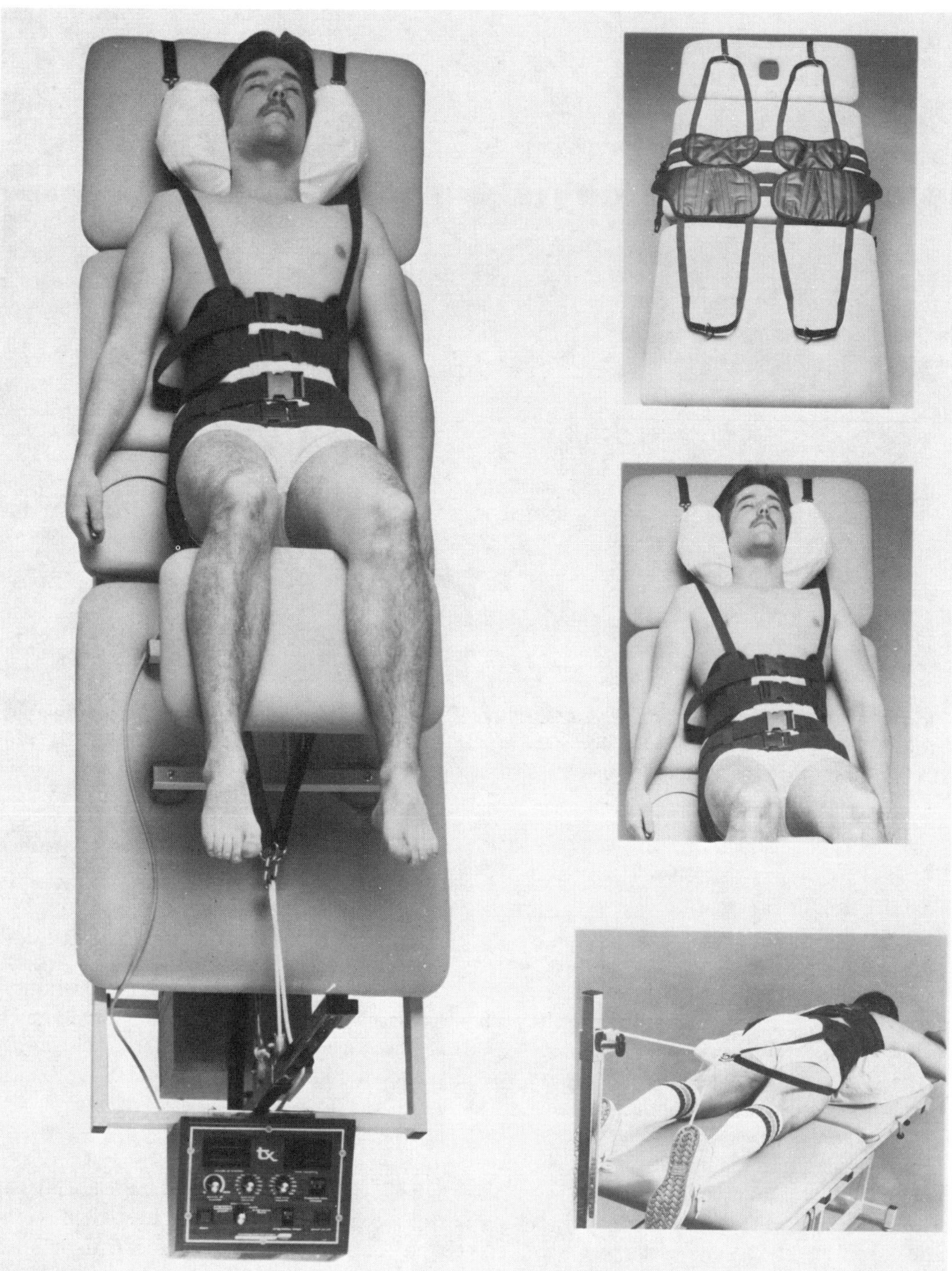

Figure 11.7. *Left,* note support of patient's legs during lumbopelvic traction. *Right top and middle,* heavy-duty traction belts are being utilized. *Right bottom,* traction with the patient in the prone position. Note pillow under the patient's abdomen (courtesy of the Chattanooga Corporation).

GENERAL RULES

The following rules apply under common circumstances:[14,15,16]

1. Place the patient in a position that will best affect the area of treatment. Pads, pillows, rolls, and other devices are helpful.

2. Secure attachment halters, straps, or other traction connections firmly but with ample padding to the skin, underlying soft tissues, and osseous structures. Excessive traction will easily result in skin damage, thus careful monitoring must be done on proper padding, strapping, poundage, and angulation.

3. Traction weight should be increased and/or decreased slowly to avoid abrupt reactions and adjusted to meet the conditions at hand. The amount of poundage utilized should be measured by a superimposed scale.

4. The duration of therapy must be adjusted to the circumstances present. Undertreatment is better than excessive poundage or duration, as these factors can always be increased after a trial period.

5. Assure that the patient is well attended and frequently monitored. Discontinue treatment immediately if untoward symptoms or signs appear; then seek and appraise the cause.

6. Hot, cold, manipulation, and/or massage can usually be applied simultaneously with cervical or lumbopelvic traction if such applications would be indicated.

PRECAUTIONS

At the least, several standard precautions should be taken whenever cervical or lumbar traction is applied.[17,18]

Cervical Traction. The patient should be instructed to remove dentures, earrings, glasses, or a wig before being harnessed. All apparatus should be kept in a sanitary condition. Care must be taken not to fasten halter straps too tight, assure that the halter straps are not twisted, and carefully avoid jerking the rope when slack is removed from it. Assure that pressure points on the skin do not become irritated; eg, use facial tissue in the chin portion of the halter. When the patient is placed in the horizontal position, the patient's feet should not be allowed to dangle in the air; be sure that the legs are well supported. Patients undergoing traction should not be allowed to read during treatment, and, during cervical traction in the seated position, the patient's arms should be placed on a lap pillow or cushion to relieve tension on the neck.

Lumbopelvic Traction. Secure the pelvic harness firmly, and see that the top of the belt can be seen to extend just barely over the iliac crests. Assure that the counter-stabilizer belt is securely fastened and that slack does not exist or arise later in the rope.

Gravity Inversion. Although gravity inversion is gaining continuing acceptance, the practitioner should be fully aware of its potential contraindications, which especially include uncontrolled hypertension, uncompensated congestive heart failure, carotid artery stenosis, and hiatal hernia. There have also been reports of patients who have experienced faintness, periorbital petechiae, headaches, and vague sensations of head pressure.[19] In a recent review of the effects of gravity inversion, Klatz and his associates report a marked increase in systemic blood pressure, pulse rate, central retinal arterial pressure, and intraocular pressure following only a 3-minute period of inversion. See Table 11.1.[20]

General Indications for Spinal Traction

The primary indications for intersegmental spinal traction are IVD protrusion, degenerative disc disease, joint hypomobility, spinal nerve root impingement, muscle spasm, and compression fractures. A general rule, but one that must always be reconsidered in individual cases, holds that static traction is used in acute conditions and intermittent traction is applicable to subacute and chronic disorders. Other indications are listed in Table 11.2.

Basically, traction encourages length, alignment, and functional stability. These goals become a priority in cases of mild structural compression that result in ischemia and pain sited either locally and/or distally, resulting in muscle spasm producing functional contraction. The associated nerve irritation, which may be sensory, motor, or both, may exhibit signs of pain, flaccidity, and diminished reflexes.[21]

Continuous moderate traction tends to immobilize and "splint" strained musculoskeletal tissue, to relieve spasms by placing them in physiologic rest, and to stimulate proprioceptive reflexes, thus relieving associated pain and tenderness. It stretches fibrotic tissues and adhesions (anticontracture factor) and relieves compression effects on articular tissues (eg, cartilage, discs) due to muscular spasm, gravity, or other compression forces (commonly seen in chronic subluxations) to restore connective tissue resiliency and contour. Traction can reduce edema in an extremity if the traction unit elevates the affected part above the heart.

In the spine, traction reduces the circumference of intervertebral discs, thus helping to restore normal positioning (eg, from suction, molding, axial pull) and relieves compression effects of foraminal distortion and/or narrowing; ie, it increases the intervertebral foramen's diameter. A by-product of these effects is the dissipation of congestion, stasis, edema, and dural-sleeve adhesions in associated tissues.

Intermittent traction effects include increased vascular and lymphatic flow (suction aspiration effect), which tends to reduce stasis, edema, and coagulates in chronic congestions. It tends to stretch and free periarticular and articular adhesions and fibrotic infiltrations, is an efficient supplement to manual adjustments, stimulates proprioceptive reflexes, and helps to tone muscles which tends to reduce fatigue and restore elasticity and resiliency. In the spine, it encourages the expansion and contraction of disc tissues, thus improving their nutrition.

DISC HERNIATION WITH PROTRUSION

Some evidence exists that indicates that an intervertebral disc protrusion can be reduced and spinal nerve root symptoms relieved to some extent when spinal traction is applied. For example, Mathews recommends sustained traction of 120 lbs for 20 minutes,[22] and several others suggest using 60—80 lbs every 3 or 4 hours until acute symptoms subside.

The effects of traction are often dramatic but sometimes short lived if a herniated disc is involved. Extreme care must be taken in posttraumatic cases to eliminate the possibility of instability prior to traction. For example, the use of traction following traumatic spondylolisthesis in which the anterior longitudinal ligament has been separated can produce severe displacement with catastrophic effects.[23]

In any occipital, vertebral, or pelvic subluxation, physiotherapy, traction, muscle relaxants, gross manipulation, muscle stretching, injections, or other methods will not offer much relief by themselves unless the fixated articulation is correctly mobilized so that intrinsic function can be normalized.[24] If traction is to be successful, conservative treatment mandates a total management program, thorough patient education, and a gradual/cautious return to normal activity.[25]

DEGENERATIVE DISC DISEASE

We have observed that many cases of degenerative disc disease show periods of relieved symptomatology for months or years following a series of treatments with traction. Other patients, for reasons unknown, do not respond, and a small percentage of patients with spondylosis report an aggravation of symptoms.

Table 11.1. Effects of Inversion on Systemic and Ocular Pressures

Pressure (mm Hg)	*Average Preinversion Pressure (seated)*	*Average Inverted Pressure (3 minutes)*	*Average Postinversion Pressure (seated)*
Systolic blood pressure	119	148	123
Diastolic blood pressure	74	90	75
Intraocular pressure	19	35	19
Central retinal systolic pressure	45	105	51
Central retinal diastolic pressure	26	62	32

Table 11.2. General Indications in the Use of Traction

CONTINUOUS TRACTION

Articular jamming
Brachial neuritis
Compression fractures
Degenerative disc disease
IVD syndrome (early stages)
IVF narrowing
Joint hypomobility
Kyphosis
Lordosis
Occipital neuralgia
Osteoarthritis
Perivertebral adhesions, contractures, and fixations
Scalenus anticus syndrome
Scoliosis
Spasticity
Spinal nerve root impingement
Spondylolisthesis
Sprains (splinting effect)
Steinbrocker's syndrome
Stimulation of mechanoreceptors
Torticollis (subacute)
Vertebral subluxation (subacute, chronic)
Whiplash syndrome (uncomplicated)

INTERMITTENT TRACTION

Deficient IVD hydration
Joint hypomobility
Kyphosis (chronic)
Lordosis (chronic)
Occipital neuralgia
Osteoarthritis
Perivertebral adhesions, contractures, and fixations
Perivertebral congestion
Perivertebral hypotonicity
Posttraumatic edema
Scoliosis (chronic)
Stimulation of mechanoreceptors
Vascular and lymphatic stasis
Vertebral subluxation (chronic)

JOINT HYPOMOBILITY AND MUSCLE SPASM

Almost any situation where hypomobilization is present may respond favorably to traction. Traction in chronic arthritis, for example, often encourages a greater range of motion.[26] Muscle spasm and antalgic guarding frequently respond to traction.

ROOT IMPINGEMENT

Spinal nerve root impingement caused by spondylolisthesis, spinal nerve root swelling, osteophyte encroachment, narrowing of the intervertebral disc, ligamentous encroachment, hyperlordosis, or herniated disc may respond favorably to traction.

If traction is used on a lordotic spine where the sacral angle is increased, care must be taken that the angle of pull is correct. Traction applied to the legs is a most inadequate method when compared to the effectiveness of pelvic traction. Direct horizontal pull on the legs tends to rotate the pelvis forward and increase the sacral angle and lordosis. To correct this, the pelvic pull must be inferoanterior from the posterior with the hips and knees flexed so that body weight will tend to flatten the lumbar curve and the pelvis will curl into slight extension.[27] See Figure 11.8.

SPINAL DEFORMITY

Lawson/Crawford and several others report that traction can be used as a major tool in the treatment of spinal deformities such as scoliosis. A majority of spinal surgeons use preoperative traction when curves are greater than 80°. Halo-femoral traction is considered to be indicated in curves greater than 80° and/or associated with pelvic obliquity and in paralytic/neuromuscular curves.[28,29,30]

Halo-pelvic traction is reported to have poor results in "collapsing spines" and has generally been replaced by halo-gravity procedures (eg, circoelectric bed, specialized wheelchair). A halo-cast is widely accepted as an effective method to treat severe cervicothoracic curves or posttraumatic cervical injuries (eg, fracture/dislocations).[31,32,33]

The clinical objectives of traction in scoliosis, especially during youth, are based upon Wolff's law and the Heuter-Volkmann theory. The major principles are described below:[34]

Axial Loading. Continuous and intermittent axial traction has proven helpful in many cases of scoliosis. The typical mechanism is opposite stretching forces that are applied cephally and caudally to elongate the spine. The actual correction of the angular distortion, however, is *not* produced by the axial tensile forces created. It is produced by the bending moments produced at the wedged

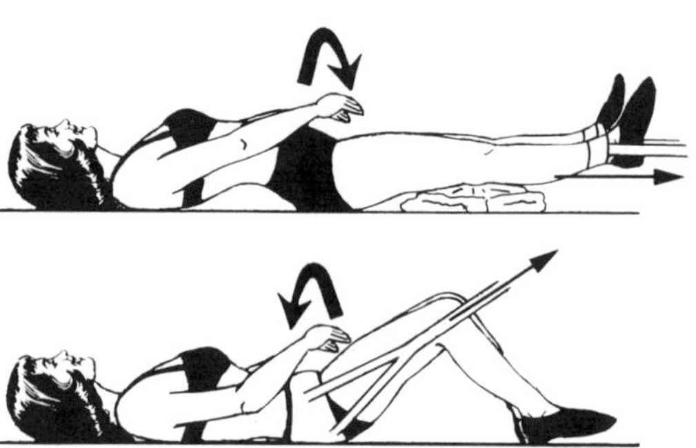

Figure 11.8. *Top,* improper horizontal traction tends to anteriorly rotate the pelvis clockwise in this illustration and produce a hyperlordosis. Excessive stress is also placed on the knees and hips. *Bottom,* diagonal pelvic traction, directed counterclockwise on the pelvis in this illustration, produces posterior rotation, and the lumbar curve flattens. For simplicity only, counterforce harnesses are not shown in the above drawings (courtesy of Associated Chiropractic Academic Press).

disc spaces. See Figure 11.9.

Computing Axial Loads. When applying axial stress to the spine, the corrective bending moment at the farthest lateral point of the curve can be computed by multiplying the axial force by its perpendicular distance from the midline to the apex of the curve. Thus, a given axial force that would increase corrective bending moments in a severe deformity would not be as helpful to a mild deformity. This is important to consider when adjusting the magnitude of traction forces.

Transverse Loading. Transverse loading is also beneficial but more difficult to apply. Attempts have been made by using a lateral pad within a spinal corset. Another method is to apply broad transverse pressure by some means during axial traction. A shoe lift creates transverse spinal loading by shifting the body's center of gravity unless these forces are absorbed in lower segments such as in a supple spine. As in applying axial stresses, the corrective forces are the bending moments created at the wedged disc spaces. See Figure 11.10.

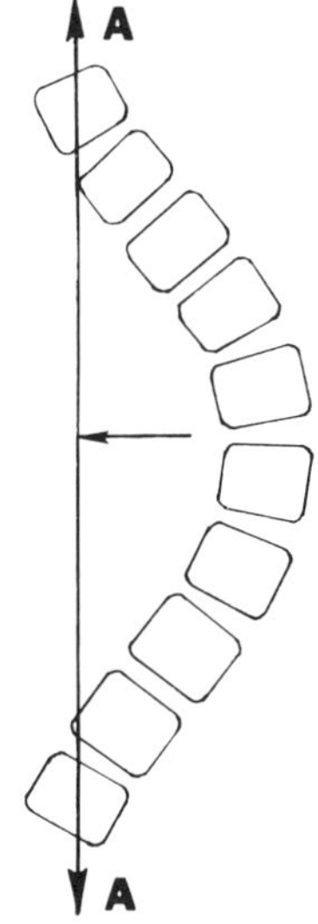

Figure 11.9. Diagram of a scoliotic spine under two-point load from typical traction along the longitudinal axis, *A,* (courtesy of Associated Chiropractic Academic Press).

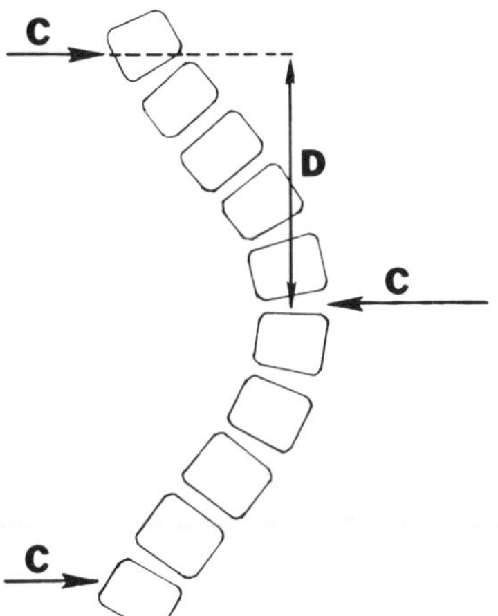

Figure 11.10. Diagram of a scoliotic spine under three-point transverse loading: *C,* transverse forces; *D,* distance between opposing forces. Note that orthopedic braces are usually designed to provide some transverse forces or to provide cutaneous stimulation to produce corrective intrinsic (proprioceptive) reactions (courtesy of Associated Chiropractic Academic Press).

Computing Transverse Loads. When applying transverse stress to the spine, the correcting bending moment at the farthest lateral point of the curve can be computed by multiplying *half* of the axial force by its perpendicular distance from the midline to the apex of the curve. In contrast to axial stress, the corrective bending moments in transverse loading decrease as the deformity increases from the midline.

Axial vs Transverse Loading. The basic facts just described point out that axial traction is most beneficial in cases of severe deformity and transverse loading is most beneficial in mild deformities. In all instances, however, combined axial and transverse loading is the ideal biomechanical approach. For example, if axial forces are being applied with the patient supine, some means of applying transverse pressure should be applied laterally to the apex of the curve while contralateral aspects above and below the curve are fixed by some padded device.

Mensuration. Since its introduction to the field just a few years ago, the Scoliometer has received wide reception in measuring spinal curves. Invented by a chiropractic physician, Dr. Michael Sabia, it accurately measures six areas to detect scoliosis and three measurements to detect abnormal anteroposterior curves. The instrument gives measurements in centimeters, millimeters, and degrees.[35] See Figures 11.11 and 11.12.

Contraindications to Traction

Whenever a patient under traction complains of dizziness, nausea, undue discomfort, or other adverse sensory changes (eg, numbness), the therapy should be discontinued immediately. A number of contraindications or areas that require special precaution

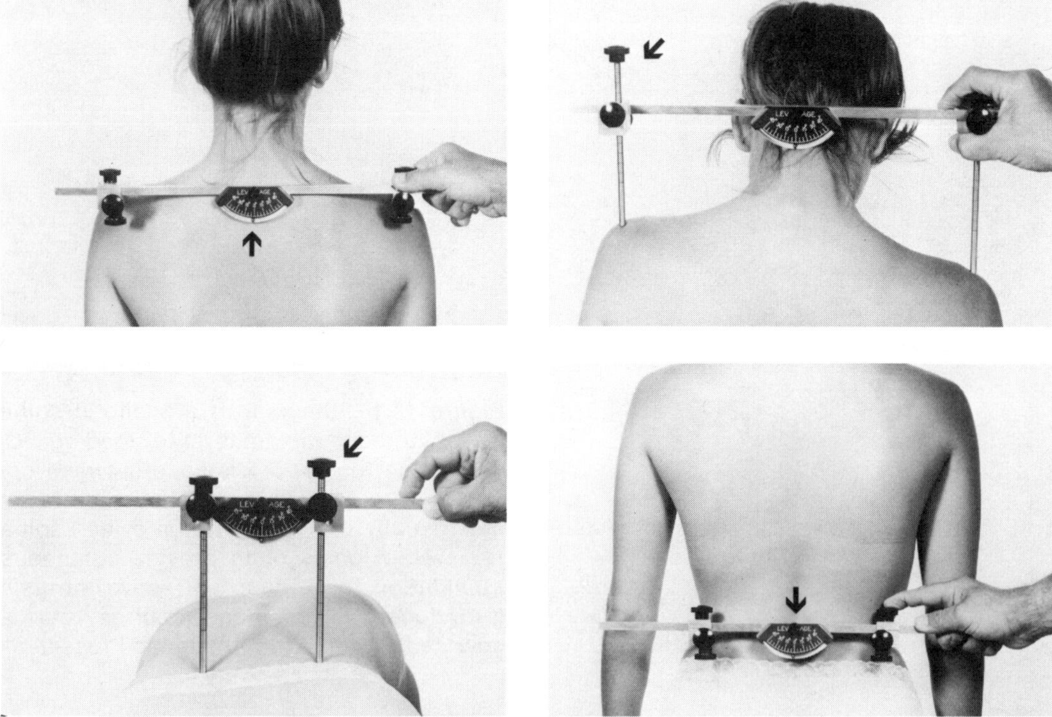

Figure 11.11. Applications of the Scoliometer (courtesy of Dr. M. Sabia).

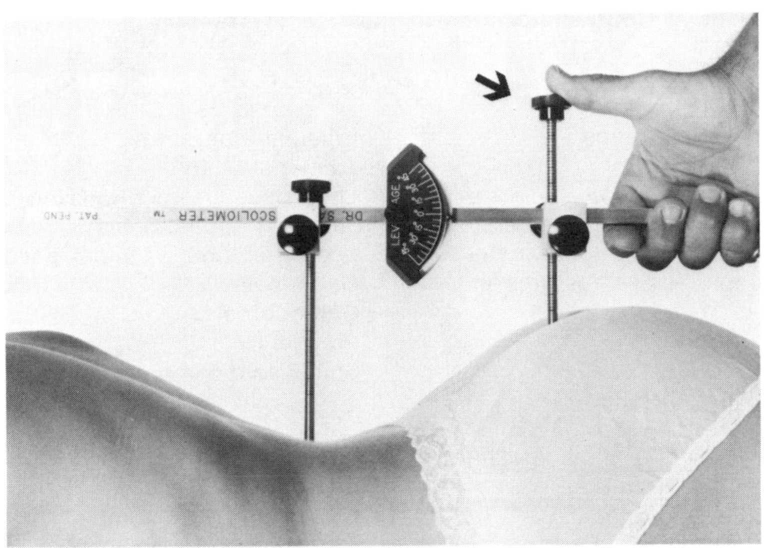

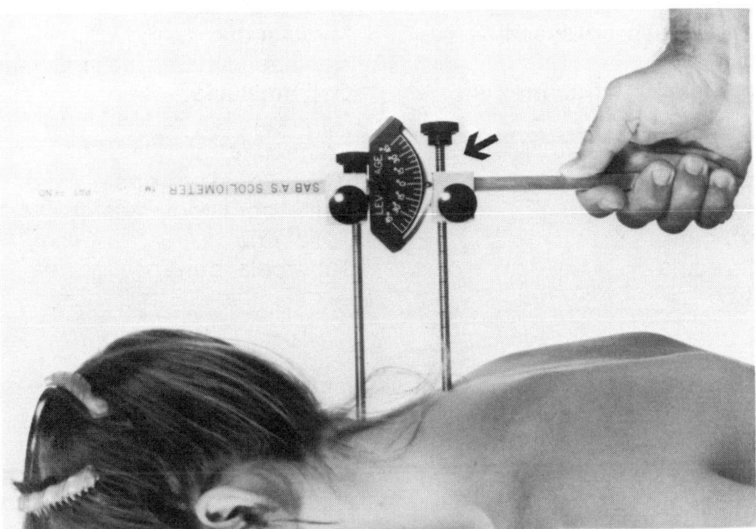

Figure 11.12. Further applications of the Scoliometer (courtesy of Dr. M. Sabia).

are listed in Table 11.3. In general, any condition for which immobilization would be indicated would have traction contraindicated. Spinal traction may easily aggravate acute musculoskeletal complaints and is considered by some to represent an absolute contraindication.[36]

STRETCHING THERAPY

Therapeutic stretching refers to any maneuver designed to lengthen abnormally shortened soft tissues, producing an increase in joint range of motion. It may or may not involve pure traction forces. The tissues affect-

Table 11.3. General Contraindications in the Use of Traction

CONTINUOUS TRACTION	
Acute traumatic syndromes	Inflammation, acute
Cachexia, advanced	Joint instability
Cancer	Local osseous infections (eg, osteomyelitis, tuberculosis)
Cardiovascular disease, advanced	Local peripheral vascular disease
Claustrophobia	Osteomalacia
Healing noncompressive fractures and dislocations	Osteoporosis
Hemorrhagic states	Pregnancy*
Hiatal hernia*	Spinal cord compression or pathology
Hypertension (uncontrolled)	
INTERMITTENT TRACTION	
Acute traumatic syndromes	Local osseous infections
Arthritis, acute inflammatory	Local peripheral vascular disease
Bursitis	Muscle spasm, severe
Cachexia, advanced	Musculoskeletal inflammation, acute
Cardiovascular disease, advanced	Myofascitis
Claustrophobia	Neoplastic states (eg, malignancy)
Healing noncompressive fractures and dislocations	Osteomalacia
Hemorrhagic states	Osteoporosis
Hiatal hernia*	Pregnancy*
Hypertension (uncontrolled)	Rheumatoid arthritis
Inflammation, acute	Spinal cord compression or pathology
IVD syndrome, acute	Tendinitis
Joint instability	Tubercular bone

*Thoracolumbar traction would be contraindicated in advanced states, cervical or extremity traction would not be.

ed may be skin, fascia, ligaments, and/or muscles and tendons, and the indication may be (1) trauma, (2) any infection or degenerative pathology that results in fibrosis, adhesions, or contractures, (3) a connective-tissue disorder, or (4) restricted mobility of physiologic (eg, spasticity), postural, neuromyogenic (eg, scoliosis), or disuse (eg, immobilization) etiologies.[37,38]

General Considerations

The physiologic effects of stretching therapy are similar to those of soft-tissue traction. Besides manual application, various devices are available for this purpose. See Figures 11.13 and 11.14.

Stretching therapy may be applied (1) passively by a therapist (with or without me-

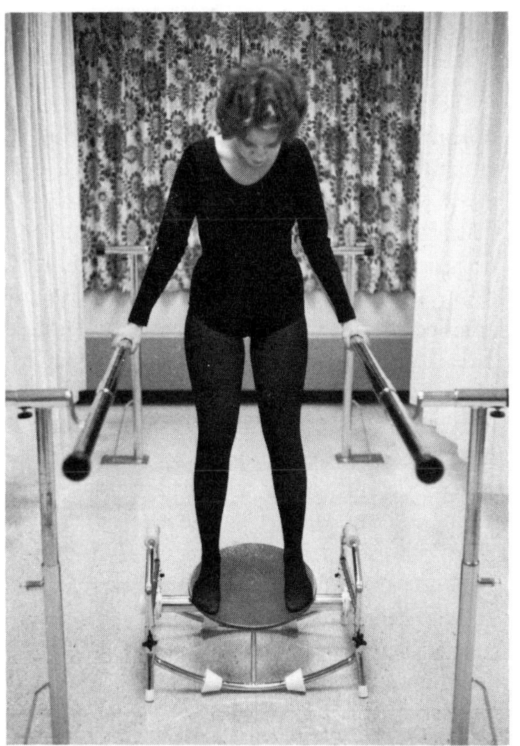

Figure 11.13. Adapto-Disc, for controlled angle motion in the development and rehabilitation of ankle joints and leg muscles (courtesy of Widen Tool & Stamping, Inc).

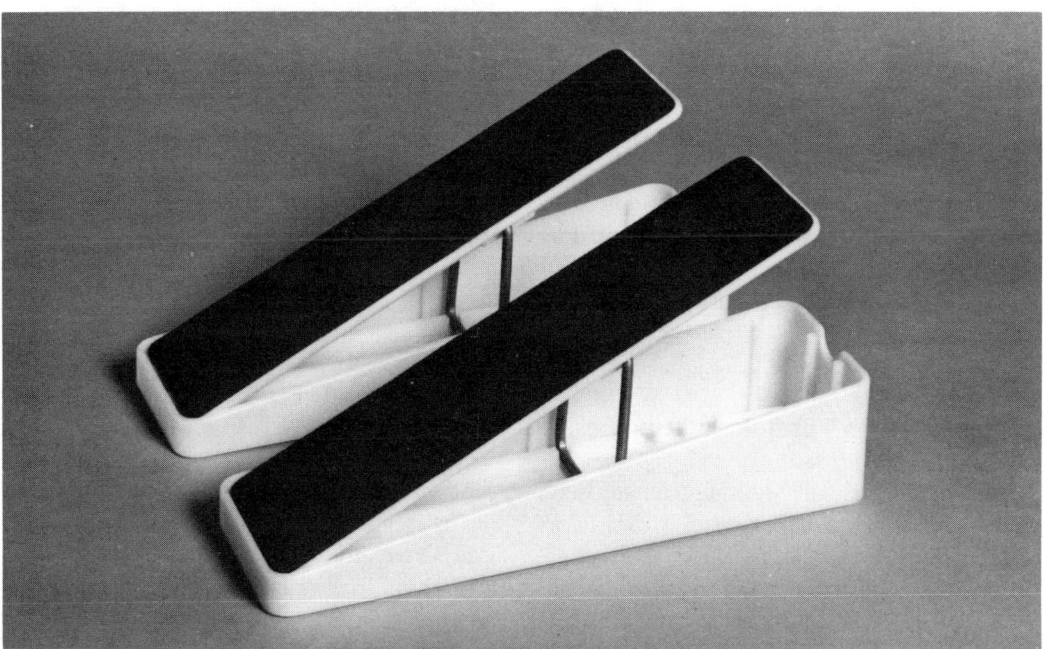

Figure 11.14. Flex-Wedge apparatus, for actively stretching lower extremity muscles and tendons in the standing position by body weight (courtesy of the Flex-Wedge Company).

chanical advantage such as a pulley or lever apparatus), (2) actively by the patient (with or without mechanical assistance), or (3) actively assisted. Passive stretch is invariably indicated in such situations as profound weakness or paralysis.

ASSOCIATED THERAPIES

Heat is helpful during stretching therapy, but cold and vapocoolant sprays have shown to be more effective in acute cases. In addition, mild isotonic exercises are useful for improving circulation and inducing the stretch reflex, especially in the cervical extensors. These exercises should be done supine to reduce exteroceptive influences on the central nervous system. In chronic cases, relaxation training with biofeedback is helpful.

ADVERSE AUTONOMIC REACTIONS

Autonomic hyperreflexia is a common complication occurring in patients with spinal cord injuries of the cervical and upper thoracic regions. Regardless of the cause, the syndrome features episodes of rapidly rising hypertension, bradycardia, hyperhidrosis, vasodilation in the head and neck, lower extremity vasoconstriction, and a characteristic "pounding" headache. It can be provoked by visceral abnormalities or manipulation, a wide variety of cutaneous stimuli, bladder distension, and proprioceptive reflexes initiated below the lesion. McGarry reports three cases that were related to passive stretching of the hip joints.[39]

Indications and Contraindications

Stretching is usually indicated in any state of abnormal soft-tissue shortening that interferes with normal function (eg, adhesions, contractures, spasticity, myogenic or ligamentous articular fixation, IVD thinning, paralytic or immobilization atrophy, lack of exercise, etc).

ABNORMALLY SHORTENED TISSUES

The reduction of spasm and/or the easing of contractures are often necessary prior to structural correction and to maintain a corrected position after adjustment.

Mild passive stretch is an excellent method of reducing spasm in the long muscles. Heavy passive stretch, however, destroys the beneficial reflexes. One technique in cervical spasticity, for example, is to place the patient prone on an adjusting table in which the headpiece has been slightly lowered. The patient's head is then turned toward the side of the spastic muscle. With head weight alone serving as the stretching tensile force, the spasm should relax within 2—3 minutes. Moderate thumb pressure placed on a trigger area is then directed toward the muscle's bony attachment. This pressure is held for a few moments until relaxation is complete.[40] The same principles will apply to most spastic muscles in other areas of the body.

LOW BACK PAIN

Cox has successfully applied a form of stretching flexion distraction manipulation in cases of acute disc lesions. The effect is to increase IVD height, allow the disc to assume its central position, restore normal apophyseal relationships, relieve the associated pain, and improve segmental biomechanics.[41]

VIBRATORY AND RELATED THERAPIES

Mechanical vibration to stimulate proprioceptive functions has gained increasing interest in recent years, essentially because of advanced technology. It may be applied manually or mechanically, superficially with relatively horizontal oscillations, or to deeper tissues via percussion strokes.

Historical Perspective

Deep mechanical stimulation is not a new modality. It was recommended by several prominent allopaths and chiropractors near the turn of the century to affect various reflex and interpretative levels (neuromeres) of the spinal cord, which, in turn, influenced relatively specific internal organs in a manner similar to the effect of sinusoidal current applied to the spine.[42]

Physiologic Effects

GENERAL EFFECTS

The primary action of vibration, under whose general classification one can include forms of percussion and concussion, is kinetic, which effects an increase in circulation and lymphatic flow, and a decrease in systemic nervous tension and general or local muscle spasm.

STIMULATION OF SPINAL CENTERS

Deep, rapid, short-duration percussion, applied either by hand or by a percussion-type vibrator, upon spinous processes at a rate of 1—2 impulses per second for about 20 seconds with 30-second rest intervals can be used to stimulate a spinal center. Prolonged stimulation such as for 3 minutes or longer appears to fatigue excitability and produces an inhibitory effect.[43]

Certain spinal segments have been mapped out empirically to produce the highest degree of physiologic response. These appear to involve the effects summarized in Table 11.4.[44,45,46]

Types of Machines and Applicators

Several excellent types of professional vibrators are available. The G-5, Genie Rub, and Vibratoner are just three examples. The description which follows will concentrate on the G-5 unit; but, in most instances, the principles will generally apply to competitive units of this caliber. See Figure 11.15.

There are 15 applicators for the G-5 unit. Most are designed for relatively specific purposes but all can be used to achieve a wide variety of goals or to suit the user's procedural preference. For example, there are round, cone, flat, contoured, multiple-ball, multiple-cup, multiple-prong, etc, shaped applicators. Figure 11.16 shows a G-5 unit utilizing a multiple-ball attachment.

For hot or cold massage, a hollow applicator attachment is also available that can be filled with hot water or ice water. If slightly deflated, this type of applicator will also produce a cupping action. Hot or cold vibratory massage should be conducted at a low-speed setting.

Indications and Contraindications

A large number of musculoskeletal ailments can be effectively treated with vibratory therapy. See Table 11.5.[47]

Several practitioners report excellent results with high-speed vibratory therapy in treating palpable trigger points. A fairly firm cone-shaped attachment with a small diameter is used for this purpose, which can be specifically directed and rolled beneath a congested or taut muscle or ligament if necessary. See Figure 11.17.

Effects of Velocity

See Table 11.6.

Angle of Application

On most professional vibrators, placement of the applicator parallel to the body surface produces a superficial *oscillatory* effect, while placement of the edge of the applicator perpendicular to the body surface produces a deeper *percussive* effect. Thus, if the angle at the applicator-skin interface is varied, a vibratory mixture of superficial oscillation and deep percussion can be achieved.

Table 11.4. Effects of Spinal Center Stimulation

Spinal Level	*Effect Initiated by Stimulation*
C1—C2	Vagal responses of increased gastric secretion and peristalsis; increase nasal, buccal, and pulmonary mucosal secretions.
C3	Phrenic influence to increase depth of diaphragmatic excursions. Note that C3 inhibition is helpful in chronic cough, hiccups.
C4—C5	Lung reflex contraction (eg, used in expiratory dyspnea, emphysema) and pulmonary vascular vasoconstriction.
C6—C7	Reflex center for increasing generalized vasoconstriction and myocardial tone.
T1—T3	Lung reflex dilation (eg, inspiratory dyspnea), relax the stomach body, and contract the pylorus; inhibit heart action (ie, antitachycardia reflex) and gastric hypermotility.
T4	Cardiac and aortic dilation and inhibit viscerospasms.
T5	Pyloric and duodenal dilation when applied to the right side.
T6	Gallbladder contraction when applied to the right side.
T7	Slight visceromotor renal dilation when applied bilaterally and stimulate hepatic function.
T8—T9	Gall duct dilation.
T10—T11	Slight visceromotor renal contraction, enhance pancreatic secretion, relax intestines and colon, and stimulate adrenals when applied bilaterally; to initiate splenic contraction (and circulatory red blood cells) when applied on the left.
T12	Prostate contraction and tone of the cecum and bladder sphincter.
L1—L3	Uterine body, round ligament, and bladder contraction; pelvic vasoconstriction; vesicular sphincter relaxation.
L4—L5	Sigmoidal and rectal contraction; increase tone of lower bowel.

Table 11.5. General Indications and Contraindications of Vibratory Therapy

GENERAL INDICATIONS	
Adhesions (superficial)	Lymphatic flow impairment
Brachial neuralgia	Myalgia
Bronchial congestion	Mild nervous tension
Circulatory stasis	Occipital headaches
Congestion	Paralysis
Constipation	Postexertion muscle fatigue and stiffness
Depression	Reflex sciatica
Edema	Sinus congestion
Hypomyotonia	Spasticity
Intestinal stasis	Trigger points
Joint swelling	
GENERAL CONTRAINDICATIONS	
Acute local inflammation	Malignant lesions
Acute low back syndromes	Near damaged organs
Advanced heart disease	Over eyes
Cervical spondylosis	Over sensitive skin lesions
Chest wall pathology	Pneumothorax
Hemorrhaging areas	Pulmonary abscess or tumor
Hyperanxiety states	Pulmonary tuberculosis
Lymphangitis	Thrombophlebitis

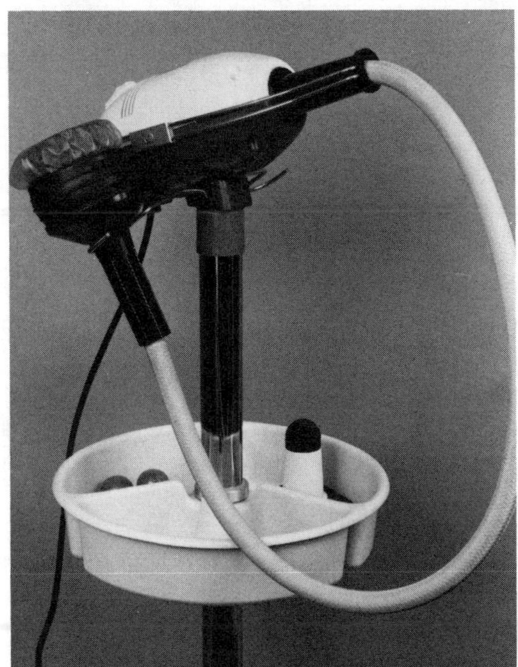

Figure 11.15. A G-5, Model K-3, vibration unit.

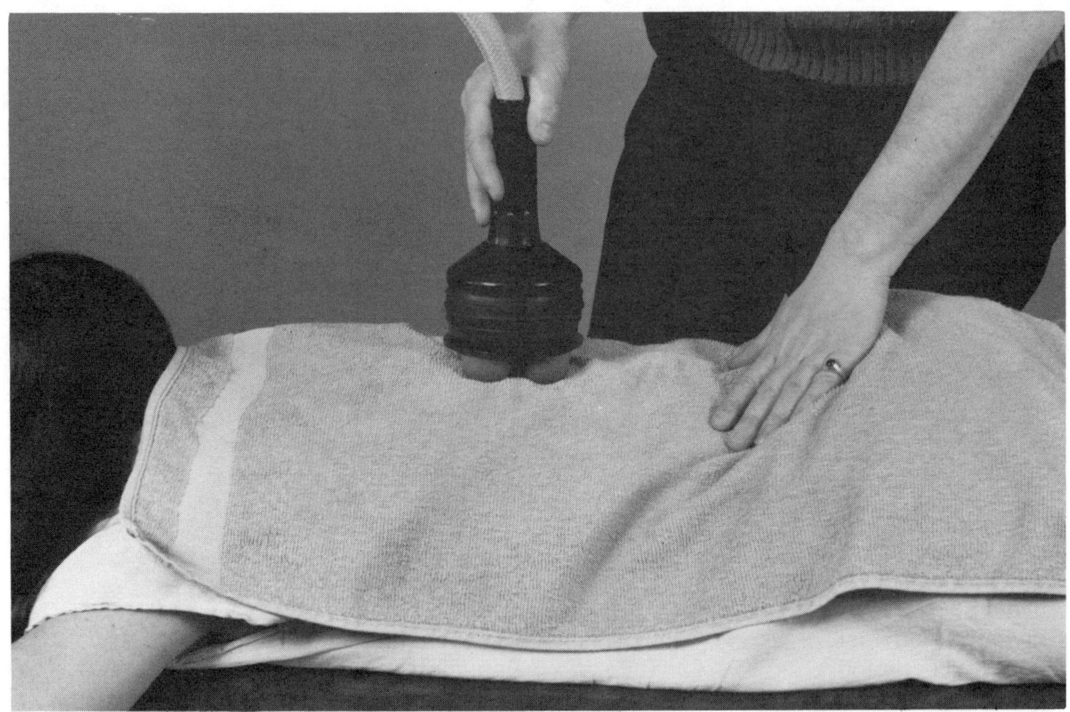

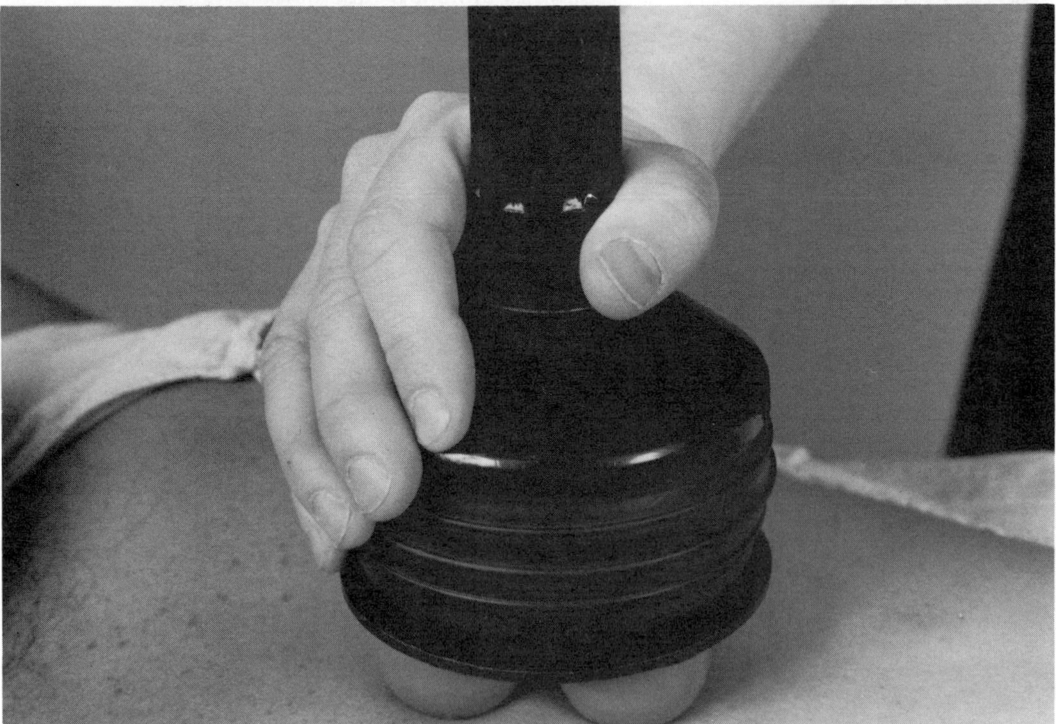

Figure 11.16. *Top,* application of vibratory therapy utilizing a multiple-ball attachment over the lower thoracic spine. *Bottom,* similar therapy to the midthoracic spine without an intervening towel.

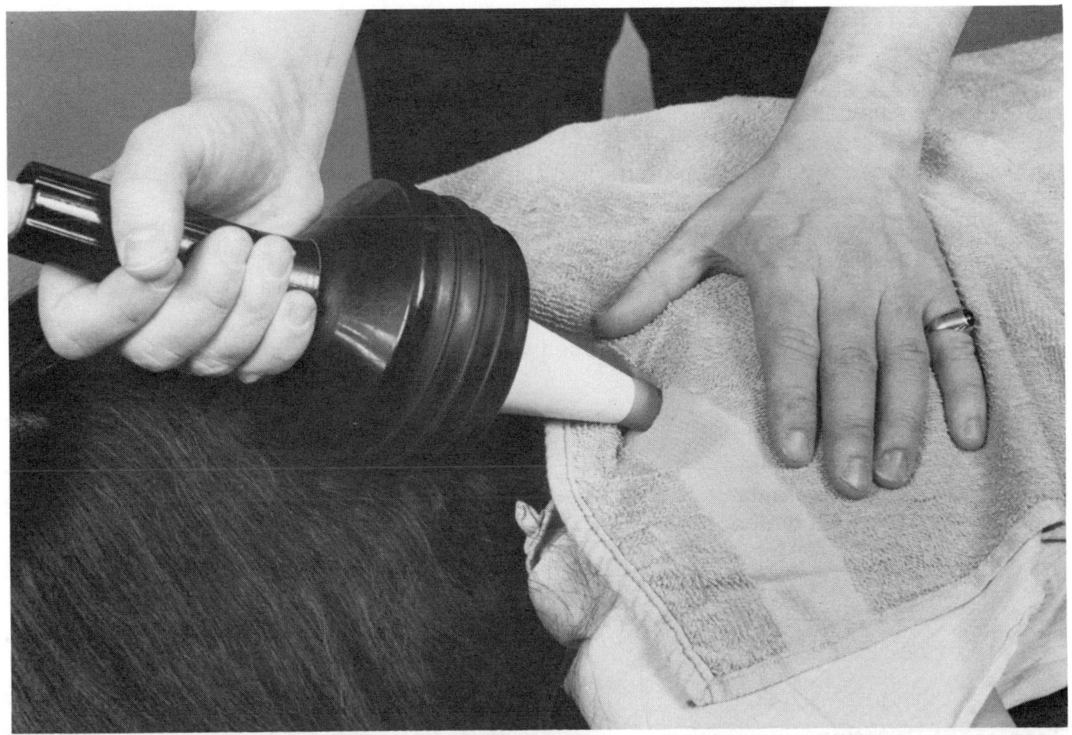

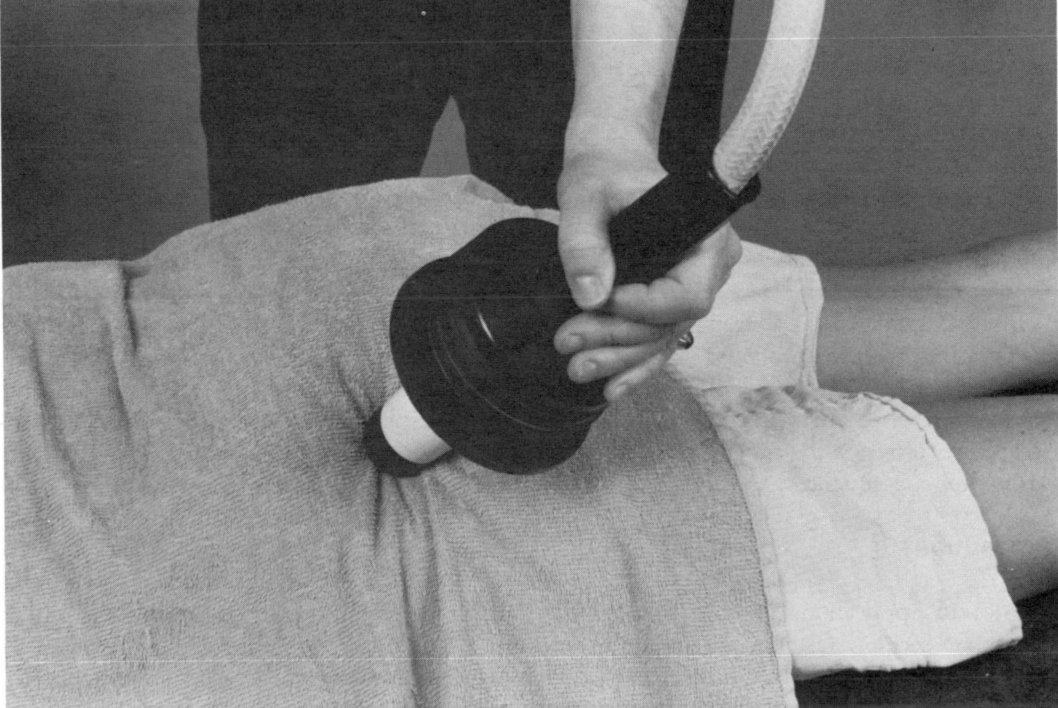

Figure 11.17. *Top,* application of vibratory therapy to a shoulder girdle trigger point, utilizing a fairly hard-tipped attachment. *Bottom,* trigger-point therapy near the sciatic notch.

Table 11.6. Effects of Vibratory Speed

Velocity	*Effects*
High	Analgesia Decrease trigger points Goad muscle and periarticular tissues Hypesthesia Pre-exercise warm-up Relax spasticity Superficial circulatory stimulation
Medium	Same effects as high, but used when a milder effect is desired.
Low	Congestion Edema Hyperesthesia Hypomyotonia Postural drainage Stasis

Treatment Duration

Because of the G-5's strong effect and deep penetration, it is not advisable to use the unit too long over an isolated site. Overuse can produce tissue inflammation and symptoms of soreness. As with most therapies, proper therapy duration depends on the patient's condition and tolerance to the modality. General guidelines for treatment time are shown in Table 11.7.

If the patient reports a strong ''itchy'' sensation, the treatment should be stopped. This sensation is invariably due to excessive stimulation of cutaneous and subcutaneous receptors, often with progressively adverse vasomotor consequences.

Precautions

Prior to application, be sure that attachments are securely fastened to the applicator head so that they will not disconnect during therapy, and assure that the cable does not become kinked. Because the unit is designed to operate against pressure, it should not be allowed to run extensively when not applied. Avoid sliding the applicator back and forth over the spinal column or bony prominences, and don't move the applicator too fast. Always work toward the heart, in the direction of venous and lymph flow, when the extremities are being treated.

Because of the deep penetration produced by the unit, there is no need to apply heavy pressure while moving the applicator. Excessive pressure or moving the unit too rapidly may cause patient discomfort and/or bruise the patient's skin. Use of a dry towel at the applicator-skin interface prevents body oils and perspiration from contaminating the attachment and prolongs the life of the attachment. It also contributes a dispersive cushioning factor. See Figure 11.18.

Note: It is not good procedure to allow excessive vibration to the operator's active hand over prolonged periods, day after day. We have witnessed several cases of unilateral hypertrophic arthritis in barbers who routinely used a small hand-attached vibrator to stimulate customers' scalps after shampooing.

Table 11.7. Guidelines for Vibratory Therapy

Concern	*Time (min)*	*Comments*
Localized treatments	10 or less	Use more time for chronic conditions, less time for acute and subacute disorders.
Reducing trigger points	6—8	Too long or too strong treatment can retraumatize the site and possibly bruise the surrounding area.
Relaxing muscles	2—10	
Postural drainage	3—15	Duration varies considerably, depending upon the particular condition being treated.
General body relaxation	3—5	
Cold massage	10—12	Duration varies considerably, depending upon the particular condition being treated.

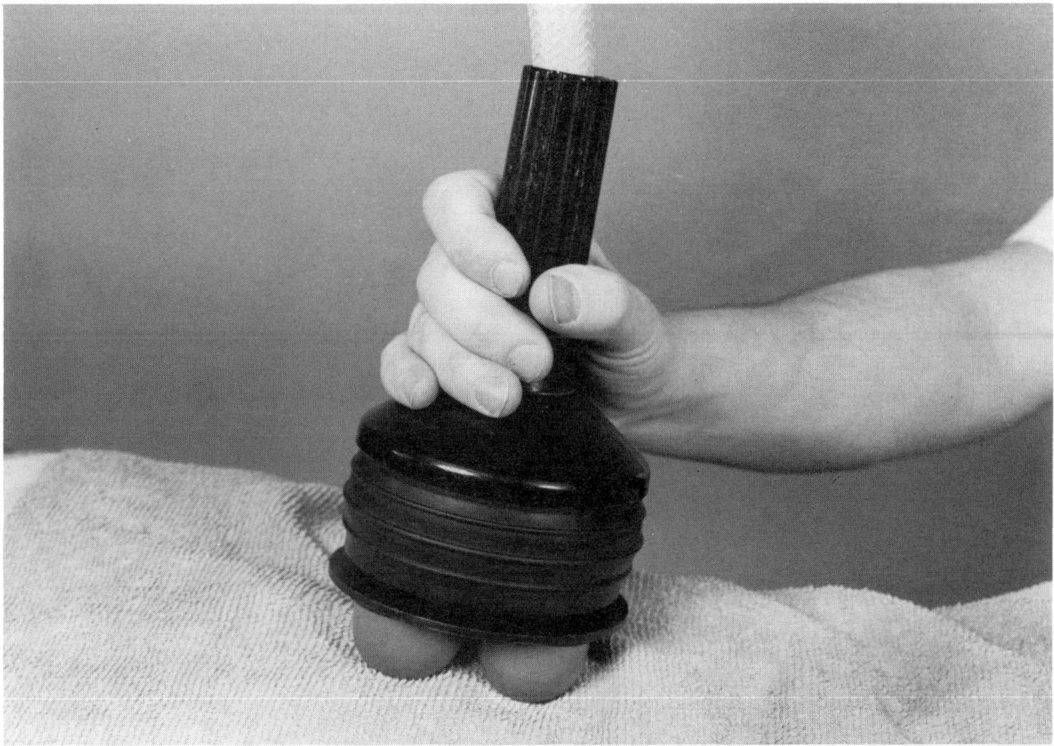

Figure 11.18. At the completion of therapy, turn the machine off and remove the towel. It may be helpful to massage the area to encourage circulatory flow.

Associated Therapies

Experience has shown that sinusoidal current is an excellent method to contract involuntary muscle without irritation, but pulsating ultrasound is also effective in stimulating spinal centers. Therapeutic heat in almost any form increases nerve conductivity; thus, it may benefit vibratory, percussion, sinusoidal, and ultrasound therapies to spinal centers. Interspaced heat and cold can also be used in conjunction with vibratory therapy, depending upon the effect to be achieved. See Figure 11.19.

Voss reports that the tonic vibration reflex is stronger under isotonic conditions and that the reflex response induced is sustained contraction of the vibrated muscle with simultaneous relaxation of the prime antagonist.[48] An active vibrator placed over a muscle belly appears to serve as a further stretch stimulus, producing an increased response and further range of motion of the involved joint.

COMMON MECHANICAL SUPPORTS AND IMMOBILIZATION PROCEDURES

Mechanical supports include such items as strapping, taping, braces, casts, corsets, collars, canes, crutches, slings, shoe lifts, and certain bandages. In general practice, most of these appliances and procedures can be divided into four major classifications of purpose: (1) immobilizing, (2) supportive, (3) corrective, and (4) protective. See Figures 11.20 and 11.21.

Physiologic Effects

Most mechanical supports are designed to relieve weight bearing or motion stress on bones and joints, and to immobilize structures in a sustained position to assist healing. A by-product of these features is to relieve muscle spasm and pain. Shoe lifts and some other supports allow for contraction of and/or encourage stretching of musculoskeletal tissues to aid desirable structural changes. In either acquired or congenital malformations, such supports may help to relieve poorly compensated structural and funtional inadequacies.[49]

Spinal bracing offers the following basic effects:[50]

1. Decreased abdominal muscle activity.
2. Decreased intradisc pressure.
3. Decreased lower extremity venous return.
4. Increased intra-abdominal pressure.
5. Increased or decreased spinal muscle activity.
6. Increased segmental motion above and below the area immobilized.
7. IVD immobilization.
8. Placebo effect.
9. Some reverse of abnormal functional spinal curvatures.
10. Transfer of some vertical axis compression load of the spine to other structures.

General Indications and Contraindications

The goals of bracing vary according to the patient's problem, thus the use of supportive appliances is a matter of clinical judgment. When used wisely with a thorough knowledge of the biomechanics involved and corrective case management, recovery can be greatly enhanced.

Indications. Mechanical support is usually indicated in situations of pain, weakness, deformity, function assistance, or paralysis of a part of the body. See Figure 11.22. In fact, it can generally be said that any patient with a musculoskeletal disorder or congenital defect (eg, traumatically aggravated spondylolisthesis, hyperlordosis) that would benefit from a degree of spinal unloading (compression or shear forces), immobilization, and/or postural correction should be considered as a candidate for an appliance.[51] Inasmuch as sprains and strains are aggravated by motion and activity, it is logical that such conditions

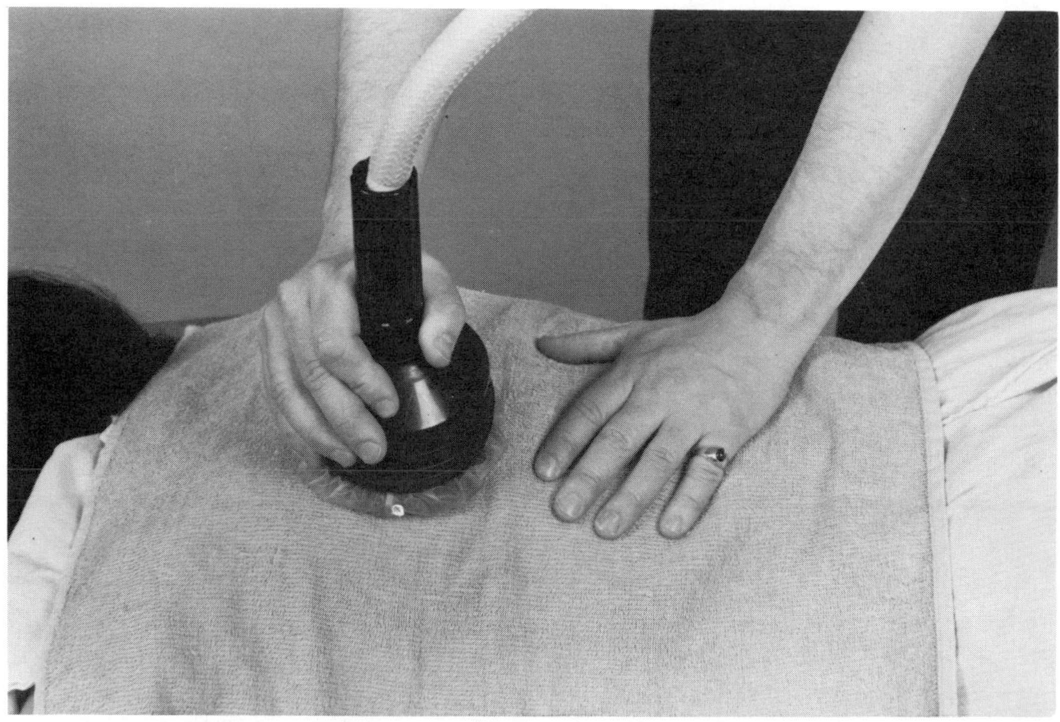

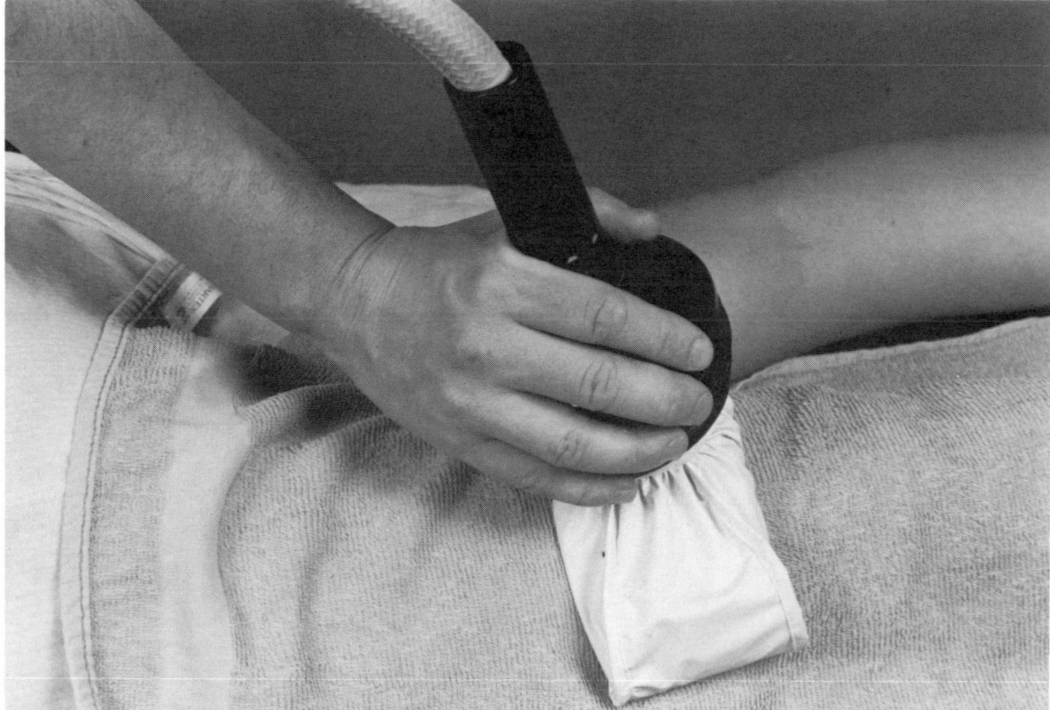

Figure 11.19. Vibratory therapy being applied over a small hot water bag, *top,* and over an ice pack, *bottom.*

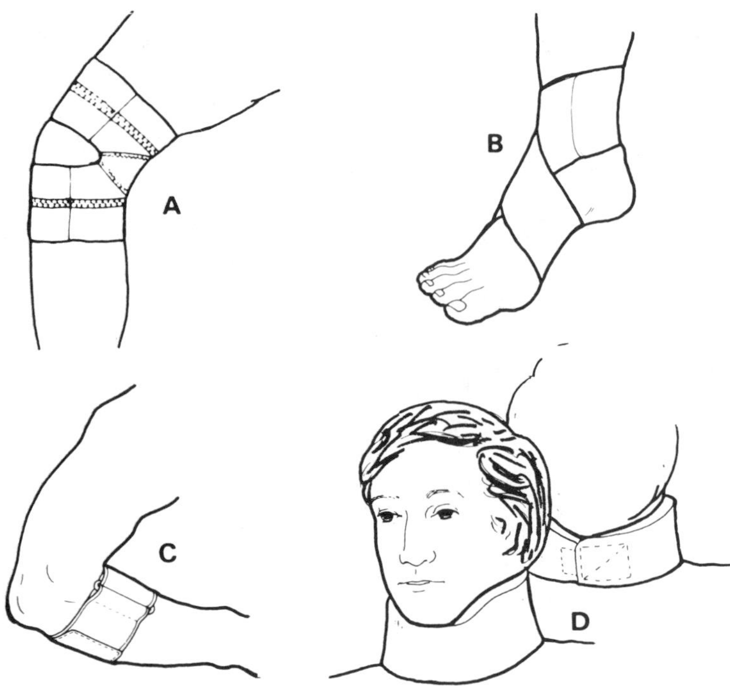

Figure 11.20. Various types of supports. *A,* knee support; *B,* ankle wrap support; *C,* tennis elbow support; *D,* foam cervical collar (courtesy of STC, Inc).

Figure 11.21. Back-Hugger cushion, for supportive relief of resistant or recurring back pain (courtesy of the Contour Comfort Company).

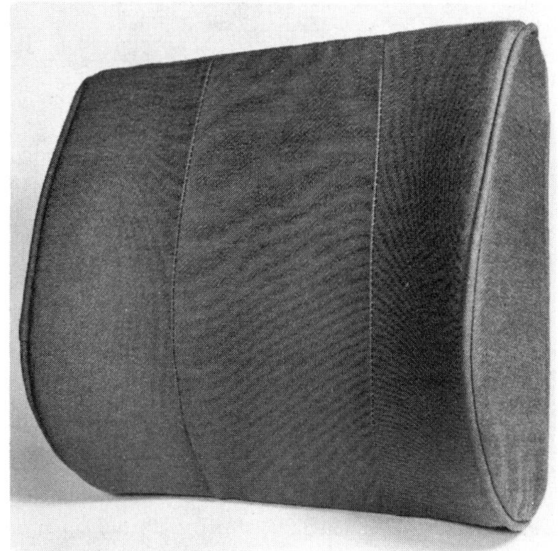

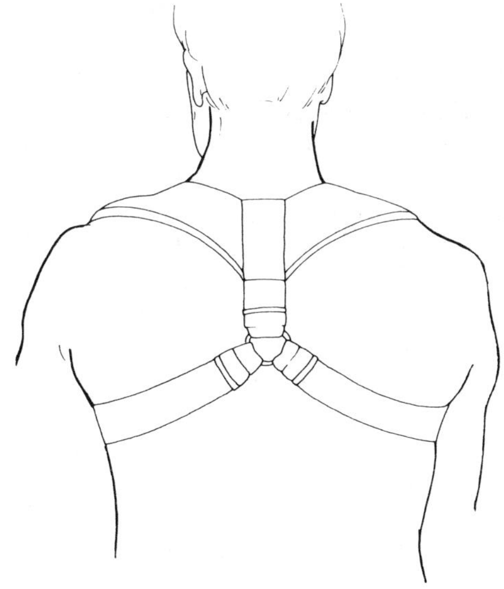

Figure 11.22. Stretch type, adjustable, clavicle splint with padded shoulder straps (courtesy of STC, Inc).

would benefit from protection, rest, and immobilization for a short duration; ie, days—weeks, until the healing of torn tissue fibers advances.

The indications for spinal bracing include:

- Acute IVD syndrome
- Acute sprains and strains
- Degenerative joint disease
- Hyperkyphosis
- Hyperlordosis
- Joint instability
- Muscle spasm and guarding
- Postural backache
- Scoliosis
- Spinal fractures
- Vertebral collapse.

Contraindications. Mechanical supports are contraindicated whenever immobilization tends to promote muscular atrophy and weakness or when immobilization tends to promote the organization of inflammatory coagulant and consequent adhesions and/or fibrotic infiltration, depending upon the nature and stage of the condition. Support is also contraindicated whenever immobilization may produce congestion, ischemia, or vascular stasis, or when immobilization or a fixed position may induce unsatisfactory stretching and/or contracture changes. These contraindications depend greatly upon such variables as overall patient status and the nature and stage of the condition.[52]

Cervical Supports

No cervical support, including the skeletal-fixed Halo appliance, completely restricts *all* possible types of cervical motion. The commonly seen "soft" cervical collars do little to limit motion and only serve to produce a reminder or placebo effect. The greater the rigidity and length of the appliance, the greater is its efficiency in restricting motion; but, even then, upper cervical flexion-extension and lateral bending are difficult to restrict with the typical appliances available.[53,54] However, even some support and mobility restriction may be sufficient in minor cervical sprains and strains if some loading is removed from the cervical spine and delivered to the shoulders. This appears to be especially true with those appliances that tend to "lift" the occiput and mandible.

See Table 11.8 and Figure 11.23.

Thoracic Supports

A large number of studies have been undertaken to appraise the ability of spinal braces to restrict thoracolumbosacral rotation.[55-60] With the exception of the modified chairback brace, few supports adequately limit rotation at the lumbosacral articulations. Several of the long stiff corsets and braces, however, tend to reduce spinal muscle activity during gait and effect good thoracic and upper lumbar motion restriction; and those supports that increase intra-abdominal pressure, especially inflatable corsets, tend to reduce the axial load on the spine. Unfortunately, while such increased abdominal pressure anteriorly reduces some intradiscal pressure, there is some corresponding inhibition of venous return and lymphatic drainage from the lower extremities whether the patient is seated or standing. This is especially true with those garments that extend to the groin or thighs.

See Table 11.8 and Figure 11.24.

Lumbopelvic and Sacroiliac Supports

One of the most commonly used yet one of the most inefficient supports is the so-called sacroiliac belt or strap, which offers some circumferential pressure around the pelvis and a pressure pad against the sacral base. This inefficiency is because isolated sacroiliac sprain (ie, that without lumbar involvement) is extremely rare and the immobilization effect is relatively inadequate even for the sacroiliac joints.

See Table 11.8 and Figure 11.25.

FITTING LUMBOPELVIC SUPPORTS

If a brace or more restrictive corset is advisable during the acute stage, several objectives must be obtained in fitting: (1) the support should contain a firm anterior abdominal lift to raise and keep the viscera well within the pelvic basin and minimize the lumbar lordosis; (2) the support should contain several flat steel stays to replace the need for splinted muscles and to restrict motion to the hips; (3) the support must be long enough to extend from the sacrum to the midthoracic area posteriorly and from just below the pubis to the upper abdomen anteriorly; and (4) bony prominences should be well padded. Short-waisted elastic supports that compress tissues but do not restrict motion or support weakened muscles or ligaments have little more than a psychologic benefit. See Figure 11.26.

SCOLIOSIS

When using braces, corsets, and other supports in the treatment of scoliosis, at least four objectives should be kept in mind: (1) to prevent progression, (2) to hold the improvement gained by minimizing adverse forces, (3) to apply corrective mechanical forces, and last but not least, (4) to stimulate corrective neuromuscular forces. Success is usually relative to tissue flexibility and plasticity properties and to sensory excitement on the convexity of the curve to stimulate corrective muscular reactions. This latter point refers to the patient moving away from a site of irritation by straightening the spine such as the tracheal and abdominal pads of a Milwaukee brace.[61] See Figure 11.27.

Several studies have pointed out that braces and casts have little effect in idiopathic scoliosis if there is a strong neurologic defect present or if the curve is extreme.[62,63] If paraspinal muscles cannot respond to the irritation of the appliance, there is no corrective neuromuscular action. As described earlier, the more the spine is curved, the more the

Table 11.8. Common Spinal Supports

Type of Support	*Measuring Guidelines*
	CERVICAL SUPPORTS
Firm cervical collar	Neck circumference and necessary height to position and support the cranium as desired.
Philadelphia collar	Neck circumference and necessary height to position and support the cranium as desired.
Soft foam collar	Neck circumference and necessary height to position and support the cranium as desired.
Somi brace	Standard sizes of large, medium, and small, selected according to the dimensions of the patient.
Two- and four-poster	Standard sizes of large, medium, and small, selected according to the dimensions of the patient.
	THORACOLUMBOSACRAL SUPPORTS
Dorsolumbar corset	Anterior height from hip angle to comfortable clearance below breasts when seated, hip circumference, posterior height from superior angle of shoulder blade to sacrococcygeal joint, and waist circumference.
Jewett brace	Anterior height from 1 inch below sternal notch to symphysis pubis, hip circumference, and thorax circumference.
Knight-Taylor brace	Posterior height from mid-sacrum to 1 inch below the superior angle of the shoulder blade and hip circumference.
Taylor brace	Posterior height from mid-sacrum to 1 inch below the superior angle of the shoulder blade and hip circumference.
	LUMBAR AND SACROILIAC SUPPORTS
Chairback brace	Posterior height from mid-sacrum to lower thoracic region, according to patient's comfort, and hip circumference.
Knight spinal brace	Posterior height from mid-sacrum to lower thoracic region, according to patient's comfort, and hip circumference.
Lumbosacral corset	Anterior height from hip angle to comfortable clearance below breasts when seated, hip circumference, posterior height from lower thoracic area to sacrococcygeal joint, and waist circumference.
Sacroiliac girdle	Hip circumference.
Williams brace	Posterior height to mid-sacrum to lower thoracic region, according to patient's comfort, and hip circumference.

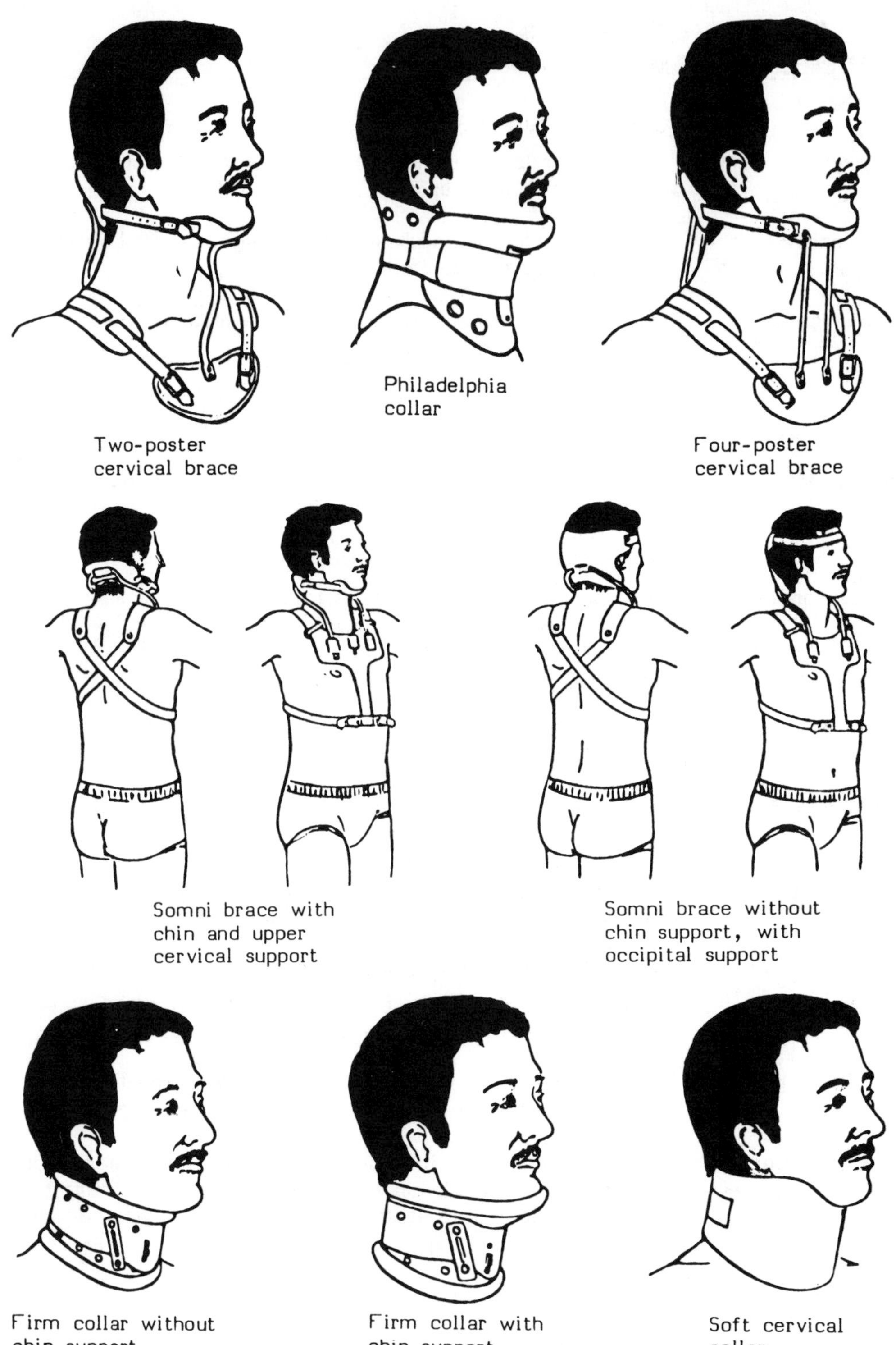

Figure 11.23. Common cervical supports.

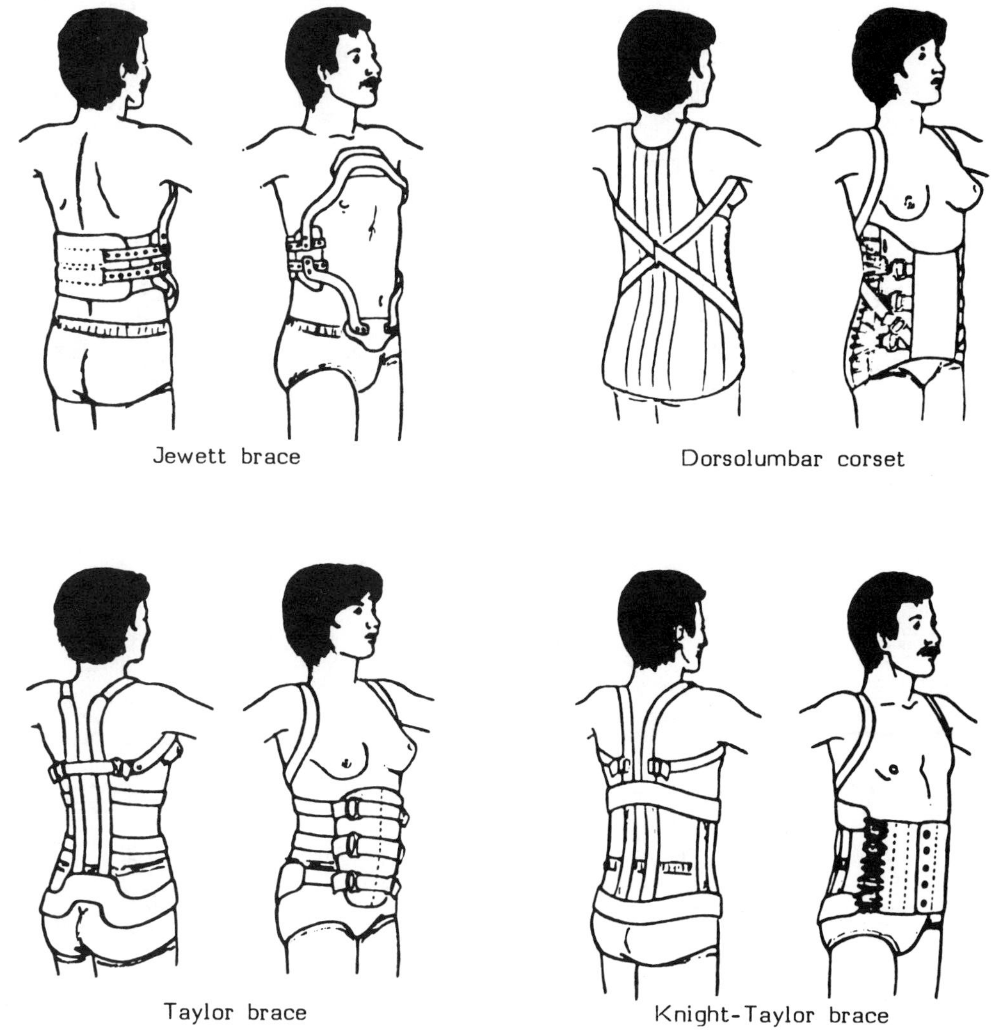

Figure 11.24. Common thoracolumbosacral supports.

spinal segments are subjected to lateral bending moments than to axial forces. In curves greater than 40°, typical braces have little effect because such curves are invariably associated with severe muscle weakness and frequently exhibit the lack of optimal mechanoreceptor input. Always keep in mind that overtly *static* structural faults invariably have a large covertly *dynamic* (physiologically responsive) factor involved.

Extremity Pressure Supports

In any musculoskeletal injury, enhanced circulation is almost always a benefit and this is especially true if immobilization is required. The use of hot packs, ultrasound, massage, and sometimes whirlpools have been of some, but not excellent, benefit in this regard. There also has been a problem obtaining lightweight but strong supports

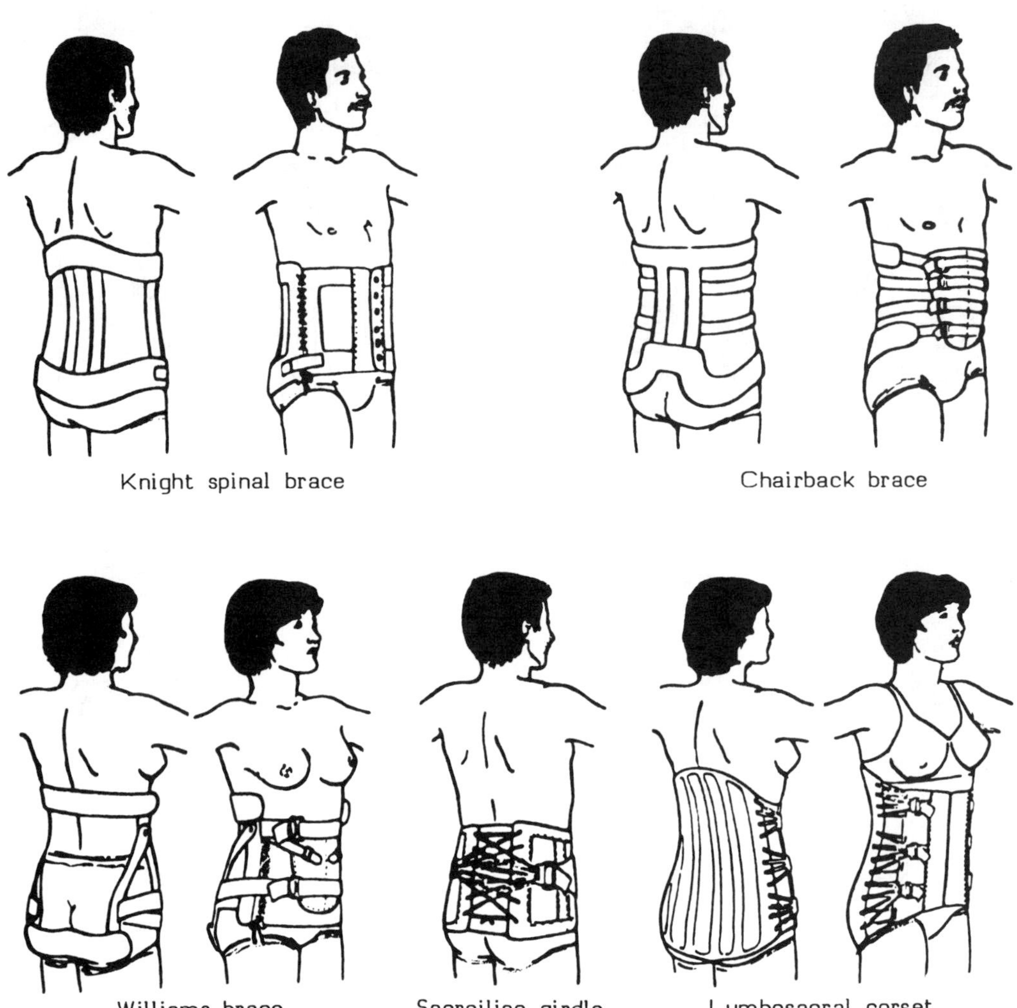

Figure 11.25. Common lumbar and sacroiliac supports.

that restrict motion in some ranges but still allow some type of activity (eg, locomotion). New technology appears to have solved some of these problems.

THE HYDROPULSE AND THE PRESSION UNITS

In recent years, to meet the need for immobilization and support without the venous and lymphatic circulatory deficit, new therapies have been introduced that pulsate warm water or air within specially designed cuffs. Two examples are the Hydropulse and Pression units. See Figure 11.28. Such units, which optimally offer a unidirectional action towards the heart, are efficient in treating sprains, strains, spasticity, cramps, diabetic complications, decreased circulation, local edema, and other types of pain or discomfort from a degree of anoxia and/or circulatory stasis.

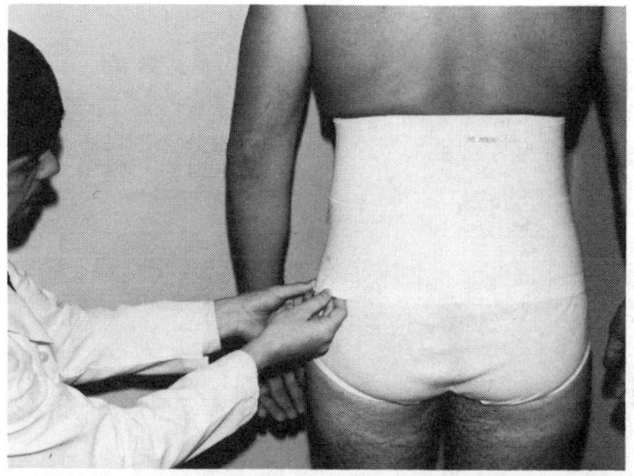

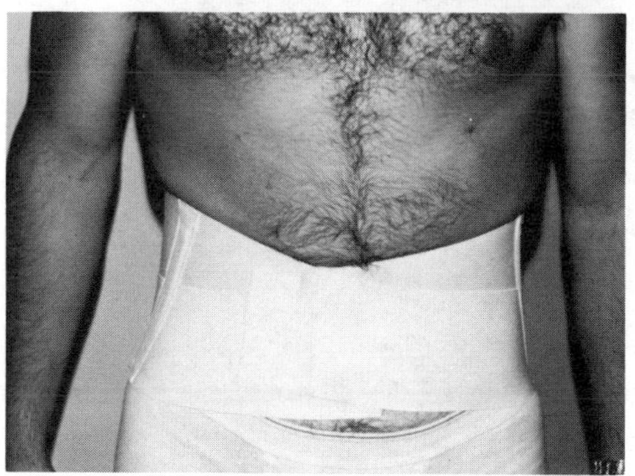

Figure 11.26. Simple lumbosacral support (courtesy of Associated Chiropractic Academic Press).

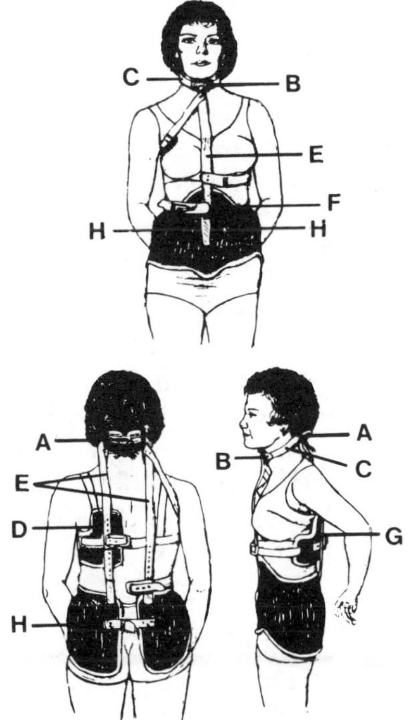

Figure 11.27. Diagrams of a Milwaukee brace as viewed from the front, back, and side: *A,* occipital pad, which tends to straighten the cervical and lumbar lordosis; *B,* anterior trachial pad; *C,* cervical ring; *D,* lower thoracic apex transverse pressure pad; *E,* vertical bars; *F,* abdominal pad; *G,* upper lumbar apex transverse pressure pad; *H,* molded pads over the iliac crests.

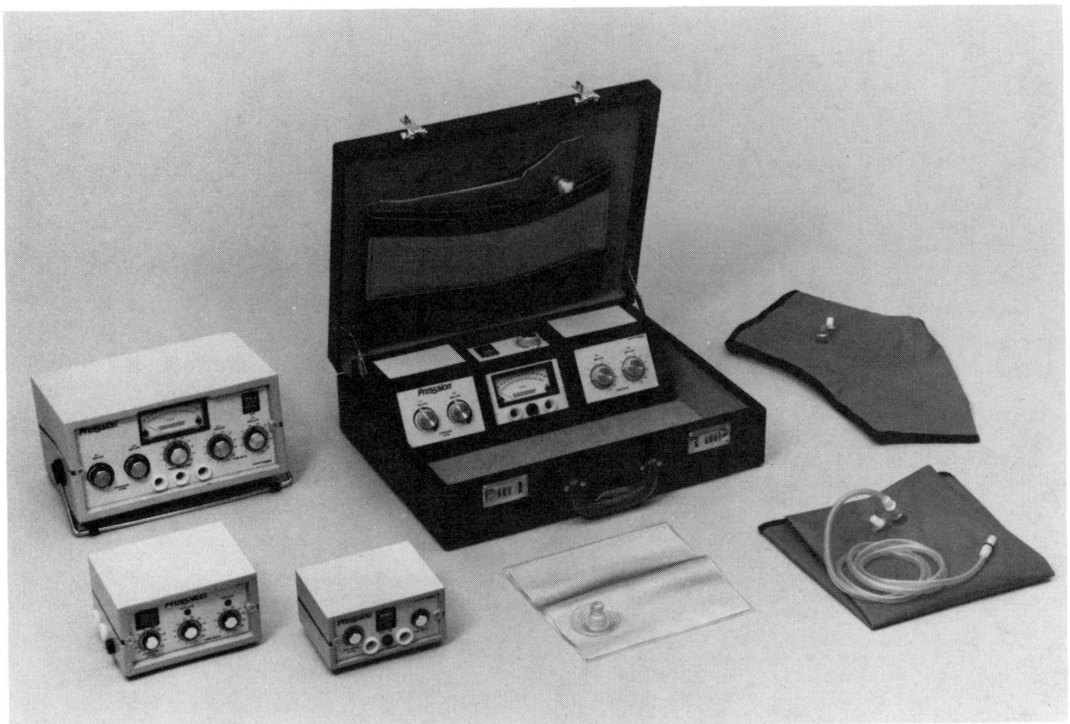

Figure 11.28. Pression intermittent compression units.

THE AIRCAST/AIRSTIRRUP SYSTEM

Aircasts and Airstirrups have proved themselves excellent innovations in the treatment of extremity injuries and have overcome many of the disadvantages of conventional plaster casting. An Aircast consists of two plastic half shells that are connected by Velcro straps, and two or more self-inflated/self-sealing air bags are attached to the inner surface of the shells. See Figure 11.29. Similar AirStirrups are U-shaped appliances for the lower extremity.

In many instances, an athlete with a sprained ankle, for example, can continue running almost immediately when the appliance has been applied. Such appliances also allow normal, gradual recuperative functions to take place, prevent recurrence of injury during rehabilitation, and eliminate motion pain while still allowing motion in nonpainful directions. They appear to efficiently bridge the gap between immovable plaster casts and inefficient flexible supports.[64-67]

Adhesive Strapping

Adhesive taping or strapping can be used for prevention against reinjury and treatment to limit joint motion, secure protective devices and padding, support and stabilize a part, and hold dressings secure. The rule of thumb is: the larger the part, the wider the tape; eg, 2- or 3-inch tape is best for thighs or shoulders, and half-inch tape for fingers and toes. In athletics, heavy backed tape (85 longitudinal fibers per square inch) with a rubber-base adhesive is usually preferred for

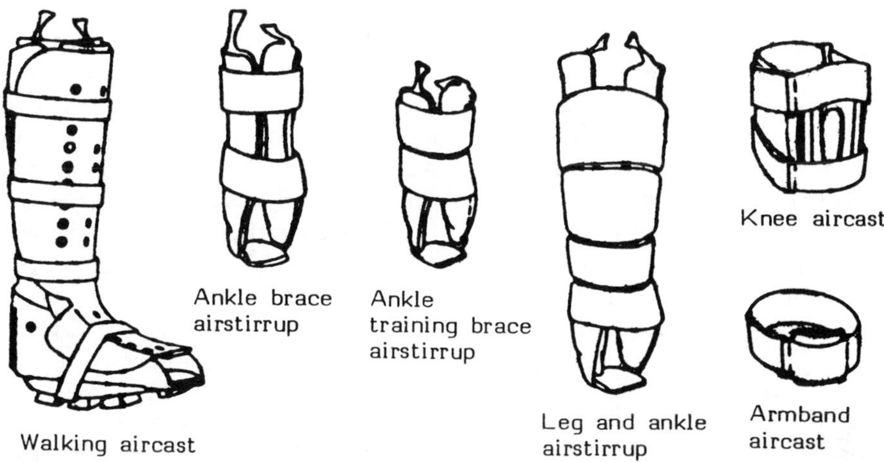

Figure 11.29. Various types of Aircasts and Airstirrups.

greater backing strength and superior adhesion as opposed to the acrylic adhesives and lighter backing used in surgery. Before tape is positioned, the skin should be cleaned and dried, cuts should be treated, hair should be shaved, and a nonallergenic skin adherent should be applied.[68]

APPLICATION

Strips of adhesive tape are used, rather than one continuous winding, to avoid constriction. After one turn of the tape, the tape is torn. Further strips are then overlapped about an inch at the ends and at least a half inch above or below. The tape should be carefully smoothed and molded to fit the natural contour of the part as it is laid on the skin with equal tension.

PRECAUTIONS

Most irritation is seen in the mechanical irritation caused by tape removal, but the reddened area disappears quickly. Allergic reactions are rarely seen and are characterized by erythema, papules, vesicles, and edema. A patch test will indicate a positive reaction within 48 hours if a sensitivity exists. The irritative effects of inhibited sweating beneath tape may be relieved by using a porous nonocclusive-type tape.

Bandaging

Bandaging is used to secure dressings and splints, to limit motion of a part, and to apply compression to a wound to control hemorrhage. Cotton cloth is commonly used over a dressing or to secure splints. Rolled gauze secures dressings and serves as a protective support beneath strappings. Elastic bandages provide compression.

Mobilization After Support

To minimize strength loss, improve nutrition of the part, and reduce atrophy, exercise of adjacent joints should be advised when support is provided as well as thereafter. Both progressive passive manipulation and active exercise are the keys to fast recovery.

However, joint movement should not be made whenever it increases pain, muscle spasm, or involuntary splinting.

Postinjury edema soon becomes filled with fibroblasts ("joint glue"), and excessive collagen formation produces stiffness, especially when collateral ligaments are immobilized in a position shorter than that for the functional position. However, a normal joint can tolerate a long session of immobilization without ill effects, such as that seen in fracture healing. Degenerative changes, intra-articular adhesions, and periarticular stiffness are more of a concern in the elderly patient in short-term immobilization than the young athlete in long-term immobilization. It is not abnormal to have some swelling after removal of a lower-extremity support, but this may be minimized by elastic stockings and contrast baths followed by elevation.[69]

Shoe Lifts

Shoe lifts generally refer to heel and/or sole inserts or attachments that are applied for the purpose of correcting abnormal biomechanics of the axial skeleton.

APPLICATION

A lift should be considered a clinical brace, with all its implications. In addition to being an adjunct to basic therapy, it can be an important modality. Functional leg deficiencies and pelvic distortions should never be fully corrected by a mechanical appliance if disuse atrophy is to be avoided. The body should always be allowed to make some correction by itself. The neuromusculoskeletal system readily adapts to its requirements and outside stimuli unless mechanical restrictions exist. If prolonged standing or walking does not aggravate a low back pain syndrome, it is unlikely that a small difference in femur height is a significant factor in the syndrome.

Studies by Logan, Steinbach, and others have shown that a 1:2:4 ratio, from above downward, exists between the lumbar spine, the sacrum, and the plantar surface of the heel. Thus, a ¼-inch heel lift will raise the ipsilateral sacral base ⅛ inch and the lumbar spine 1/16 inch. See Figure 11.30. This general rule has been applied within chiropractic with excellent results since the 1930s, with adaptations taken for an unusually narrow male pelvis or unusually wide female pelvis. Other investigators have reported an average 3:1 ratio between leg deficiency and L5 tilt; ie, a 9-mm femoral head height deficiency would be related to a 3-mm L5 tilt from the horizontal plane that averages a lumboscoliosis angle of 10°—15° by Cobb's system of measurement. The difference between these two ratios is clinically insignificant unless a severe anatomic deficiency is involved.[70]

COMMON TYPES OF LIFTS

This section refers to inserts within the patient's shoes (bilateral or unilateral) because their use is usually temporary. When a permanent shoe lift is necessary, it is best done

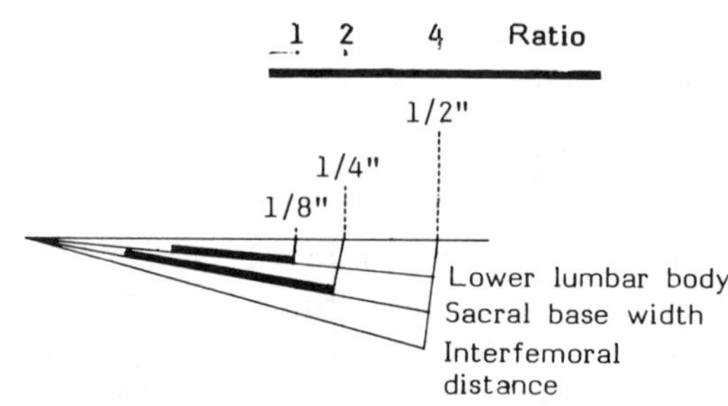

Figure 11.30. The 1-2-4 ratio between the lower lumbar level and a unilateral heel lift (courtesy of the Associated Chiropractic Academic Press).

exteriorly by shoe reconstruction: ipsilateral heel lengthening or contralateral heel shortening. A heel drop (heel-height reduction) generally has the same effect as a heel lift on the opposite side or an ipsilateral sole lift.

Heel Lifts. Structurally, a heel lift does nothing more than raise the heel, yet its biomechanical and biologic effects are manifested as far as the atlantooccipital joint. When the heel is raised, the pelvis is raised *and* rotated anteriorly. The ilium rotates anterosuperiorly and lateral, and the ischium posteroinferiorly and medial. As the sacrum is lifted and rotated anteriorly, the base of support for L5 is altered accordingly. Thus, the body of L5 will tend to rotate away from the side of lift.

Bilateral heel lifts tend to increase the lumbar lordosis. This is compensated for by an increase in the thoracic kyphosis, which may be of benefit in cases of lumbar flattening or the rigid "military" spine. Such lifts also decrease stress from minor cases of posterior lumbar sprain (eg, the so-called sprung back).

Sole Lifts. A unilateral or bilateral sole-only lift or a reduction in shoe heel height is sometimes applied. Sole lifts have no effect upon functional extremity length, but they tend to place a stretch on the posterior ankle, calf, thigh, and pelvic extensors. When applied bilaterally, such lifts are beneficial in reducing the lumbosacral angle in cases of anterior pelvic rotation, lumbar hyperlordosis, thoracic hyperkyphosis, or lumbar spinous process impingement.

To avoid possible tendinitis, a sole lift or heel height reduction is contraindicated in patients whose Achilles tendons have contracted. Gradual reduction in heel height, along with progressive stretching exercises of the calf, has been beneficial in many of these cases. Heel height reduction would also be inadvisable in any condition where stretching the posterior musculature of the leg, posterior rotation of the pelvis, or flattening the lumbar lordosis would be contraindicated.

Full Plantar Lifts. A plantar lift extending from the heel to the toe tends to raise the femoral head without altering pelvic rotation. This is most helpful when it is desirable to shift weight laterally but not alter ipsilateral iliac posture. Examples of this are often seen following poliomyelitis in youth, severe fractures of the femoral shaft or acetabular neck, and sometimes following epipyseal disorders of the femur that alter linear growth and cause a unilateral leg-length deficiency.

Ischial Lifts. If the axial measurements of the ischia are asymmetrical and aggravating a sacroiliac dysfunction or lumbar scoliosis in the sitting position, a supportive lift under the deficient ischium is sometimes advisable. See Figure 11.31. This is especially true with patients whose occupations require prolonged sitting on a firm surface (eg, typists, computer operators, students).

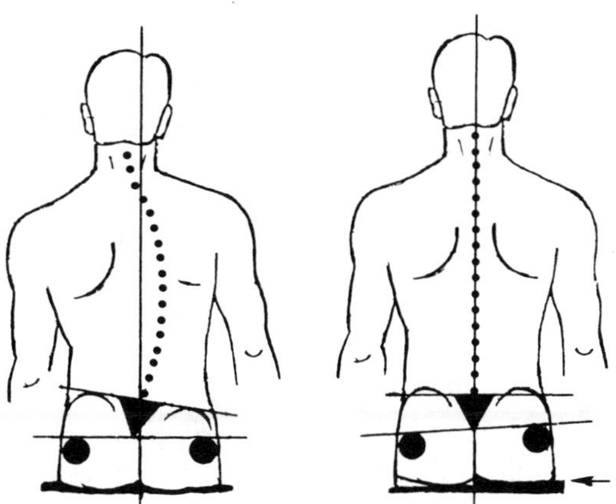

Figure 11.31. *Left,* sitting functional scoliosis due to structural deficiency in length of the right side of the pelvis. *Right,* postural correction through use of a right ischial lift. Correction would not be this ideal if structural changes in the spine had occurred (courtesy of Associated Chiropractic Academic Press).

HEEL LIFT INDICATIONS AND CONTRAINDICATIONS

When used correctly, heel lifts are beneficial in aiding faulty body mechanics, improving static balance, creating a corrective force, and supporting the benefits gained from articular or soft-tissue adjustments. Once structural changes have occurred, full correction cannot be expected. In applications where the biomechanics involved are not fully appreciated or individual reactions are not carefully monitored, lifts can aggravate the symptomatology.

Indications. There are four basic reasons for the use of a temporary unilateral heel lift:

1. To raise the ipsilateral pelvis up and forward.
2. To raise an inferoposteriorly rotated lumbar segment that is contributing to a lumbar scoliosis. If there is inferiority without posteriority (wedge tilt), a plantar lift would be more appropriate.
3. To shift body weight contralaterally with the goal of balancing body weight or shifting weight temporarily away from the side of acute irritation. Application in the latter example is for the same reason that the acute sciatic or hip case will lift the heel and stand on the toe of the painful side.
4. To force mobility of a contralateral hypomobile area. In this case, enough lift must be provided to shift more weight contralaterally as judged by dual weight scales.

Contraindications. Due to the mechanics involved, a heel lift would be inadvisable whenever a shift in body weight contralaterally or an ipsilateral anterior rotation of the ilium on the same side would be contraindicated. The use of a lift without articular correction and comprehensive case management can lead to the aggravation of symptoms.

PRESCRIPTION OF LIFTS

Periodic assessment of biomechanical changes must be evaluated and the applied forces altered as necessary for the particular situation at hand. For general reference, lift applications related to common distortions are outlined in Table 11.9.[71]

The exact amount of initial lift is a clinical judgment based upon patient adaptability as exhibited by signs and symptoms. Thus, a degree of trial and error is always involved even by the experienced practitioner. Acute and minimal conditions can usually adapt to immediate 50% correction. Chronic and gross distortions, undoubtedly presenting with fibrosis, require progressive changes of no more than ⅛-inch at a time. Some patients will respond dramatically to a ⅛-inch lift, while others will show little change with an immediate ⅜-inch correction.

Monitoring. A lift should never be prescribed and its effects left unchecked. Likewise, the effects of a lift cannot be appreciated immediately. This is essentially due to the biomechanical phenomena of tissue creep, relaxation, and fatigue, as well as the new patterns of mechanoreceptor excitation produced.

Overcorrection. Structural overcorrection should be avoided unless there is a special clinical reason for its employment. In a flexible spine, overcorrection can lead to instability. On rare occasions, it may be temporarily desirable to move gravitational forces away from an ipsilateral irritation. In a stiff spine, overcorrection may be carefully employed to stretch contralateral tissues that have shortened (eg, scoliotic concavity) if pain or new symptoms are not produced. When in doubt, it is always better to undercorrect rather than overcorrect.

Permanent Applications. The only time a permanent heel lift is necessary is in cases of anatomic (eg, growth deficiency, fracture) or stubborn functional shortening over ¼ inch (eg, hemiplegia). Keep in mind that a functional deficiency may be superimposed on an anatomic deficiency, and the contribution of each should be differentiated before a permanent lift is prescribed. If a permanent heel lift of over ⅜ inch is necessary, it is best to have half the amount added to the ipsilateral heel and half the amount removed from the contralateral heel.

Table 11.9. Common Distortions and Related Shoe Lift Applications

LATERAL DISTORTIONS

Type	*Ipsilateral Application*	*Contralateral Application*
Lumbar scoliosis (convexity)....	Heel lift	Sole lift or heel drop
Sacral anteroinferiority	Heel lift	Sole lift or heel drop
Sacral posterosuperiority	Sole lift or heel drop	Heel lift
Iliac anterosuperiority	Sole lift or heel drop	Heel lift
Iliac posteroinferiority	Heel lift	Sole lift or heel drop
Unilateral pelvic anteriority	Sole lift or heel drop	Heel lift
Unilateral pelvic posteriority....	Heel lift	Sole lift or heel drop
Unilateral low femur head	Plantar lift	
Unilateral short ischium........	Ischial lift	

ANTERIOR-POSTERIOR DISTORTIONS

Type	*Application*
Sprung back (lumbar sprain)..............	Bilateral heel lifts
Kissing spines (lumbar)..................	Bilateral sole lifts or heel drops
Lumbar hyperlordosis...................	Bilateral sole lifts or heel drops
Lumbar flattening	Bilateral heel lifts
Fixed pelvic anterior tilt	Bilateral sole lifts or heel drops
Fixed pelvic posterior tilt	Bilateral heel lifts

REFERENCES

1. Basmajian JV (ed): *Manipulation, Traction, and Massage,* ed 3. Baltimore, Williams & Wilkins, 1985, p 172.
2. Schafer RC: *Chiropractic Health Care,* ed 3. Des Moines, IA, Foundation for Chiropractic Education and Research, 1979.
3. Saunders HD: *Orthopaedic Physical Therapy: Evaluation and Treatment of Musculoskeletal Disorders.* Minneapolis, MN, published by author, 1982, p 143.
4. Voss DE, et al: Traction and approximation. *Proprioceptive Neuromuscular Facilitation: Patterns and Techniques,* ed 3. Philadelphia, Harper & Row, 1985, p 294.
5. Back specialists hit "inversion" fad. *Medical World News,* 28 March 1983, pp 49-50.
6. Rogoff JB (ed): *Manipulation, Traction, and Massage,* ed 2. Baltimore, Williams & Wilkins, 1980, p 191-198.
7. Lawson GA, Godfrey CM: A report on studies of spinal traction. *Journal of Medical Services* (Canada), 14:762-771, 1958.
8. Judovich BD: Herniated cervical disc: a new form of traction therapy. *American Journal of Surgery,* 84: 646-656, 1952.
9. McFarland JW, Krusen FH: Use of the Sayre head sling in osteoarthritis of cervical portion of spinal column. *Archives of Physical Therapy,* 24:263-269, 1943.
10. Basmajian JV (ed): *Manipulation, Traction, and*

Massage, ed 3. Baltimore, Williams & Wilkins, 1985, pp 184-187.

11. Hill LL: *Parameters of Physiotherapy Modalities.* Lombard, IL, National Chiropractic College, class notes, date not shown, p 78.
12. Saunders HD: *Orthopaedic Physical Therapy: Evaluation and Treatment of Musculoskeletal Disorders.* Minneapolis, MN, published by author, 1982, pp 157-160.
13. Hill LL: *Parameters of Physiotherapy Modalities.* Lombard, IL, National Chiropractic College, class notes, date not shown, p 77.
14. ACA Council on Physiological Therapeutics: Physiotherapy guidelines for the chiropractic profession, *ACA Journal of Chiropractic,* p S-68, June 1975.
15. Rogoff JB (ed): *Manipulation, Traction, and Massage,* ed 2. Baltimore, Williams & Wilkins, 1980, p 199.
16. Downer AH: *Physical Therapy Procedures: Selected Techniques,* ed 2. Springfield, IL, Charles C. Thomas, pp 155-164.
17. Ibid.
18. Hill LL: *Parameters of Physiotherapy Modalities.* Lombard, IL, National Chiropractic College, class notes, date not shown, pp 78-79.
19. Plocher DW: Inversion petechiae. *New England Journal of Medicine,* 307:1406-1407, 25 November, 1982.
20. Klatz RM, et al: The effects of gravity inversion procedures on systemic blood pressure, intraocular pressure, and central retinal arterial pressure. *Journal of the American Osteopathic Association,* 82 (11), July 1983.
21. Schafer RC: *Chiropractic Management of Sports and Recreational Injuries.* Baltimore, Williams & Wilkins, 1982, p 203.
22. Mathews JA: The effects of spinal traction. *Physiotherapy,* 58:64-66, 1972.
23. Schafer RC: *Clinical Biomechanics: Musculoskeletal Actions and Reactions.* Baltimore, Williams & Wilkins, 1983, p 263.
24. Ibid: pp 263-264.
25. Saunders HD: *Orthopaedic Physical Therapy: Evaluation and Treatment of Musculoskeletal Disorders.* Minneapolis, MN, published by author, 1982, p 146.
26. Voss DE, et al: Traction and approximation. *Proprioceptive Neuromuscular Facilitation: Patterns and Techniques,* ed 3. Philadelphia, Harper & Row, 1985, p 294.
27. Schafer RC: *Clinical Biomechanics: Musculoskeletal Actions and Reactions.* Baltimore, Williams & Wilkins, 1983, p 438.
28. Lawson SM, Crawford AH: Traction in the treatment of spinal deformity. *Orthopedics,* 6(4):447-451, April 1983.
29. Cotrel Y: Proceedings: Traction in the treatment of vertebral deformity. *Journal of Bone and Joint Surgery,* 57B:260, 1975.
30. Dewald A, Ray RD: Skeletal traction for the treatment of severe scoliosis. *Journal of Bone and Joint Surgery,* 52A:233-238, 1970.
31. Garrett A, et al: Stabilization of the collapsing spine. *Journal of Bone and Joint Surgery,* 43A:474-484, 1961.
32. Letts RM, Bobechko WP: Preoperative skeletal traction in scoliosis. *Journal of Bone and Joint Surgery,* 57A:616-619, 1975.
33. Moe JH, et al: *Scoliosis and Other Spinal Deformities.* Philadelphia, W.B. Saunders, 1978, p 467.
34. Schafer RC: *Clinical Biomechanics: Musculoskeletal Actions and Reactions.* Baltimore, Williams & Wilkins, 1983, pp 254-255.
35. Dr. Sabia's Scoliometer: *Handbook of Instruction.* Little Silver, NJ, Dr. Sabia's Scoliometer, Inc, 1983.
36. Basmajian JV (ed): *Manipulation, Traction, and Massage,* ed 3. Baltimore, Williams & Wilkins, 1985, pp 191-192.
37. Ibid: pp 157-163.
38. Rogoff JB (ed): *Manipulation, Traction, and Massage,* ed 2. Baltimore, Williams & Wilkins, 1980, pp 170-178.
39. McGarry J, et al: Autonomic hyperreflexia following passive stretching to the hip joint. *Physical Therapy,* 62(1):30-31, January 1982.
40. Schafer RC: *Clinical Biomechanics: Musculoskeletal Actions and Reactions.* Baltimore, Williams & Wilkins, 1983, p 263.
41. Cox JM: *Low Back Pain: Mechanism, Diagnosis and Treatment,* ed 4. Baltimore, Williams & Wilkins, 1985, pp 186-190.
42. Janse J, et al: *Chiropractic Principles and Technic.* Chicago, National College of Chiropractic, 1947, pp 512-515.
43. Johnson AC: *Chiropractic Physiological Therapeutics,* ed 5. Palm Springs, CA, published by author, 1977, pp 34-39.
44. Schafer RC: *Clinical Biomechanics: Musculoskeletal Actions and Reactions.* Baltimore, Williams & Wilkins, 1983, p 371.
45. Janse J, et al: *Chiropractic Principles and Technic.* Chicago, National College of Chiropractic, 1947, pp 516-518.
46. Johnson AC: *Chiropractic Physiological Therapeutics,* ed 5. Palm Springs, CA, published by author, 1977, p 40.
47. Hill LL: *Parameters of Physiotherapy Modalities.* Lombard, IL, National Chiropractic College, class notes, date not shown, pp 42-43.
48. Voss DE, et al: Traction and approximation. *Proprioceptive Neuromuscular Facilitation: Patterns and Techniques,* ed 3. Philadelphia, Harper & Row, 1985, p 314.
49. Schafer RC: *Chiropractic Management of Sports and*

Recreational Injuries. Baltimore, Williams & Wilkins, 1982, p 204.

50. Saunders HD: *Orthopaedic Physical Therapy: Evaluation and Treatment of Musculoskeletal Disorders.* Minneapolis, MN, published by author, 1982, p 167.
51. Watts H: Bracing in spinal deformities. *Orthopedic Clinics of North America,* 10:769-785, 1979.
52. Schafer RC: *Chiropractic Management of Sports and Recreational Injuries.* Baltimore, Williams & Wilkins, 1982, pp 205-206.
53. Johnson R, et al: Cervical orthosis. *Journal of Bone and Joint Surgery,* 59A:332-339, 1977.
54. Colachis S, et al: Cervical spine motion in normal women: Radiographic study of effect of cervical collars. *Archives of Physical Medicine and Rehabilitation,* 54:161-169, 1973.
55. Wasserman J, McNamee M: Engineering evaluation of lumbosacral orthosis using in vivo noninvasive testing. *Proceeding of the Tenth Southeast Conference of Theoretical and Applied Mechanics,* 1980.
56. Waters R, Morris J: Effect of spinal supports on the electrical activity of muscles of the trunk. *Journal of Bone and Joint Surgery,* 52A:51-60, 1970.
57. Lumsden R, Morris J: An in vivo study of axial rotation and immobilization at the lumbosacral joint. *Journal of Bone and Joint Surgery,* 50A:1591-1602, 1968.
58. Nachemson A, Morris J: In vivo measurements of intradiscal pressure. *Journal of Bone and Joint Surgery,* 46A:1077-1092, July 1964.
59. Morris J, et al: Role of the trunk in stability of the spine. *Journal of Bone and Joint Surgery,* 43A:327-351, April 1961.
60. Norton P, Brown T: The immobilizing efficiency of back braces. *Journal of Bone and Joint Surgery,* 39A:111-139, 1957.
61. Schafer RC: *Clinical Biomechanics: Musculoskeletal Actions and Reactions.* Baltimore, Williams & Wilkins, 1983, pp 355-356.
62. Black J, Dumbleton JH (eds): *Clinical Biomechanics.* New York, Churchill-Livingston, 1980.
63. MacEwen GD, et al: Acute neurological complications in the treatment of scoliosis. *Journal of Bone and Joint Surgery,* 57A:404-408, 1975.
64. Raemy H, and Jakob RP: Functional treatment of fresh fibula ligament lesions using the Aircast splint. *Swiss Journal of Sports Medicine,* January 1983.
65. Stover CN, York JM: The Aircast/AirStirrup system for graduated management of lower extremity injuries. Monograph published by Aircast, Inc, Summit, NJ, no date shown.
66. Hamilton WG: Sprained ankles in ballet dancers. *Foot & Ankle,* September-October 1982, pp 99-102.
67. Nirschi RP: The etiology and treatment of tennis elbow. *Journal of Sports Medicine,* 2:308-323, 1974.
68. Schafer RC: *Chiropractic Management of Sports and Recreational Injuries.* Baltimore, Williams & Wilkins, 1982, p 207.
69. Ibid: p 206.
70. Schafer RC: *Clinical Biomechanics: Musculoskeletal Actions and Reactions.* Baltimore, Williams & Wilkins, 1983, pp 484-486.
71. Ibid: p 487.

POSTSCRIPT

To any circumspect practitioner, it is obvious that no single therapy offers a panacea. However, one therapy may be better suited to the problem than another, or a combined effort might be advisable. The ancient but still valid axioms of the healing arts, *Primo Non Nocere* (The First Principle Is —Do No Harm) and *Salus Aegroti Suprema Lex* (The Welfare of the Ailing is the Supreme Law) places an enormous responsibility upon the physician since he or she has to decide which therapy or therapies are indicated for the individual patient.

The authors of this manual have endeavored to give the reader a comprehensive review of the more popular procedures utilized in physical therapy. It must be emphasized, however, that the application of therapy as described must always be tempered by those clinical findings exhibited by each patient. Many factors—including age, weight, sex, physical status, emotional temperament, general health and resistance, and the working diagnosis—must play a part in the decision-making process. The general parameters provided in this manual are only that—general parameters.

It should also be re-emphasized that every patient who presents with neuromusculoskeletal symptomatologies represents *a condition in kinetic flux.* As the patient's pain eases, as healing evolves, the approach should change to meet the patient's structural, physiological, and psychological needs at hand.

Due to length restrictions that any book must maintain along with other priorities, this book has not reviewed the lengthy subjects of therapeutic exercise or nutrition, which fall under the general category of *physiological therapeutics,* and the many techniques of rehabilitation and immobilization have been restricted to their "core" substance. However, these procedures often play an integral part in the care of the patient. The reader is therefore encouraged to refer to specific texts on these subjects, and study the procedures carefully, so that they may be wisely incorporated in case management when warranted by the diagnosis.

> *There are only two sorts of doctors; those who practice with their brains, and those who practice with their tongues.* —Sir William Osler

Glossary Of Physiotherapeutic Terms

Absorption. The taking in, reception, or incorporation of gases, fluids, heat, or light.

ac. Abbreviation of alternating current.

ACC. Anode closing current during galvanic therapy.

Actinic. Pertaining to radiant energy, especially the photochemical effects; capable of producing chemical changes as applied to radiant energy.

Actinotherapy. Treatment of disease by rays of light, especially actinic rays, chemical light, radium, or x-rays.

Action potential. The change in electric potential of nerve or muscle fiber when stimulated; action current.

Acupuncture. A technique for treating certain painful conditions, various dysfunctions, and for producing regional anesthesia by passing thin needles through the skin to certain specific points.

Adjustment. A change made to improve function or a specific condition.

Adsorption. The attraction and holding (sucking up) of a gas or liquid on the surface of a substance in solution or suspension.

Agonist. A muscle or muscle group that is a prime mover, directly engaged in contraction.

Algesiometer. An instrument used to measure the degree of sensitivity to a painful stimulus; also, algesimeter, algometer, odynometer.

All-or-none law. When an individual muscle fiber is stimulated sufficiently to produce contraction, it acts to its fullest extent. This applies to the motor unit only and not to the entire muscle.

Alternating current. A current that periodically flows in opposite directions at regular intervals.

Alternator. An electrical generator that produces alternating current.

Altherm. A device containing heat-producing chemicals for applying heat to the eye or a sinus; altherm pad.

AMF. Amplitude modulation frequency, an acronym commonly associated with interferential therapy.

Ammeter. An instrument calibrated in amperes to measure the strength of an electric current. An ampere is usually too large to be used for medical purposes, thus it is divided into a thousand parts (milliamperes).

Ampere. The unit of intensity (strength) of electric current that is produced by 1 volt acting through the resistance of 1 ohm.

Amplifier. An instrument used to enlarge, magnify, extend, or increase electronic impulses such as high-frequency currents, and its output is of greater amplitude than the input; an electronic device for increasing current or a signal.

Amplitude. The size (height of maximum displacement) of a wave; the measure of the maximum deviation from zero to normal axis.

Analgesia. Complete absence of sensitivity to a painful stimulus.

Anaphoresis. Transmission of charged ions into tissues (toward a positive pole) by passage of electric current; insufficient sweat gland activity.

Angle of incidence. The angle formed between a ray incident on a surface and a line drawn perpendicular to that surface at the point of incidence.

Anelectrotonus. The state of diminished irritability of a nerve or muscle that is produced in the region near the anode during the passage of an electric current.

Angstrom. The international unit of wavelength of light that is equal to 1/10,000 micron (0.1 nanometer), used especially to specify radiation wavelengths.

Anion. An ion carrying a negative charge and thus attracted to a positive pole such as an acid radical.

Anode. The positive pole on an electrical source,

serving as a collector nor electrons emitted from a hot filament when rectified or designed as part of a battery.

Anode current. The current passing between an anode and cathode through a vacuum or a partially evacuated space.

Anode voltage. The voltage between an anode and some specified point of a cathode.

AOC. Anode opening current during galvanic therapy.

Arc lamp. A source of light consisting of gaseous particles from the electrodes of an electric arc that are raised to a temperature of incandescence by an electric current.

Arc light. Light emitted from glowing electrodes of an arc lamp or luminous particles between two electrodes of carbon, tungsten, or other material when an electric current is applied and the electrodes are separated a short distance to produce a spark.

Arc reflex. The path followed by a nerve impulse to produce a reflex action.

Atom. The smallest particle of an element that can exist alone or in combination with like particles or other elements.

Auriculotherapy. Acupuncture of the ear.

Autotransformer. A transformer that has some of its turns common to both the primary and secondary circuits.

Base. An alkaline compound in solution that is capable of reacting with an acid to form a salt and water; specifically, the hydroxide of a positive element or radical. Strong bases are corrosive to human tissue.

Bias. The voltage that is impressed on a grid which is relative to the cathode filament (usually negative).

Bipolar. Referring to the use of two poles in electrotherapeutics, especially when direct current is used.

Biterminal. Referring to the two poles utilized in electrotherapeutics, especially when alternating current is used.

Black light lamp. An apparatus producing Wood's rays to detect ultraviolet-fluorescent materials.

Booster. A device for increasing the electromotive force of an ac circuit of a device in series (eg, dynamo) to increase the voltage of a direct current circuit. A booster essentially consists of a small induction coil with an adjustable core.

Breakdown voltage. That quantity of voltage at which a discharge device (eg, a spark gap or grid-glow tube) begins to pass an electric current.

Brush discharge. The discharge from an electrotherapeutic static machine.

Capacitance. That property of an electric nonconductor that permits the storage of energy as a result of electric displacement when opposite surfaces of the nonconductor are maintained at a different potential; the measure of this property equal to the ratio of the charge on either surface to the potential difference between the surfaces.

Capacitor. A device giving capacitance and usually consisting of conducting coils separated by thin layers of dielectric (eg, air, mica) with the plates on opposite sides of the dielectric layers oppositely charged by a source of voltage and the electrical energy of the charged system stored in the polarized dielectric; a condenser.

Capacity. The quantity of electric energy a condenser can store; a measure of electric output of a generator; capacitance.

Cataphoresis. The transmission of electronegative ions or drugs into tissues or through a membrane by using an electric current.

Catelectrotonus. The state of increased excitability produced in a nerve or muscle in the region near the cathode during the passage of an electric current.

Cathode. The negative pole or electrode of any electrical device; an emitter of electrons; the electrode source of the electronic stream in a vacuum tube.

Cathode current. The energy flow passing from a negatively charged electrode; cathode stream.

Causalgia. An agonizing burning pain that is essentially a reflex vasomotor dystrophy, consisting chiefly of sympathetic phenomena. invariably following trauma, involving one or more limbs.

Cavitation. The formation of a cavity or blind cyst within tissue such as from gas formation (eg, gangrene, ultrasound) or pathologic destruction (eg, pulmonary tuberculosis, bone tumor).

CCC. Cathode closing current during galvanic therapy.

Celsius. Centigrade; 100 divisions between freezing and boiling.

Chronaxie. Time intensity (measured in seconds) relation of electric stimuli; the minimal time for a current having twice the intensity of the rheobasic current; the sensitivity index of a nerve to electrical stimulation.

Circuit breaker. A special switch that functions like a fuse to open or close a circuit, manually or automatically during overload.

Claudication. A cramping, severely distressing pain due to ischemia.

Cobb's angle. A measurement of segmental position in scoliosis, arrived at by drawing a line through the upper border of the cephalad vertebra that tilts the most to the concavity of the curve and the same is done at the inferior border of the caudad vertebra that tilts the most to the convexity. The angle is measured where these two lines transect.

COC. Cathode opening current during galvanic therapy.

Colic. A nondiagnostic term referring to any symptom complex whose major feature is acute paroxysmal pain.

Colloid. An apparently dissolved substance that diffuses extremely slowly through a membrane or is indiffusable. They are usually glue-like, gelatinous compounds such as albumen, gelatin, or starch.

Commutator. A device that reverses the direction of an electric current such as a segmental ring attached to a dynamo on which brushes slide.

Condenser. See Capacitor.

Conductance. The ability of a substance to conduct a form of energy such as electricity or heat; the reciprocal of unit resistance, ohm/cm.

Conduction. The transfer of heat, ions, or sound waves through a conductor or conducting medium.

Conduction heat. Heat transmitted by transference through a medium such as from a hot pack or poultice.

Conductivity. See Conductance.

Constant current. Direct (galvanic) current; continuous current.

Convection. Energy (eg, heat) transferred through a medium such as currents of air or water.

Converse heat. Heat generated in tissues because of an application of electric current or radiant energy.

Conversion. The process of transforming one form of energy into another such as the change of electrical energy into heat within body tissues.

Co-planar. In the same plane, such as electrode positioning.

Coulomb. That quantity of electricity transferred by a current of 1 ampere in 1 second.

Coupler. A device that transfers energy from one circuit to another.

Coupling medium. A relatively air-less fluid used between the applicator (sound head) and the skin during ultrasound therapy.

Counterirritation. Superficial irritation applied to relieve some other irritation of deeper tissues.

cps. Abbreviation for cycles per second; same as Hertz (Hz) when applied to alternating current.

Cryesthesia. Abnormal sensitivity to cold.

Crymoanesthesia. Anesthesia produced by thermosteresis.

Crymotherapy. The use of cold in treating a disease or disorder.

Cryocautery. An instrument that uses cold to a degree sufficient to kill tissue (eg, -20 °C).

Cryokinetics. Therapeutic cold combined with exercise.

Cryotherapy. The use of therapuetic cold in any form; crymotherapy.

Cupping. Application to the skin of a glass vessel (usually) from which air has been exhausted by heat or suction to draw blood to the surface; a form of counterirritation often used in Europe and the Orient.

Current breaker. A special in-line switch (usually for safety purposes) that quickly disrupts a circuit during overload. It can usually be re-set manually.

Cycle. One period of alternating current, which represents the complete change from zero to positive maximum, to zero, to negative maximum, and then back to zero.

Damped current. A series of electrical oscillating waves that has a gradually decreasing amplitude.

dc. Abbreviation of direct current.

Deep heat therapy. Microwave, shortwave, or ultrasonic therapy; therapy utilizing high frequency currents.

Depolarize. To cause to become wholly or partially unpolarized; to prevent or remove polarization of a cell membrane or battery.

Dermatome. The topographic area of skin that is supplied by afferent cutaneous fibers from a single posterior spinal root, usually overlapped considerably by neighboring dermatomes.

Desiccation. The process of drying, demoisturizing, or dehydrating.

Desquammation. Epithelial shedding, especially of the skin, in scales or sheets.

Diapulse. Pulsed diathermy with 25 ms off for

every 1 ms of power on, thus allowing some time for the dissipation of the heat produced.

Diathermy. The therapeutic use of high-frequency electric current to generate deep heat within some part of the body; transtherma; thermopenetration.

Dielectric. A nonconductor of direct electric current; an insulator that has been placed between two electrically charged plates of a condenser (capacitor).

Dielectric heating. The rapid and uniform heating throughout a nonconducting material by means of a high-frequency electromagnetic field.

Diode. A thermionic tube that contains two electrodes which pass current essentially in one direction.

Diplode. A diathermy induction-coil drum with flexible hinges.

Direct current. A current that flows continuously in one direction only; galvanic current.

Distraction. The act of drawing or pulling along the long axis of a joint to the degree that articular facets separate, without injury to the joint(s), and the involved fibrocartilages (eg, IVDs) increase in thickness. Also see Traction.

Dosage. The product of intensity X duration, such as in electrotherapy.

Drum. A diathermy induction coil enclosed in a container, which serves as the applicator.

Dry cell. A zinc container lined with thin blotting paper, which serves as the negative electrode, and a centrally located carbon rod, which serves as the positive electrode. Typically, a paste made up of ammonium chloride. zinc chloride, manganese dioxide, water,and granulated carbon fills the space between the electrodes.

Dry heat. Dehumidified heat; the application of heat without accompanying moisture such as with the use of an electric heating pad, a hot water bottle, or an infra-red lamp.

DuBois-Reymond's law. The intensity of a stimulus and the following muscular contraction are directly proportional to the magnitude and change in current strength, or, in the presence of the same current strength, the intensity is proportional to the rate of fluctuation.

Edema. An abnormal (local or generalized) accumulation of an excessive amount of watery fluid in cells, intercellular spaces, or serous cavities.

Effleurage. The use of the whole palmar surface to administer slow, longitudinal, deep or gentle strokes to the skin.

Elastic bandage. Bandage that can be stretched to exert continuous pressure.

Electricity. A type of energy formed by the interaction of positive and negative charges that exhibits chemical, magnetic, mechanical, and thermal effects; electromotive force.

Electrization. The act of charging or treating by the use of electricity.

Electroanalgesia. The relief of pain by using low intensity electrical currents applied locally or through implanted electrodes.

Electrocauterization. The process of cauterizing tissue by an electric instrument, using either direct or alternating current, that heats a wire to extremely high temperatures.

Electrocoagulation. Coagulation of tissue by means of a high-frequency current, where the heat that produces the coagulation is generated within the tissue to be destroyed.

Electrocution. The destruction of living cells by means of an electric current.

Electrode. An instrument with a point or a surface from which an electric current is discharged to a part of the body.

Electrodesiccation. The destructive drying of cells or tissues by means of short, high-frequency sparks.

Electrodiagnosis. The determination of functional states of various tissues and organs according to their response to electrical stimulation.

Electrolysis. The electrical decomposition of a chemical compound such as the separation of an electrolyte into its constituents by an electric current; the destruction of hair follicles by using electricity.

Electrolyte. A solution that conducts electricity; a substance in solution that conducts an electric current and is decomposed by the passage of an electric current.

Electromassage. Massage combined with electrical therapy.

Electromotive force. The effect of differences of potential that causes a flow of electricity in a closed circuit from one site to another.

Electron. An extremely minute particle or charge of electricity.

Electronization. The use of radiation to restore electrical equilibrium to diseased cells.

Electrophoresis. The movement of charged colloidal particles through the medium in which they are dispersed as a result of changes in electrical potential.

Electropyrexia. The use of electricity to produce a fever.

Electrotherapy. The use of electricity therapeutically; electrotherapeutics.

Electrothermotherapy. The therapeutic production of heat within living tissues created by tissue resistance to the passage of electricity.

Electrotonus. The change in the irritability of a nerve or muscle during passage of an electric current.

EMF. Shortened form for electromotive force.

Endogenous. Arising from or on the inside; originating within the body.

Endorphin. One of a variety of opioid-like polypeptides found in the brain and other tissues. In the brain, it binds to the same receptors that bind exogenous opiates. Different types (eg, alpha-endorphin and beta-endorphin) have different physical and chemical properties and physiologic actions.

Enkephalin. A pentapeptide, hypothesized to be an endogenous neurotransmitter, that is found in many parts of the brain, which binds to specific receptor sites. Many of these sites are considered to be pain-related opiate receptors.

Epilation. The destruction or removal of hair; depilation.

Erythema ab igne. Localized erythema due to exposure to heat.

Erythema dose. The amount of radiant energy sufficient to evoke a perceptible diffuse redness of the skin.

Excitable. Capable of being excited, activated, or able to respond to a stimulus.

Exogenous. Originating from or due to an external cause or causes; introduced from or produced outside the organism.

Exponentially progressive current. A gradually increasing current.

Farad. One farad represents the capacity of a condenser which charged with 1 coulomb gives a difference of potential of 1 volt.

Faradic coil. A device for producing an induced (faradic) current from a direct current source.

Faradic current. An intermittent alternating current induced in the secondary winding or an induction cell.

Far ultraviolet. Ultraviolet radiation with a short wavelength, which is farthest from the visible spectrum.

Fatigue theory of pain. Repeated contractions with short rest intervals (1—2 seconds) produce a decrease in contraction amplitude accompanied by fatigue, which results in an inability to achieve complete relaxation and leads to spasm.

FCC. Federal Communications Commission.

Filament. The cathode (negative pole) in a thermionic or roentgen ray tube.

Fluidotherapy. A dry heat modality that uses a finely pulverized solid suspended in an air stream, the pressurized mixture of which has the properties of a liquid.

Fluorescence. Luminescence of a substance when acted on by short-wave radiation (eg, ultraviolet light).

Flux. The electromagnetic lines of force (eg, of a magnetic field) that are produced by a current passing through a coil.

Fortis. Strong; produced with unusual force.

Frequency. The rate of oscillation or alternation in ac current; sometimes used to refer to the periodicity of interrupted direct current.

Friction massage. The use of fingertips to strongly move superficial skin over subjacent structures in a circular manner, which should always be followed by centripetal stroking.

Fulguration. The destruction of cells by means of long, high-frequency sparks.

Fuse. An in-line current-limiting (safety) device to prevent circuit overload, usually consisting of an easily meltable metallic alloy of specified thickness that has a low melting point and which opens the circuit during an overload.

Galvanic current. An uninterrupted unidirectional electric current; galvanism.

Gate theory. Large myelinated nerve fibers of the skin, when stimulated, have an inhibitory effect on the small pain-bearing fibers that enter the same segment of the spinal cord.

Generator (electric). An apparatus that converts mechanical energy into electric power. It is made of the following components: a magnetic field, an armature, metallic brushes, slip rings (in ac generators) or a commutator (in DC generators), and the activating power source.

Gildemeister effect. The depolarization of nerve fibers, according to the summation principle.

Grid. An electrode that has openings through which ions or electrons may pass.

Ground. An electrical connection with the earth or any conductor of large capacity.

Halo cast. A cast applied to the shoulders in which metal bars are set that extend over the head like a halo, from which traction may be applied to the head by means of tongs or a halter.

Head's law. When a painful stimulus is applied to a part of low sensibility (eg, viscus) in close central connection with a part of much greater sensibility (eg, skin), the pain produced is felt in the part of higher sensibility rather than in the part of lower sensibility to which the stimulus was actually applied.

Heliotherapy. The therapeutic application of radiation from the sun.

Henry. A unit of inductance; a circuit of 1 henry refers to a current changing rate where 1 ampere per second produces 1 volt back.

Hertz. A unit of frequency equal to 1 cycle per second, usually restricted to that of alternating current.

Heterotopic sensation. A referred perception (eg, pain or tenderness) sensed to arise from an area other than its origin.

Heuter-Volkmann theory. Increased pressure across an epiphyseal plate inhibits growth, while decreased pressure tends to accelerate growth.

High frequency. A current having a frequency interruption or change of direction sufficiently high enough to avoid tetany when the current is passed through contractile tissue; a therapeutic frequency sufficient to produce heat within tissues.

High-volt therapy. High voltage monophasic pulsed electrical stimulation.

Homotopic sensation. A perception sensed at the point of injury; ie, not referred or radiated.

Hydrocollator. Trade name for a type of hot moist packs.

Hydroelectric bath. A quantity of water through which electricity is administered to tissues for therapeutic purposes.

Hydrotherapy. The scientific application of water in the treatment of disease.

Hygienics. Any system for promoting health.

Hypalgesia. A diminution of sensitivity to a painful stimulus; hypoalgesia.

Hyperalgesia. An exaggerated sensitivity to a painful stimulus.

Impedence. The ratio of voltage to current flow in a circuit; a measure of the opposition to current flow such as capacity, reactance, inductance, and resistance, or a combination of such factors; the apparent opposition in an electrical circuit to the flow of an alternating current that is analogous to the actual resistance to a direct current and that is the ratio of effective electromotive force to the effective current.

Indication. A sign or circumstance that indicates the proper treatment of a disease.

Induction (electrical). The process by which a magnetizable body becomes magnetized when in a magnetic field or in the magnetic flux set up by a magnetomotive force, or by which an electromotive force is produced in a circuit by varying the magnetic field linked with the circuit.

Induction coil. A device for obtaining intermittent high voltage, consisting of a primary coil through which the direct current flows; an interrupter; a secondary coil of a larger number of turns in which high voltage is induced.

Induction heating. Heating a substance by means of an electric current that is caused to flow through the material or its container by electromagnetic induction.

Infrared rays. Radiations just beyond the red end of the spectrum, with wavelengths between 7,700 and 500,000 Angstroms; therapeutic wavelengths between 7,700 and 14,000 Angstroms.

Insulation. The protection of the body, a body part, or an electrical conductor with a nonconducting medium to prevent the transfer of electricity, heat, or sound.

Interferential. Interference; in physiotherapy, a modality that crosses two medium frequency alternating currents within the body.

Interrupted circuit. A current that is periodically opened and closed.

Interrupted current. A flow of electricity (usually dc) that is frequently opened and closed.

Inverse square law. The intensity of radiation at any distance is inversely proportional to the square of the distance between the source point and the irradiated surface.

Invisible spectrum. The part of the spectrum which is imperceivable by the eye; spectrum wavelengths below the red (infrared) or above the violet (ultraviolet); wavelengths beyond visual perception such as cosmic, gamma, and roentgen rays.

Ion. An electrified particle derived from an atom or group of atoms into which the molecules of an electrolyte are divided; an electrical particle into which the molecules of a gas are divided by an ionizing agent (eg, gamma, roentgen, or ultraviolet rays).

Ionization. The process by which neutral atoms or molecules become charged positively or negatively.

Ion transfer. The therapuetic introduction of chemical ions into superficial tissues by means of a direct current; iontophoresis.

Iontophoresis. The therapeutic introduction of ionized substances into superficial tissues by means of a carefully controlled low-volt direct current that transfers positive ions to a cathode and negative ions to an anode; ionic medication; ionotherapy; iontotherapy.

Irradiation. The exposure to some form of radiation (eg, microwaves, roentgen rays, radium, sunlight, ultraviolet rays, or infrared light).

Ischemia. Local, usually temporary, anemia due to functional or mechanical obstruction (eg, lumen narrowing or blocking); inadequate circulation; hypoemia.

Joule. A unit of electrical energy equivalent to work expended when 1 ampere flows for 1 second against a resistance of 1 ohm; 10,000,000 ergs.

Joule's laws. (1) heat is produced in direct proportion to the square of current strength; (2) heat produced by a given amount of current is directly proportional to the resistance of the conductor, and (3) the heat produced is directly proportional to the duration of current flow.

Kilocycle. 1000 cycles.

Kirchhoff's law. The greatest level of heat is produced in the area of greatest current density.

Kneading. A type of massage in which the palmar surface is used to produce a rotary pressure to superficial tissues; pressing, grasping, wringing, lifting, or rolling a part of a muscle or muscle group; petrissage.

Kromayer lamp. Trade name for a hot quartz, water-cooled, ultraviolet radiating apparatus.

Laser. Acronym for light amplification by stimulated emission of radiation.

Latent period. The time interval between a stimulus and the response.

Light. The sensation produced by electromagnetic radiations between 4,000 and 7,000 Angstroms that fall on the retina to effect vision.

Light therapy. The therapeutic application of radiations whose wavelengths are within the visible spectrum. Note: some authorities also relate infrared and ultraviolet radiation with this term.

Low frequency. Alternating currents that have relatively few cycles per second such as those which produce tetany.

ma. Abbreviation for milliampere.

Magnet. A body having the property of attracting ions and producing a magnetic field external to itself.

Magnetic field. The portion of space permeated by detectable magnetic lines of force surrounding a permanent magnet or coil of wire carrying an electric current.

Magneto. A magnetoelectric machine; an alternator with permanent magnets used to generate current for the ignition in an internal-combustion engine.

Magnetotherapy. The application of magnets or magnetism in treating disease.

Magnetron. A diode vacuum tube in which the flow of electrons is controlled by an externally applied magnetic field to generate power at microwave frequencies.

Malpractice. An act of professional negligence; a dereliction from duty or a failure to exercise an acceptable degree of professional skill or learning by one rendering professional services which result in injury, loss, or damage to an individual.

Massage. Manipulation, kneading, pinching, pressure, or friction applied to the bare skin.

Massotherapy. The use of massage in treating disease.

Mechanoreceptor. A neuroreceptor that is activated by mechanical pressure or distortion; mechanicoreceptor.

Mechanotherapy. Treatment of disease by means of apparatus or mechanical appliances.

MED. Minimal (tonic) erythemal dose.

Megaohm. 1,000,000 ohms.

Meridian. A theoretical pathway (circuit) of energy (eg, that of Oriental medicine); a group of acupuncture points.

MHz. Megahertz; a frequency of 1,000,000 cycles per second.

Microfarad. 1,000,000th of a farad.

Micromassage. A mechanically induced vibratory effect at the molecular level (eg, as in ultrasound therapy).

Micron. 1,000,000th of a meter.

Milliammeter. An electronic meter calibrated to read in milliamperes.

Milliampere. 1,000th of an ampere; ma.

Millimicron. 1,000,000th of a millimeter.

Mitis. Mild.

Modality. A method of therapeutic application or the use of a therapeutic agent, especially a physical agent; a physical mode.

Mode. A manner in which a thing is done; a control setting on electrotherapeutic apparatus.

Modulate. To vary the amplitude, frequency, or phase of a carrier wave.

Monode. An inflexible helical induction-coil diathermy applicator.

Monoterminal. An electrotherapeutic arrangement where one terminal is used as the active electrode and the ground acts as the second terminal to complete the circuit.

Motion unit. An articular segment and its contiguous structures.

Motorpathy. Treatment of a condition by prescribed movements; kinesitherapy; kinetotherapy.

Motor point. The point where a motor nerve enters a muscle and where visible contraction can be produced by minimal stimulation.

Motor unit. A motor neuron, its various parts, and the many muscle fibers innervated by the neuron.

Movement. Any manipulation or stroke used to provoke reflex or mechanical effects on soft tissue.

Moxibustion. Cauterization by means of an inflammable substance that is fired at the top to produce counterirritation.

ms. Abbreviation for millisecond.

mv. Abbreviation for millivolt.

Myotome. A group of skeletal muscles derived from one somite (embryonic muscle plate) and innervated by a single segmental spinal nerve. The sensory innervation of muscle follows the motor innervation and not that of the cutaneous zones.

Nernst's postulate. Muscle or nerve stimulation is triggered by changes in ionic concentration at the cell membrane. Ions migrate at different velocities through the two media of the body (interstitial fluid and cellular protoplasm) in which they are soluble, according to the strength and duration of the current applied.

Nerve tracing. The palpable act of following the course of tenderness over nerves that are irritated or impinged; used to assist in locating the focus of pain, tenderness, or headache.

Nociceptor. A sensory receptor for pain; a pain-oriented receptor stimulated by trauma or irritation.

Normalis. Normal, typical.

Ohm. Unit of electrical resistance equal to that of a conductor in which a current of 1 ampere is produced by a potential of 1 volt across the terminals.

Ohm's law. In an electrical circuit, the flow of current (amperage) is in direct proportion to the electromotive force (voltage) of the generator and inversely proportional to the resistance (ohms) of the circuit.

Open circuit. A circuit that is not complete; a broken circuit.

Oscillating current. An alternating current with either a constant wave amplitude or a gradually diminishing amplitude.

Oscilloscope. A device that indirectly demonstrates (eg, visibly graphs) the nature and form of electrical oscillations.

Pain. The complex mind-body experience characterized by physical or emotional suffering, distress, or discomfort due to sensory provocation; a basic bodily sensation induced by a noxious stimulus, received by naked nerve endings, characterized by physical discomfort (as pricking, throbbing, or aching), and typically leading to evasive action.

Paraffin therapy. The therapeutic application of melted paraffin wax that has been diluted with mineral oil at a predetermined ratio (eg, 7:1).

Parameter. An arbitrary constant, measurement, property, boundary, or factor.

Percussion. Tapotement, tapping, or thumping.

Periarticular. Around a joint.

Period. The time required for one cycle of ac to pass through all of its positive and negative values.

Periodicity. The rate of rise and fall or interruption of a direct current.

Petrissage. A form of kneading massage in which superficial tissues are picked up and twisted.

Pfluger's law. The closing ("make") of a galvanic current on a nerve triggers an increase in irritability at the negative pole, called *catelectrotonus,* and a decrease in nerve irritability at the positive pole, called *analectrotonus.*

Phonophoresis. The act of introducing chemicals

into the skin via ultrasonic waves.

Phoresis. A suffix referring to the migration of ions through a membrane by means of an electric current such as in anaphoresis or cataphoresis.

Phosphorescence. The induced luminescence that persists after the irradiation that caused it has ceased.

Photometer. An instrument for measuring the intensity of light.

Physiatrics. The science of physiotherapeutic applications; the treatment of disease by natural methods; physical therapy.

Physical therapy. Application of specific modalities such as rehabilitative procedures concerned with the restoration of function and prevention of disability following disease, injury, or loss of a body part; the therapeutic use of physical agents.

Physiotherapy. A shortened form for physiologic therapeutics; treatment by physical or mechanical means; physical therapy.

Piezoelectric effect. The transformation of mechanical energy into electrical energy; electric currents generated by pressure upon certain crystals.

Plate. The anode of a thermionic tube; the positively charged element that collects electrons emitted by the filament.

Polarity. The status of having poles; the exhibition of opposite states or conditions; the orientation or direction of negativity relative to positivity.

Pole changing switch. An electrical device by which the polarity of a circuit may be reversed.

Potential. In electrophysics, a condition by which current tends to flow from a place of higher to lower potential, which is measured in volts.

Poultice. A hot moist substance applied to the skin to act as a counterirritant, relieve congestion or pain, or stimulate absorption of inflammatory products.

pps. Acronym for pulses per second.

Prescribe. To lay down as a guide, recommendation, or suggested action.

Prime mover. A muscle or muscle group that is essential for a particular movement; an agonist.

Prone. Laying in the face-down recumbent position.

Pulsating current. An electric current with a regular rhythm, usually a unidirectional current; regularly interrupted alternating or direct current.

Pulsed current. An electrical current that is regularly interrupted; electromagnetic waves of brief duration.

Pulse duration. Pulse width, from starting point to finishing point.

Quartz glass. Crystalline glass used for prisms and lenses, and through which ultraviolet radiations are easily transmitted.

Radiant energy. A form of energy that is readily transmitted through space without the support of a sensible medium such as cosmic rays, gamma rays, incandescent light, infrared rays, radio waves, sunlight, ultraviolet rays, and x-rays.

Radiation. A general term for any type of radiant energy, emission or divergence such as that being distributed in all directions from antennae, fluorescent substances, luminous bodies, radioactive elements, and x-ray tubes.

Radio frequency. Wavelengths with frequencies above 10,000 cycles per second.

RD. Shortened form of reaction of degeneration.

Reactance. Resistance due to the inductive and condenser characteristics of a circuit; the ratio between voltage and that component of a circuit which is 90° out of phase with the voltage.

Reaction component. Central modification of peripherally generated impulses (eg, pain).

Reaction of degeneration. The change in muscle reactivity to electricity, seen in lower motor neuron paralysis.

Rebound tenderness. The sensation or intensification of discomfort when pressure is released.

Recruiting response. The bringing into action of additional motor neurons to cause greater activity in response to increased duration of the stimulus applied to a given receptor or afferent nerve.

Rectified. Corrected; purified; when applied to an electrical current, an alternating current made unidirectional.

Rectifier. A device for converting alternating current into direct (unidirectional, galvanic) current.

Reduction. The act of restoring, repositioning; in chemistry, the gain of one or more electrons by an ion or compound (eg, the reverse of oxidation).

Reflection. The bending or throwing back of a light ray, sound wave, electric current, or radiant energy after striking a surface (eg, as light striking a mirror).

Refraction. The deflection of a light ray when it passes from one medium to another of different optical density (denser or rarer) so that it is deflected away from a line that is perpendicular to the surface of the refracting medium.

Refractory period. During nerve cell fiber stimulation, the period of depolarization and return to the normal resting voltage.

Relay. A device by which contacts in one circuit are operated by a change in conditions in the same circuit or in one or more related circuits.

Resistance. The opposing factors in a medium to the passage of an electric current, the typical effect of which is to generate heat.

Rheobase. The voltage just barely sufficient for a minimal response during galvanic stimulation; threshold of stimulation.

Rheostat. A device for regulating a current by means of electrical resistance.

Ripple current. A pulsating current that is superimposed on a direct current, and in which the constant component is usually large relative to the sum of the amplitudes of the harmonic components.

Ryodoraku. A form of meridian-point analysis and treatment utilizing 24 cutaneous electroconductive points on the wrists and feet, where hyper- and hypo-electroconductivity values are calculated.

Sclerotome. The area of bone innervated from a single spinal segment.

Series. A mode of arranging the parts of a circuit by connecting them successively end-to-end to form a single path (in-series) for the current.

Short circuit. An accidental overload of current due to the establishment of a low resistance bypass.

Shortwave. A wavelength between 3 and 100 meters.

Shunt. A device for dividing current.

Sine wave. A wave form that represents periodic oscillations in which the amplitude of displacement at each point is proportional to the sine of the phase angle of the displacement.

Sinusoidal current. An alternating current consisting of sine waves to produce separate (clonic) muscular contractions; a surging type current; alternating induced electric current, the two strokes of which are equal.

Solarium. A room design for heliotherapy or the application of artificial light.

Solenoid. A coil where the wire is spaced equally between the turns and where the length of the coil is greater than its diameter; an electromagnet.

Space plate. A diathermy air-spaced condenser-field applicator.

Spacers. Wooden or other types of nonconducting devices used to separate a shortwave diathermy induction cable.

Spasm. An involuntary, often painful, muscular contraction (tonic or clonic) of either striated or smooth muscle; a cramp.

Spasm theory of pain. Exercise to the level where capillaries are occluded by muscle contraction produces intrinsic ischemia and potassium leakage into extracellular tissues which, in turn, elevate osmotic pressure. This increased pressure irritates pain receptors that initiate a reflex tonic contraction which, in turn, enhances the ischemia; thus, a pathologic cycle is created.

Spectrum. The charted band of wavelengths of electromagnetic energy obtained by reflection and diffraction; in interferential therapy, the range of frequency through which the alternating current can be made to swing rhythmically above a present base frequency.

Splint. Any appliance, movable or immovable, used to fixate, unite, or protect an injured part of the body.

Splinting. An involuntary tonic spasm to prevent movement (temporary fixation) of an injured part; a reflex spasm of agonists and antagonists.

Spondylotherapy. Spinal therapeutics; the application of vertebral manipulation or percussion/stimulation of spinal centers in the treatment of disease.

Static electricity. Electricity that is mechanically produced by friction.

Stroking movements. Superficial and deep effleurage.

Summation principle. The process by which a sequence of stimuli that are individually inadequate to produce a response are cummulatively able to induce a nerve impulse.

Superimposition. The process of placing or laying over or above something; in interferential therapy, the act of one current crossing another.

Supine. Laying in the face-up position.

Surge. An electric current that suddenly rises and falls (like waves).

Surgical diathermy. The use of high frequency electrical current to destroy tissue.

Switch rate. A control setting, usually on a high-volt unit, that permits the activation of one (or one set) of electrodes and then another on an alternating basis.

Tapotement. A type of massage where relaxed fingers, palms, or fists are used to administer a rhythmic series of blows to the skin.

Tenderness. A frequently encountered sensory symptom characterized by pain produced by (usually extrinsic) pressure or contact.

TENS. Acronym for transcutaneous electric nerve stimulation.

Tension. Tautness; long-axis stress; voltage.

Tetanizing current. An electrical current that induces tonic muscular spasm.

Thermal. Pertaining to heat.

Thermaerotherapy. Treatment by the application of hot air.

Thermesthesia. The perception of heat or cold.

Thermokinetics. Therapeutic heat combined with exercise.

Thermophore. A flat bag, used as a substitute for a hot water bag, containing salts that produce heat when moistened.

Thermophile. A thermoelectric battery used in measuring slight variation of heat.

Thermosteresis. The deprivation or removal of heat; eg, as in cryotherapy, refrigeration.

Thermotherapy. The therapeutic application of heat.

Threshold. The point where a stimulus begins to produce a sensation; the minimal stimulus necessary to elicit a sensory or motor response.

Traction. The act of drawing or pulling along a predetermined axis of a joint (usually the long axis) to the degree that muscle and ligamentous fibers are stretched but not injured. Also see Distraction.

Transcerebral application. The passage of a high frequency current through the cranium.

Transducer. A device that is activated by power from one system and supplies power usually in another form to a second system.

Transformer. A device, incorporating a coarsely wound coil of thick wire and a finely wound coil of thin wire that are placed side-by-side, for changing the voltage (step-up or step-down) in alternating currents.

Treatment. The techniques or actions customarily applied in a specified situation; an act to care for, alter, improve, or deal with.

Trigger points. Small nodules of spastic or degenerated muscle tissue that serve as focal points for referred pain and other noxious reflexes, usually the result of prolonged hypertonicity and stasis.

Ultrasound. Inaudible sound in the high frequency range of from 17,000 to 10 billion cycles/second.

Ultraviolet radiation. Radiation possessing strong actinic and chemical properties, characterized by powerful invisible actinic rays in the electromagnetic spectrum between the violet rays and roentgen rays, ranging approximately between 1,800 and 4,000 Angstroms.

Undamped current. An oscillating current maintaining a constant amplitude.

Unidirectional. Transmission in one direction such as direct (galvanic) current.

Unipolar. Monoterminal.

Utilization time. The minimum time below which the efficiency of a stimulus to a nerve decreases.

Vapocoolant. A cooling agent administered in the form of a mist; eg, ethyl chloride or fluorimethane.

Vectoring. To guide; to change direction.

Vertebral motion unit. The structures, especially the articulations, of two contiguous vertebrae.

Vibration. The use of fingers or a mechanical device to administer taps in rapid succession.

Visible spectrum. Colors from red to violet.

Volt. The unit of electromotive force; the electrical pressure required to send a current of 1 ampere through the resistance of 1 ohm.

Watt. The unit of electrical power: 1 watt represents the power delivered when the current flows at the rate of 1 ampere with a pressure of 1 volt.

Wave. One wavelength; a single electrical impulse.

Wavelength. The distance between corresponding points in two adjacent waves.

Wedensky inhibition. The phenomenon in which continuous stimulation with a medium frequency current leads to inhibition of the reaction or a complete blockage through the duration of the stimulation.

Wolff's law. Bones in their external contour and internal architecture conform to the intensity and the stresses to which they are habitually subjected.

Wood's filter. A screen that permits ultraviolet rays to be transmitted but absorbs visible rays.

Index